Basics of Anesthesia

Basics of Anesthesia

Robert K. Stoelting, M.D.

Professor and Chairman
Department of Anesthesia
Indiana University School of Medicine
Indianapolis, Indiana

Ronald D. Miller, M.D.

Professor and Chairman of Anesthesia
Professor of Pharmacology
Department of Anesthesia
University of California, San Francisco
School of Medicine
San Francisco, California

CHURCHILL LIVINGSTONE
New York, Edinburgh, London, and Melbourne   1984

Acquisitions editor: Lewis Reines
Copy editor: Donna C. Balopole
Production editor: Fred L. Kantrowitz
Production supervisor: Joe Sita
Compositor: Maryland Composition Company, Inc.
Printer/Binder: The Maple-Vail Book Manufacturing Group

© Churchill Livingstone Inc. 1984

Distributed in the United Kingdom by Churchill Livingstone, Robert Stevenson House, 1-3 Baxter's Place, Leith Walk, Edinburgh EH1 3AF and by associated companies, branches and representatives throughout the world.

First published 1984

Printed in U.S.A.

ISBN 0-443-08281-2
9 8 7 6 5 4 3 2 1

Library of Congress Cataloging in Publication Data

Stoelting, Robert K.
  Basics of anesthesia.

  Includes bibliographies and index.
  1. Anesthesia. I. Miller, Ronald D., 1939–
II. Title. [DNLM: 1. Anesthesia. WO 200 S872b]
RD81.S86 1984 617'.96 84-12084
ISBN 0-443-08281-2

Manufactured in the United States of America

Preface

Basics of Anesthesia is intended to provide the student and beginning trainee with introductory information pertinent to the wide spectrum (operating room, intensive care, pain management, cardiopulmonary resuscitation) of the practice of anesthesiology. Likewise, the advanced trainee and practitioner should find the concise but thorough description of anesthetic practice a useful review as well as a reference source for fundamental questions.

An in-depth and highly referenced presentation is not the goal of *Basics of Anesthesia*. Nevertheless, we believe it is possible, in a concise manner, to achieve an accurate and pertinent presentation of essential information for the practice of anesthesiology. References are limited in number but should direct the reader to classic articles or more detailed discussions of the specific topic.

The editors wish to acknowledge the superb editorial and technical assistance of Ms. Deanna Walker (Indiana University) and Ms. Susan M. S. Ishida (University of California, San Francisco). The staff of Churchill Livingstone provided the necessary encouragement and flexibility to ensure timely progression of the textbook to its final form. In particular, Ms. Donna Balopole guided this project through the important publication steps.

Robert K. Stoelting, M.D.
Ronald D. Miller, M.D.

Contents

Section I
Introduction

1

History and Scope of Anesthesia

Since its beginning in 1842, anesthesiology has evolved into a recognized medical specialty providing continuing improvement in patient care based on the introduction of new drugs and techniques made possible in large part by research in the basic and clinical sciences (Table 1-1). The scope of anesthesiology extends beyond the operating room to include respiratory therapy, management of chronic pain problems and the care of acutely ill patients in Intensive Care Units. As for other medical specialties, anesthesiology is represented by professional societies, scientific journals, and a Board that establishes criteria for becoming a certified specialist in anesthesiology (Table 1-1).

DISCOVERY OF ANESTHESIA

Discovery of anesthesia represents a totally American contribution to medicine.[1] Dr. Crawford W. Long, a medical practitioner in rural Georgia, was the first physician known to administer the vapor of ether by inhalation to produce surgical anesthesia, in 1842. This finding was not publicized. Thus four years later a dentist, Dr. William T. Morton, from Hartford, Connecticut, administered the vapor of ether to Mr. Gilbert Abbott for the removal of a tumor from below the mandible by the well-known surgeon Dr. John C. Warren. The successful anesthesia and surgery took place at Massachusetts General Hospital on Friday, October 16, 1846 in front of an audience that included surgeons, medical students, and a newspaper reporter. Indeed, an account of the "ether demonstration" appeared the next day in the *Boston Daily Journal*. Within a few weeks, the entire civilized world knew the discovery of surgical anesthesia.

In England, Dr. James Y. Simpson, a highly respected obstetrician, administered ether to a parturient in 1847 to relieve the pain of labor. The use of chloroform in England for obstetrical analgesia gained public acceptance when Simpson administered this drug to Queen Victoria during the birth of Prince Leopold in 1853. Another London physician, Dr. John Snow, qualifies as the first anesthesiologist because he was the first to devote his medical practice to the administration of anesthetics.

Another American dentist, Dr. Horace Wells, was the first to recognize the potential of nitrous oxide as an anesthetic. Although nitrous oxide was isolated in 1772 and its anesthetic properties described in 1799, it was not until 1844—when Dr. Wells allowed nitrous oxide to be administered to him by Gardner C. Colton (an itinerant

1

Table 1-1. History of Anesthesia

1842	Diethyl ether used by Long to produce surgical anesthesia
1844	Nitrous oxide used by Wells to produce dental analgesia
1846	Diethyl ether used publicly by Morton to produce surgical anesthesia
1847	Chloroform popularized for surgical anesthesia in England
1853	Chloroform administered by Simpson to Queen Victoria for the birth of Prince Leopold; this removed the stigma attached to pain relief for child birth
1854	Hollow metallic needle invented by Wood
1868	Administration of nitrous oxide with oxygen introduced by Andrews
1871	Cylinders of compressed nitrous oxide introduced by Brothers
1884	Cocaine used by Koller to produce topical anesthesia
1885	Nerve block and infiltration anesthesia by injection of cocaine introduced by Halstead
	Epidural block anesthesia introduced by Corning
1893	London Society of Anaesthetists founded
1898	Spinal block anesthesia introduced by Bier
1904	Buchanan appointed first professor of anesthesia in the United States at the New York Medical College
1905	Procaine synthesized by Einhorn
	Long Island Society of Anesthetists founded by Erdmann
1911	Long Island Society of Anesthetists becomes the New York Society of Anesthetists
1914	*Americal Journal of Anesthesia and Analgesia* first published as a quarterly supplement to the *American Journal of Surgery*
1917	Oxygen mask developed by Poulton
1919	National Anesthesia Research Society founded by McMechan
1920	Gudel published data on signs of anesthesia
	Tracheal tubes for delivery of inhaled anesthetics introduced by Magill
1922	The journal, *Current Researches in Anesthesia and Analgesia* first published
1923	Mary A. Ross, M.D. becomes the first postgraduate trainee (Iowa) in anesthesiology in the United States
	British Journal of Anaesthesia first published
1924	Lundy organized a Department of Anesthesia at the Mayo Clinic
1925	National Anesthesia Research Society becomes the International Anesthesia Research Society
1926	*American Journal of Anesthesia and Analgesia* ceases publication
1927	Waters appointed as the first university professor of anesthesia in the United States at the University of Wisconsin
	Anesthetists' Travel Club founded
1930	Circle anesthetic breathing and carbon dioxide absorption system described by Sword
1932	Association of Anaesthetists of Great Britain and Ireland founded
1933	Cyclopropane used by Waters to produce surgical anesthesia
1934	Thiopental used by Lundy for induction of anesthesia
1935	Rovenstine organized a Department of Anesthesia at Bellevue Hospital in New York
	New York Society of Anesthetists becomes the American Society of Anesthetists
1938	American Board of Anesthesiology founded
1940	The journal *Anesthesiology* first published
1942	d-Tubocurarine used by Griffith and Johnson to produce skeletal muscle relaxation during general anesthesia
1943	Lidocaine synthesized by Lofgren
1945	American Society of Anesthetists becomes the American Society of Anesthesiologists
1946	The journal *Anaesthesia* first published
1949	Succinylcholine used clinically by Phillips and Fusco
1952	The journal *Der Anaesthetist* first published
1953	Association of University Anesthetists founded
	Residency Review Committee in Anesthesiology established

Continued

Table 1-1. (*continued*)

1954	*Canadian Anaesthetists' Society Journal* first published
	Anesthetists' Travel Club becomes the Academy of Anesthesiology
1956	Halothane used clinically by Johnson
1957	The journal *Survey of Anesthesiology* first published
	The journal *Acta Anesthesiologica Scandinavica* first published
	Current Researches in Anesthesia and Analgesia becomes *Anesthesia and Analgesia, Current Researches*
1958	"Audio Digest Anesthesiology" first recorded
1959	Methoxyflurane used clinically by Artusio and Van Poznak
1968	Society of Academic Anesthesia Chairman founded
1972	Enflurane used clinically
1973	The journal *Critical Care Medicine* first published
1975	In-Training Examination in Anesthesiology initiated
	American Society of Regional Anesthesia refounded
1976	The journal *Regional Anesthesia* first published
1979	*Anesthesia and Analgesia, Current Researches* becomes *Anesthesia and Analgesia*
1981	Isoflurane used clinically

(Information in part derived from a chart prepared by William H. G. Dornette, M.D., for the Ohio Chemical and Surgical Equipment Company, 1962.)

showman) while a fellow dentist painlessly extracted one of Dr. Well's teeth—that the anesthetic potential of this gas was realized. Unfortunately, the use of nitrous oxide for medical purposes temporarily fell into disrepute when Dr. Wells, who did not appreciate the lack of potency of nitrous oxide, failed in an attempt to produce anesthesia for surgery during a demonstration before a group of his colleagues at the Massachusetts General Hospital. It was not until 1868 when a Chicago surgeon, Dr. Edmund W. Andrews, popularized the use of nitrous oxide with oxygen that the full value of this gas as an anesthetic began to be appreciated. Between 1844 and 1868 nitrous oxide continued to be used by itinerant showmen who staged public displays of the exhilarating effects of this gas on the sensorium. Likewise, ether was often used for nonmedical purposes described as "ether frolics." Indeed, it is likely that Dr. Long saw ether used in this way during his medical student days in Philadelphia prior to 1842.

ANESTHESIA AFTER ETHER

The discovery of the anesthetic properties of ether, chloroform, and nitrous oxide satisfied the immediate needs to provide an-algesia during surgery. Indeed, no significant new inhaled anesthetics were introduced during the next 80 years (Fig. 1-1).[2] The search for new inhaled anesthetics began in the 1920s when the expanding scientific basis of anesthesia and surgery demanded drugs with greater flexibility and fewer side effects than currently provided by ether and chloroform. As such, cyclopropane, because of its low blood solubility and support of the circulation, became the most important new inhaled anesthetic in the 1930s.

Until the 1950s, all the available anesthetics possessed at least one of two defects: either being explosive in oxygen (ether, ethylene, vinethene, cyclopropane) or toxic (chloroform, vinethene, trichloroethylene). The evolution of fluorine technology stimulated originally by the need to separate uranium isotopes for the development of the atomic bomb served to lead to a new generation of fluorinated inhaled anesthetics in the 1950s. For example, combining fluorine with carbon decreased flammability while the stability of this bond tended to reduce metabolism and thus organ toxicity. The first of the new fluorinated inhaled anesthetics introduced in 1954 was

Anesthetics Used In
Clinical Practice
(Cumulative)

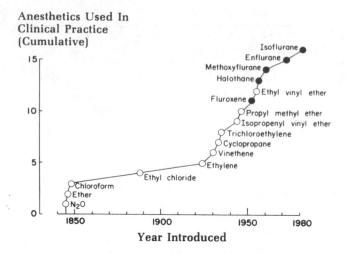

Figure 1-1. The history of anesthesia began with the introduction of nitrous oxide, ether and chloroform. After 1950, all introduced drugs with the exception of ethyl vinyl ether have contained fluorine (closed circles) (Eger EI, Isoflurane (Forane). A compendium and reference. Madison, Wisconsin, Ohio Medical Products, 1981:4-7.)

fluroxene. Fluroxene had several desirable characteristics, including low blood solubility and a minimal tendency to depress cardiovascular function or to sensitize the heart to exogenous epinephrine. However, fluroxene frequently caused nausea and vomiting and at higher anesthetic concentrations was flammable. Later work also suggested this inhaled anesthetic could on rare occasions be hepatotoxic and might also be carcinogenic.[3] Fluroxene was voluntarily withdrawn from the market in 1975 mainly because of its flammability.

Modern Inhaled Anesthetics

In the 1980s, one gas (nitrous oxide) and the vapors of three volatile liquids (halothane, enflurane, isoflurane) represent the commonly used inhaled anesthetics. These drugs differ in physical and chemical characteristics (see Chapter 2) and their pharmacology (see Chapters 4 and 5).

Halothane was introduced in 1956 after pharmacologists had predicted that its halogenated chemical structure would provide nonflammability, low blood solubility, molecular stability (trifluorocarbon molecule), and anesthetic potency (chlorine and bromine) (Fig. 1-2).[4] This drug was found to produce a rapid and pleasant induction of

anesthesia, bronchodilatation, skeletal muscle relaxation, a prompt return to consciousness, and minimal postoperative nausea and vomiting. These attributes and the subsequent clinical popularity of halothane temporarily halted the search for new inhaled anesthetics. With continued use of halothane, however, its limitations (depression of ventilation and circulation, enhanced arrhythmogenic effects of epinephrine, rare potential to produce hepatotoxicity) led to renewed interest in the search for other inhaled anesthetics.[5]

Methoxyflurane. The search for new inhaled anesthetics focused on methyl ethyl ethers, since ether derivatives do not increase the incidence of cardiac dysrhyth-

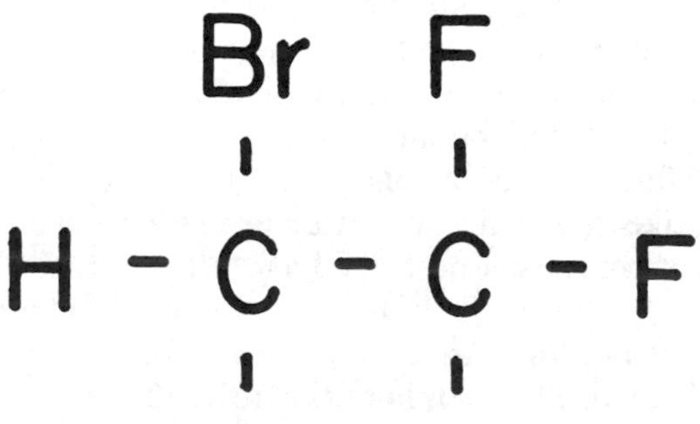

Figure 1-2. Chemical structure of halothane.

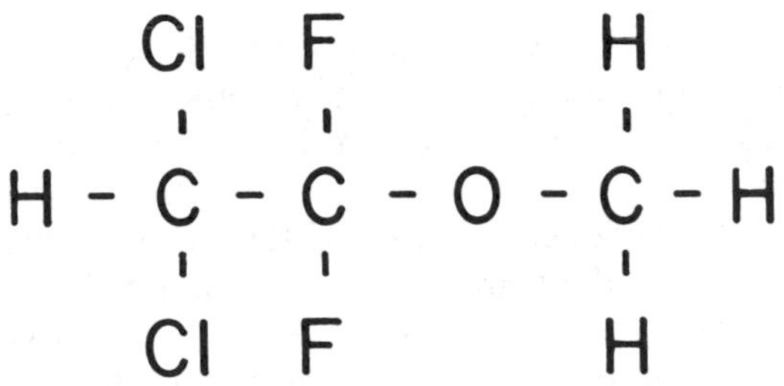

Cl   F   H
 | | |
H — C — C — O — C — H
 | | |
Cl   F   H

Figure 1-3. Chemical structure of methoxyflurane, the first halogenated methyl ethyl ether derivative introduced for use as an inhaled anesthetic.

mias. Methoxyflurane, introduced in 1959, was the first of the methyl ethyl ethers to be used clinically (Fig. 1-3).[6] This drug did not increase myocardial irritability and seemed to be less depressant to the circulation than halothane. Methoxyflurane was, however, extensively metabolized (up to 50 percent of the absorbed dose) particularly to fluoride, introducing the potential for fluoride nephrotoxicity (see Chapter 5). In addition, its high blood and tissue solubility resulted in slow induction of anesthesia and in the potential for delayed awakening especially after prolonged administration. These undesirable characteristics have led to the infrequent use of methoxyflurane despite its continued clinical availability.

Enflurane, introduced in 1972, was the next methyl ethyl ether derivative to become available for use as an inhaled anesthetic (Fig. 1-4).[7] This drug provided stable cardiac rhythm, produced excellent skeletal muscle relaxation, and underwent minimal

Cl   F   F
 | | |
H — C — C — O — C — H
 | | |
 F   F   F

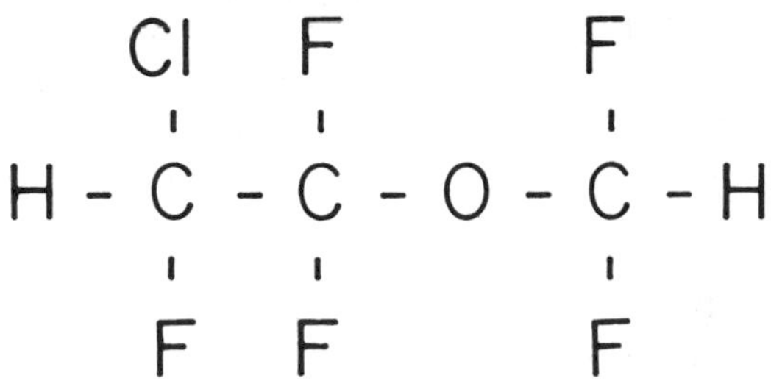

Figure 1-4. Chemical structure of enflurane, a halogenated methyl ethyl ether.

metabolism which made organ toxicity unlikely. Rapid induction and recovery from anesthesia was predictable because of the low blood solubility of enflurane. As a result of these desirable characteristics, enflurane has become a popular and frequently administered anesthetic.

Isoflurane was introduced for patient use in 1981 (Fig. 1-5).[8] This inhaled anesthetic is the chemical isomer of enflurane but in contrast to enflurane undergoes less metabolism, does not stimulate the central nervous system, and is less soluble in blood. In many respects, isoflurane possesses the characteristics considered important for the ideal inhaled anesthetic (Table 1-2).

Regional Anesthesia

The introduction of regional anesthesia awaited the development of a hollow metal needle in 1854 and the discovery of local

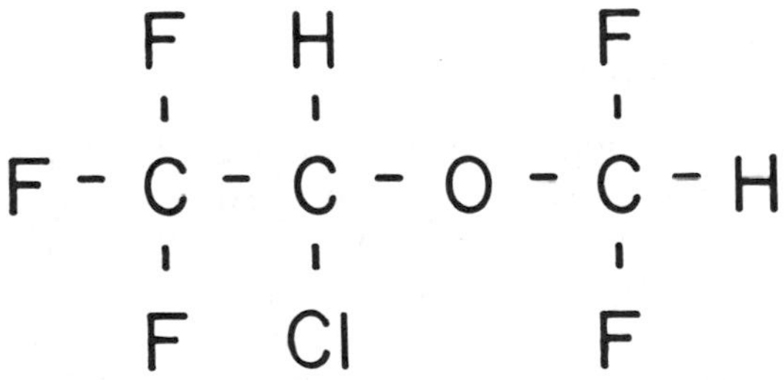

F   H   F
 | | |
F — C — C — O — C — H
 | | |
 F   Cl   F

Figure 1-5. Chemical structure of isoflurane, the isomer of enflurane.

Table 1-2. Characteristics of an Ideal Inhaled Anesthetic

Absence of flammability
Easily vaporized at ambient temperature
Potent
Low blood solubility to assure induction and recovery
Minimal metabolism
Compatible with epinephrine
Skeletal muscle relaxation
Suppresses excessive sympathetic nervous system activity
Not irritating to airways
Bronchodilation
Absence of excessive myocardial depression
Absence of cerebral vasodilation
Absence of hepatic and renal toxicity

anesthetics. Dr. Carl Koller in 1884 discovered the local anesthetic effects of cocaine when applied topically to the eye. In 1885, Dr. William S. Halstead, a surgeon, introduced the concept of nerve block and infiltration anesthesia by the injection of cocaine. Also, in 1885, Dr. Leonard Corning, a neurologist, was the first to produce lumbar epidural block by the injection of cocaine. Dr. August Bier in 1898 demonstrated the feasibility of spinal block by the injection of cocaine into the subarachnoid space of a patient undergoing a foot amputation. Procaine, synthesized in 1905 by Einhorn, replaced cocaine for use in producing regional anesthesia. Today, the most frequently used local anesthetics are tetracaine (topical anesthesia, spinal block), lidocaine (topical anesthesia, infiltration anesthesia, peripheral nerve block, epidural block, spinal block) and bupivacaine (peripheral nerve block, epidural block) (see Chapter 7).

Injected Drugs

Induction of anesthesia with the intravenous injection of thiopental was introduced by Dr. John S. Lundy in 1934. Subsequently, the introduction of d-tubocurarine into clinical anesthesia in 1942 revolutionized the methods by which skeletal muscle relaxation during surgery was produced.[9] Finally, narcotics used for many years in combination with nitrous oxide to produce general anesthesia have been recently proposed for use as the sole anesthetic (high-dose fentanyl) for critically ill patients who cannot tolerate even minimal cardiac depression produced by inhaled drugs.[10]

ANESTHESIA AS A MEDICAL SPECIALTY

Anesthesia as a medical specialty evolved differently in England and the United States. Chloroform, the standard anesthetic in England, was a potent ventilatory and cardiac depressant requiring great skills in its administration. As a result, only physicians were considered competent to administer chloroform. In contrast, ether remained the dominant anesthetic in the United States. Unlike chloroform, ether stimulated ventilation and maintained the circulation. For these reasons, ether was thought to have a built-in protection for the patient and its administration was often regulated to an inexperienced physician or nurse. Indeed, it was more than 60 years after the demonstration of ether anesthesia by Dr. Morton before American physicians began to devote their full-time medical practice to the administration of anesthetics. For example, the first Department of Anesthesia was created in 1904 at the New York Medical College with Dr. Thomas D. Buchanan as Professor and Chairman. Dr. Arthur E. Gudel, a 1908 graduate of Indiana University School of Medicine, described the stages and planes of anesthesia in a monograph published in 1920. In 1923, Dr. Mary A. Ross became the first formal postgraduate trainee in anesthesiology in the United States receiving a certificate from the University of Iowa for her year of training following graduation from medical school. Dr. John S. Lundy organized a Department of Anesthesia at the Mayo Clinic in 1924 while Dr. Ralph M. Waters arrived at the University of Wisconsin for the same purpose in 1927. Graduates of the training programs directed by Drs. Lundy and Waters continued to expand the scope of anesthesiology. Among these graduates was Dr. Emory A. Rovenstine who in 1935 left Wisconsin to develop a Department of Anesthesia at Bellevue, the teaching hospital of New York University. During the next 25 years over 30 graduates of Dr. Rovenstine's program became chairmans of Departments of Anesthesia.

American Society of Anesthesiologists (ASA)

The first anesthesia organization in the United States was the Long Island Society of Anesthetists started in 1905 by Dr. A.

Frederick Erdmann and eight physician colleagues from the Brooklyn, New York area. The stated goal of this society was to "promote the art and science of anesthesia" and annual dues were established as $1.00. Only the London Society of Anaesthetists founded in 1893 preceded this first society in America. The Long Island Society of Anesthetists grew in membership, becoming the New York Society of Anesthetists in 1911. This society became the American Society of Anesthetists in 1935 with 487 members and annual dues of $5.00. In 1945, the name was changed to the American Society of Anesthesiologists. This name change was intended to more accurately reflect the background of the membership of the society which is physicians with postgraduate training in anesthesia (anesthesiologists) in contrast to nonphysicians (anesthetists) who also administer anesthesia (see the section *Certified Registered Nurse Anesthetists (CRNA)*). This semantic distinction is observed most consistently in the United States while in other areas of the world the terms tend to be used interchangeably. Today, the American Society of Anesthesiologists has over 20,000 members, making anesthesia the sixth largest among the American medical specialties.

Anesthesiology, the official journal of the American Society of Anesthesiologists, was first published in July 1940 with Dr. Henry S. Ruth as the Editor. This initial issue was sent to 568 members of the society and 300 additional nonmember subscribers. Today, this highly respected journal has a monthly worldwide circulation that exceeds 30,000.

International Anesthesia Research Society (IARS)

At the same time the New York Society of Anesthetists was evolving into the American Society of Anesthesiologists, another important organization was developing under the direction of Dr. Francis H. McMechan, a physician practicing in Cincinnati, Ohio. In 1919, Dr. McMechan established the National Anesthesia Research Society. This society held annual meetings, and in August, 1922 the first medical journal devoted entirely to the specialty of anesthesiology, *Current Researches in Anesthesia and Analgesia* appeared with Dr. McMechan as editor. Previously, the only other source of scientific information for anesthesiology was the *American Journal of Anesthesia and Analgesia*, published since 1914 as a quarterly supplement to the *American Journal of Surgery*. In 1925, the National Anesthesia Research Society was renamed the International Anesthesia Research Society, which today continues to sponsor an annual scientific meeting and publish the journal, *Anesthesia and Analgesia*.

American Society of Regional Anesthesia (ASRA)

The American Society of Regional Anesthesia was founded in 1923 to provide a forum for those physicians interested in regional anesthesia. This society was absorbed into the American Society of Anesthetists in 1941 only to again become an independent organization in 1975. The official journal of this society, *Regional Anesthesia*, was first published in October 1976.

American Board of Anesthesiology (ABA)

The American Board of Anesthesiology was incorporated as an affiliate of the American Board of Surgery in 1938. Following the first voluntary examinations, there were 87 physicians certified as Diplomates of the American Board of Anesthesiology. The American Board of Anesthesiology was recognized as an independent board by the American Board of Medical Specialties in 1941. To date, over 11,000 anesthesiologists have been certified as Diplomates of the American Board of Anesthesiology.

Certified Registered Nurse Anesthetists (CRNA)

In the past, nearly 50 percent of the anesthetics given in the United States each year were administered by certified registered nurse anesthetists. To become a nurse anesthetist, the candidate must earn a Registered Nurse degree followed by 2 years of anesthesia training in an approved nurse anesthesia training program. At present, the American Association of Nurse Anesthetists (AANA) remains responsible for the curriculum of the majority of nurse anesthesia training programs as well as establishment of criteria for certification as a nurse anesthetist. The activities of nurse anesthetists are usually confined to the operating room, where they often work under the supervision of an anesthesiologist. This supervised approach is consistent with the concept that the administration of anesthesia is the practice of medicine.

Postgraduate (residency) Training in Anesthesiology

Postgraduate training in anesthesiology consists of 4 years of supervised experience in an approved program after the degree of Doctor of Medicine or Osteopathy has been obtained. The first year of postgraduate training in anesthesiology consists of nonanesthesia experience (Clinical Base Year) in patient care related specialties such as internal medicine, surgery, or pediatrics. The second and third years of postgraduate training (Clinical Anesthesia Years 2 and 3) are spent in learning all aspects of clinical anesthesia. The fourth year of postgraduate training (Specialized Year) is spent in gaining advanced experience in specific areas of clinical anesthesia (obstetrical anesthesia, pediatric anesthesia, cardiac anesthesia, neuroanesthesia, pain management, critical care medicine) or in pursuing research interests. In lieu of the Specialized Year, the physician may elect the Practice Credit Pathway which requires 2 years of clinical practice. After May 1, 1986, the Specialized Year and Practice Credit Pathway will no longer be available and all postgraduate training in anesthesiology will consist of a Clinical Base Year followed by 3 years of Clinical Anesthesia.

The content of the educational experience during the Clinical Anesthesia Years reflects the wide-ranging scope of anesthesiology as a medical specialty. At present, anesthesiology is defined in the booklet of information of the American Board of Anesthesiology as a practice of medicine dealing with but not limited to:

A. The provision of insensibility to pain during surgical, obstetrical, therapeutic and diagnostic procedures, and the management of patients so affected.

B. The monitoring and restoration of homeostasis during the perioperative period, as well as homeostasis in the critically ill, injured, or otherwise seriously ill patient.

C. The diagnosis and treatment of painful syndromes.

D. The clinical management and teaching of cardiac and pulmonary resuscitation.

E. The evaluation of respiratory function and application of respiratory therapy in all its forms.

F. The supervision, teaching, and evaluation of performance of both medical and paramedical personnel involved in anesthesia, respiratory, and critical care.

G. The conduct of research at the clinical and basic science levels to explain and improve the care of patients insofar as physiologic function and the response to drugs is concerned.

H. The administrative involvement in hospitals, medical schools, and outpatient facilities necessary to implement these responsibilities.

This definition emphasizes the continued major role of the anesthesiologist in the operating room. Indeed, the anesthesiologist should function as the clinical pharmacologist and internist or pediatrician in the operating room. Furthermore, this definition emphasizes that the scope of anesthesiology extends beyond the operating room to include pain management (see Chapter 33), cardiopulmonary resuscitation (see Chapter 34), respiratory therapy (see Chapter 31), critical care medicine (see Chapter 32), and research. Indeed, much remains to be learned, for even the mechanism of general anesthesia remains unknown.

Approximately 160 postgraduate training programs in anesthesiology are approved by the Accreditation Council for Graduate Medical Education of the American Medical Association. These training programs offer about 3200 postgraduate positions in anesthesiology. Approved postgraduate training programs are visited periodically by a representative of the Residency Review Committee to assure continued adherence to the high standards of quality medical education. The Residency Review Committee consists of members appointed by the American Medical Association, American Society of Anesthesiologists, and American Board of Anesthesiology.

Following completion of the required postgraduate training in anesthesiology, the physician can voluntarily enter the examination system of the American Board of Anesthesiology. Successful completion of a written and then oral examination results in the issuance of a certificate confirming the physician is a Diplomate ("Board certified") of the American Board of Anesthesiology.

REFERENCES

1. Greene NM. Anesthesia and the development of surgery (1846–1896). Anesth Analg 1979;58:5–12.
2. Eger EI. Isoflurane (Forane). A compendium and reference. Madison, Wisconsin, Ohio Medical Products, 1981:4–7.
3. Baden JM, Kelley M, Wharton RS, Hitt BA, Simmon VF, Mazze RI. Mutagenicity of halogenated ether anesthetics. Anesthesiology 1977;46:346–50.
4. Raventos J. Action of Fluothane—New volatile anesthetic. Br J Pharmacol 1956;11:394–410.
5. Summary of the national halothane study. JAMA 1966;197:775–88.
6. Artusio JF, VanPoznak A, Hunt RE, Tiers FM, Alexander M. A clinical evaluation of methoxyflurane in man. Anesthesiology 1960;21:512–7.
7. Dobkin AB, Heinrich RG, Israel JS, Levy AA, Neville JF, Ounkasem K. Clinical and laboratory evaluation of a new inhalation agent. Compound 347 (CHF_2OCF_2CHFC1). Anesthesiology 1968;29:275–87.
8. Vitcha JF. A history of Forane. Anesthesiology 1971;35:4–7.
9. Griffith HR, Johnson GG. Use of curare in general anesthesia. Anesthesiology 1942;3:418–20.
10. Stanley TH, Webster LR. Anesthetic requirements and cardiovascular effects of fentanyl-oxygen and fentanyl-diazepam-oxygen anesthesia in man. Anesth Analg 1978;57:411–6.

Section II
Pharmacology

2

Basic Principles

To understand the basic pharmacologic principles of both inhaled and intravenously administered anesthetics, the principles of pharmacokinetics and pharmacodynamics should be appreciated. *Pharmacokinetics* describes how a drug is absorbed, distributed within the body, and eliminated from the body. Conversely, *pharmacodynamics* refers to the relative potency of a particular drug, and often is expressed by the concentration of drug in blood or tissue required to evoke a given pharmacologic response. Crucial to the pharmacodynamic response to a drug is the receptor, which is the component of a cell or organism that interacts with the drug and initiates a chain of events leading to the drug's pharmacologic effect. Receptors determine the quantitative relationship between a dose or concentration of drug and its pharmacologic effect. Also, receptors are responsible for selectivity of drug action. The molecular size, shape, and electrical charge of a drug usually determines with which receptor it will bind, both from a qualitative and quantitative point of view. Assuming a fundamental relationship between the pharmacologic or toxic effect of a drug and the concentration of drug in blood, a knowledge of pharmacokinetics will allow the clinician to administer a drug in a manner most likely to achieve the desired blood concentration.

TERMINOLOGY AND DEFINITIONS

A drug which regulates the function of a receptor macromolecule or changes the function of the receptor as a direct result of binding to it is called an *agonist*. Isoproterenol is an example of a beta receptor agonist. Conversely, an *antagonist* binds to a receptor without directly altering the receptor's function, but prevents an agonist from stimulating the receptor to function. There are two separate types of antagonism. *Competitive antagonism* is present when increasing concentrations of the antagonist progressively inhibit the response to a fixed concentration of agonist. High antagonist concentrations prevent the response completely. Conversely, *noncompetitive antagonism* is present when, after administration of an antagonist, even high concentrations of agonists cannot completely overcome antagonism.

An *idiosyncratic* drug response is one that is infrequently observed in most patients. Idiosyncratic responses are usually caused by genetic differences in metabolism of a drug or by immunologic mechanisms, including allergic reactions. If a patient is hyporeactive or hyper-reactive to a drug, the inference is that the intensity of effect of a given dose of drug is diminished or increased in comparison to the effects seen in most individuals. This should be separated from the term *hypersensitivity*, which refers to an allergic or other immunologic response to a drug. With some drugs, the intensity of response to a given dose may change during the course of therapy. When the responsiveness decreases as a consequence of continued drug administration, a state of relative *tolerance* to the drug's effect exists. When the responsiveness diminishes rapidly after administration of a drug, the response is said to be subject to *tachyphylaxis*.

The difference between the terms *additive, synergistic* and *antagonism* should be understood when describing a drug interaction (Fig. 2-1). An *additive* effect means that a second drug acting with the first will produce an effect equal to a simple algebraic summation. For example, inhaled anesthetics are additive (e.g., 0.5 MAC of nitrous oxide plus 0.5 MAC of halothane produces 1.0 MAC of anesthetic effect). *Synergistic* means that two drugs interact to produce an effect more than simple algebraic summation. For example, certain antibiotics do not produce a significant neuromuscular blockade alone, but markedly enhance that produced by nondepolarizing muscle relaxants. *Antagonism* means that two drugs interact to produce an effect less than simple algebraic summation.

The fundamentals of a dose-response curve should be understood (Fig. 2-2). When two dose-response curves are *parallel* with each other, then a potency ratio can be derived. For example, the relationship between the ED_{90}'s of two drugs (dose of drug which produces a 90 percent response) is the same as the relationship between the ED_{20}'s of these drugs (dose of drug which produces a 20 percent response). Such a convenient relationship does not exist, however, when two dose-response curves deviate from parallelism. Therefore, it is only appropriate to describe the potencies between two drugs when the dose-response curves are parallel. When the dose-response curves deviate from parallelism, then the potency must be described individually at each level of response.

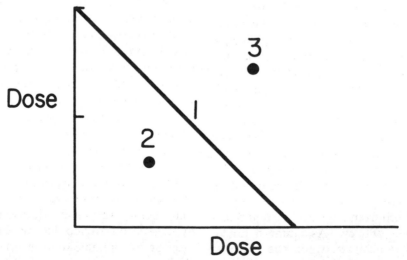

Figure 2-1. An illustration of additive, synergistic, or antagonistic interactions. The vertical and horizontal axes refer to those doses of drug required to produce a given effect. When a drug interaction follows the straight line, an additive effect occurs, as illustrated by curve number 1. When the curve is shifted to the left (number 2) a synergistic effect exists. Conversely, when the curve is shifted to the right (number 3) antagonism exists.

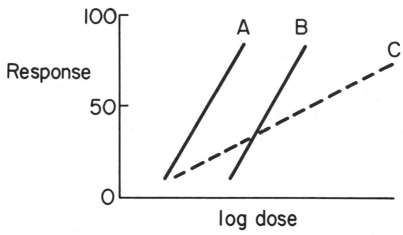

Figure 2-2. Schematic dose response curves that illustrate parallelism (curves A and B) and deviation from parallelism (curve C compared with A or B). A potency ratio can be derived only when the dose response curves for two drugs are parallel. Conversely, when the curves deviate from parallelism, a potency ratio cannot be derived. For example, at 20 percent response, the drug represented by curve C is more potent than the drug represented by curve B. At 90 percent response, however, the potency of these two drugs is reversed.

PHARMACOKINETICS OF INHALED ANESTHETICS

Pharmacokinetics of inhaled anesthetics describes their uptake (absorption) from alveoli into the systemic circulation, distribution in the body, and eventual elimination via the lungs.[1] By controlling the inspired partial pressure (PI) (same as concentration when referring to the gas phase) of the inhaled anesthetics, a gradient is created such that the anesthetic is delivered from the anesthetic machine to its site of action, the brain. *The primary objective of inhalation anesthesia is to achieve a constant and optimal partial pressure of the anesthetic in the brain (Pbr).*

The brain and all other tissues equilibrate with the partial pressure of the inhaled anesthetic delivered to them by the arterial blood (Pa) (Fig. 2-3). Likewise, the blood equilibrates with the alveolar partial pressure (PA) of the anesthetic (Fig. 2-3). Therefore, maintaining a constant and optimal PA becomes an indirect but reliable method for controlling the Pbr. The fact that the PA of an inhaled anesthetic mirrors its Pbr is the reason the PA is used as an index of anesthetic depth, reflection of the rate of induction and recovery from anesthesia, and measure of equal potency (see the section *Minimum Alveolar Concentration*).

Understanding those factors that determine the PA and thus the Pbr allows the anesthesiologist to skillfully control the dose of inhaled anesthetic delivered to the brain.

Factors that Determine the Alveolar Partial Pressure (PA)

The PA and ultimately Pbr of an inhaled anesthetic is determined by input (delivery) into the alveoli minus uptake (loss) of the drug from the alveoli into the arterial blood (Table 2-1). Input of the inhaled anesthetic is dependent on three factors: PI, alveolar ventilation (VA), and characteristics of the anesthetic breathing system. Likewise, uptake of the inhaled anesthetic is dependent

Table 2-1. Summary of Factors Determining Partial Pressure Gradients Necessary for Establishment of Anesthesia

Transfer of inhaled anesthetic from anesthetic machine to alveoli
  Inspired partial pressure
  Alveolar ventilation
  Characteristics of anesthetic breathing system
Transfer of inhaled anesthetic from alveoli to arterial blood
  Blood:gas partition coefficient
  Cardiac output
  Alveolar to venous partial pressure difference
Transfer of inhaled anesthetic from arterial blood to brain
  Brain:blood partition coefficient
  Cerebral blood flow
  Arterial to venous partial pressure difference

on three factors: solubility, cardiac output (CO), and the alveolar to venous partial pressure diffference (A − vD). These six factors act simultaneously to determine the PA. Metabolism and percutaneous loss of the inhaled anesthetic do not significantly influence PA.

Inspired Anesthetic Partial Pressure (PI). A high PI is necessary during initial administration of an inhaled anesthetic. This initial high PI (e.g., input) offsets the impact of uptake and thus accelerates induction of anesthesia as reflected by the rate of rise in the PA. This effect of the PI is known as the *concentration effect*.

With time, as uptake into the blood decreases, the PI should be decreased to match the reduced anesthetic uptake. Indeed, decreasing the PI to match decreasing uptake with time is crucial if one is to achieve the goal of maintaining a constant and optimal Pbr. For example, if the PI were maintained constant with time (e.g.,

input constant), the PA (and Pbr) would progressively increase as uptake diminished.

Second Gas Effect. The second gas effect is a distinct phenomenon that occurs independently of the concentration effect.[2] The ability of the large volume uptake of one gas (first gas) to accelerate the rate of rise of the PA of a concurrently administrated companion gas (second gas) is known as the second gas effect. For example, the initial large volume uptake of nitrous oxide accelerates the uptake of companion gases such as a volatile anesthetic and oxygen. Indeed, the transient increase (about 10 percent) in PaO_2 that accompanies the early phases of nitrous oxide administration reflects the second gas effect. This increase in PaO_2 has been designated as *alveolar hyperoxygenation*. Increased tracheal inflow of all inhaled gases (e.g., first and second gases) and concentration of the second gases in a smaller lung volume (*concentrating effect*) due to the high volume uptake of the first gas are the explanations for the second gas effect.[3] Although the second gas effect may produce detectable alterations in the PA, it probably should not be considered clinically significant.

Alveolar Ventilation (VA). Increased VA, like PI, promotes input of the inhaled anesthetic to offset uptake. The net effect is a more rapid rate of rise in the PA and induction of anesthesia. Predictably, hypoventilation has the opposite effect, acting to slow the induction of anesthesia.

Controlled ventilation of the lungs that results in hyperventilation and decreased ven-

PA ⇌ Pa ⇌ Pbr

Figure 2-3. The alveolar partial pressure (PA) of an inhaled anesthetic is in equilibrium with the arterial blood (Pa) and brain (Pbr). Therefore, the PA is an indirect measure of the anesthetic partial pressure at the site of action, the brain.

ous return accelerates the rate of rise of the PA by virtue of increased input (e.g., increased VA) and decreased uptake (e.g., decreased CO, see the section *Cardiac Output*). As a result, the risk of anesthetic overdose may be increased during controlled ventilation of the lungs. For this reason, it may be appropriate to reduce the PI of a volatile anesthetic when ventilation of the lungs is changed from spontaneous to controlled so as to maintain the PA similar to that present during spontaneous ventilation.

Another effect of hyperventilation is decreased cerebral blood flow due to reductions in the $PaCO_2$. Conceivably, the impact of increased input on the rate of rise of the PA would be offset by decreased delivery of anesthetic to the brain. Furthermore, coronary blood flow may remain unchanged, such that increased input produces myocardial depression while decreased cerebral blood flow prevents a concomitant onset of anesthesia.

Anesthetic Breathing System. Characteristics of the anesthetic breathing system that influence the rate of rise of the PA include the (1) volume of the system; (2) solubility of the inhaled anesthetic in the rubber or plastic components of the system; and (3) gas inflow from the anesthetic machine. The volume of the anesthetic breathing system acts as a buffer to slow achievement of the PA. High gas inflow from the anesthetic machine negates this buffer effect. Solubility of inhaled anesthetics in the components of the anesthetic breathing system initially slows the rate at which the PA rises. At the conclusion of an anesthetic, reversal of the partial pressure gradient in the anesthetic breathing system results in elution of the anesthetic that slows the rate at which the PA decreases. Furthermore, reuse of the same anesthetic breathing system results in exposure of the patient to that anesthetic, even if another drug or technique has been selected.

Solubility of an inhaled anesthetic in blood and tissues is denoted by its partition coefficient (Table 2-2). A partition coefficient is a distribution ratio describing how the inhaled anesthetic distributes itself between two phases at equilibrium (e.g., when the partial pressures are identical). For example, a blood:gas partition coefficient of 10 means that the concentration of the inhaled anesthetic is 10 in the blood and 1 in the alveolar gas when the partial pressures of that anesthetic in these two phases are identical. It is important to recognize that partition coefficients are temperature dependent. For example, solubility of a gas in a liquid is increased when the temperature of the liquid decreases. Unless otherwise stated, partition coefficients are for 37 Celsius.

Blood:Gas Partition Coefficient. Based on their blood:gas partition coefficients (e.g., solubilities), inhaled anesthetics are traditionally considered as soluble (methoxyflurane), of intermediate solubility (halothane, enflurane, isofurane), and poorly soluble (nitrous oxide) (Table 2-2). High blood solubility means that a large amount of inhaled anesthetic must be dissolved in the blood before equilibrium is reached with the gas phase. For example, the high solubility of a methoxyflurane slows the rate at which the PA and Pa rise such that the induction of anesthesia is slow (Fig. 2-4). The blood can be considered a pharmacologically inactive reservoir, the size of which is determined by the solubility of the anesthetic in the blood. When the blood:gas partition coefficient is high, a large amount of anesthetic must be dissolved in the blood before the Pa equilibrates with the PA. Clinically, the impact of high blood solubility on the rate of rise of the PA can be offset to some extent by increasing the PI. When blood solubility is poor, as with nitrous oxide, minimal amounts of the anesthetic have to be dissolved before equilibrium is reached such

Table 2-2. Comparative Characteristics of Inhaled Anesthetics

	Methoxyflurane	Halothane	Enflurane	Isoflurane	Nitrous Oxide
Blood:gas partition coefficient[a]	12	2.4	1.9	1.4	0.47
Brain:blood partition coefficient[a]	2	2.6	2.6	3.7	1.1
Oil:gas partition coefficient[a]	970	224	98	98	1.4
MAC (volumes percent, 30–55 years old)	0.16	0.75	1.68	1.15	105–110
Vapor pressure (mmHg)					
18 Celsius	20	224	156	219	
20 Celsius	23	244	172	240	
22 Celsius	26	267	189	262	
Molecular weight	165	197.4	184.5	184.5	
Commercial preparation contains preservative	Yes	Yes	No	No	
Stable in soda lime	No	No	Yes	Yes	
Reacts with metal	Yes	Yes	No	No	

[a] 37 Celsius

that the rate of rise of the PA and Pa, and thus the induction of anesthesia, is rapid (Fig. 2-4).

Tissue:blood partition coefficients determine the time necessary for equilibration of the tissue with the Pa. This time can be predicted by calculating a time constant (amount of inhaled anesthetic that can be dissolved in the tissue divided by tissue blood flow) for each tissue. Brain:blood partition coefficients for volatile anesthetics are approximately 2.5, resulting in a time constant equal to roughly 5 minutes (Table 2-2). Complete equilibration of any tissue, including the brain, with the Pa requires at least three time constants. This is the rationale for maintaining the PA of a volatile drug constant for about 15 minutes before assuming the Pbr is similar. Three time constants for nitrous oxide amount to about 6 minutes, reflecting its low brain solubility (Table 2-2).

Nitrous Oxide Transfer to Closed Gas Spaces. The blood:gas partition coefficient of nitrous oxide (0.47) is 34 times greater than nitrogen (0.014). This differential solubility means nitrous oxide can leave the blood to enter an air-filled cavity 34 times more rapidly than nitrogen can leave the cavity to enter the blood.[4] As a result of this preferential transfer of nitrous oxide, the volume or pressure of the air-filled cavity increases. The entrance of nitrous oxide into an air-filled cavity surrounded by a compliant wall (intestinal gas, pneumothorax, pulmonary blebs, air embolism) causes the gas space to expand. Conversely, entrance of nitrous oxide into an air-filled cavity surrounded by a noncompliant wall (middle ear, cerebral ventricles,

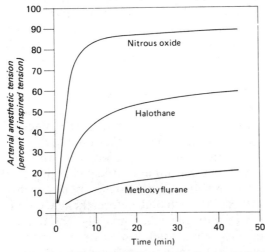

Figure 2-4. The rate of rise of the Pa (e.g., PA) as a percent of the PI is slow with a soluble anesthetic (methoxyflurane), intermediate with halothane and rapid with a poorly soluble anesthetic (nitrous oxide).

supratentorial subdural space) causes an increase in pressure.

The magnitude of volume or pressure increase is influenced by the PA of nitrous oxide, blood flow to the air-filled cavity, and duration of nitrous oxide administration. In an animal model, the inhalation of 75 percent nitrous oxide doubled the volume of a pneumothorax in 10 minutes.[4] Therefore, the presence of a closed pneumothorax is a contraindication to the administration of nitrous oxide. Indeed, decreasing pulmonary compliance during administration of nitrous oxide to a patient with a history of chest trauma may reflect nitrous oxide-induced expansion of a previously unrecognized pneumothorax. Increased intracranial pressure due to the accumulation of nitrous oxide in an air-filled cavity in the cranium is known as a tension penumocephalus (see Chapter 24).

In contrast to the rapid expansion of a pneumothorax, the increase in bowel gas volume produced by nitrous oxide is slow. The question of whether or not to administer nitrous oxide to a patient with a bowel obstruction is of little importance if the operation is short. Limiting the inhaled concentration of nitrous oxide to 50 percent, however, may be a prudent recommendation when bowel gas volume is increased preoperatively. Following this guideline, bowel gas volume, at most, would double even with prolonged operations.

Postoperative manifestations of nitrous oxide passage into the middle ear include altered hearing acuity, serous otitis, tympanic membrane rupture, disruption of prior ossicle reconstructive surgery (see Chapter 25), and possibly nausea and vomiting due to altered middle ear pressures.

Cardiac output (CO) influences uptake and, therefore, PA by carrying away more or less anesthetic from the alveoli. A high CO (fear) results in more rapid uptake such that the rate of rise in the PA, and thus the induction of anesthesia, is slowed. A low CO (shock) speeds the rate of rise of the PA since there is less uptake to oppose input. Indeed, it is a common clinical impression that the induction of anesthesia in a patient in shock is rapid.

Right-to-Left Shunt. A right-to-left intracardiac or intrapulmonary shunt slows the rate of induction of anesthesia. This slowing reflects the dilutional effect of shunted blood containing no anesthetic on the partial pressure of anesthetic in blood coming from ventilated alveoli. Although shunt will slow the induction of anesthesia, the magnitude of this change is small and probably would not be apparent clinically.

Alveolar to Venous Partial Pressure Difference (A − vD). The A − vD reflects tissue uptake of the inhaled anesthetic. Highly perfused tissues (brain, heart, kidneys) account for less than 10 percent of body mass but receive about 75 percent of the CO. As a result, these tissues equilibrate rapidly with the Pa. Indeed, after three time constants (15 minutes for volatile anesthetics) about 75 percent of the returning venous blood is at the same partial pressure as the PA. For this reason, uptake of anesthetic from the alveoli is greatly decreased after 15 minutes, as reflected by a narrowing of the inspired to alveolar partial pressure difference. After this time, the inhaled concentration of anesthetic should be reduced so as to maintain a constant PA in the presence of decreased uptake.

Muscle and fat represent about 70 percent of the body mass but receive less than 25 percent of the CO. Therefore, these tissues continue to act as an inactive reservoir for anesthetic uptake for several hours. Indeed, equilibration of fat with an inhaled anesthetic in the arterial blood probably never occurs.

Recovery from Anesthesia

Recovery from anesthesia can be defined as the rate at which the PA decreases with time. In many respects, recovery is the inverse of induction of anesthesia. For example, VA, solubility, and CO determine the rate at which the PA decreases.

Duration of Anesthesia. A factor that is important in the rate of recovery but not induction is the duration of anesthesia (see Chapter 30). The influence of duration of anesthesia on rate of recovery reflects the solubility of the inhaled anesthetic in blood and tissues. Storage of an inhaled anesthetic in tissues increases with time. At the conclusion of the anesthetic when the partial pressure gradient is reversed by decreasing the PI to near zero, anesthetic dissolved in tissues acts as a reservoir to maintain the PA and slow recovery. The impact of duration of anesthesia is most important when a soluble drug is administered and of minimal importance when a poorly soluble drug is utilized. This is the reason nitrous oxide can be administered to near the end of the anesthetic without delaying recovery as reflected by the rate of decrease of the PA.

Diffusion hypoxia is a possibility at the conclusion of nitrous oxide administration if the patient is allowed to inhale room air. The initial high volume outpouring of nitrous oxide from the blood into the alveoli when inhalation of this gas is discontinued can so dilute the PAO_2 that the PaO_2 decreases.[1] The occurrence of diffusion hypoxia is prevented by filling the patient's lungs with oxygen at the conclusion of nitrous oxide administration.

PHARMACODYNAMICS OF INHALED ANESTHETICS

Minimum Alveolar Concentration (MAC)

MAC is the minimum alveolar concentration (partial pressure) of an inhaled anesthetic at 1 atmosphere which prevents skeletal muscle movement in response to a noxious stimulus (surgical skin incision) in 50 percent of patients.[5] As such, MAC represents one point on the dose response curve of effects produced by inhaled anesthetics. The fact that MAC reflects the partial pressure at the anesthetic site of action (e.g., Pbr) has made MAC the most important index of anesthetic equal potency.

Use of equal potent doses (e.g., comparable MAC concentrations) of inhaled anesthetics is mandatory for comparing effects of these drugs on vital organ function. For example, 1 MAC enflurane (1.68 percent) depresses cardiac output more than an equally potent concentration of isoflurane (1.15 percent) (see Chapter 4). The fact that the dose response curves for different inhaled anesthetics are not parallel with respect to vital organ depression is an important observation. Specifically, a therapeutic index may be characterized for the inhaled anesthetics with respect to any untoward or desired side effect (e.g., respiratory or cardiac depression, neuromuscular blockade, cerebral, renal, hepatic, or coronary blood flow). The denominator in this ratio is MAC. Each anesthetic possesses unique qualities with respect to these anesthetic side effects, yet similar MAC concentrations all produce equivalent depression of the central nervous system. Such information is vital for the safe and rational selection of specific inhaled anesthetics for individual patients as well as the dose of drug that is administered.

MAC values for combinations of inhaled anesthetics are probably additive. For example, 0.5 MAC nitrous oxide plus 0.5 MAC isoflurane has the same effect at the brain as either drug alone at a 1 MAC concentration. The fact that nitrous oxide MAC is above 100 percent, however, means that this anesthetic cannot be used alone at 1 atmosphere and still provide a minimum of 21 percent oxygen. Therefore, 50 to 75 percent inhaled nitrous oxide is commonly administered with the remaining anesthetic requirement being provided by a volatile anesthetic and/or narcotic (see Chapter 9). A guideline is that MAC for a volatile anesthetic is reduced about 1 percent for every

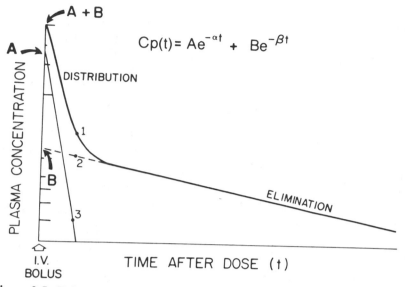

$$Cp(t) = Ae^{-\alpha t} + Be^{-\beta t}$$

A + B

A

DISTRIBUTION

PLASMA CONCENTRATION

B

1

2

3

ELIMINATION

I.V. BOLUS

TIME AFTER DOSE (t)

Figure 2-5. Following the intravenous bolus administration of a drug, the plasma concentration decreases with time. The initial rapid decrease in plasma concentration reflects distribution of drug to tissues while the subsequent slow decline in plasma concentration reflects elimination of the drug by the liver and kidneys. The time necessary for the plasma concentration to decrease 50 percent during the distribution or elimination phase is the corresponding half-life for that drug.

bound to protein is readily available to interact with receptors and, thus, elicit a pharmacologic response, changes in the protein binding of drugs may change the availability of drugs to receptors. Also, in long-term diseases and in the aged, debilitative changes often occur. Furthermore, most drugs distribute and bind in tissues in extravascular compartments. As a result, decreases in skeletal muscle mass and subsequent changes in lean body-to-fat ratios as occur with aging may result in significant changes in drug pharmacokinetics.

Biotransformation and Elimination from the Body

Kidneys. The extent to which drugs are excreted into the urine is subject to considerable variation between individuals. The three mechanisms involved in urinary excretion are (1) glomerular filtration, (2) tubular secretion, and (3) tubular reabsorption.

The rate at which a drug enters the glomerular filtrate depends on its molecular weight and its concentration in plasma. Binding to plasma protein retards the rate of filtration, and displacement from protein facilitates filtration. As far as tubular secretion is concerned, the cells of the proximal convoluted tubules actively transport a wide range of substances from the plasma into the tubular urine. Unlike glomerular filtration, the extent to which a drug is actively transported into the urine is not necessarily related to the degree of binding to plasma protein.

The urine is concentrated to a considerable extent by the time it reaches the distal renal tubules. Thus, a concentration gradient exists from tubular urine to plasma for drugs that were initially in equilibrium with plasma in the glomerular filtrate. For drugs that are actively transported into the urine, the concentration gradient already established in a proximal renal tubule is in-

1 percent alveolar nitrous oxide concentration. An important reason for administering nitrous oxide with a volatile anesthetic is the observation that depression of ventilation and circulation is less when nitrous oxide is substituted for an equivalent MAC dose of the volatile drug (see Chapter 4).

Clinically, greater than a 1 MAC concentration of inhaled anesthetic is necessary, remembering that 50 percent of patients would move with surgical stimulation at a 1 MAC concentration. Administration of approximately 1.3 MAC prevents movement in nearly all patients during surgery (see Chapter 9).

In addition to its value as an index of equal potency, the MAC concept also allows a quantitative analysis of the impact of various pharmacologic and physiologic factors on anesthetic requirements (Table 2-3).[6] Likewise, factors that do not influence MAC can be determined (Table 2-3).[6] Lastly, MAC is being utilized as a tool to better understand the mechanism by which anesthetics produce anesthesia.

THEORIES OF ANESTHESIA

Inhaled anesthetics produce reversible inhibition of synaptic transmission in several areas of the central nervous system. A decrease in dorsal horn activity produced by low partial pressures of inhaled anesthetics interferes with synaptic transmission in the spinothalamic tract and presumably produces some degree of analgesia (Stage 1). At a higher brain partial pressure, blockade of inhibitory neurons plus facilitation of excitatory transmission accounts for the disinhibitory effects of inhaled anesthetics, manifesting as patient excitement prior to the onset of unconsciousness (Stage 2). The ascending pathways in the reticular activating system are progressively depressed with further increases in the brain partial pressures of the inhaled drugs, leading to unconsciousness (Stage 3). Occurring at the same time as unconsciousness is

Table 2-3. Impact of Physiologic and Pharmacologic Factors on Minimum Alveolar Concentration (MAC)

No change in MAC
  Duration of anesthesia
  Hyperkalemia or hypokalemia
  Magnitude of anesthetic metabolism
  Thyroid gland dysfunction
  Male or female
  Arterial $PaCO_2$ 15–95 mmHg
  Arterial PaO_2 above 38 mmHg
  Blood pressure above 40 mmHg

Increase MAC
  Hyperthermia
  Hypernatremia
  Drugs that increase CNS catecholamine levels
    (monoamine oxidase inhibitors, tricyclic
    antidepressants, acute cocaine ingestion,
    acute amphetamine ingestion)
  Chronic ethanol abuse

Decrease MAC
  Hypothermia
  Hyponatremia
  Pregnancy
  Lithium
  Pancuronium
  Magnesium
  Lidocaine
  Physostigmine
  Arterial PO_2 below 38 mmHg
  Blood pressure below 40 mmHg
  Increasing age
  Preoperative medication
  Drugs that decrease CNS catecholamine levels
    (alpha-methyldopa, clonidine, chronic
    amphetamine ingestion)
  Acute ethanol ingestion

suppression of spinal reflex activity which produces skeletal muscle relaxation. At an even higher brain partial pressure (e.g., overdose), there is depression of vital medullary centers, manifesting as profound cardiorespiratory depression (Stage 4).

Proposed Theories of Anesthesia

The mechanism by which inhaled anesthetics produce progressive and sometimes selective depression of the central nervous system (e.g., anesthesia) is not known. Most evidence is consistent with inhibition of synaptic transmission produced by an action of inhaled anesthetics at a hydrophobic (e.g., lipophilic) site on biologic membranes. A single theory, however, to explain the mechanism of anesthesia seems unlikely. Nevertheless, several unitary theories have been proposed to explain the production of anesthesia by inhaled drugs.[7]

Meyer-Overton Theory (Critical-Volume Hypothesis). This theory recognizes the close correlation between the lipid solubility of inhaled anesthetics (oil:gas partition coefficient) and their potencies (e.g., MAC) (Table 2-2). Such a correlation suggests that anesthesia occurs when a sufficient number of anesthetic molecules dissolve (critical-volume) in a crucial hydrophobic site, such as lipid cell membranes. Conceptually, expansion of this hydrophobic membrane by dissolved anesthetic molecules could exert pressure on ionic channels necessary for sodium flux and the subsequent development of an action potential necessary for synaptic transmission. Indeed, membrane expansion by a critical volume of 0.4 percent results in anesthesia. Furthermore, high pressures (40 to 100 atmospheres) partially antagonize the action of inhaled anesthetics (pressure reversal), presumably by returning (compressing) the lipid membranes to their "awake" contour.[8] Universal acceptance of this theory, however, is prevented by the observation that some lipid soluble compounds are not anesthetics, and, in fact, may be convulsants.

Protein (Receptor) Hypothesis. This theory proposes hydrophobic regions of specific proteins (receptors) in the central nervous system as the site and mechanism of action of inhaled anesthetics. Evidence to support this theory includes the steep nature of the anesthetic does response curve (e.g., 1 MAC prevents movement in 50 percent of subjects while 1.3 MAC is effective in 95 percent), suggesting a crucial receptor occupancy. Receptor specificity is also suggested by conversion of an anesthetic to a nonanesthetic by increasing the molecular weight despite corresponding increases in lipid solubility.

Endogenous Endorphin Release. Recognition that there is an endogenous pain suppression system has led to the speculation that inhaled anesthetics could act by evoking the release of endogenous opiate-like substances. Indeed, beta-endorphin injected directly into the cerebral ventricles of animals produces unconsciousness.[9] Furthermore, naloxone, a specific narcotic antagonist partially antagonizes the circulatory and central nervous system effects of the volatile anesthetic, halothane.[10] Nevertheless, in another report, pretreatment of animals with large doses of naloxone did not alter halothane MAC.[11] The current consensus is that, although anesthetics may produce some degree of analgesia by stimulating the release of endogenous opiates, they do not produce anesthesia by this mechanism.

PHARMACOKINETICS OF INTRAVENOUS ANESTHETICS

Many of the same principles which govern the pharmacokinetics of inhaled anesthetics also apply to anesthetics given intravenously.[12] Volume of distribution (Vd) and clearance (CL) of a drug from the body are important determinants of pharmacokinetics of intravenous anesthetics.

Volume of Distribution (Vd)

Vd relates the total amount of drug in the body (Q) to the concentration of drug in blood or plasma (C) as illustrated by the following equation:

$$Vd = Q - C$$

Vd can be described in a variety of ways, including Vd at steady state and/or initial volume of distribution. Of prime importance is that Vd does not represent a real volume, but is a mathematical estimate of the size of the pool of body fluids that would be required if the drug was distributed equally throughout all portions of the body. Pooly lipid soluble and highly ionized drugs, such as nondepolarizing muscle relaxants, have a small Vd similar to the extracellular fluid volume. Conversely, lipid soluble and un-ionized drugs, such as thiobarbiturates and narcotics, have a large Vd. The Vd is influenced by the (1) pKa of a drug; (2) degree of plasma protein binding; (3) the solubility (partition coefficient) of the drug in various tissues; and (4) the degree of binding to other tissues in the body.

Clearance (CL)

The factors which influence drug CL are similar to those regulating renal physiology, in which creatinine or urea clearance is defined as the rate of elimination of a compound in the urine, relative to the plasma drug concentration. CL of a drug from the blood or plasma is equal to the rate of elimination (ER) by all routes, especially liver and kidney, divided by the concentration (C) of drug.

$$CL = ER/C$$

CL is one of the most important pharmacokinetic variables to be considered when defining a constant drug infusion regime. To maintain a steady-state therapeutic drug concentration during constant drug infusion requires the infusion rate to be equal to ER. Therefore, if the desired steady-state concentration is known, the CL in that patient will dictate the infusion rate. This concept will be increasingly important in anesthesia when administering short-acting drugs, such as the muscle relaxants, atracurium and vecuronium, and the narcotic, alfentanil.

Half-Life

Half-life of a drug is illustrated by plotting the plasma concentration of a drug (on a log scale) following its bolus intravenous injection versus time (Fig. 2-5). The time nec-

essary for the plasma drug concentration to decrease 50 percent is the half-life for that drug. The initial rapid decline in plasma concentration following intravenous injection reflects distribution of drug from the systemic circulation to tissues. This rapid decline is known as the distribution or alpha half-life. Following this phase, the plasma drug concentration decreases gradually, reflecting elimination of drug from the body. The time necessary for the plasma drug concentration to decrease 50 percent during this phase is known as the elimination or beta half-life. Knowledge of the beta half-life of a drug is crucial for achieving steady state therapeutic concentrations during constant drug infusion regimes. It must be recognized that individual variations in Vd and CL may alter the elimination half-life of a drug in an individual patient as compared with values calculated in normal patients.

Effects of Diseases

Diseases which alter the manner in which drugs are distributed and eliminated will influence the final concentration which reaches the receptor or active site. For example, renal failure allows an accumulation of drugs by preventing their normal elimination from plasma. This has been exemplified by the prolonged neuromuscular blockade from nondepolarizing muscle relaxants in patients with renal failure. Furthermore, diseases which impair the liver's ability to metabolize and excrete drugs also will have an influence on the final concentration of drug which reaches the receptor site and how long the effect of this drug will last. Diseases, such as congestive heart failure, can compromise cardiac function and reduce perfusion of tissues such as the liver and kidney which are responsible for absorption, distribution, and elimination of drugs. As a result, the time course and disposition of a number of drugs can be significantly altered. Since only a drug not

creased. Since the tubular epithelium has properties of a lipid membrane, only the unionized fraction of drugs contributes to the concentration gradient.

The renal clearance value of a drug is expressed by the following equation:

renal clearance
$$= \frac{Cu \times \text{rate of urine formation}}{Cp}$$

where Cu represents concentration in urine, and Cp represents concentration in plasma.

Liver. The main organ concerned with drug metabolism is the liver, and many drugs are substrates for the microsomal enzyme systems of hepatocytes. The kidney, lung, intestinal mucosa, plasma, and nerves also contain important drug-metabolizing enzymes. Generally, the metabolism of a drug decreases its lipid solubility; therefore, it becomes more hydrophilic, thereby facilitating its renal excretion. Drugs which are water soluble, but not lipid soluble, are usually excreted unchanged (e.g., before metabolism) in the urine, and have only a short persistence in the body.

Many drug-metabolizing enzymes are located in the lipophilic membranes of the endoplasmic reticulum of the liver and other tissues. When these membranes are isolated and have undergone various biochemical transformations, vesicles called *microsomes* result. The microsomes are involved with protein synthesis and oxidative drug metabolism. In the oxidative-reductive process, cytochrome P-450 microsomal enzymes play key roles.

The ability of a drug to stimulate synthesis of cytochrome P-450 enzymes is designated as *enzyme induction*. This change results in an acceleration of metabolism of other drugs. For example, administration of phenobarbital can accelerate the rate of halothane metabolism. Conversely, *enzyme inhibition* refers to drugs that inhibit cytochrome P-450 enzyme activity.

PHARMACODYNAMICS OF INTRAVENOUS DRUGS

Characteristics of Receptors

The observed effects of injected drugs result from their interaction with specific macromolecules called *receptors*. The existence of receptors for most clinically useful drugs has been only inferred from the chemical structures of the drugs themselves and the resulting pharmacologic effects. Also, the complimentary shape and distribution of electrical charge of the receptor site can be imagined. Because drug receptors can now be isolated and characterized, they are being described in biochemical terms. Receptors are usually proteins, presumably because their polypeptide structure provides the necessary diversity and specificity of shape and charge, allowing specific drugs to attach to them.

Classification of Receptors

Regulatory proteins are the best described drug receptors which mediate the action of endogenous chemical signals produced by neurotransmitters and hormones. These receptors also mediate the effects of most useful drugs, which either mimic actions of the endogenous agonists or act as antagonists to prevent response to endogenous chemical signals. *Enzymes* represent another class of proteins that have been identified as drug receptors, which may be inhibited by binding with a drug. *Transport proteins* represent still another type of membrane receptor for drugs such as the cardioactive aspects of digitalis. Of the membrane-bound proteins that function as receptors for hormones and drugs, the nicotinic receptor is a classic example. When this receptor binds with acetylcholine, a transmembrane channel is opened through which sodium ions penetrate from the extracellular fluid into the cell. This action initiates an action potential in nerves or muscles that are targets for nicotinic stimulation. Finally, the adrenergic receptors are probably among the most intensely studied receptors (see Chapter 3).

Relationship between Drug Concentration and Response

To best characterize a pharmacodynamic response, correlation between the drug concentration at the receptor site and the pharmacologic response is required. The drug concentration, however, at the receptor site usually cannot be measured from a technical point of view. Therefore, pharmacodynamics are usually expressed by relating the plasma concentration of drug to the pharmacologic response. The plasma concentration of drug probably reflects the receptor concentration of drug, so long as a steady-state exists. When a drug is given by a bolus injection intravenously, the plasma concentration is fluctuating so widely that a steady-state probably never exists. In the initial time following a bolus intravenous injection of a drug, the plasma concentration is probably higher than that at the actual receptor site. Conversely, at a later time, the gradient probably has been reversed; that is, the drug concentration at the receptor site is probably higher than that which exists in the blood. This temporal dysequilibrium between the blood concentration of drug and the drug effect, which has also been termed *hysteresis*, is characteristic for many drugs. Furthermore, if the site of action is a highly perfused organ, such as the brain or heart, equilibrium between the blood/drug concentration and the site of actual action will be rapid. If the site of action, however, is a poorly perfused tissue, such as muscle or fat, onset of effect will be delayed and the dysequilibrium will be greater. Several pharmacokinetic and pharmacodynamic models have utilized the relationship between blood concentration and pharmacologic effect when hysteresis exists.[12] From these models, drug sensitivity or potency is measured by the ED_{50} or CP_{ss50} which refers to that plasma concentration of drug which results in a 50 percent effect at steady state.[13]

VARIATION IN RESPONSE TO A DRUG

Several factors may be responsible for a variable response to a drug. Most of these variables can be categorized into one of the four following categories.

Alteration in Concentration of Drug that Reaches a Receptor

In essence, any alteration in the pharmacokinetics of a drug alters not only the concentration of drug that reaches the receptor, but the rate at which the drug disassociates from the receptor. These pharmacokinetic influences can often be predicted on the basis of age, weight, sex, disease state, and liver and/or kidney function.

Variation in Concentration of Endogenous Receptor Ligand

This mechanism contributes significantly to the variability of drug effect in individual patients as well as the response to pharmacologic antagonists. For example, propranolol, a beta antagonist, slows the heart rate of a patient in whom endogenous catecholamines are elevated, such as in heart failure, but does not affect the resting heart rate of a well-trained runner. Another example is that when acetylcholine concentrations are abnormally high at the neuromuscular junction due to recent neostigmine administration, much less succinylcholine is required to produce a given degree of neuromuscular blockade.

Variation in Number or Function of Receptors

Certainly, changes in drug response can be caused by increases (up-regulation) or decreases (down-regulation) in the number

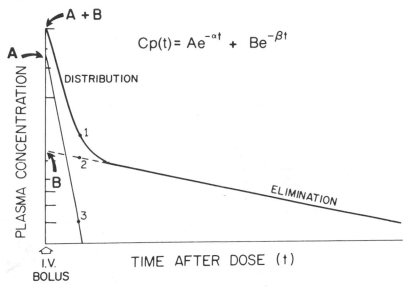

Figure 2-5. Following the intravenous bolus administration of a drug, the plasma concentration decreases with time. The initial rapid decrease in plasma concentration reflects distribution of drug to tissues while the subsequent slow decline in plasma concentration reflects elimination of the drug by the liver and kidneys. The time necessary for the plasma concentration to decrease 50 percent during the distribution or elimination phase is the corresponding half-life for that drug.

bound to protein is readily available to interact with receptors and, thus, elicit a pharmacologic response, changes in the protein binding of drugs may change the availability of drugs to receptors. Also, in long-term diseases and in the aged, dcbilitative changes often occur. Furthermore, most drugs distribute and bind in tissues in extravascular compartments. As a result, decreases in skeletal muscle mass and subsequent changes in lean body-to-fat ratios as occur with aging may result in significant changes in drug pharmacokinetics.

Biotransformation and Elimination from the Body

Kidneys. The extent to which drugs are excreted into the urine is subject to considerable variation between individuals. The three mechanisms involved in urinary excretion are (1) glomerular filtration, (2) tubular secretion, and (3) tubular reabsorption.

The rate at which a drug enters the glomerular filtrate depends on its molecular weight and its concentration in plasma. Binding to plasma protein retards the rate of filtration, and displacement from protein facilitates filtration. As far as tubular secretion is concerned, the cells of the proximal convoluted tubules actively transport a wide range of substances from the plasma into the tubular urine. Unlike glomerular filtration, the extent to which a drug is actively transported into the urine is not necessarily related to the degree of binding to plasma protein.

The urine is concentrated to a considerable extent by the time it reaches the distal renal tubules. Thus, a concentration gradient exists from tubular urine to plasma for drugs that were initially in equilibrium with plasma in the glomerular filtrate. For drugs that are actively transported into the urine, the concentration gradient already established in a proximal renal tubule is in-be required if the drug was distributed equally throughout all portions of the body. Pooly lipid soluble and highly ionized drugs, such as nondepolarizing muscle relaxants, have a small Vd similar to the extracellular fluid volume. Conversely, lipid soluble and un-ionized drugs, such as thiobarbiturates and narcotics, have a large Vd. The Vd is influenced by the (1) pKa of a drug; (2) degree of plasma protein binding; (3) the solubility (partition coefficient) of the drug in various tissues; and (4) the degree of binding to other tissues in the body.

Clearance (CL)

The factors which influence drug CL are similar to those regulating renal physiology, in which creatinine or urea clearance is defined as the rate of elimination of a compound in the urine, relative to the plasma drug concentration. CL of a drug from the blood or plasma is equal to the rate of elimination (ER) by all routes, especially liver and kidney, divided by the concentration (C) of drug.

$$CL = ER/C$$

CL is one of the most important pharmacokinetic variables to be considered when defining a constant drug infusion regime. To maintain a steady-state therapeutic drug concentration during constant drug infusion requires the infusion rate to be equal to ER. Therefore, if the desired steady-state concentration is known, the CL in that patient will dictate the infusion rate. This concept will be increasingly important in anesthesia when administering short-acting drugs, such as the muscle relaxants, atracurium and vecuronium, and the narcotic, alfentanil.

Half-Life

Half-life of a drug is illustrated by plotting the plasma concentration of a drug (on a log scale) following its bolus intravenous injection versus time (Fig. 2-5). The time nec-essary for the plasma drug concentration to decrease 50 percent is the half-life for that drug. The initial rapid decline in plasma concentration following intravenous injection reflects distribution of drug from the systemic circulation to tissues. This rapid decline is known as the distribution or alpha half-life. Following this phase, the plasma drug concentration decreases gradually, reflecting elimination of drug from the body. The time necessary for the plasma drug concentration to decrease 50 percent during this phase is known as the elimination or beta half-life. Knowledge of the beta half-life of a drug is crucial for achieving steady state therapeutic concentrations during constant drug infusion regimes. It must be recognized that individual variations in Vd and CL may alter the elimination half-life of a drug in an individual patient as compared with values calculated in normal patients.

Effects of Diseases

Diseases which alter the manner in which drugs are distributed and eliminated will influence the final concentration which reaches the receptor or active site. For example, renal failure allows an accumulation of drugs by preventing their normal elimination from plasma. This has been exemplified by the prolonged neuromuscular blockade from nondepolarizing muscle relaxants in patients with renal failure. Furthermore, diseases which impair the liver's ability to metabolize and excrete drugs also will have an influence on the final concentration of drug which reaches the receptor site and how long the effect of this drug will last. Diseases, such as congestive heart failure, can compromise cardiac function and reduce perfusion of tissues such as the liver and kidney which are responsible for absorption, distribution, and elimination of drugs. As a result, the time course and disposition of a number of drugs can be significantly altered. Since only a drug not

plain the mechanism of anesthesia seems unlikely. Nevertheless, several unitary theories have been proposed to explain the production of anesthesia by inhaled drugs.[7]

Meyer-Overton Theory (Critical-Volume Hypothesis). This theory recognizes the close correlation between the lipid solubility of inhaled anesthetics (oil:gas partition coefficient) and their potencies (e.g., MAC) (Table 2-2). Such a correlation suggests that anesthesia occurs when a sufficient number of anesthetic molecules dissolve (critical-volume) in a crucial hydrophobic site, such as lipid cell membranes. Conceptually, expansion of this hydrophobic membrane by dissolved anesthetic molecules could exert pressure on ionic channels necessary for sodium flux and the subsequent development of an action potential necessary for synaptic transmission. Indeed, membrane expansion by a critical volume of 0.4 percent results in anesthesia. Furthermore, high pressures (40 to 100 atmospheres) partially antagonize the action of inhaled anesthetics (pressure reversal), presumably by returning (compressing) the lipid membranes to their "awake" contour.[8] Universal acceptance of this theory, however, is prevented by the observation that some lipid soluble compounds are not anesthetics, and, in fact, may be convulsants.

Protein (Receptor) Hypothesis. This theory proposes hydrophobic regions of specific proteins (receptors) in the central nervous system as the site and mechanism of action of inhaled anesthetics. Evidence to support this theory includes the steep nature of the anesthetic does response curve (e.g., 1 MAC prevents movement in 50 percent of subjects while 1.3 MAC is effective in 95 percent), suggesting a crucial receptor occupancy. Receptor specificity is also suggested by conversion of an anesthetic to a nonanesthetic by increasing the molecular weight despite corresponding increases in lipid solubility.

Endogenous Endorphin Release. Recognition that there is an endogenous pain suppression system has led to the speculation that inhaled anesthetics could act by evoking the release of endogenous opiate-like substances. Indeed, beta-endorphin injected directly into the cerebral ventricles of animals produces unconsciousness.[9] Furthermore, naloxone, a specific narcotic antagonist partially antagonizes the circulatory and central nervous system effects of the volatile anesthetic, halothane.[10] Nevertheless, in another report, pretreatment of animals with large doses of naloxone did not alter halothane MAC.[11] The current consensus is that, although anesthetics may produce some degree of analgesia by stimulating the release of endogenous opiates, they do not produce anesthesia by this mechanism.

PHARMACOKINETICS OF INTRAVENOUS ANESTHETICS

Many of the same principles which govern the pharmacokinetics of inhaled anesthetics also apply to anesthetics given intravenously.[12] Volume of distribution (Vd) and clearance (CL) of a drug from the body are important determinants of pharmacokinetics of intravenous anesthetics.

Volume of Distribution (Vd)

Vd relates the total amount of drug in the body (Q) to the concentration of drug in blood or plasma (C) as illustrated by the following equation:

$$Vd = Q - C$$

Vd can be described in a variety of ways, including Vd at steady state and/or initial volume of distribution. Of prime importance is that Vd does not represent a real volume, but is a mathematical estimate of the size of the pool of body fluids that would

1 percent alveolar nitrous oxide concentration. An important reason for administering nitrous oxide with a volatile anesthetic is the observation that depression of ventilation and circulation is less when nitrous oxide is substituted for an equivalent MAC dose of the volatile drug (see Chapter 4).

Clinically, greater than a 1 MAC concentration of inhaled anesthetic is necessary, remembering that 50 percent of patients would move with surgical stimulation at a 1 MAC concentration. Administration of approximately 1.3 MAC prevents movement in nearly all patients during surgery (see Chapter 9).

In addition to its value as an index of equal potency, the MAC concept also allows a quantitative analysis of the impact of various pharmacologic and physiologic factors on anesthetic requirements (Table 2-3).[6] Likewise, factors that do not influence MAC can be determined (Table 2-3).[6] Lastly, MAC is being utilized as a tool to better understand the mechanism by which anesthetics produce anesthesia.

THEORIES OF ANESTHESIA

Inhaled anesthetics produce reversible inhibition of synaptic transmission in several areas of the central nervous system. A decrease in dorsal horn activity produced by low partial pressures of inhaled anesthetics interferes with synaptic transmission in the spinothalamic tract and presumably produces some degree of analgesia (Stage 1). At a higher brain partial pressure, blockade of inhibitory neurons plus facilitation of excitatory transmission accounts for the disinhibitory effects of inhaled anesthetics, manifesting as patient excitement prior to the onset of unconsciousness (Stage 2). The ascending pathways in the reticular activating system are progressively depressed with further increases in the brain partial pressures of the inhaled drugs, leading to unconsciousness (Stage 3). Occurring at the same time as unconsciousness is

Table 2-3. Impact of Physiologic and Pharmacologic Factors on Minimum Alveolar Concentration (MAC)

No change in MAC
  Duration of anesthesia
  Hyperkalemia or hypokalemia
  Magnitude of anesthetic metabolism
  Thyroid gland dysfunction
  Male or female
  Arterial $PaCO_2$ 15–95 mmHg
  Arterial PaO_2 above 38 mmHg
  Blood pressure above 40 mmHg

Increase MAC
  Hyperthermia
  Hypernatremia
  Drugs that increase CNS catecholamine levels
    (monoamine oxidase inhibitors, tricyclic
    antidepressants, acute cocaine ingestion,
    acute amphetamine ingestion)
  Chronic ethanol abuse

Decrease MAC
  Hypothermia
  Hyponatremia
  Pregnancy
  Lithium
  Pancuronium
  Magnesium
  Lidocaine
  Physostigmine
  Arterial PO_2 below 38 mmHg
  Blood pressure below 40 mmHg
  Increasing age
  Preoperative medication
  Drugs that decrease CNS catecholamine levels
    (alpha-methyldopa, clonidine, chronic
    amphetamine ingestion)
  Acute ethanol ingestion

suppression of spinal reflex activity which produces skeletal muscle relaxation. At an even higher brain partial pressure (e.g., overdose), there is depression of vital medullary centers, manifesting as profound cardiorespiratory depression (Stage 4).

Proposed Theories of Anesthesia

The mechanism by which inhaled anesthetics produce progressive and sometimes selective depression of the central nervous system (e.g., anesthesia) is not known. Most evidence is consistent with inhibition of synaptic transmission produced by an action of inhaled anesthetics at a hydrophobic (e.g., lipophilic) site on biologic membranes. A single theory, however, to ex-

creased. Since the tubular epithelium has properties of a lipid membrane, only the un-ionized fraction of drugs contributes to the concentration gradient.

The renal clearance value of a drug is expressed by the following equation:

renal clearance
$$= \frac{Cu \times \text{rate of urine formation}}{Cp}$$

where Cu represents concentration in urine, and Cp represents concentration in plasma.

Liver. The main organ concerned with drug metabolism is the liver, and many drugs are substrates for the microsomal enzyme systems of hepatocytes. The kidney, lung, intestinal mucosa, plasma, and nerves also contain important drug-metabolizing enzymes. Generally, the metabolism of a drug decreases its lipid solubility; therefore, it becomes more hydrophilic, thereby facilitating its renal excretion. Drugs which are water soluble, but not lipid soluble, are usually excreted unchanged (e.g., before metabolism) in the urine, and have only a short persistence in the body.

Many drug-metabolizing enzymes are located in the lipophilic membranes of the endoplasmic reticulum of the liver and other tissues. When these membranes are isolated and have undergone various biochemical transformations, vesicles called *microsomes* result. The microsomes are involved with protein synthesis and oxidative drug metabolism. In the oxidative-reductive process, cytochrome P-450 microsomal enzymes play key roles.

The ability of a drug to stimulate synthesis of cytochrome P-450 enzymes is designated as *enzyme induction*. This change results in an acceleration of metabolism of other drugs. For example, administration of phenobarbital can accelerate the rate of halothane metabolism. Conversely, *enzyme inhibition* refers to drugs that inhibit cytochrome P-450 enzyme activity.

PHARMACODYNAMICS OF INTRAVENOUS DRUGS

Characteristics of Receptors

The observed effects of injected drugs result from their interaction with specific macromolecules called *receptors*. The existence of receptors for most clinically useful drugs has been only inferred from the chemical structures of the drugs themselves and the resulting pharmacologic effects. Also, the complimentary shape and distribution of electrical charge of the receptor site can be imagined. Because drug receptors can now be isolated and characterized, they are being described in biochemical terms. Receptors are usually proteins, presumably because their polypeptide structure provides the necessary diversity and specificity of shape and charge, allowing specific drugs to attach to them.

Classification of Receptors

Regulatory proteins are the best described drug receptors which mediate the action of endogenous chemical signals produced by neurotransmitters and hormones. These receptors also mediate the effects of most useful drugs, which either mimic actions of the endogenous agonists or act as antagonists to prevent response to endogenous chemical signals. *Enzymes* represent another class of proteins that have been identified as drug receptors, which may be inhibited by binding with a drug. *Transport proteins* represent still another type of membrane receptor for drugs such as the cardioactive aspects of digitalis. Of the membrane-bound proteins that function as receptors for hormones and drugs, the nicotinic receptor is a classic example. When this receptor binds with acetylcholine, a transmembrane channel is opened through which sodium ions penetrate from the extracellular fluid into the cell. This action initiates an action potential in nerves or muscles that are targets for nicotinic stimulation. Finally, the adrenergic receptors are probably among the most intensely studied receptors (see Chapter 3).

Relationship between Drug Concentration and Response

To best characterize a pharmacodynamic response, correlation between the drug concentration at the receptor site and the pharmacologic response is required. The drug concentration, however, at the receptor site usually cannot be measured from a technical point of view. Therefore, pharmacodynamics are usually expressed by relating the plasma concentration of drug to the pharmacologic response. The plasma concentration of drug probably reflects the receptor concentration of drug, so long as a steady-state exists. When a drug is given by a bolus injection intravenously, the plasma concentration is fluctuating so widely that a steady-state probably never exists. In the initial time following a bolus intravenous injection of a drug, the plasma concentration is probably higher than that at the actual receptor site. Conversely, at a later time, the gradient probably has been reversed; that is, the drug concentration at the receptor site is probably higher than that which exists in the blood. This temporal dysequilibrium between the blood concentration of drug and the drug effect, which has also been termed *hysteresis*, is characteristic for many drugs. Furthermore, if the site of action is a highly perfused organ, such as the brain or heart, equilibrium between the blood/drug concentration and the site of actual action will be rapid. If the site of action, however, is a poorly perfused tissue, such as muscle or fat, onset of effect will be delayed and the dysequilibrium will be greater. Several pharmacokinetic and pharmacodynamic models have utilized the relationship between blood concentration and pharmacologic effect when hysteresis exists.[12] From these models, drug sensitivity or potency is measured by the ED_{50} or CP_{ss50} which refers to that plasma concentration of drug which results in a 50 percent effect at steady state.[13]

VARIATION IN RESPONSE TO A DRUG

Several factors may be responsible for a variable response to a drug. Most of these variables can be categorized into one of the four following categories.

Alteration in Concentration of Drug that Reaches a Receptor

In essence, any alteration in the pharmacokinetics of a drug alters not only the concentration of drug that reaches the receptor, but the rate at which the drug disassociates from the receptor. These pharmacokinetic influences can often be predicted on the basis of age, weight, sex, disease state, and liver and/or kidney function.

Variation in Concentration of Endogenous Receptor Ligand

This mechanism contributes significantly to the variability of drug effect in individual patients as well as the response to pharmacologic antagonists. For example, propranolol, a beta antagonist, slows the heart rate of a patient in whom endogenous catecholamines are elevated, such as in heart failure, but does not affect the resting heart rate of a well-trained runner. Another example is that when acetylcholine concentrations are abnormally high at the neuromuscular junction due to recent neostigmine administration, much less succinylcholine is required to produce a given degree of neuromuscular blockade.

Variation in Number or Function of Receptors

Certainly, changes in drug response can be caused by increases (up-regulation) or decreases (down-regulation) in the number

3

Autonomic Nervous System

The pharmacologic effects of catecholamines, sympathomimetics, antihypertensives, beta-adrenergic agonists, beta-adrenergic antagonists, anticholinergics, and anticholinesterases involve the actions of these drugs on the central and peripheral autonomic nervous system. An appreciation of the anatomy and physiology of the peripheral autonomic nervous system is important for understanding the effects of these drugs and predicting potential adverse drug interactions in the perioperative period.

ANATOMY AND PHYSIOLOGY OF THE PERIPHERAL AUTONOMIC NERVOUS SYSTEM

The peripheral autonomic nervous system is divided into the sympathetic and parasympathetic nervous systems (Fig. 3-1).[1] Preganglionic fibers of the sympathetic nervous system arise from cells in the thoracolumbar portions of the spinal cord, while craniosacral cells are the origin of preganglionic fibers of the parasympathetic nervous system. A number of cell bodies form the autonomic ganglion which acts as the site of synapse between preganglionic and postganglionic fibers. The preganglionic fibers are myelinated. The postganglionic fibers of the sympathetic nervous system are distributed throughout the body, while distribution of parasympathetic nervous system postganglionic fibers is more limited. The parasympathetic nervous system has its terminal ganglia near the organs innervated and thus is more discrete in its discharge of impulses than is the sympathetic nervous system (Fig. 3-1).

Sympathetic Nervous System

Postganglionic fibers of the sympathetic nervous system that release norepinephrine as the neurotransmitter are adrenergic, and receptors that respond to norepinephrine are adrenoceptive (Table 3-1). Postsynaptic adrenoceptive receptors are classified as beta-1, beta-2, and alpha-1 (Fig. 3-2).[1] Alpha-2 receptors are presynaptic (Fig. 3-2).[1] Stimulation of alpha and beta-adrenergic receptors by endogenous catecholamines or synthetic adrenergic agonists produces predictable pharmacologic responses (Table 3-1). Likewise, the effects of alpha- and beta-adrenergic antagonists are predictable based on a knowledge of responses evoked by stimulation of these receptors.

Adrenoceptive receptors have not been isolated chemically, but the enzyme adenylate cyclase probably is an important component of beta-adrenergic receptors (Fig. 3-3).[2] Activation of adenylate cyclase cata-

27

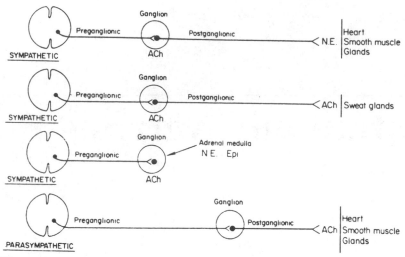

Figure 3-1. Anatomy of the peripheral autonomic nervous system ACh-acetylcholine, NE-norepinephrine. (Miller RD, Stoelting RK. Pharmacology of the autonomic nervous system. In: Miller RD, ed. Anesthesia. New York, Churchill Livingstone, 1981;539–60.)

lyzes the conversion of adenosine triphosphate (ATP) to cyclic adenosine monophosphate (cAMP). It is cAMP which acts as the second messenger to stimulate events characterized as beta-adrenergic stimulation (Table 3-1). Hydrolysis of cAMP by phosphodiesterase results in inactivation of this second messenger. Alpha-adrenergic receptors have not been well characterized but it is thought that cyclic guanosine monophosphate (cGMP) may act as the second messenger at these sites.

Termination of the action of norepinephrine on adenoceptive receptors is by uptake (reuptake) of this neurotransmitter from the receptors back into the postganglionic nerve ending. Following uptake, a small amount of norepinephrine is deaminated in the cytoplasm by the enzyme monoamine oxidase (MAO). Most of the norepinephrine, however, escapes breakdown and can be stored for subsequent release.

Parasympathetic Nervous System

Postganglionic fibers of the parasympathetic nervous system release acetylcholine as the neurotransmitter. Receptors that re-

spond to acetylcholine are cholinoceptive. These receptors are classified as nicotinic and muscarinic (Table 3-1). Stimulation of nicotinic or muscarinic receptors by acetylcholine or synthetic cholinergic agonists produces predictable pharmacologic responses (Table 3-1). Likewise, the effects of cholinergic antagonists are predictable based on a knowledge of responses evoked by stimulation of cholinoceptive receptors. The action of acetylcholine at cholinoceptive receptors is terminated by hydrolysis of this neurotransmitter by the enzyme acetylcholinesterase.

CATECHOLAMINES

Catecholamines are compounds with hydroxyl groups on the 3 and 4 positions of the benzene ring of phenylethylamine (Fig. 3-4).[3] Endogenous catecholamines are dopamine, norepinephrine, and epinephrine. Catecholamines that do not occur endogenously are isoproterenol and dobutamine. Pharmacologic effects produced by catecholamines reflect the ability of these substances to stimulate adrenoceptive recep-

PRESYNAPTIC   POSTSYNAPTIC

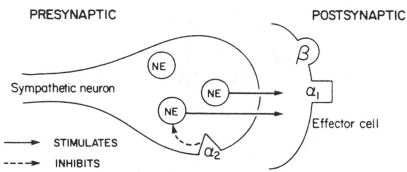

Figure 3-2. Schematic representation of the synapse between the postganglionic sympathetic neuron and postsynaptic receptors (effector cells). Stimulation of presynaptic receptors by previously released neurotransmitter, norepinephrine (NE) results in inhibition of further release of NE from the sympathetic neuron. (Reproduced with permission from Ram CVS, Kaplan NM: Alpha- and beta-receptor blocking drugs in the treatment of hypertension. In Harvey WP, et al, eds. Current problems in cardiology. Copyright 1979 by Year Book Medical Publishers, Inc, Chicago, as modified in Miller RD, Stoelting RK. Pharmacology of the autonomic nervous system. In: Miller RD, ed. Anesthesia. New York, Churchill Livingstone, 1981;539–60.)

tors. Clinically, catecholamines are administered as continuous intravenous infusions to produce desirable pharmacologic effects manifesting predominately on the cardiovascular system (Table 3-2).

Dopamine

Dopamine, depending on the dose, directly stimulates postsynaptic dopaminergic, beta and alpha-adrenergic receptors.[4] This catecholamine is unique among this class of drugs in its ability to stimulate dopaminergic receptors and redistribute blood flow to the kidneys. These renal effects predominate when the rate of continuous intravenous infusion of dopamine is less than 3 μg/kg/min. This dose can inhibit secretion of aldosterone, which, along with dopaminergic stimulation, results in increased urine output. Beta-adrenergic stimulation characterized by increased myocardial contractility without marked changes in heart rate and blood pressure occurs when the rate of dopamine infusion is 3 to 10 μg/kg/min. Some residual dopaminergic stimulation persists up to doses of 5 μg/kg/min.

Dopamine also exerts part of its inotropic effect by releasing endogenous stores of norepinephrine which predisposes to cardiac dysrhythmias. Furthermore, this indirect stimulation may be an unreliable mechanism when cardiac catecholamine stores are depleted as with chronic congestive heart failure. Beta and alpha-adrenergic agonist effects occur with dopamine infusion rates between 10 and 20 μg/kg/min, while alpha-adrenergic effects of dopamine predominate with doses above 20 μg/kg/min. High doses of dopamine can inhibit release of insulin, leading to hyperglycemia.

Dopamine is most often used in clinical situations characterized by decreased cardiac output, reduced blood pressure, increased left ventricular end-diastolic pressure, and oliguria. It should be recognized, however, that infusion rates of dopamine (above 8 μg/kg/min) may increase pulmonary artery occlusion pressure. The ability of dopamine to exert positive inotropic effects and concomitantly increase pulmonary artery occlusion pressure is not shared by other catecholamines. The speculated mechanism for this paradoxical response is

β - ADRENERGIC RECEPTOR

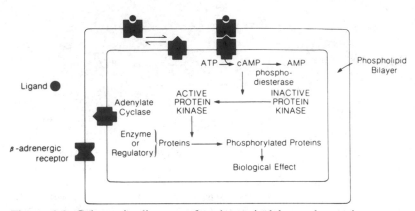

Figure 3-3. Schematic diagram of a theoretical beta-adrenergic receptor consisting of two components in the membrane of the target cell. The component facing the exterior of the cell recognizes the neurotransmitter (ligand). After binding, the ligand-receptor complex diffuses laterally along the membrane until it couples to the component facing the interior of the cell. It is presumed that the component facing the interior of the cell is the enzyme adenylate cyclase. Activation of adenylate cyclase catalyzes the conversion of adenosine triphosphate (ATP) to cyclic adenosine monophosphate (cAMP) which functions as the second messenger to stimulate other reactions culminating in a biological (beta-adrenergic) effect. The intracellular concentration of cAMP is also influenced by phosphodiesterase, which hydrolyzes the second messenger to an inactive molecule. For example, inhibition of phosphodiesterase activity allows cAMP to accumulate and produce a beta-adrenergic effect in the absence of a prior ligand-receptor interaction. (Maze M. Clinical implications of membrane receptor function in anesthesia. Anesthesiology 1981;55:160–71.)

redistribution of blood volume from the periphery to the central circulation due to alpha-adrenergic induced venoconstriction. In addition, dopamine may increase filling pressure by reducing left ventricular compliance.

Dopamine is prepared in a solution of 5 percent dextrose in water. More alkaline intravenous solutions may inactivate dopamine.

Norepinephrine

Norepinephrine, as the endogenous neurotransmitter for adrenoceptive receptors, is responsible for maintaining blood pressure by appropriate adjustments in systemic vascular resistance. Vasoconstriction induced by norepinephrine produces increased systemic vascular resistance re-

flected by increases in systolic, diastolic, and mean arterial pressure. Beta-1 agonist effects of norepinephrine on the heart are overshadowed by the alpha-1 agonist effects of this catecholamine on the peripheral vasculature. Cardiac output may be reduced despite the increased blood pressure, reflecting the effect of increased ventricular afterload and baroreceptor-mediated reflex bradycardia. Beta-2 agonist effects of norepinephrine are minimal. Clinically, norepinephrine is seldom used to treat cardiovascular collapse.

Epinephrine

Epinephrine stimulates alpha-1, beta-1, and beta-2 receptors. Low doses of epinephrine stimulate alpha-1 receptors in the skin, mucosa, and hepatorenal vasculature,

Table 3-1. Characteristics of the Autonomic Nervous System

Receptors	Effector Organ	Response to Stimulation	Synthetic Drugs	
			Agonist	Antagonist
		Adrenoceptive (postsynaptic)		
Beta-1	Heart	Increased heart rate Increased contractility Increased automaticity Increased conduction velocity	Dobutamine Dopamine Isoproterenol[a]	Metoprolol Propranolol[a] Timolol[a] Alprenolol[a] Oxprenolol[a]
	Fat cells	Lipolysis		Pindolol[a] Atenolol[a] Sotalol[a]
Beta-2	Blood vessels (especially skeletal and coronary arteries)	Dilatation	Terbutaline Ritoridine Salbutamol Isoproterenol[a]	Propranolol[a] Timolol[a] Alprenolol[a] Oxprenolol[a] Pindolol[a] Atenolol[a] Sotalol[a]
	Bronchioles	Dilatation		
	Uterus	Relaxation		
	Kidney	Renin secretion		
	Liver	Glycogenolysis Gluconeogenesis		
	Pancreas	Insulin secretion		
Alpha-1	Blood vessels	Constriction	Phenylephrine Methoxamine	Prazosin Phentolamine[b]
	Pancreas	Inhibit insulin secretion		Phenoxy-benzamine[b]
	Intestine and bladder	Relaxation Constriction of sphincters		
		Adrenoceptive (presynaptic)		
Alpha-2	Postganglionic sympathetic nerve ending	Inhibit norepinephrine release	Clonidine	Yohimbine Phentolamine[b]
		Cholinoceptive (postsynaptic)		
Muscarinic	Heart	Decreased heart rate Decreased contractility Decreased conduction velocity	Methacholine Carbachol	Atropine Glycopyrrolate Scopolamine
	Bronchioles	Constriction		
	Salivary glands	Stimulate secretions		
	Intestine	Contraction Relaxation of sphincters Stimulate secretions		
	Bladder	Contraction Relaxation of sphincter		
Nicotinic	Autonomic ganglia	Sympathetic nervous system stimulation		Hexamethonium
	Neuromuscular junction	Skeletal muscle contraction	Succinylcholine[c]	d-Tubocurarine Metocurine Gallamine Pancuronium Atracurium Vecuronium

[a] Produces mixed beta-1 and beta-2 effects.
[b] Produces mixed alpha-1 and alpha-2 effects.
[c] Initial stimulation (fasiculation) followed by inhibition of contractions due to proloned depolarization.

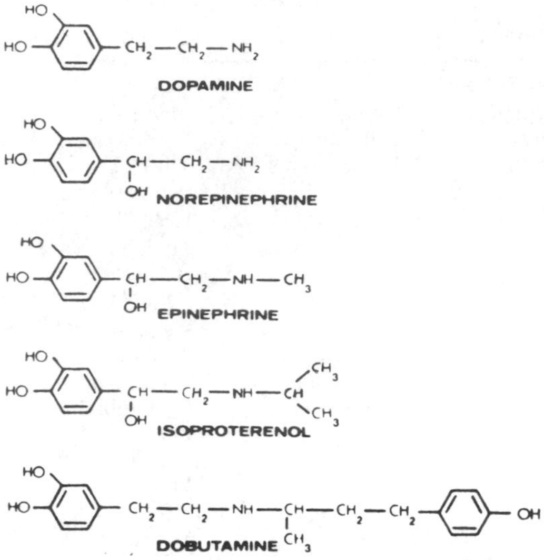

Figure 3-4. Chemical structure of the endogenous and synthetic (isoproterenol, dobutamine) catecholamines. A catecholamine is defined as any compound with hydroxyl groups on the 3 and 4 positions of the benzene ring of phenylethylamine. The first endogenous catecholamine, dopamine, is 3,4-dihydroxyphenylethylamine. (Sonnenblick EH, Frishman WH, LeJemtel TH. Dobutamine: a new synthetic cardioactive sympathetic amine. N Engl J Med 1979;300:17–22.)

producing vasoconstriction, while beta-2 induced vasodilation predominates in skeletal muscle. The net effect is decreased systemic vascular resistance and a preferential distribution of cardiac output to skeletal muscle. Renal blood flow is greatly reduced during infusion of epinephrine even with an unchanged blood pressure. Stimulation of

beta-1 receptors increases heart rate and myocardial contractility, resulting in an increased cardiac output. Since the blood pressure is not greatly elevated, compensatory baroreceptor reflexes are not elicited and the cardiac output is increased. Beta-1 stimulation also increases automaticity of the heart, which manifests as cardiac irritability, most often in the form of ventricular premature contractions.

Of all the catecholamines, epinephrine has the most significant effects on metabolism. For example, beta-adrenergic stimulation from epinephrine increases adipose tissue lipolysis and liver glycogenolysis, while alpha-1 stimulation inhibits release of insulin from the pancreas (Table 3-1). Epinephrine release in response to surgical stimulation is the most likely explanation for the characteristic hyperglycemia observed in the perioperative period.

Epinephrine is occasionally used as a continuous intravenous infusion to treat reduced myocardial contractility. Subcutaneous epinephrine is also used in combination with local anesthetics to reduce systemic absorption and to provide local hemostasis. In addition, epinephrine is administered during cardiopulmonary resuscitaion to produce ventricular fibrillation that is more likely to be responsive to external defibrillation (see Chapter 34). Finally, epinephrine is indicated in the treatment of life-threatening allergic reactions.

Table 3-2. Pharmacologic Effects and Therapeutic Doses of Catecholamines

Catecholamine	MAP	HR	CO	SVR	RBF	Preparation (mg/500 ml)	Intravenous Dose (μg/kg/min)
Dopamine	+	+ +	+ + +	+	+ + +	400	2–20
Norepinephrine	+ + +	−	−	+ + +	− − −	8	0.05–0.2
Epinephrine	+ +	+ +	+ +	+ +	− −	8	0.05–0.2
Isoproterenol	−	+ + +	+ + +	− −	−	2	0.03–0.3
Dobutamine	+	+	+ + +	±	±	500	2–20

Abbreviations: MAP, mean arterial pressure; HR, heart rate; CO, cardiac output; SVR, systemic vascular resistance; RBF, renal blood flow.
Symbols: + = mild increase; + + = moderate increase; + + + = severe increase; − = mild decrease; − − = moderate decrease; − − − = severe decrease.

Isoproterenol

Isoproterenol is a synthetic catecholamine with potent stimulant effects on beta-1 and beta-2 receptors and no effect on alpha-1 receptors. Myocardial contractility, heart rate, systolic blood pressure, and cardiac automaticity are increased, while sytemic vascular resistance and diastolic blood pressure are decreased. The net effect is an increase in cardiac output and occasionally a reduction in mean arterial pressure. Bronchodilation is accompanied by significant cardiovascular effects, since isoproterenol does not discriminate between beta-1 and beta-2 receptors (Table 3-1).

Excessive tachycardia and simultaneous diastolic hypotension may reduce coronary blood flow at the time myocardial oxygen requirements are increased by tachycardia. These events, combined with a high incidence of cardiac dysrhythmias and diversion of blood flow to skeletal muscle, detract from the value of this catecholamine, particularly in patients with coronary artery disease. The major clinical use of isoproterenol is in patients with valvular heart disease associated with pulmonary hypertension. Such patients may benefit from isoproterenol-induced increases in heart rate and reductions in systemic and pulmonary vascular resistance.

Dobutamine

Dobutamine is a synthetic catecholamine with structural characteristics of dopamine and isoproterenol.[3] Removal of the side-chain hydroxyl groups from the isoproterenol portion decreases cardiac arrhythmogenicity but retains the inotropic properties. Dobutamine acts selectively on beta-1 receptors without significant effects on beta-2 or alpha-1 receptors. Unlike dopamine, this catecholamine does not act indirectly by stimulating endogenous norepinephrine release, nor does it stimulate dopaminergic receptors to increase renal blood flow. The most prominent effect during the infusion of dobutamine (2 to 20 µg/kg/min) is a dose-dependent increase in cardiac output without marked changes in heart rate or systemic vascular resistance. This ability to increase myocardial contractility with minimal chronotropic or alpha-1 stimulation is unique to dobutamine. Dobutamine may be ineffective for those patients who need increased systemic vascular resistance to elevate blood pressure. Drug-induced increases in the rate of atrioventricular conduction of the cardiac impulse detracts from the use of dobutamine in patients with atrial fibrillation. Since dobutamine lacks dopaminergic stimulating effects, it is reasonable to consider infusing this catecholamine with dopamine to the patient who is hypotensive and oliguric. Dobutamine, like dopamine, can be inactivated when prepared in alkaline intravenous solutions—emphasizing the importance of preparing this drug in a 5 percent dextrose in water solution.

SYMPATHOMIMETICS

Sympathomimetics are synthetic drugs that are used as vasopressors to reverse downward trends in blood pressure as may accompany vasodilation produced by spinal or epidural blockade. Likewise, hypotension produced by inhaled anesthetics may be treated with a sympathomimetic to assure maintenance of an adequate perfusion pressure during the time needed to eliminate the excess inhaled drug. Structurally, sympathomimetics resemble catecholamines except that hydroxyl groups are not present on both the 3 and 4 positions of the benzene ring.

Classification

Sympathomimetics are classified according to their selectivity for stimulating alpha and/or beta-adrenergic receptors (Table 3-3). Knowing the selectivity for either receptor permits selection of a drug specifically to elevate blood pressure by periph-

Table 3-3. Classification and Therapeutic Doses of Sympathomimetics

Sympathomimetic[a]	Alpha	Beta-1	Beta-2	Direct (D) Indirect (I)	Intravenous Dose for an Adult (mg)
Ephedrine	+ +	+ + +	+ +	I (some D)	10–25
Metaraminol (Aramine)	+ + +	+ +	+ +	I (some D)	0.5–5
Mephentermine (Wyamine)	+	+ +	+ + +	I	5–15
Phenylephrine (Neo-Synephrine)	+ + + +	+	0	D	0.1–0.5
Methoxamine (Vasoxyl)	+ + + +	0	0	D	5–10

Symbols: 0 = none; + = minimal; + + = mild; + + + = moderate; + + + + = marked.
[a] Trade names in parentheses.

eral vasoconstriction, increased myocardial contractility, or a combination of these effects. Most sympathomimetics are mixed, producing both alpha and beta agonist effects.[5]

Alternatively, sympathomimetics may be classified as direct- or indirect-acting drugs (Table 3-3). Direct-acting drugs produce effects similar to the sympathetic nervous system neurotransmitter, norepinephrine, such that depletion of norepinephrine or denervation does not reduce the efficacy of these drugs. In contrast, indirect-acting drugs act by evoking the release of endogenous norepinephrine, and their efficacy is reduced by depletion of the neurotransmitter. This classification permits prediction of altered responses to sympathomimetics. For example, antihypertensives that reduce sympathetic nervous system activity will also decrease the pressor response elicited by indirect-acting sympathomimetics (Fig. 3-5).[6] Conversely, the pressor response elicited by direct-acting drugs may be exaggerated as the receptors are sensitized (denervation hypersensitivity) by a lack of tonic impulses (Fig. 3-5).[6]

Treatment of patients with tricyclic antidepressants or monoamine oxidase inhibitors introduces the potential for adverse drug interactions with sympathomimetics as well as other undesirable responses.

Tricyclic antidepressants inhibit uptake of previously released norepinephrine back into postganglionic sympathetic nerve ending, resulting in increased availability of this neurotransmitter. Therefore, administration of an indirect-acting drug such as ephedrine is likely to evoke an exaggerated blood pressure response. Furthermore, administration of pancuronium to halothane-anesthetized dogs who have been pretreated with a tricyclic antidepressant is associated with an increased incidence of cardiac dysrhythmias. Finally, tricyclic antidepressant therapy is associated with anticholinergic effects (dry mouth, central nervous system dysfunction, urinary retention) and, occasionally, changes in conduction of the cardiac impulse that manifest on the electrocardiogram as prolongation of the QRS complex, prolongation of the PR interval, and bundle branch block.

Monoamine oxidase inhibitors prevent the breakdown of norepinephrine in the postganglionic nerve ending and peripheral tissues by monoamine oxidase, resulting in increased availability of this neurotransmitter. Therefore, administration of an indirect-acting drug such as ephedrine is likely to evoke an exaggerated blood pressure response. Should treatment of hypotension require administration of a sympa-

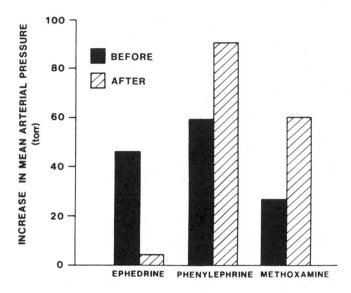

Figure 3-5. The increase in mean arterial pressure in response to injection of various sympathomimetics was determined before and after the administration of a centrally acting antihypertensive, reserpine, to anesthetized dogs. The blood pressure response evoked by an indirect-acting sympathomimetic, ephedrine, was attenuated in the presence of the antihypertensive. Conversely, the blood pressure response produced by the direct-acting sympathomimetics, phenylephrine and methoxamine was exaggerated following administration of the antihypertensive. (Goodloe SL. Essential hypertension. In Stoelting RK, Dierdorf SF, eds. Anesthesia and co-existing disease. New York, Churchill Livingstone, 983: 99–117, based on data in ref. 6.)

thomimetic, the best selection is a reduced dose of a direct-acting drug such as phenylephrine. Administration of even small doses of narcotics to patients being treated with monoamine oxidase inhibitors can result in dangerous elevations in body temperature, seizures, depression of ventilation, and cardiovascular collapse. In view of these potential adverse perioperative drug interactions and the prolonged effect of monoamine oxidase inhibitors, it is recommended that this class of drugs be discontinued 14 to 21 days prior to elective surgery.

Ephedrine

Ephedrine is an indirect-acting sympathomimetic that exerts its blood pressure effects by stimulating the release of norepinephrine. In addition, ephedrine has some direct-acting effects. Clinically, ephedrine produces responses consistent with alpha (vasoconstriction) and beta-adrenergic (increased myocardial contractility) stimulation. The systolic and diastolic blood pressures are typically increased and the cardiac output is improved, providing there is adequate venous return to the heart. Increased heart rate is consistent with beta-adrenergic stimulation. Cardiac dysrhythmias have been demonstrated in the dog anesthetized with halothane and treated with ephedrine.[8] Placental blood flow is preserved by ephedrine, making this drug the best choice for treating anesthetic-induced hypotension in the parturient (see Chapter 26).[7]

The cardiovascular stimulating effects of ephedrine diminish with repeated doses. The mechanism of this tachyphylaxis is not known, but depletion of catecholamine stores is a consideration.

Metaraminol

Metaraminol has both indirect and direct actions and overall effects similar to those of norepinephrine. Its vasoconstrictive action is of longer duration than its cardiac stimulating action such that alpha agonist effects predominate. It may be useful to think of metaraminol as a potent ephedrine.

Metaraminol depletes and replaces norepinephrine from its storage sites and then acts as a false neurotransmitter. The release of metaraminol rather than norepinephrine in response to an adrenergic stimulus results in less alpha agonist stimulation, since this false neurotransmitter is about one-tenth as potent as the endogenous neurotransmitter. Therefore, continued infusion of metaraminol for longer than 3 hours may result in hypotension.

Mephentermine

Mephentermine, like ephedrine and metaraminol, acts in part by stimulating the release of catecholamines. In contrast to metaraminol, the cardiac stimulating effects of mephentermine predominate over its peripheral vascular effects. Hence, cardiac output is increased while changes in systemic vascular resistance are variable. Cardiac dysrhythmias are less likely to occur with this drug as compared with other sympathomimetics that stimulate alpha and beta-adrenergic receptors.

Phenylephrine and Methoxamine

Phenylephrine and methoxamine are direct-acting sympathomimetics that increase systemic vascular resistance and blood pressure by selective stimulation of alpha-adrenergic receptors. These drugs are devoid of clinically significant cardiac stimulating effects. Reflex bradycardia is a predictable response when blood pressure is elevated by phenylephrine and methoxamine.

Choice of phenylephrine or methoxamine to treat hypotension due to volatile anesthetics must consider the possible detrimental cardiac effects of drug-induced vasoconstriction on the anesthetic depressed heart.[8] Hypotension due to spinal or epidural block is logically treated with a drug such as phenylephrine or methoxamine that offsets anesthetic-induced reductions in systemic vascular resistance by producing

Table 3–4. Antihypertensives Used in the Ambulatory Treatment of Essential Hypertension

Central sympatholytics
  Alpha-methyldopa (Aldomet)
  Clonidine (Catapres)
Peripheral sympatholytics
  Guanethidine (Ismelin)
Peripheral vasodilators
  Hydralizine (Apresoline)
  Minoxidil (Loniten)
  Diazoxide (Hyperstat)[a]
  Nitroprusside (Nipride)[a]
  Nitroglycerin (Tridil)[a]
Alpha-adrenergic antagonists
  Prazosin (Minipress)
  Phentolamine (Regitine)[a]
Beta-adrenergic antagonists
  Propranolol (Inderal)
  Metoprolol (Lopressor)
  Nadolol (Corgard)
  Atenolol (Tenormin)
  Timolol (Blocadren)
Alpha- beta-adrenergic antagonists
  Labetalol (Normodyne)
Ganglionic blocking drugs
  Trimetaphan (Arfonad)[a]

Trade names in paretheses.
[a] Not used for ambulatory treatment of essential hypertension because of extreme potency. Instead, administered intravenously to rapidly lower blood pressure to normal levels in patients experiencing hypertensive crises.

alpha-adrenergic stimulation. Nevertheless, ephedrine is also a useful drug to treat this form of hypotension.

ANTIHYPERTENSIVES

Antihypertensives are used in the treatment of ambulatory essential hypertension to reduce blood pressure toward normal levels by selectively impairing sympathetic nervous system function at the heart and/or peripheral vasculature (Table 3-4). Attenuation of sympathetic nervous system activity is reflected by orthostatic hypotension. During anesthesia, exaggerated reductions in blood pressure (as associated with hemorrhage, positive airway pressure, or sudden changes in body position) may reflect an impaired degree of compensatory peripheral vascular vasoconstriction due to inhibitory effects of antihypertensives on sympathetic nervous system activity. The response to sympathomimetics may be modified by prior treatment with antihypertensives (see the section *Sympathomimetics*). Selective impairment of sympathetic nervous system activity by antihypertensives results in a predominance of parasympathetic nervous system tone, manifesting as bradycardia. Finally, antihypertensives that reduce central nervous system sympathetic activity are associated with sedation and reduced anesthetic requirements (MAC).[9] Despite interference of antihypertensives with normal sympathetic nervous system activity it is agreed that these drugs should be continued during the perioperative period so as to maintain optimal control of the blood pressure.

Alpha-Methyldopa

The most likely explanation for the antihypertensive effect of alpha-methyldopa is the accumulation of alpha-methylated amines in the central nervous system, resulting in a reduced outflow of sympathetic nervous system impulses. Methyldopa decreases blood pressure by reducing both the cardiac output and systemic vascular resistance. The plasma half-time of this drug is only 1 to 2 hours but its hypotensive effect can last as long as 24 hours, probably because the active metabolite, alpha-methylnorepinephrine, has a long half-time in the brain.

A major side effect of alpha-methyldopa is depression of the central nervous system and drowsiness. In animals, this effect is associated with a dose-dependent 15 to 30 percent decrease in MAC (Fig. 3-6).[9] Decreased blood pressure responses following the administration of ephedrine also occurred in these animals. About 20 percent of patients treated with alpha-methyldopa develop a positive Coombs' test which may result in difficulty in cross-matching whole blood for that patient. As many as 5 percent of patients with a positive Coombs' test sec-

ondary to alpha-methyldopa develop hemolytic anemia, necessitating the cessation of treatment with this drug. A rare but important side effect of treatment with this drug is fever and hepatic dysfunction. Patients who are receiving alpha-methyldopa may develop hypertension following administration of propranolol. This hypertensive response presumably reflects the ability of propranolol to block the vasodilating effects of alpha-methylnorepinephrine. As a result, only the potent alpha stimulating effects of this metabolite are apparent. Alpha-methyldopa is a logical choice in patients with renal disease, since this drug maintains or increases renal blood flow.

Clonidine

Clonidine is a centrally acting antihypertensive that stimulates alpha-2 receptors in the depressor area of the vasomotor center, leading to a decreased outflow of sympathetic nervous system impulses to the periphery. The net effect of this decreased sympathetic nervous system activity is a reduction in cardiac output, systemic vascular resistance, and blood pressure. Sedation is a common side effect of treatment, and reductions in MAC have been documented in animals treated with this drug.[10] Bradycardia and dry mouth may accompany treatment with clonidine. The duration of action of a single dose of clonidine is 6 to 24 hours.

The most important adverse effect of clonidine is rebound hypertension when the drug is discontinued. Indeed, discontinuation of treatment with clonidine has been associated with the development of adverse increases in blood pressure before the induction of anesthesia, as well as in the early postoperative period.[11] The speculated mechanism for this rebound hypertension is an abrupt increase in systemic vascular resistance due to release of catecholamines and/or activation of the renin angiotensin system. Continuation of clonidine throughout the perioperative period is difficult be-

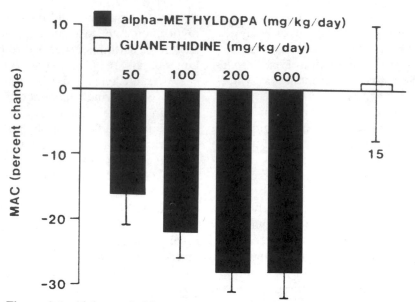

Figure 3-6. Alpha-methyldopa, a centrally acting antihypertensive produced a dose dependent reduction in anesthetic requirements (MAC) for halothane in dogs. Conversely, guanethidine, which does not cross the blood brain barrier, did not alter MAC. (Goodloe SL. Essential hypertension. In Stoelting RK, Dierdorf SF, eds. Anesthesia and co-existing disease. New York, Churchill Livingstone 1983: 99–117, based on data in ref. 9.)

cause a parenteral form of this drug is not available. Therefore, consideration should be given to replacing clonidine before elective surgery with an alternative antihypertensive such as hydralazine.

Clonidine has been shown to be effective in suppressing the signs and symptoms of withdrawal from narcotics. It is speculated that clonidine replaces opiate-mediated inhibition with alpha-2 mediated inhibition of central nervous system sympathetic activity.

Guanethidine

Guanethidine lacks significant effects on the central nervous system (MAC not altered) because its guanidine group prevents easy passage across the blood brain barrier (Fig. 3-6).[9] This drug acts selectively on the peripheral sympathetic nervous system to depress function of postganglionic sympa-

thetic nerves by causing the release and subsequent depletion of norepinephrine from the nerve ending as well as by inhibiting depolarization produced by nerve stimulation. Resulting reductions in peripheral sympathetic nervous system activity are responsible for a decrease in venous return that leads to a reduction in cardiac output and a subsequent decline in blood pressure. Decreased responsiveness of resistance and capacitance blood vessels to sympathetic nervous system stimulation manifests as orthostatic hypotension. Predominance of parasympathetic nervous system activity is often manifested as bradycardia. Drugs (cocaine, tricyclic antidepressants, ketamine) that block uptake of norepinephrine into the postganglionic sympathetic nerve ending may antagonize the antihypertensive effects of guanethidine as both substances depend on the same transport mechanism to gain access into the nerve ending. The elimination half-time of guanethidine is prolonged, requiring about 5 days.

Hydralazine

Hydralazine probably interferes with calcium transport at the arterial vascular smooth muscle and thus lowers blood pressure by vasodilation. Activity of the baroreceptor reflex remains intact, leading to an increased outflow of sympathetic nervous system activity from the central nervous system. This maintenance of sympathetic nervous system activity prevents orthostatic hypotension but may offset the desired antihypertensive effect of hydralazine by increasing the heart rate. Baroreceptor-mediated reflex stimulation of heart rate can be prevented by combining hydralazine with other antihypertensives such as guanethidine or a beta-adrenergic antagonist. Hydralazine is a good choice for patients with renal disease, since this drug maintains renal blood flow. A lupus erythematosus-like syndrome is likely when the daily dose of hydralazine exceeds 200 mg.

Minoxidil

Minoxidil reduces blood pressure by direct vascular smooth muscle relaxation. As with any peripheral vasodilator, minoxidil is associated with reflex tachycardia, salt retention, and water retention. For these reasons, minoxidil is often administered in combination with a beta-adrenergic antagonist and diuretic. Pulmonary hypertension associated with minoxidil is more likely due to fluid retention than a unique effect of this drug on pulmonary vasculature. Growth of facial hair is a harmless but unpleasant side effect of minoxidil.

Prazosin

Prazosin lowers blood pressure by decreasing systemic vascular resistance due to selective alpha-1 receptor blockade. If alpha-2 receptor blockade was also present, the associated release of norepinephrine due to loss of feedback inhibition would manifest as renin release and tachycardia, tending to offset the effects of alpha-1 receptor blockade.

Prazosin, like other alpha-1 antagonists, can cause orthostatic hypotension. This effect is particularly prominent during the first few days of treatment and may manifest as syncope. Prazosin is indicated primarily in patients who do not tolerate hydralazine.

Labetalol

Labetalol is a prototype of a new class of antihypertensives that competitively blocks peripheral alpha- and beta-adrenergic receptors. Dose-dependent orthostatic hypotension is the major adverse side effect.

BETA-ADRENERGIC AGONISTS

Catecholamines are examples of beta-1 agonists used to increase heart rate and myocardial contractility (Table 3-1) (see the section *Catecholamines*). Beta-2 agonists produce relaxation of bronchial, uterine, and vascular smooth muscle, reflecting selective stimulation of beta-2 receptors (Table 3-1). Beta-2 agonists are used to treat bronchial asthma and to stop premature labor.

Drugs that are selective for beta-2 receptors are less likely than beta-1 agonists to produce adverse cardiac effects such as tachycardia or cardiac dysrhythmias. Nevertheless, reflex tachycardia, presumably due to beta-2 mediated vasodilation and subsequent hypotension, has been observed after administration of these drugs.[12] Another serious hazard of continuous intravenous infusion of a beta-2 agonist as used to stop premature labor is hypokalemia.[13] Hypokalemia most likely reflects sustained beta-2 stimulation of the sodium pump with transfer of potassium intracellularly. Tachyphylaxis to the effects of beta-2 agonists is attributed to a decreased number of beta receptors (down-regulation) that occurs with chronic stimulation of these receptors.[2]

Drug-induced inhibition of phosphodiesterase enzyme activity results in the accumulation of cAMP, leading to beta agonist effects in the absence of activation of adenylate cyclase (Fig. 3-3) (Table 3-1). Aminophylline is an example of a useful drug that produces beta-adrenergic stimulation in part by this mechanism. In addition, aminophylline stimulates the release of norepinephrine. Patients receiving a continuous intravenous infusion of aminophylline to treat bronchial asthma may be at increased risk for developing cardiac dysrhythmias during halothane anesthesia.[14] For this reason, an inhaled anesthetic such as enflurane or isoflurane, which is less likely to evoke cardiac dysrhythmias, may be a better choice than halothane when patients who are being treated with aminophylline require surgery.

BETA-ADRENERGIC ANTAGONISTS

Beta antagonists may produce selective beta-1 blockade (decreased heart rate and myocardial contractility) or mixed responses reflecting drug effects at beta-2 receptors (bronchial and vascular smooth muscle constriction) (Table 3-1). Examples of cardioselective beta antagonists are alprenolol and metoprolol. Beta antagonists may also possess membrane stabilizing activity (sotalol and propranolol) and intrinsic sympathomimetic activity (alprenolol, oxprenolol, pindolol).

Beta antagonists probably decrease blood pressure by reducing cardiac output. Inhibition of the release of renin from the kidneys may also contribute to the antihypertensive effects of these drugs, particularly in patients with high plasma renin activity. Since reductions in secretion of renin will lead to a decreased release of aldosterone, the beta antagonists will prevent compensatory sodium and water retention that often accompanies treatment of essential hypertension with a vasodilator. Furthermore, beta blockade attenuates the baroreceptor-mediated increase in heart rate associated with vasodilator therapy. An important advantage of beta antagonists as used to treat essential hypertension is the absence of orthostatic hypotension. In addition, these drugs do not produce sedation and MAC is not altered.

In addition to treatment of essential hypertension, beta antagonists are effective in reducing myocardial oxygen requirements by virtue of reductions in heart rate and myocardial contractility. These beta-1 antagonist effects more than offset any adverse effect of an increase in coronary vascular resistance due to concomitant beta-2 receptor blockade. Evidence of reduced myocardial oxygen requirements in patients treated with beta antagonists is relief of angina pectoris. Recently beta antagonists have been shown to be effective in reducing postmyocardial infarction mortality.

The major hazards of beta blockade include excessive myocardial depression and bronchoconstriction. Additive myocardial depression with volatile anesthetics can occur, but this has not proven to be a clinically significant problem. When bronchoconstriction is a likely response, as in the patient with bronchial asthma or chronic obstructive airway disease, it is important to select a beta antagonist with selective beta-1 blocking effects. Likewise, a cardioselective drug would be a logical selection in the patient with peripheral vascular disease so as to minimize the occurrence of vasoconstriction that accompanies beta-1 blockade (Table 3-1). A drug with intrinsic sympathomimetic activity may be a logical selection for treatment of patients with depressed left ventricular function or bradycardia. Indeed, beta-adrenergic blockade may produce atrioventricular heart block. Finally, warning signs and symptoms of hypoglycemia are blunted by beta-adrenergic blockade, suggesting caution in the use of these drugs in insulin-dependent patients with diabetes mellitus. A cardioselective drug would be a logical selection when diabetes mellitus is present since suppression of insulin secretion is produced by beta-2 blockade (Table 3-1).

Atropine is the initial drug recommended for treatment of signs of excessive beta blockade manifesting as bradycardia or atrioventricular heart block. If signs of excessive beta blockade persist, a specific pharmacologic treatment is administration of a beta agonist such as isoproterenol or dobutamine. However, large doses of these drugs may be required to antagonize excessive beta blockade. Alternatively, calcium chloride administered intravenously antagonizes excessive beta blockade independently of any known effect mediated via beta-adrenergic receptors. As such, conventional doses of calcium chloride (5 to 10 mg/kg) are likely to be effective.

It must be recognized that abrupt discontinuation of treatment with a beta antagonist can be associated with excessive sympathetic nervous system activity manifesting as hypertension and myocardial ischemia. Therefore, treatment with these drugs should be maintained throughout the perioperative period. Continuous intravenous infusion of propranolol 3 mg/hr is effective in maintaining therapeutic plasma concentrations in adult patients who cannot take oral medications during the perioperative period.[15]

ANTICHOLINERGICS

Anticholinergics (atropine, scopolamine, glycopyrrolate) prevent the muscarinic effects of acetylcholine by competing for the same receptor as normally occupied by the neurotransmitter. Atropine and scopolamine are tertiary amines and can cross lipid barriers such as the blood brain barrier and placenta. In contrast, glycopyrrolate acts only on peripheral cholinergic receptors because its quaternary ammonium structure prevents it from crossing lipid barriers in significant amounts.

Responses produced by anticholinergics include (1) inhibition of salivation (antisialagogue effect), (2) decreased gastric hydrogen ion secretion, (3) increased heart rate, (4) mydriasis, and (5) relaxation of the lower esophageal sphincter. The sensitivity of peripheral cholinergic receptors differs such that low doses of an anticholinergic may be sufficient to inhibit salivation but large doses are necessary for cardiac of gastrointestinal effects. Furthermore, the magnitude of anticholinergic effects may differ between drugs despite similar doses. For example, scopolamine is a potent antisialagogue, sedative, and amnesic, but has minimal effects on heart rate. Conversely, atropine is a less potent antisialagogue than scopolamine but produces significant cardiac vagolytic effects. As an antisialagogue, glycopyrrolate is more potent and longer lasting than atropine, but the heart rate effects of glycopyrrolate are minimal. Central nervous system toxicity (central anticholinergic syndrome) is more likely following administration of scopolamine than atropine and is unlikely after glycopyrrolate, since this drug is unable to easily cross the blood brain barrier.

ANTICHOLINESTERASES

Anticholinesterases are represented by quaternary ammonium (neostigmine, pyridostigmine and edrophonium) and tertiary amine drugs (physostigmine). These drugs inhibit the enzyme acetylcholinesterase (true cholinesterase) which is normally responsible for the rapid hydrolysis of acetylcholine following its release from cholinergic nerve endings. Therefore, in the presence of an anticholinesterase, there is accumulation of acetylcholine at nicotinic and muscarinic sites. Quaternary ammonium drugs cannot easily cross the blood brain barrier such that accumulation of acetylcholine is predominantly at peripheral sites such as the nicotinic neuromuscular junction. Indeed, this is the mechanism for pharmacologic reversal of nondepolarizing muscle relaxants (see Chapter 8). Conversely, physostigmine with its tertiary amine structure can cross the blood brain barrier, making this an effective drug for treatment of the central anticholinergic syndrome that manifests as emergence delerium in the recovery room (see Chapter 30).

Organophosphates produce prolonged inhibition of acetylcholinesterase activity. These substances are used as insecticides and are a frequent cause of poisoning (bradycardia, salivation, bronchoconstriction, skeletal muscle weakness) among agricultural workers, emphasizing the potential for their rapid absorption through intact skin. Pralidoxime is a specific antidote for organophosphate poisoning. Medically, organophosphate drugs (echothiophate, isoflurophate) are applied topically to the cornea to produce sustained miosis in the treatment of glaucoma (see Chapter 25). These drugs also inhibit the enzyme activity of pseudocholinesterase (serum cholinesterase) which introduces the potential for a prolonged response to succinylcholine, as this drug is normally hydrolyzed by pseudocholinesterase.

REFERENCES

1. Miller RD, Stoelting RK. Pharmacology of the autonomic nervous system. In: Miller RD, ed., Anesthesia. New York, Churchill Livingstone, 1981:539–60.
2. Maze M. Clinical implications of membrane receptor function in anesthesia. Anesthesiology 1981;55:160–71.
3. Sonnenblick EH, Frishman WH, LeJemtel TH. Dobutamine. A new synthetic cardioactive sympathetic amine. N Engl J Med 1979;300:17–22.
4. Chernow B, Rainey TG, Lake R. Endogenous and exogenous catecholamines in critical care medicine. Crit Care Med 1981;10:409–17.
5. Smith NT, Corbascio AN. The use and misuse of pressor agents. Anesthesiology 1970;33:58–101.
6. Eger EI, Hamilton WK. The effect of reserpine on the action of various vasopressors. Anesthesiology 1959;20:641–5.
7. Ralston DH, Shnider SM, deLorimer AA. Effects of equipotent ephedrine, metaraminol, mephentermine and methoxamine on uterine blood flow in the pregnant ewe. Anesthesiology 1974;40:354–70.
8. Filner BE, Karliner JS. Alterations of normal left ventricular performance by general anesthesia. Anesthesiology 1976;45:610–21.
9. Miller RD, Way WL, Eger EI. The effects of alpha-methyldopa, reserpine, guanethidine, and iproniazid on minimum alveolar anesthetic requirement (MAC). Anesthesiology 1968;29:1153–8.
10. Bloor BC, Flacke WE, Randall F. Clonidine potentiation of halothane anesthesia and reversal. Anesthesiology 1980;53:S13.
11. Bruce DL, Croley TF, Lee JS. Preoperative clonidine withdrawal syndrome. Anesthesiology 1979;5:90–2.
12. Ravindran R, Viegas OJ, Padilla LM, LaBlonde P. Anesthetic considerations in pregnant patients receiving terbutaline therapy. Anesth Analg 1980;59:391–2.
13. Moravec MA, Hurlbert BJ. Hypokalemia associated with terbutaline administration in obstetrical patients. Anesth Analg 1980;59:917–20.
14. Roizen MF, Stevens WC. Multiform ventricular tachycardia due to interaction of aminophylline and halothane. Anesth Analg 1978;57:738–41.
15. Smulyan H, Weinberg SE, Howanitz PJ. Continuous propranolol infusion following abdominal surgery. JAMA 1982;247:2539–42.

4

Inhaled Anesthetics

Currently used inhaled anesthetics, represented by one gas (nitrous oxide) and three volatile drugs (halothane, enflurane, isoflurane), have important and often differing pharmacologic effects on ventilation and circulation. Data from healthy volunteers exposed to equal potent concentrations of these drugs have provided the foundation for establishing comparative differences of inhaled anesthetics on ventilation and circulation in the absence of extraneous influences.[1] It must always be appreciated, however, that the surgical patient with other variables (co-existing disease, drug therapy that influences the function of the autonomic nervous system, preoperative medication, surgical stimulation, altered intravascular fluid volume, extremes of age) can respond differently from the healthy volunteer.

VENTILATION

Inhaled anesthetics produce dose-dependent and drug-specific effects on ventilation.[1] The respiratory pattern during inhalation of anesthetic concentrations of volatile drugs becomes regular, in contrast to the awake pattern characterized by intermittent deep breaths (sighs) and varying intervals between breaths. Typically, the respiratory rate is increased and the tidal volume decreased during anesthesia. The net effect of these drug-induced changes is a decrease in alveolar ventilation and increase in $PaCO_2$. The normal stimulation to ventilation produced by increased $PaCO_2$ or decreased PaO_2 is blunted by inhaled drugs. Airway resistance may be decreased by volatile anesthetics. Inhaled anesthetics may attenuate reflex hypoxic pulmonary vasoconstriction, contributing to a maldistribution of ventilation to perfusion and a decrease in PaO_2. Finally, surgical stimulation and duration of administration of the inhaled anesthetics may influence the impact of these drugs on ventilation.

The mechanism of rapid and shallow ventilation produced by volatile anesthetics remains obscure. Previous suggestions that the stimulation of pulmonary stretch receptors was an explanation for this ventilatory pattern in man have not been substantiated. Conversely, stretch receptors responsible for mediating intermittent deep breaths are inhibited by inhaled anesthetics. The diminished ventilatory response to carbon dioxide presumably reflects anesthetic-induced depression of the medullary ventilatory center response to changes in hydrogen ion concentration.

Arterial Partial Pressure of Carbon Dioxide

The resting $PaCO_2$ is the most frequently used index of the dose-dependent depression of ventilation produced by inhaled anesthetics. In healthy volunteers breathing equal potent concentrations of volatile anesthetics, the $PaCO_2$ is increased most by enflurane and less by isoflurane and halothane (Fig. 4-1).[1,2] The presence of chronic obstructive airway disease may accentuate the magnitude of increase in $PaCO_2$ produced by a volatile anesthetic such as halothane (Fig. 4-2).[3] Nitrous oxide administered to volunteers in a hyperbaric chamber does not alter $PaCO_2$ from awake levels. Indeed, substitution of nitrous oxide for an equivalent portion of the volatile anesthetic results in less elevation of the $PaCO_2$ than that produced by the volatile anesthetic alone. Likewise, the addition of nitrous oxide without changing the inhaled concentration of volatile anesthetic does not further increase the $PaCO_2$ despite the greater depth of anesthesia in the presence of both inhaled groups.[4] The beneficial effect of nitrous oxide on limiting the increase in $PaCO_2$ is seen with all three volatile anesthetics, but the greatest impact is present when nitrous oxide is used to replace an equivalent amount of enflurane.

In addition to nitrous oxide, surgical stimulation and duration of administration may influence the magnitude of increase in $PaCO_2$ associated with the inhalation of a volatile anesthetic. For example, surgical stimulation increases the tidal volume and respiratory rate such that minute ventilation increases about 40 percent.[1] However, the $PaCO_2$ declines only about 5 mmHg (10 percent) in response to surgical stimulation (Fig. 4-3).[1] This discrepancy is presumed to reflect increased production of carbon dioxide by activation of the sympathetic nervous system in response to surgical stimulation. This increased production of carbon dioxide prevents the increase in ventilation from reducing the $PaCO_2$ by the same magnitude. Finally, the magnitude of $PaCO_2$ elevation produced by the same dose of volatile anesthetic is less after 5 to 6 hours of administration than after 1 to 3 hours of administration (Table 4-1).[2] The reason for this apparent lessening of depression of ventilation with time is not known.

Assisted ventilation of the lungs is not greatly effective in lowering the $PaCO_2$ because the apneic threshold (maximum $PaCO_2$ which does not initiate spontaneous ventilation) is only about 5 mmHg below the resting $PaCO_2$, regardless of the level of the

P_aCO_2 (torr)

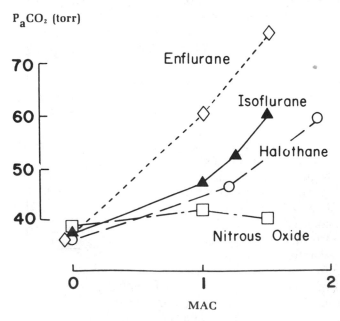

Figure 4-1. Increasing MAC levels of enflurane, isoflurane, and halothane produce dose-dependent elevations in the $PaCO_2$ when administered to healthy volunteers. Nitrous oxide was given in a pressure chamber and did not increase the $PaCO_2$. (Eger EI. Isoflurane (Forane). A compendium and reference. Madison, Wisconsin, Ohio Medical Products, 1981;24–31.)

resting $PaCO_2$. For example, a patient inhaling a volatile anesthetic at a dose sufficient to elevate the $PaCO_2$ to 55 mmHg would likely become apneic when assisted ventilation of the lungs lowered the $PaCO_2$ to about 50 mmHg. For this reason, assisted ventilation of the lungs is not a highly effective method to reduce the $PaCO_2$ during general anesthesia. Controlled ventilation of the lungs is the most predictable method for maintaining a normal $PaCO_2$ during inhalation of volatile anesthetics.

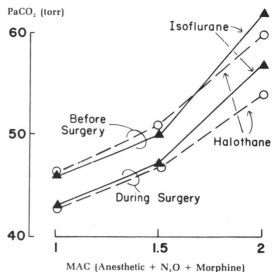

Figure 4-3. The increase in $PaCO_2$ in patients that accompanies increasing MAC levels of isoflurane or halothane is partially offset by the stimulus of surgery. (Eger EI. Isoflurane (Forane). A compendium and reference. Madison, Wisconsin, Ohio Medical Products, 1981, 24–31.)

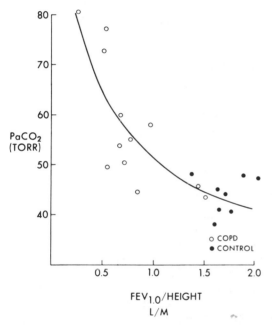

Figure 4-2. The effects of halothane (1 percent alveolar concentration) on the $PaCO_2$ (torr, mmHg) were measured during spontaneous ventilation in patients with chronic obstructive pulmonary disease (COPD) and in normal patients of similar age. During halothane anesthesia, the $PaCO_2$ was increased more (depression of ventilation was greater) in patients with co-existing pulmonary disease compared with normal patients. The magnitude of the elevation of $PaCO_2$ was best related to a preoperative measurement of the forced exhaled volume in 1 second (FEV_1) expressed in terms of body height (Pietak S, Weenig CS, Hickey RF, Fairley HB. Anesthetic effects of ventilation in patients with chronic obstructive pulmonary disease. Anesthesiology 1975;42:160–6.)

Ventilatory Response to Carbon Dioxide

Plotting the volume of ventilation at increasing levels of $PaCO_2$ (carbon dioxide response curve) is a sensitive method for quantitating the effects of drugs on ventilation (Fig. 4-4). In the normal man, inhalation of carbon dioxide increases minute ventilation 1 to 3 L/min/mmHg increase in $PaCO_2$. Inhaled anesthetics, including nitrous oxide, produce dose-dependent

Table 4-1. Recovery from Drug-Induced Ventilatory Depression with Time

	PaCO₂	
Enflurane	One Hour of Administration	Five Hours of Administration
1 MAC	61 mmHg	46 mmHg
2 MAC	Apnea	67 mmHg

(Data from Calverley RK, Smith NT, Jones CW, Prys-Roberts C, Eger EI. Ventilatory and cardiovascular effects of enflurane anesthesia during spontaneous ventilation in man. Anesth Analg 1978;57:610–8.)

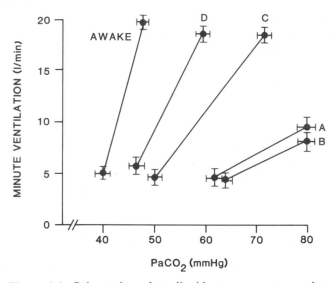

Figure 4-4. Schematic carbon dioxide response curves plotting the minute ventilation (L/min) versus $PaCO_2$ (mmHg). In the awake state minute ventilation increases 1 to 3 L/min/mmHg increase in $PaCO_2$ (curve AWAKE). The carbon dioxide response curve is dramatically shifted to the right and the slope decreased during the first 2 to 3 hours of inhalation of a 1.1 MAC concentration of a volatile anesthetic (curve A). Addition of 70 percent nitrous oxide to a 1.1 MAC concentration of a volatile anesthetic does not significantly alter the position or slope of the carbon dioxide response curve despite the increased anesthetic depth produced by the drug combination (curve B). The combination of 70 percent nitrous oxide with a sufficient concentration of volatile anesthetic to result in a 1.1 MAC concentration produces less depression of ventilation than seen with a 1.1 MAC concentration of the volatile anesthetic alone (curve C). Recovery from the ventilatory depressant effects produced by a 1.1 MAC concentration of a volatile anesthetic occurs after 5 to 6 hours of administration (curve D).

depression of the slope of the carbon dioxide response curve. In addition, the position of the carbon dioxide response curve is shifted to the right as compared with the awake curve. A decreased slope reflects reduced sensitivity to the ventilatory stimulant effects of carbon dioxide while rightward displacement depicts an attenuated responsiveness to carbon dioxide. Substitution of nitrous oxide for a portion of the volatile anesthetic (while maintaining the same total dose of anesthetic) results in a return of the slope and position of the carbon dioxide response curve toward the awake level.[4] This effect of nitrous oxide is present with all three volatile anesthetics, but the impact is most apparent when nitrous oxide is substituted for an equivalent amount of enflurane. The slope and position of the carbon dioxide response curve during inhalation of volatile anesthetics returns toward normal (like the $PaCO_2$) after 5 to 6 hours of administration of these drugs. The depression of the ventilatory response to

Table 4-2. Ventilatory Responses to Arterial Hypoxemia or Hypercapnia during Administration of Halothane to Humans

Halothane Concentration (MAC)	Percent of Awake Response	
	Arterial Hypoxemia (%)	Hypercapnia (%)
0.1	31	100
1.1	zero	36
2.0	zero	17

(Data from Knill RL, Gelb AW. Ventilatory response to hypoxia and hypercapnia during halothane sedation and anesthesia in man. Anesthesiology 1978;49:244–51.)

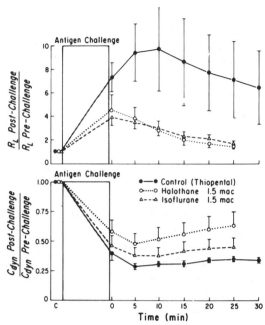

Figure 4-5. The increase in airway resistance (R_L) and decrease in pulmonary compliance (Cdyn) following Ascaris antigen challenge was measured during thiopental, halothane, and isoflurane anesthesia in dogs. The horizontal axis shows elapsed time from the conclusion of antigen administration. Halothane and isoflurane were equally effective in attenuating the antigen-induced increase in R_L as compared with thiopental. Conversely, halothane was somewhat more effective than isoflurane in minimizing a concomitant decrease in Cdyn. (Hirshman CA, Edelstein G, Peetz S, Wayne R, Downes H. Mechanism of action of inhalational anesthesia on airways. Anesthesiology 1982;56:107–11.)

carbon dioxide implies that the drive to overcome resistance to breathing (upper airway obstruction, kinked endotracheal tube, airway secretions) will be reduced during inhalation of these drugs.

Ventilatory Response to Arterial Hypoxemia

Reductions in the PaO_2 below 60 mmHg normally produce increases in minute ventilation. This response in man is mediated by the peripheral chemoreceptors known as the carotid bodies. Subanesthetic concentrations (0.1 MAC) of inhaled anesthetics greatly attenuate, while anesthetic concentrations (1 MAC) abolish, the ventilatory response to arterial hypoxemia (Table 4-2).[5] Conversely, subanesthetic concentrations of inhaled anesthetics do not depress the ventilatory response to carbon dioxide to the same degree (Table 4-2).[5] Inhaled anesthetics also attenuate the usual synergistic effect of arterial hypoxemia and hypercapnia on stimulation of ventilation. The depression of hypoxic responsiveness by subanesthetic concentrations of inhaled drugs suggests that patients would manifest a diminished ventilatory response to arterial hypoxemia in the recovery room (see Chapter 30).

Bronchodilation

Volatile anesthetics administered at 1 MAC concentrations produce similar attenuation of antigen-induced bronchospasm in dogs (Fig. 4-5).[6] Halothane has also been shown to reduce airway resistance in patients with bronchoconstriction provoked by ultrasonic aerosols. Conversely, halothane has little or no impact on airway resistance in normal patients.

The relaxant effect of volatile anesthetics on bronchial smooth muscle most likely reflects anesthetic-induced reductions in afferent nerve traffic or central medullary depression of bronchoconstriction reflexes. In addition, volatile anesthetics may produce bronchial smooth muscle relaxation by direct effects. Indeed, it has been suggested that halothane exerts beta agonist effects on bronchial smooth muscle leading to bronchodilation.

Hypoxic Pulmonary Vasoconstriction

Hypoxic pulmonary vasoconstriction is the reflex constriction of pulmonary arterioles in areas of atelectasis in an attempt to reduce or prevent perfusion of unventilated alveoli. This reflex vasoconstriction is protective and its inhibition by inhaled anesthetics could adversely affect the PaO_2. To date, however, the effect of inhaled anesthetics on hypoxic pulmonary vasoconstriction are inconclusive.[7] Halothane has been demonstrated to inhibit this reflex response in man. In the dog, isoflurane, but not enflurane, produced inhibition. Nitrous oxide has been reported to produce no effect, inhibition, and enhancement of hypoxic pulmonary vasoconstriction. Based on available data, it would seem premature to select one inhaled anesthetic over another based on presumed effects on hypoxic pulmonary vasoconstriction.

Mucociliary Function

Halothane produces a dose-dependent decrease in mucociliary function, manifesting as a decreased rate of mucus travel towards the glottic opening. A similar depression occurs with enflurane and when nitrous oxide is added to halothane. Decreased mucociliary activity can persist up to 6 hours following discontinuation of halothane. The importance of this decreased activity is its potential role in retention of secretions leading to atelectasis and pneumonia. The mechanism by which inhaled anesthetics inhibit mucociliary activity is not known.

Respiratory Muscle Function

Optimal respiratory muscle function occurs when descent of the diaphragm is coupled with expansion of the rib cage produced by contraction of the intercostal muscles. Halothane produces preferential suppression of intercostal muscle function with relative sparing of the diaphragm.[8] Depression of intercostal muscle function interferes with rib cage expansion in response to chemical stimuli such as arterial hypoxemia or hypercapnia. Furthermore, depression of intercostal muscle function means that stabilization of the rib cage is reduced such that descent of the diaphragm tends to cause the chest to collapse inward, contributing to reductions in lung volumes, particularly the functional residual capacity. It is concluded that, in addition to depression of central nervous system respiratory drive, halothane also produces depression of ventilation by virtue of interfering with normal intercostal muscle function. The effects of other inhaled anesthetics on intercostal muscle function have not been reported.

CIRCULATION

Inhaled anesthetics produce dose-dependent and drug-specific effects on the circulation.[1] Data obtained from healthy volunteers during controlled ventilation of the lungs to maintain normocarbia permits isolation of circulatory changes due solely to the inhaled anesthetic. Again, the surgical patient with other variables that influence circulatory responses can respond differently from the healthy volunteer.

Arterial Blood Pressure

Dose-dependent reductions of arterial blood pressure are produced by halothane, enflurane, and isoflurane while nitrous oxide alone usually does not alter the blood pressure (Fig. 4-6).[1] The decrease in blood pressure is similar for isoflurane and enflurane and greater than that produced by halothane. Substitution of nitrous oxide for an equivalent portion of the volatile anesthetic results in less blood pressure decrease at the same anesthetic dose. Re-

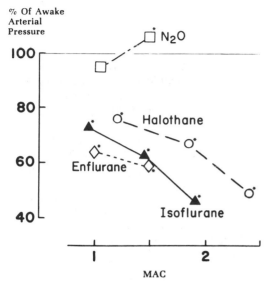

Figure 4-6. Isoflurane, halothane, and enflurane, but not nitrous oxide, administered to healthy volunteers decreases arterial blood pressure from the awake value in a dose-dependent manner. Asterisks indicate significant changes from awake values. (Eger EI. Isoflurane (Forane). A compendium and reference. Madison, Wisconsin, Ohio Medical Products, 1981:32–55.)

placement of a portion of enflurane with nitrous oxide, however, offers less attenuation of the blood pressure decrease than when nitrous oxide is substituted for halothane or isoflurane.

Heart Rate

Heart rate is unchanged by halothane and only minimally increased by nitrous oxide (Fig. 4-7).[1] Isoflurane increases heart rate 20 percent above awake levels but not in a dose-dependent manner, which may reflect the ability of this anesthetic to depress parasympathetic nervous system activity more than sympathetic nervous system activity. Others have speculated that isoflurane has mild beta agonist properties which would be consistent with the heart rate effects of this drug. Nevertheless, the increased heart rate found during isoflurane administered to volunteers does not always occur in older surgical patients or those receiving narcotics in the preoperative medication. Enflurane is the only inhaled anesthetic that manifests dose-dependent elevations in heart rate with a 40 percent increase produced by 1.5 MAC.

An anesthetic-induced reduction in blood pressure would tend to increase heart rate via stimulation of the carotid sinus baroreceptors. The presence of this reflex response is suggested by the increased heart rate that accompanies isoflurane- and enflurane-induced reductions in blood pressure. By contrast, halothane inhibits the baroreceptor reflex response and heart rate usually remains unchanged despite halothane-induced reductions in blood pressure.

Cardiac Output

Volatile anesthetics produce dose-dependent reductions in cardiac output (Fig. 4-8).[1] Isoflurane produces the least depression, and at a 1 MAC concentration of this drug the cardiac output is not reduced below awake values. The depression of cardiac output produced by halothane and enflurane parallels the reduction in blood pressure produced by these drugs. In contrast to volatile anesthetics, nitrous oxide is associated with a mild increase in cardiac output, presumably reflecting a weak sympathomimetic effect of this drug.[9]

Stroke Volume

Halothane, enflurane, and isoflurane produce dose-dependent reductions in calculated stroke volume (cardiac output divided by heart rate) with the greatest decrease occurring during inhalation of enflurane (Fig. 4-9).[1] Stroke volume is not changed by nitrous oxide. A reduction in stroke volume is consistent with decreased myocardial contractility manifesting as a lowered cardiac output. The increased heart rate during inhalation of isoflurane offsets the decreased stroke volume, and cardiac output is unchanged. The increased heart rate as-

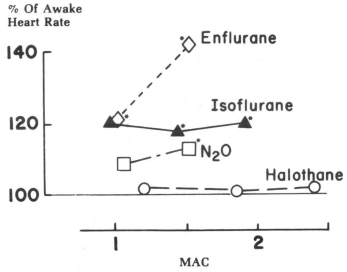

% Of Awake
Heart Rate

Figure 4-7. Halothane and nitrous oxide produce minimal to no change in heart rate when administered to healthy volunteers. Heart rate is increased about 20 percent by 1 and 2 MAC isoflurane. Enflurane produces a dose-dependent increase in heart rate. Asterisks indicate significant changes from awake values. (Eger EI. Isoflurane (Forane). A compendium and reference. Madison, Wisconsin, Ohio Medical Products, 1981:32–55.)

sociated with inhalation of enflurane is insufficient to offset the reduction in stroke volume, and cardiac output decreases.

Myocardial Contractility

Inhaled anesthetics studied in vitro (isolated papillary muscle preparations) produce dose-dependent direct myocardial depression. The depression produced by nitrous oxide, however, is less than that produced by comparable concentrations of volatile anesthetics. Depression of myocardial contractility is greater in papillary muscle taken from animals in congestive heart failure as compared with measurements in muscle taken from normal animals. Therefore, a patient with impaired myocardial contractility due to congestive heart failure

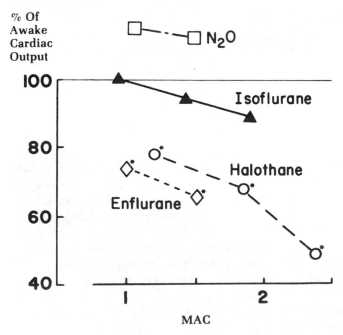

% Of
Awake
Cardiac
Output

Figure 4-8. Cardiac output during inhalation of nitrous oxide is increased above awake levels, while 1 MAC isoflurane produces no change and higher concentrations result in only small decreases. Conversely, halothane and enflurane produce dose-dependent reductions in cardiac output. Asterisks indicate significant changes from awake values. (Eger EI. Isoflurane (Forane). A compendium and reference. Madison, Wisconsin, Ohio Medical Products, 1981;32–55.)

Nevertheless, discontinuation of beta antagonists before anesthesia is not recommended, as this practice may accentuate the patient's hypertension or provoke myocardial ischemia.

Surgical Stimulation

Surgical stimulation modifies the circulatory effects produced by inhaled anesthetics. Indeed, sympathetic nervous system stimulation produced by the surgical incision often results in increased blood pressure and heart rate. Volatile anesthetics oppose this response in a dose-dependent manner. For example, 1.47 MAC halothane or 1.63 MAC enflurane prevents the blood pressure and heart rate response evoked by surgical skin incision in 50 percent of patients.[16]

Duration of Administration

Inhalation of volatile anesthetics for 5 to 6 hours is associated with an increased heart rate, cardiac output, right atrial pressure, and decreased systemic vascular resistance compared with similar measurements after 1 hour of administration. Despite the increased cardiac output, the blood pressure is unchanged with time, reflecting the decrease in systemic vascular resistance. This recovery from the depressant effects of volatile anesthetics with time is most apparent during inhalation of halothane, intermediate with enflurane, and minimal with isoflurane. Prior administration of propranolol prevents these time-related changes, suggesting increased sympathetic nervous system activity as the mechanism.[17]

Co-Existing Disease

Co-existing disease, particularly of the heart, can influence the circulatory effects produced by inhaled anesthetics. For example, patients with coronary artery disease can experience exaggerated cardiac depression during inhalation of nitrous oxide or halothane, presumably reflecting decreased cardiac reserve in these individuals. Anesthetic-produced direct myocardial depression is greater in the presence of congestive heart failure. Patients with stenotic lesions of the aortic or mitral valve tolerate poorly changes in blood pressure and systemic vascular resistance produced by inhaled anesthetics (see Chapter 19).

REFERENCES

1. Eger EI. Isoflurane (Forane). A compendium and reference. Madison, Wisconsin, Ohio Medical Products, 1981;1–110.
2. Calverley RK, Smith NT, Jones CW, Prys-Roberts C, Eger EI. Ventilatory and cardiovascular effects of enflurane anesthesia during spontaneous ventilation in man. Anesth Analg 1978;57:610–8.
3. Pietak S, Weenig CS, Hickey RF, Fairley HB. Anesthetic effects of ventilation in patients with chronic obstructive pulmonary disease. Anesthesiology 1975;42:160–6.
4. Lam AM, Clement JL, Chung DC, Knill RL. Respiratory effects of nitrous oxide during enflurane anesthesia in humans. Anesthesiology 1982;56:298–303.
5. Knill RL, Gelb AW. Ventilatory response to hypoxia and hypercapnia during halothane sedation and anesthesia in man. Anesthesiology 1978;49:244–51.
6. Hirshman CA, Edelstein G, Peetz S, Wayne R, Downes H. Mechanism of action of inhalational anesthesia on airways. Anesthesiology 1982;56:107–11.
7. Pavlin EG. Respiratory pharmacology of inhaled anesthetic agents. In: Miller RD, ed. Anesthesia. New York, Churchill Livingstone 1981:349–82.
8. Tusiewicz K, Bryan AC, Froese AB. Contributions of changing rib cage-diaphragm interactions to the ventilatory depression of halothane anesthesia. Anesthesiology 1977;47:327–37.
9. Smith NT, Eger EI, Stoelting RK, Whayne TF, Cullen D, Kadis LB. The cardiovascular and sympathomimetic responses to the addition of nitrous oxide to halothane in man. Anesthesiology 1970;32:410–21.

10. Reiz S, Balfors E, Sorensen MB, Ariola S, Friedman A, Truedsson H. Isoflurane—a powerful coronary vasodilator in patients with coronary artery disease. Anesthesiology 1983;59:91–7.
11. Kotrly KJ, Ebert TJ, Vucins E, Igler FO, Barney JA, Kampine JP. Baroreceptor reflex control of heart rate during isoflurane anesthesia in humans. Anesthesiology 1984;60:173–9.
12. Johnston RR, Eger EI, Wilson C. A comparative interaction of epinephrine with enflurane, isoflurane and halothane in man. Anesth Analg 1976;55:709–12.
13. Maze M, Smith CM. Identification of receptor mechanism mediating epinephrine induced arrhythmias during halothane anesthesia in the dog. Anesthesiology 1983;59:322–6.
14. Schulte-Sasse U, Hess W, Tarnow J. Pulmonary vascular responses to nitrous oxide in patients with normal and high pulmonary vascular resistance. Anesthesiology 1982;57:9–13.
15. Horan BF, Prys-Roberts C, Hamilton WK, Roberts JG. Haemodynamic responses to enflurane anaesthesia and hypovolemia in the dog, and their modification by propranolol. Br J Anaesth 1977;49:1189–97.
16. Roizen MF, Horrigan RW, Frazer BM. Anesthetic doses blocking adrenergic (stress) and cardiovascular responses to incision—MAC BAR. Anesthesiology 1981;54:390–8.
17. Price HL, Skovsted P, Pauca AW, Cooperman LW. Evidence for B-receptor activation produced by halothane in normal man. Anesthesiology 1970;32:389–95.

5

Metabolism and Toxicity of Inhaled Anesthetics

Inhaled anesthetics were for many years considered to be chemically inert and thus resistant to even minimal metabolism (biotransformation). It is now recognized that inhaled anesthetics can undergo varying degrees of metabolism in the liver and to a lesser extent in the lungs, kidneys, and gastrointestinal tract (see Tables 5-1 and 5-2).[1–3] The significance of this metabolism can relate to toxic effects of metabolites on the liver, kidneys, and reproductive organs (see the section *Organ Toxicity Due to Anesthetic Metabolism*). Metabolism does not influence the rate of induction of anesthetia or the inhaled concentration of anesthetic necessary for the maintenance of anesthesia, since the inhaled anesthetics are administered in great excess of the amount metabolized.

DETERMINANTS OF METABOLISM

Metabolism of inhaled anesthetics is dependent on the activity of the cytochrome P-450 enzymes located in the endoplasmic reticulum of the hepatocyte. These enzymes mediate both oxidative and reductive metabolism of inhaled anesthetics. The cytochrome P-450 enzymes are susceptible to induction by many drugs, including the inhaled anesthetics. With the prevalence of polypharmacy, enzyme induction may be a common occurrence in patients undergoing surgery. Indeed, anesthetic-induced hepatotoxicity and nephrotoxicity are often attributed to increased production of toxic metabolites as a reflection of enzyme induction. Nevertheless, a study of surgical patients in whom enzymes were induced failed to show an increased incidence of toxic effects. Finally, genetic factors appear to be the most important determinant of drug metabolizing enzyme activity.

Chemical structure is important in determining the susceptibility of the anesthetic molecule to metabolism. The ether bond (carbon-oxygen-carbon) and carbon-halogen bond are the sites most likely to undergo oxidative metabolism mediated by the cytochrome P-450 enzymes. Two halogen atoms on a terminal carbon atom represent the optimal condition for dehalogenation, while a terminal carbon atom with three fluorine atoms (trifluorocarbon) is stable and resistant to oxidative metabolism. Oxidation of the ether bond is less likely when hydrogen atoms on the carbons surrounding the oxygen atom of this bond are replaced with halogen atoms. Reductive (anaerobic) metabolism of inhaled anesthetics is rare, having been documented to occur only with halothane. Hydrolysis of inhaled anesthetics does not occur, since these drugs do not contain ester bonds.

Table 5-1. Metabolism of Inhaled Anesthetics

Anesthetic	Percent of Absorbed Anesthetic Recovered as Metabolites
Nitrous oxide	0.004
Isoflurane	0.17
Enflurane	2.4
Halothane	20
Methoxyflurane	50

The fraction of anesthetic passing through the liver that undergoes metabolism is influenced by the concentration of anesthetic in the blood.[2] For example, high concentrations (1 MAC) saturate hepatic enzymes, reducing the fraction of anesthetic that is metabolized on passage through the liver. Conversely, subanesthetic concentrations (0.1 MAC or less) undergo extensive metabolism on passage through the liver. Inhaled anesthetics, such as nitrous oxide, isoflurane, and enflurane, that are poorly soluble in blood and lipids tend to be rapidly eliminated by ventilation of the lungs at the conclusion of their administration. As a result, less drug is available to pass through the liver at low concentrations conducive to metabolism, and the magnitude of metabolism of these drugs is likely to be minimal (Table 5-1).[1-3] Halothane and methoxyflurane are more soluble in blood and lipids and are likely to be extensively stored in tissues, providing a reservoir to maintain subanesthetic concentrations in the blood for prolonged periods following discontinuation of these drugs. Indeed, the magnitude of metabolism of these drugs is large compared to less soluble anesthetics (Table 5-1).[1-3]

Disease states such as cirrhosis of the liver or congestive heart failure may decrease the magnitude of metabolism of inhaled anesthetics by reducing hepatic blood flow and the subsequent delivery of these drugs to hepatic enzymes for metabolism. Cirrhosis of the liver may also reduce enzyme activity due to loss of hepatic parenchyma. Finally, morbid obesity, for un-known reasons, is associated with increased defluorination of volatile anesthetics (see Fig. 5-2).[5]

HALOTHANE METABOLISM

Halothane undergoes significant metabolism in man, with about 20 percent of the absorbed dose recovered as metabolites (Table 5-1).[1-3] Oxidative and reductive pathways for metabolism are present, but halothane preferentially undergoes oxidative metabolism. This is fortunate, since oxidative metabolites are not likely to be toxic, while metabolites formed during reductive metabolism of halothane may produce hepatotoxicity (see the section *Halothane-Associated Hepatic Dysfunction*).

Oxidative Metabolism

The major metabolite of oxidative metabolism of halothane is trifluoroacetic acid, which is excreted in the urine. Trifluoroacetic acid has no known adverse effects, perhaps reflecting the highly ionized characteristic of this metabolite which limits its ability to cross lipid membranes and gain access to intracellular structures. Other oxidative metabolites that appear in the urine are chloride and bromide. Based on measurements in patients, serum bromide concentrations will increase approximately 0.5 mEq/L/MAC hour of halothane administration (Fig. 5-1).[6] Since signs of bromide toxicity (somnolence, mental confusion) do not occur until serum bromide concentrations exceed 6 mEq/L, the likelihood of symptoms due to accumulation of bromide from metabolism of halothane is remote. Trifluoroethanol and trifluoroacetaldehyde, although theoretically possible, do not occur as a result of the metabolism of halothane.

Reductive Metabolism

Reductive metabolism of halothane is most likely to occur in the presence of inadequate oxygen delivery to hepatocytes

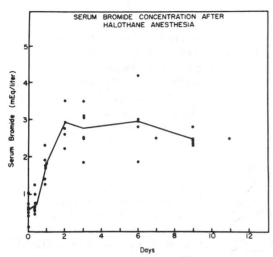

Figure 5-1. Serum bromide concentrations were measured in seven healthy male volunteers following a prolonged exposure (about 7 hours) to halothane. Mean serum bromide concentration was 2.9 mEq/L on the second day after anesthesia. Nine days after anesthesia, serum bromide was still elevated to 2.5 mEq/L. Individual values peaked on the second to sixth days with the highest concentration being 4.2 mEq/L (Johnstone RE, Kennell EM, Beher MG, Brummund W, Ebersole RC, Shaw LM. Increased serum bromide concentration after halothane anesthesia in man. Anesthesiology 1975;42:598–601).

and stimulation of hepatic microsomal enzyme activity by drugs (phenobarbital) or exposure to chemicals (polychlorobiphenyls). Metabolism of halothane by reductive pathways results in the formation of reactive intermediary metabolites and fluoride. The significance of formation of reactive intermediary metabolites is their potential to produce liver damage either by direct effects on hepatocytes or initiation of an immune-mediated hypersensitivity (allergic) reaction (see the section *Halothane-Associated Hepatic Dysfunction*).

An increase in the serum concentration of fluoride after the administration of halothane implies that reductive metabolism and the formation of potentially hepatotoxic reactive intermediary metabolites has occurred. Serum fluoride concentrations increase following the administration of halothane to obese but not to nonobese patients (Fig. 5-2).[5] Evidence of liver dysfunction, however, based on measurements of serum glutamic transaminase concentrations in these obese patients, does not occur. Likewise, peak serum fluoride concentrations (about 10 μM/L) are far below the 50 μM/L concentration likely to be associated with renal dysfunction (see the section *Fluoride-Induced Nephrotoxicity*).

ENFLURANE METABOLISM

Enflurane undergoes minimal oxidative metabolism in man, with about 2.4 percent of the absorbed dose recovered as metabolites. The most important metabolite of enflurane metabolism is fluoride which originates from the terminal carbon atom (Table 5-2).[1,2] Oxidation of the ether bond and release of additional fluorine atoms does not occur, reflecting the stability imparted to this bond by the surrounding halogens. In addition to this chemical stability, the low blood and lipid solubility of enflurane facilitates its removal by ventilation of the lungs before significant hepatic metabolism can occur.

Enzyme induction with phenobarbital does not increase the defluorination of enflurane. Conversely, defluorination of enflurane is increased in patients being treated chronically with isoniazid (Fig. 5-3).[7] Likewise, in vitro incubations of hepatic microsomes from rats pretreated with ethanol revealed increased defluorination of enflurane when compared with untreated rats. Excessive serum concentrations of fluoride from the metabolism of enflurane could result in renal dysfunction (see the section *Fluoride-Induced Nephrotoxicity*). Finally, serum fluoride concentrations are greater after administration of enflurane to obese as compared with nonobese patients. The incidence of renal dysfunction, however, has not been reported to be increased in obese patients following administration of enflurane.

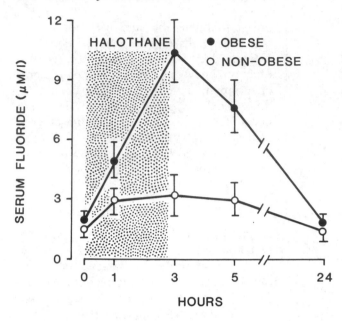

Figure 5-2. Serum fluoride concentrations (mean ± SE) were measured during and following a 3 hour administration of halothane to obese (143 ± 8 kg) and nonobese patients. The peak serum fluoride concentration in obese patients was 10.4 ± 1.5 μM/L at the conclusion of anesthesia. Serum fluoride concentrations did not change in nonobese patients. (Based on data in Young SR, Stoelting RK, Peterson C, Madura JA. Anesthetic biotransformation and renal function in obese patients during and after methoxyflurane or halothane anesthesia. Anesthesiology 1975;42:451–7.)

ISOFLURANE METABOLISM

Isoflurane undergoes insignificant oxidative metabolism in man with about 0.17 percent of the absorbed dose recovered as metabolites (Table 5-1).[1-3] Chemical stability of isoflurane is assured by the trifluorocarbon molecule and the presence of halogen atoms on three sides of the ether bond. Likewise, the low blood and lipid solubility of isoflurane favors its elimination by ventilation of the lungs before significant metabolism can occur.

Table 5-2. Comparative Serum Fluoride Concentrations

Anesthetic	Peak Fluoride (μM/L)	Time to Peak Fluoride after Anesthesia (hr)	Dose[a] (MAC hr)
Halothane	No change		4.7
Isoflurane	4.4	6	4.9
Enflurane	22.2	4	2.7
Methoxyflurane	61	48	2.5

[a] MAC hour is calculated as the MAC concentration × duration of administration in hours. Administration of a 1 MAC concentration for 2.5 hours is a 2.5 MAC hour dose.

The primary pathway of isoflurane metabolism most likely begins with the oxidation of the ethyl alpha carbon atom, ultimately resulting in the formation of difluoromethanol and trifluoroacetic acid. Difluoromethanol is unstable, leading to the production of formic acid and the release of fluoride.

The resistance of isoflurane to metabolism is evidenced by the minimal increase in serum fluoride concentration that accompanies prolonged administration of this anesthetic (Table 5-2).[1,2] Enzyme induction with drugs including isoniazid does not significantly increase the metabolism of isoflurane. The insignificant metabolism of isoflurane makes hepatic or renal toxicity following the administration of this drug unlikely.

METHOXYFLURANE METABOLISM

Methoxyflurane undergoes substantial oxidative metabolism in man, with up to 50 percent of the absorbed dose recovered as metabolites (Table 5-1).[1-3] Methoxyflurane can be dehalogenated at the dichloro-

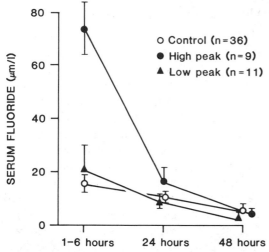

Figure 5-3. Serum fluoride concentrations were measured in 36 control patients taking no drugs and 20 patients treated with 300 mg of isoniazid daily for periods of up to 1 year. Anesthesia was maintained in all patients using enflurane with or without nitrous oxide. Nine isoniazid-treated patients (high peak) had serum fluoride concentrations significantly higher ($P < 0.001$) than either the 11 other isoniazid-treated patients (low peaks) or the control patients. These high peak serum fluoride concentrations occurred 1 to 6 hours after anesthesia. It is speculated that isoniazid resulted in enzyme induction and accelerated defluorination in these nine patients, presumably reflecting a genetically determined ability for rapid acetylation. (Based on data in Mazze RI, Woodruff RE, Heerdt ME. Isoniazid-induced enflurane defluorination in humans. Anesthesiology 1982;57:5–8.)

methyl carbon atom or at the ether bond. The most significant metabolite of methoxyflurane is fluoride (Table 5-2).[1,2] Other metabolites are oxalic acid, dichloroacetic acid, and probably methoxydifluoroacetic acid. Methoxydifluoroacetic acid is labile and would be expected to break down in the acid environment of the kidneys to release oxalic acid and fluoride. Metabolism of methoxyflurane is increased by enzyme induction. As with enflurane, the serum fluoride concentrations are greater following administration of methoxyflurane to obese compared with nonobese patients.[5] Serum fluoride concentrations are lower in pediatric patients compared with adults receiving methoxyflurane, presumably due to avid uptake of fluoride by metabolically active bone.[20]

ORGAN TOXICITY DUE TO ANESTHETIC METABOLISM

Organ toxicity due to toxic metabolites of inhaled anesthetics may manifest postoperatively as halothane-associated hepatic dysfunction or fluoride-induced nephrotoxicity. In addition, adverse responses may occur in personnel who are chronically exposed to trace concentrations of inhaled anesthetics present in the operating room atmosphere.

Halothane-Associated Hepatic Dysfunction

The mechanism responsible for halothane-associated hepatic dysfunction is unknown. The most frequently invoked theories include metabolism of halothane to an hepatotoxic reactive intermediary metabolite or the occurrence of an allergic reaction. With respect to toxic metabolites, it is speculated that products of reductive metabolism can bind irreversibly (covalently) to intracellular constituents of hepatocytes and cause their destruction. Conversely, evidence of an allergic reaction as the cause of liver damage produced by halothane includes the rarity of the response, the occurrence of eosinophilia, and accelerated liver dysfunction following a second or repeat exposure to halothane. It is possible that halothane or one of its metabolites alters the antigenicity of liver cell constituents, leading to the production of antibodies that initiate an allergic reaction with the liver as a target organ. Indeed, genetic factors could be important in determining the likelihood that patients will form antibodies or utilize reductive pathways of metabolism for halothane.

Hypoxia alone has been shown to produce a mild degree of hepatic dysfunction following administration of halothane, enflurane, or isoflurane.[8,9] These observations suggest liver damage previously attributed to halothane metabolism may have been caused by hepatocyte hypoxia. Indeed, it has been proposed that halothane-associated hepatic dysfunction is two entities.[10] One entity is a mild and transient form of hepatic dysfunction unrelated to the anesthetic but rather reflecting unrecognized hepatocyte hypoxia during or following anesthesia. This unrecognized hypoxia may directly damage hepatocytes and/or favor the production of reductive metabolites that are toxic to the liver. Perhaps reductions in hepatic blood flow during anesthesia and surgery contribute to inadequate delivery of oxygen to the hepatocyte regardless of the drug used for anesthesia. The other more rare but fulminant variety of halothane-associated hepatic dysfunction is speculated to be due to an allergic reaction.

The diagnosis of liver dysfunction due to halothane depends on the elimination of other possible causes as likely explanations. Undoubtedly, halothane has been wrongfully incriminated in the past as a cause for hepatic dysfunction when a more detailed investigation would have exonerated the anesthetic. Nevertheless, most cases of alleged halothane-associated hepatic dysfunction have occurred in middle-aged obese females, especially with repeat administration of halothane within 4 weeks of a previous halothane anesthetic. Laboratory measurements in these patients suggest hepatocellular damage (markedly elevated serum transaminase enzyme concentrations) and eosinophilia may be present. Finally, the pediatric patient seems less likely than the adult to experience halothane-associated hepatic dysfunction even with re-exposure to the drug at short intervals.

Fluoride-Induced Nephrotoxicity

Metabolism of methoxyflurane, and to a lesser extent enflurane, to fluoride may result in nephrotoxicity. Fluoride-induced nephrotoxicity is characterized by an inability to concentrate urine. The resulting polyuria leads to dehydration with hypernatremia and increased serum osmolarity. Inability to concentrate urine may reflect fluoride-induced inhibition of adenylate cyclase activity necessary for the normal action of antidiuretic hormone on the distal convoluted renal tubule. Alternatively, fluoride may produce intrarenal vasodilation with increased medullary blood flow which interferes with the counter current mechanism in the kidney necessary for optimal concentration of urine.

Detectable renal dysfunction is likely when the administered dose of methoxyflurane results in a serum fluoride concentration that exceeds 50 μM/L.[11] This level of fluoride elevation is likely when the duration of methoxyflurane administration to adult patients exceeds 2.5 MAC hours (Table 5-2).[1,2] The nephrotoxic potential of methoxyflurane has led to the almost total abandonment of the use of this drug to produce general anesthesia.

The metabolism of enflurane to fluoride, although much less than with methoxyflurane, is potentially great enough to produce transient decreases in urine concentrating ability, particularly after prolonged administration (1 MAC for 9.6 hours).[11] Nevertheless, short administration (1 MAC for 2.7 hours) does not reveal a difference between enflurane or halothane with respect to urine concentrating ability. Indeed, the likelihood of fluoride-induced nephrotoxicity due to metabolism of enflurane seems remote, since serum concentrations of fluoride after clinical use of this drug are about one-half the speculated toxic level of 50 μM/L (Table 5-2).[1,2] Nevertheless, the advisability of administration of enflurane to patients with known renal disease or undergoing operations likely to be associated with renal dysfunction is questionable. This concern is based on the realization that elimination of fluoride depends on glomerular filtration rate. Therefore, it is likely that patients with decreased glomerular filtration rates will maintain elevated circulating levels of fluoride for longer periods of time than normal patients. Fluoride-induced nephrotoxicity depends on the duration of the exposure of the renal tubules to fluoride as well as on the absolute increase of the serum fluoride concentration. As a result, it is possible that patients with decreased glomerular filtration rates are at an increased risk in the presence of fluoride concentrations usually considered to be nontoxic (e.g., below 50 μM/L). Nevertheless, both enflurane and halothane anesthesia were associated with slight improvements in postoperative renal function in surgical patients with co-existing renal insufficiency (serum creatinine 1.5 to 3 mg/100 ml).[12]

Trace Concentrations of Inhaled Anesthetics

Approximately 225,000 operating room personnel are chronically exposed to trace concentrations of inhaled anesthetics. This is of concern because the mutagenicity, teratogenicity, and carcinogenicity of chemicals (including anesthetics) probably results from direct alteration of chromosomal proteins (DNA) by these substances. Reactive intermediary metabolites, and not the relatively stable parent molecule, are most likely to attack (adduct to) chromosomal proteins. Depending on the point in life at which adduction occurs, the result may be fetal death and spontaneous abortion, a birth defect, or cancer.

Synthesis of chromosomal protein may be inhibited by inactivation of methionine synthetase by nitrous oxide.[13] Such a mechanism may explain the anemia and polyneuropathy resembling pernicious anemia that can accompany prolonged exposure to nitrous oxide. Unlike nitrous oxide, volatile anesthetics do not inhibit methionine synthetase.

Mutagenicity. The Ames test is the most widely used in vitro test for determination of the mutagenic and carcinogenic potential of chemicals. Nitrous oxide, halothane, enflurane, and isoflurane give negative Ames test results suggesting the mutagenic, and thus carcinogenic, potential of these inhaled anesthetics is low if not nonexistent. Nevertheless, potential metabolites of halothane may give a positive Ames test. In addition, inhaled anesthetics containing vinyl groups (divinyl ether, fluroxene) give a positive Ames test. Therefore, these drugs and any new drugs with a vinyl moiety should be considered potential carcinogens.

Teratogenicity. Female operating room personnel have an increased incidence of spontaneous abortion (1.3 to 2 times) compared with matched controls not working in the operating rooms.[14] Less well documented than the increased incidence of spontaneous abortion is an increased incidence of minor and major congenital malformations in the offspring of these anesthetic-exposed females. Even less well documented is an increased incidence of spontaneous abortion among spouses of anesthetic-exposed males. Furthermore, the roles of stress or exposure to radiation have not been adequately evaluated as explanations for the increased incidence of spontaneous abortion among females working in operating rooms.

The cause of the increased incidence of spontaneous abortion or other adverse responses observed in operating room personnel is not known, but chronic exposure to trace concentrations of inhaled anesthetics, particularly nitrous oxide, has received much attention. Indeed, the rationale for scavenging systems is to reduce the trace concentrations of anesthetic gases in the operating room atmosphere and hopefully reduce any toxic effects associated with chronic exposure to these gases (see Chapter 11).

Carcinogenicity. No study has demonstrated the existence of a cause and effect relationship between inhaled anesthetics and cancer. Nevertheless, there is an increased incidence of leukemia among female, but not male, operating room personnel.[14] Additional data are needed before it can be concluded, however, that the incidence of cancer is truly increased in females chronically exposed to trace concentrations of anesthetics. As with spontaneous abortion, the possible role of stress and exposure to radiation associated with working in operating rooms will also have to be considered.

Gonadal Toxicity. Inhaled anesthetics and their metabolites may be directly toxic to the testes. Evidence for this toxicity is from animals who manifested injury to the seminiferous tubules and damage to spermatogenic cells after prolonged exposure to nitrous oxide.

RESISTANCE TO INFECTION

Inhaled anesthetics, particularly nitrous oxide, produce dose-dependent inhibition of mobilization of polymorphonuclear leukocytes and subsequent migration for phagocytosis that is necessary for the inflammatory response to infection.[15] Nevertheless, the effects produced by these drugs are probably clinically insignificant, considering the usual duration of anesthesia and the dose used. Therefore, a decrease in the resistance to infection in the postoperative period due to persistent effects of inhaled anesthetics seems remote. Inhaled anesthetics do not have a bacteriostatic effect at clinically useful concentrations.[15] Low concentrations (0.2 MAC) of volatile anesthetics inhibit replication of measles virus by 50 percent, while 0.5 to 1 MAC greatly inhibits replication. Furthermore,

volatile anesthetics have been shown to reduce mortality in mice receiving intranasal influenza virus during anesthesia.[16] These data suggests that if volatile anesthetics inhibit the body's immune defenses against infection, they may also directly inhibit growth of the infecting organism.

REFERENCES

1. VanDyke R. Biotransformation of volatile anesthetics with special emphasis on the role of metabolism in the toxicity of anaesthetics. Can Anaesth Soc J 1973;20:21–33.
2. White AE, Stevens WC, Eger EI II, Mazze RI, Hitt BA. Enflurane and methoxyflurane metabolism at anesthetic and subanesthetic concentrations. Anesth Analg 1979;58:221–4.
3. Hong K, Trudell JR, O'Neil JR, Cohen EN. Metabolism of nitrous oxide by human and rat intestinal contents. Anesthesiology 1980;52:16–9.
4. Greene NM. Halothane anesthesia and hepatitis in a high risk population. N Engl J Med 1973;289:304–7.
5. Young SR, Stoelting RK, Peterson C, Madura JA. Anesthetic biotransformation and renal function in obese patients during and after methoxyflurane or halothane anesthesia. Anesthesiology 1975;42:451–7.
6. Johnstone RE, Kennell EM, Behar MG, Brummund W, Ebersole RC, Shaw LM. Increased serum bromide concentration after halothane anesthesia in man. Anesthesiology 1975;42:598–601.
7. Mazze RI, Woodruff RE, Heerdt ME. Isoniazid-induced enflurane defluorination in humans. Anesthesiology 1982;57:5–8.
8. VanDyke RA. Hepatic centrilobular necrosis in rats after exposure to halothane, enflurane or isoflurane. Anesth Analg 1982;61:812–9.
9. Shingu K, Eger EI II, Johnson BH. Hypoxia may be more important than reductive metabolism in halothane-induced hepatic injury. Anesth Analg 1982;61:824–7.
10. Pohl LR, Gillette JR. A perspective on halothane-induced hepatotoxicity (Editorial). Anesth Analg 1982;61:809–11.
11. Cousins MJ, Greenstein LR, Hitt BA, Mazze RI. Metabolism and renal effects of

enflurane in man. Anesthesiology 1976;44: 44–53.

12. Mazze, RI, Sievenpiper, TS, Stevenson J. Renal effects of enflurane and halothane in patients with abnormal renal function. Anesthesiology 1984;60:161–3.

13. Koblin DD, Watson JE, Deady JE, Stokstad ELR, Eger EI II. Inactivation of methionine synthetase by nitrous oxide in mice. Anesthesiology 1981;54:318–24.

14. American Society of Anesthesiologists. Report of an ad hoc committee on the effect of trace anesthetics on the health of operating room personnel. Occupational disease among operating room personnel. A national study. Anesthesiology. 1974;41:321–40.

15. Duncan PG, Cullen BF. Anesthesia and immunology. Anesthesiology 1976;45:522–38.

16. Knight PR, Bedows E, Nahrwold ML, Maassab HF, Smitka CW, Busch MT. Alterations in influenza virus pulmonary pathology induced by diethyl ether, halothane, enflurane and pentobarbital in mice. Anesthesiology 1983;58:209–15.

6

Intravenous Anesthetics

Although many drugs are administered intravenously for induction and maintenance of anesthesia (usually in combination with nitrous oxide), thiopental is historically the standard to which most drugs are compared. Also, in the last 15 years, use of narcotics (especially large doses) with and without nitrous oxide have become increasingly popular. Drugs currently used as intravenous anesthetics can be classified as barbiturates, benzodiazepines, narcotics, and miscellaneous drugs such as ketamine and etomidate.[1]

BARBITURATES

Barbiturates are divided into four classes, including long-acting, intermediate-acting, short-acting, and ultrashort-acting. Ultrashort-acting barbiturates, which include thiopental, thiamylal, and methohexital, are most frequently administered intravenously to produce a rapid induction of anesthesia. Thiopental is the drug used most often for this purpose.

General Pharmacology

The parent molecule, barbituric acid, can be manipulated to form a barbiturate in any one of these four classes by substitution on the key parts of the molecule (Fig. 6-1). Substitution with a phenyl group on carbon number 5 results in anticonvulsive activity. Addition of a methyl group to nitrogen number 1 results in a compound that has a short duration of action. Lipid solubility is increased and duration of action is shortened by substitution of sulfur (e.g., a thiobarbiturate) for the oxygen (e.g., an oxybarbiturate) attached to carbon number 2.

Barbiturates have numerous sites of action in the central nervous system.[1] As with inhaled drugs the potency of barbiturates is related to their lipid solubility, suggesting a lipophilic site of action. The midbrain reticular formation appears to be one site of barbiturate action, in that the threshold for electrical stimulation is increased. The barbiturates can also suppress neuronal activities of the posterior hypothalamus, the amygdla, and limbic structures. At the synaptic level, reduced excitatory synaptic transmission has been observed with maintained synaptic inhibition, especially that involving glycine and gamma aminobutyric acid (GABA) as the endogenous inhibitory neurotransmitters. In anesthetic doses, the barbiturates probably reduce sensitivity of postsynaptic membranes to excitatory neural transmitters.

Administration of thiopental (3 to 5 mg/kg) to patients to produce a rapid induction of anesthesia typically reduces the blood pressure and increases the heart rate. Comparable doses of thiamylal (3 to 5 mg/kg) and methohexital (1 to 2 mg/kg) are likely to produce similar changes. These hemodynamic changes may be due to direct myocardial

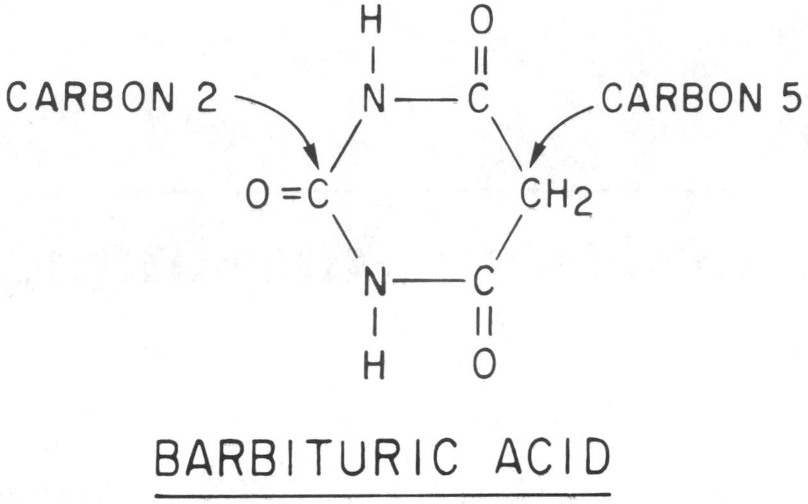

BARBITURIC ACID

Figure 6-1. The formula for barbituric acid. (Stanley TH. Pharmacology of intravenous non-narcotic anesthetics. In: Miller RD, ed., Anesthesia, New York, Churchill Livingstone, 1981:451–85.

depression, decreased systemic vascular resistance, and reduced sympathetic nervous system outflow from the central nervous system. Direct myocardial depression is readily demonstrated using isolated heart preparations after even moderate doses of barbiturates. In patients, however, negative inotropic effects may be obscured by baroreceptor reflex responses, specifically an increased heart rate in response to reductions in blood pressure. Thiopental can also increase venous compliance with resultant pooling of blood and reduced venous return to the heart.[2] This venous dilatation might also obscure any tendency for the central venous pressure to increase secondary to direct myocardial depression. The impact of reduced central nervous system sympathetic outflow is likely to be transient due to reflex increases in peripheral sympathetic nervous system activity.

The importance of reflexly mediated responses in minimizing circulatory changes after intravenous barbiturates must be remembered when administering these drugs to patients with attenuated baroreceptor activity. Conceivably, such patients would be less able to compensate for direct myocar-dial depressant and peripheral vasodilating effects of barbiturates. Baroreceptor responses are blunted in elderly patients, those with a history of essential hypertension, and patients receiving antihypertensives or beta-blockers. Inhaled anesthetics also greatly depress baroreceptor activity. It is possible that blood pressure lowering effects of barbiturates would be exaggerated in patients deprived of normal compensatory mechanisms. Although supporting data are not available, it is a clinical impression that hypotension is exaggerated when barbiturates are used for induction of anesthesia in the presence of hypovolemia. Hypotension may be minimized in susceptible patients by administering intermittent small doses of barbiturate rather than the same dose as a bolus. A slow infusion rate is more likely to permit sufficient time for compensatory reflex responses to offset direct myocardial depression and peripheral pooling that follow barbiturate administration.

Barbiturates depress ventilation by decreasing the sensitivity of the medullary respiratory center to carbon dioxide. Tidal volume is usually depressed more than respiratory rate. Intravenous administration of thiopental for induction of anesthesia is likely to produce transient apnea requiring temporary controlled ventilation of the lungs. Narcotics, as used for preoperative medication, are likely to accentuate ventilatory depressant effects of thiopental. Laryngeal reflexes are not depressed unless large doses of thiopental are administered. Indeed, stimulation of the trachea during light levels of narcosis induced by thiopental may result in laryngospasm and/or bronchospasm. This response should not be interpreted as unique to thiopental but rather as an example of an adverse response to stimulation in the absence of inadequate suppression of reflex responsiveness.

Barbiturates are potent cerebral vasoconstrictors producing predictable reductions in cerebral blood flow. Cerebral metabolism and oxygen utilization also decrease after barbiturate administration. Cerebral blood flow, however, is reduced less than oxygen consumption, making a drug such as thiopental ideal for patients undergoing neurosurgical procedures (see Chapter 24). Thiobarbiturates predictably decrease activity on the electroencephalogram. Conversely, the oxybarbiturate, methohexital, evokes electroencephalographic evidence of epileptic foci. Finally, barbiturates are contraindicated in patients with the diagnosis of porphyria (see Chapter 23).

Pharmacokinetics and Pharmacodynamics

Induction of anesthesia with thiopental is rapid (less than 60 seconds), reflecting its rapid penetration into the central nervous system despite being 70 to 80 percent bound to protein. Awakening after a single dose of thiopental (3 to 5 mg/kg) reflects redistribution of the drug from the brain to inactive tissue sites in fat and skeletal muscle. Ultimately, nearly all of an injected dose of thiopental is metabolized in the liver at a rate of about 15 to 20 percent per hour of the available drug. The volume of distribution of thiopental at steady state (Vdss) is large, reflecting this drug's high lipid solubility in tissues (Table 6-1).[3] This tissue storage plus a slow rate of clearance from plasma results in a long elimination half-time (Table 6-1).[3] Methohexital is less lipid soluble than thiopental, as reflected by a smaller Vdss (Table 6-1).[3] Furthermore, the rate of clearance of methohexital by the liver is greater, resulting in a shorter elimination half-time than thiopental. Theoretically, these pharmacokinetic characteristics of methohexital should result in recovery after a single dose that is more rapid than following thiopental. Indeed, those who recommend methohexital often cite its shorter duration of action, although this difference from thiopental has not been conclusively proven.

The relationship between the blood or brain concentration of thiopental and depth of anesthesia (e.g., pharmacodynamics) has been difficult to establish. This reflects the difficulty in achieving steady state concentrations of thiopental or an adequate measure of the drug's anesthetic effect. Nevertheless, a plasma thiopental concentration sufficient to prevent movement in response to surgical stimulation (about 1 MAC) produced less evidence of direct myocardial depression than volatile anesthetics.[4] Use of the electroencephalogram may prove ultimately to be the tool used to measure the depth of thiopental anesthesia.

Clinical Pharmacology

Thiopental is most often used for induction of anesthesia and occasionally to aid in the maintenance of anesthesia. When used for induction of anesthesia, thiopental, 3 to 5 mg/kg, is injected rapidly intravenously followed by succinylcholine to produce skeletal muscle paralysis and facilitate subsequent intubation of the trachea. This approach is referred to as "rapid sequence" induction. Anesthesia can then be maintained with an inhaled anesthetic or an in-

Table 6-1. Pharmacokinetics of Several Drugs Used for Anesthesia

Drug	Rapid Distribution Half-Time (min)	Slow Distribution Half-Time (min)	Elimination Half-Time (hr)	Clearance (ml/kg/min)	Vdss[a] (L/kg)
Thiopental	2.9	47	9	2.4	2.45
Methohexital	Not determined	6	1.5	12.1	1.13
Diazepam	12	90	30	0.4	1.25
Lorazepam	8	Not determined	15	0.9	1.00
Midazolam	10	Not determined	2	7.0	1.50

[a] Vdss, volume of distribution at steady state.

travenously administered narcotic such as fentanyl or a benzodiazepine such as diazepam. Although a rapid sequence induction is pleasant for the patient, it has associated hazards. For example, if the trachea cannot be immediately intubated, the paralyzed patient will be totally dependent upon the anesthesiologist for adequate ventilation of the lungs. Also, if a patient has unsuspected hypovolemia, hypotension may result from the rapid administration of large doses of thiopental.

Another approach for induction of anesthesia is to initially administer small doses of thiopental (0.5 to 1 mg/kg) before applying a mask to the patient's face. The prior thiopental improves patient acceptance of inhalation of pungent volatile anesthetics, such as isoflurane or enflurane. Even these small doses of thiopental, however, can induce apnea, which then may require administration of inhaled anesthetics via controlled ventilation of the lungs. This method of ventilation increases the danger of administering an excessive amount of inhaled anesthetic and also increases the risk of inflating the patient's stomach with gas, with resultant vomiting and aspiration of gastric contents.

For short surgical procedures, a combination of nitrous oxide and thiopental can be given to maintain anesthesia (e.g., dilatation and curettage or breast biopsy). Repeated injections of small doses of thiopental will be based on evidence of light anesthesia, which includes tachycardia, hypertension, sweating, tachypnea, or move-ment. Very little skeletal muscle relaxation can be achieved with the barbiturates. Therefore, the addition of a muscle relaxant and controlled ventilation of the lungs will be necessary if skeletal muscle relaxation is important for the surgical procedure.

The highly alkaline (pH about 10.6) solutions of thiopental rarely produce pain during intravenous administration. A subcutaneous injection of thiopental, however, can result in local irritation and if higher concentrations are used (greater than 2.5 percent of thiopental or 1.0 percent methohexital), tissue necrosis can occur. If thiopental is accidentally given intra-arterially, vasospasm and intense pain can result. Profound arterial vasoconstriction manifests as disappearance of distal arterial pulses and blanching of the limb followed by severe cyanosis and even gangrene. The treatment is immediate injection of a solution into the artery to dilute the thiopental. This solution can be saline, but preferably should be lidocaine or procaine to also produce vasodilation. It has been advised to inject heparin into the artery to minimize the chances of a thrombosis occurring. Finally, blockade of the sympathetic nervous system innervation to the extremity is recommended to minimize the intense pain due to vasoconstriction (e.g., stellate ganglion block).

BENZODIAZEPINES

Benzodiazepines, which include diazepam, lorazepam, and midazolam are classified as minor tranquilizers or sedative-

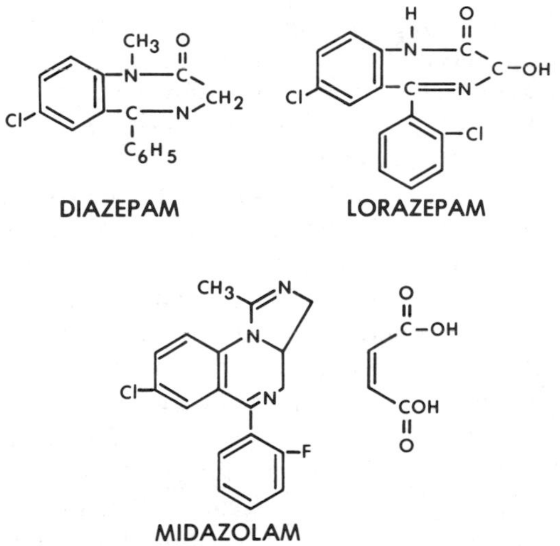

Figure 6-2. The chemical formulas for diazepam, lorazepam, and midazolam.

hypnotics (Fig. 6-2). Diazepam is the most frequently used benzodiazepine and the one with which other drugs are compared.

General Pharmacology

As with barbiturates, benzodiazepines have several sites of action in the central nervous system, including the limbic system, thalamus, and reticular formation. Benzodiazepines depress evoked potentials in each of these anatomic regions at doses which have little effect on the cortical electroencephalogram. From a biochemical point of view, benzodiazepines are speculated to attach to specific receptors that represent a regulatory site on the receptor normally occupied by the endogenous inhibitory neurotransmitter, GABA.[5] When this regulatory site is occupied by an exogenous benzodiazepine, the affinity of the receptor for GABA is enhanced, resulting in inhibition of synaptic transmission.

Induction of anesthesia with diazepam (0.3 to 1.0 mg/kg) or midazolam (0.15 to 0.3 mg/kg) produces hemodynamic changes similar to those observed during natural sleep.[1] Typically, arterial blood pressure decreases about 10 percent from the awake level while heart rate is minimally changed, even in patients with underlying coronary artery or valvular heart disease.[6] Indeed, much of the popularity of benzodiazepines for induction of anesthesia is due to the minimal circulatory effects even in patients with heart disease. Nevertheless, it is unlikely that benzodiazepines offer any advantage over barbiturates for induction of anesthesia in normovolemic patients without underlying heart disease.

Benzodiazepines probably produce less depression of ventilation than barbiturates. Nevertheless, rapid intravenous administration can, on occasion, produce transient apnea. This response is more likely in the presence of narcotics as used for preoperative medication. Benzodiazepines decrease cerebral blood flow and reduce cerebral oxygen consumption, although the magnitude of these changes may be less than with equivalent doses of thiopental.

Pharmacokinetics and Pharmacodynamics

Benzodiazepines have a longer distribution half-time than do thiopental and methohexital (Table 6-1).[3] Clearance of diazepam is exclusively via hepatic metabolism. Metabolites of diazepam possess pharmacologic activity. Conversely, metabolites of midazolam are inactive. The Vdss is large for diazepam due to its high lipid solubility. The combination of a large Vdss and low rate of hepatic clearance is responsible for the prolonged elimination half-time for diazepam. Midazolam also has a large Vdss but its high rate of hepatic clearance results in an elimination half-time that is shorter than for diazepam or lorazepam (Table 6-1).[1] This short duration of action of midazolam may be an advantage if a benzodiazepine is selected for induction of anesthesia.

Poor water solubility of diazepam requires commercial preparation of this drug in organic solvents which may be responsible for pain during intravenous injection and subsequently lead to phlebitis. In contrast, a unique pH-dependent solubility accounts for the water solubility of midazolam in vitro and conversion to a lipid soluble form when injected into the patient's more alkaline circulation. This water solubility of midazolam eliminates the need for organic solvents and decreases the incidence of burning with intravenous injection as well as the occurrence of postoperative phlebitis.

Unlike many drugs, the absorption of diazepam administered intramuscularly is unpredictable. In contrast, the oral administration of diazepam results in rapid and complete absorption with a peak plasma level achieved in 30 to 90 minutes (see Chapter 10).

Clinical Pharmacology

Benzodiazepines can produce tranquility, sedation, and, in high doses, unconsciousness. As a result, these drugs can be used for preoperative medication as well as induction of anesthesia. In addition, benzodiazepines possess anticonvulsant and muscle relaxant effects. The muscle relaxant effect is not due to action at the neuromuscular junction, but rather to specific effects on polysynaptic reflexes and internuncial transmission. This action has been useful for relaxing contracted skeletal muscles associated with muscle spasm or joint diseases. The anticonvulsant activity of diazepam is emphasized by the efficacy of this drug (0.05 to 0.1 mg/kg) in stopping seizures due to local anesthetics, presumably by virtue of a specific inhibitory effect in the limbic system.

Benzodiazepines have been utilized in preference to thiopental for induction of anesthesia. Despite rapid penetration of diazepam into the brain and cerebrospinal fluid, the rate of induction of anesthesia is slower with diazepam than with thiopental. This delayed onset and the lack of predictability of effect have made diazepam less desirable as an induction drug than thiopental. Lorazepam has a similar pharmacokinetic profile and, like diazepam, has the disadvantage of unpredictable induction of anesthesia. Furthermore, the prolonged central nervous system depression following a single dose of either diazepam or lorazepam makes them unsuitable as a primary anesthetic drug for outpatient anesthesa. Midzolam 0.2 mg/kg given intravenously can produce anesthesia within 80 seconds in an unpremedicated patient.[7] With narcotic preoperative medication, the induction time can be reduced. Although midazolam is a better induction drug than diazepam, it still is not as satisfactory as thiopental. Midazolam, however, does have advantages over diazepam in that there is less pain during injection, thrombophlebitis is rare, and onset of action is rapid.

NARCOTICS

Narcotics are used in many facets of anesthetic practice, including preoperative medication, induction and maintenance of anesthesia, and postoperative pain relief (Fig. 6-3). During the last 10 to 15 years, increasingly large doses of narcotics have been used to achieve general anesthesia, especially in patients undergoing cardiac surgery or other major surgery when circulatory reserve is minimal.[8,9] It must be appreciated, however, that even large doses of narcotics do not predictably produce unconsciousness that is considered characteristic of anesthesia.

General Pharmacology

The identification of circulating endogenous opiate-like peptides (endorphins) followed by confirmation of the presence of highly specific opiate receptors has enhanced the understanding of the mechanism of action and pharmacology of narcotics.[5] Apparently, the body can release endorphins in response to pain and other stimuli. These opiate-like peptides then bind to multiple types of opiate receptors to modify transmission along pain pathways. Several populations of opiate receptors exist.[10] The mu receptor is present in high concentra-

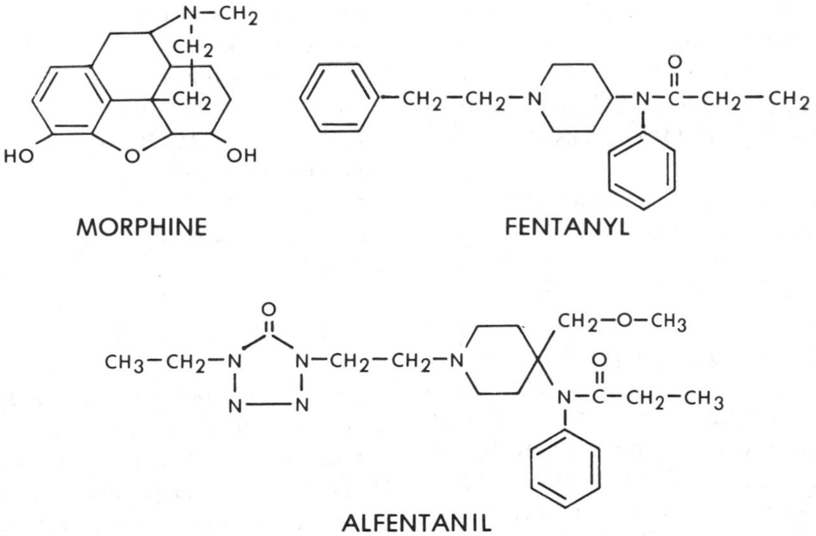

Figure 6-3. The chemical formulas for morphine, fentanyl, and alfentanil.

tions in the cerebral cortex, thalamic nuclei, and in the periaqueductal gray region. Also, there is probably a small proportion of mu receptors in the spinal cord. The mu receptor appears to mediate the traditional effects identified with narcotics including analgesia, respiratory depression, euphoria, and the ability to produce physical dependence. Ligands for the mu receptor include beta-endorphin, morphine, fentanyl, and meperidine. Kappa receptors are probably related to spinal anesthesia, sedation, and miosis. Evidence exists that the kappa receptors do not produce depression of ventilation. Apparently, the sigma receptors mediate tachycardia, tachypnea, mydriasis, and dysphoria. Delta receptors appear to modulate activity of the mu receptors. The role of the epsilon receptors has not been well delineated. Naloxone is essentially a pure mu receptor antagonist, although other receptors are also affected. Identification of opiate receptor subtypes may aid in the future development of narcotics which are more specific and lack disadvantages associated with narcotics presently available.

Narcotics, such as morphine and fentanyl (about 100 times as potent as morphine), are characterized as having benign effects on the circulation. These drugs do not sensitize

the heart to catecholamines and, with the exception of meperidine, do not produce direct myocardial depression. A prominent cardiovascular effect of narcotics is orthostatic hypotension which most likely reflects peripheral vasodilation due to histamine release and depression of central nervous system compensatory mechanisms. Indeed, blood pressure reductions produced by intravenous morphine (1 mg/kg) paralleled elevations in the plasma concentrations of histamine.[11] Conversely, intravenous fentanyl (50 μg/kg) does not evoke the release of histamine and blood pressure reductions are less likely. Furthermore, the need for intravascular fluid replacement as a reflection of histamine-induced increases in venous capacitance is greater for morphine than fentanyl. The peripheral vascular effects of narcotics suggest that blood pressure reductions are likely to be exaggerated when these drugs are administered to hypovolemic patients. Bradycardia produced by narcotics, particularly by fentanyl, reflects effects of these drugs on the brain stem. Finally, the use of other drugs to augment the central nervous system effects of narcotics may result in cardiovascular depression. For example, the combination of nitrous oxide or diazepam with morphine or fentanyl results in marked decreases in blood pressure and cardiac output.[12,13] Conversely, the addition of nitrous oxide after the administration of diazepam does not produce additional cardiovascular depression.[6]

Narcotics produce a characteristic pattern of ventilation in which the respiratory rate is slow and the tidal volume unchanged or increased. The $PaCO_2$ is predictably elevated, and the curve depicting the ventilatory response to carbon dioxide is shifted to the right and the slope depressed. Depression of the medullary ventilatory center is the presumed mechanism of narcotic-induced depression of ventilation.

Narcotics do not increase cerebral blood flow, assuming the $PaCO_2$ is not allowed to increase. In animals, extremely high doses of narcotics can produce seizures. Increased intrabiliary pressures may reflect narcotic-induced constriction of biliary tract smooth muscle and spasm of the choledochoduodenal sphincter, causing some to question the use of these drugs in patients undergoing cholecystectomies (see Chapter 21). Nausea and vomiting most likely reflect stimulation of the chemoreceptor trigger zone in the brain stem by narcotics. Finally, rapid intravenous injection of large doses of narcotics may produce skeletal muscle rigidity, especially of the abdominal and thoracic musculature. This rigidity may be so severe that ventilation of the lungs is impaired.

Sufentanil and alfentanil are chemically related to the synthetic narcotic, fentanyl. Sufentanil is five to ten times more potent than fentanyl but has a similar duration of action. Alfentanil has one-third the potency and duration of action of fentanyl. The effects of these drugs, however, on circulation, ventilation, and other organ systems are probably similar to fentanyl.

Pharmacokinetics and Pharmacodynamics

Pharmacokinetic variables for narcotics and naloxone are detailed in Table 6-2.[3] Although all the narcotics bind to proteins to varying degrees, they leave the blood rapidly and localize in tissues such as the lung, liver, kidneys, and skeletal muscle. Skeletal muscle serves as the main reservoir for narcotics because of its greater bulk. Brain concentrations of narcotics are relatively low in comparison to other organs, although the blood brain barrier is traversed readily. Narcotics are extensively metabolized, mostly to water soluble and inactive metabolites which are then readily excreted by the kidney.

Despite similar pharmacokinetic variables, morphine and fentanyl exhibit different times of onset and durations of action (Table 6-2).[3] Specifically, fentanyl has a more rapid onset and shorter duration of action than morphine. The short duration of action despite an elimination half-time similar to morphine reflects the greater lipid solubility of fentanyl compared to morphine. Highly lipid soluble fentanyl readily crosses the blood brain barrier, resulting in a rapid onset of effect after a single intravenous injection. Brain concentrations decrease rapidly, however, due to redistribution of fentanyl to inactive sites in skeletal muscle and fat. This redistribution, like thiopental, accounts for the short duration of central nervous system effect of fentanyl. After multiple doses of fentanyl or with high dose anesthetic techniques, the redistribution mechanism for terminating the central nervous system effect of fentanyl becomes less effective as inactive tissue sites become saturated and the blood and brain concentrations now become more dependent on the slow elimination half-time. Therefore, as the dose of fentanyl increases the duration of effect is likely to be prolonged similar to that of morphine.

Alfentanil is less lipid soluble than fentanyl or morphine resulting in a reduced Vdss, rapid elimination half-time, and short duration of action (Table 6-2).[3] Accumulation after repeated doses or during continuous intravenous infusion of alfentanil is minimal, making this a potentially useful drug for short operations.[14] Indeed, contin-

Table 6-2. Pharmacokinetics of Narcotics Used During Anesthesia

Drug	Rapid Distribution Half-Time (min)	Slow Distribution Half-Time (min)	Elimination Half-Time (hr)	Clearance (mg/kg/min)	Vdss[a] (L/kg)
Morphine	1.3	20	4.5	12.4	4.7
Fentanyl	1.6	13	3.7	11.6	4.2
Alfentanil	1.2	11.6	1.6	6.4	0.9
Naloxone	Not determined	2.6	1.0	30	1.8

[a] Vdss, volume of distribution at steady state.

uous intravenous infusion of alfentanil is an effective approach for maintaining desirable blood concentrations of this drug during maintenance of anesthesia.

Naloxone is a potent and specific antagonist of narcotics. Unfortunately, naloxone has a rapid clearance and short elimination half-time (Table 6-2).[3] For example, naloxone will only antagonize a narcotic effect for about 30 minutes. Furthermore, naloxone is nonselective, reversing desirable effects (analgesia) as well as undesirable effects (depression of ventilation) of narcotics (see Chapter 30).

Clinical Pharmacology

Narcotics can be used to induce and maintain anesthesia. Traditionally, "balanced anesthesia" has been defined as a combination of narcotics, sedative-hypnotics (barbiturates or benzodiazepines), nitrous oxide, and muscle relaxants utilized to produce general anesthesia and skeletal muscle relaxation. More recently, large doses of narcotics alone have been administered to achieve general anesthesia, particularly in patients undergoing cardiac surgery or major surgery when circulatory reserve is minimal.[8,9] Fentanyl (50 to 150 μg/kg) is the narcotic used most often for this purpose because it produces minimal evidence of circulatory deterioration. Despite large doses, recall or awareness during anesthesia has occurred. In addition, postoperative depression of ventilation may be a problem. Furthermore, an entity called

"biphasic respiratory depression" has been noticed with fentanyl, but it undoubtedly occurs with other narcotics (Fig. 6-4).[15] In this situation, immediately upon entering the recovery room, patients are stimulated by having their blood pressure and temperature taken, during which time evidence of depression of ventilation does not exist. Later, when stimulation is less, the ventilatory depressant effects from the narcotics reappear. Whether this is due to a pharmacokinetic effect or the absence of stimulation remains to be determined. There can, however, be no doubt that depression of ventilation lingers for a long period of time following large doses of narcotics.

KETAMINE

Ketamine produces a unique type of effect termed "dissociative anesthesia," reflecting drug-induced dissociation between the thalamic and limbic systems.[16] The unique type of anesthesia produced by ketamine is similar to a cataleptic state in which the eyes remain open and the gaze is characterized by a slow nystagmus. Skeletal muscle tone is increased and analgesia is profound. Analgesia produced by ketamine is thought to be greater for somatic than for visceral pain.

General Pharmacology

Ketamine produces evidence of sympathetic nervous system stimulation characterized by increased heart rate, blood pressure, cardiac output, and pulmonary artery

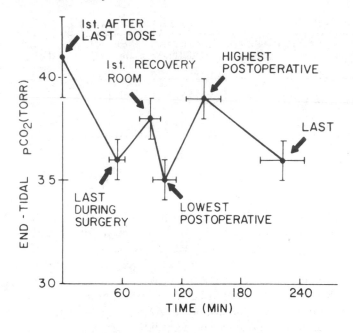

Figure 6-4. Mean resting end-tidal PCO$_2$ at the time of the last dose of fentanyl (Innovar), at the end of operation, at the time when they were the lowest, at the time when they were the highest, and at the end of the study (n = 21). (Becker LD, Paulson BA, Miller RD, Severinghaus JW, Eger EI II. Biphasic respiratory depression after fentanyl-droperidol or fentanyl alone used to supplement nitrous oxide anesthesia. Anesthesiology 1976;44: 291–6.)

pressures. The mechanisms for ketamine-induced cardiac stimulation are complex and include direct stimulation of the central nervous system to increase sympathetic nervous system outflow, impairment of baroreceptor reflexes, and inhibition of the intraneuronal uptake of norepinephrine. Furthermore, the circulatory response to ketamine depends on an intact and nondepressed central nervous system. For example, cardiovascular stimulation is reduced or eliminated by general anesthesia, high levels of epidural anesthesia, or spinal cord transection. Conversely, drugs with cardiovascular stimulant actions such as pancuronium enhance the effects of ketamine.

Maintenance of a patent upper airway is facilitated by ketamine-induced increases in skeletal muscle tone. Laryngeal reflexes are depressed only slightly. Despite relative maintenance of larygneal reflexes, the risk of inhalation of gastric fluid during anesthesia still exists, and the trachea must be protected with a cuffed tube. Minute ventilation and the ventilatory response to carbon dioxide are maintained during ketamine anesthesia. Nevertheless, an occasional patient may become apneic for a brief period immediately following an intravenous injection of ketamine. Finally, ketamine acts as bronchodilator in patients with increased airway resistance.

Ketamine is a potent cerebral vasodilator as reflected by marked increases in cerebral blood flow. Cerebral metabolic oxygen requirements are also increased. In patients with intracranial pathology, ketamine-induced changes in cerebral blood flow can adversely increase intracranial pressure. Salivary gland secretions are often increased by ketamine. This is the reason for recommending an anticholinergic in the preoperative medication of patients who will receive ketamine.

Pharmacokinetics and Pharmacodynamics

Ketamine is a lipid-soluble drug that is rapidly distributed into highly vascular organs. Subsequently, the drug is redistributed to less vascular tissues with concurrent hepatic metabolism and urinary and biliary excretion. Although pretreatment with phenobarbital, a well-known enzyme inducer, accelerates the rate at which ketamine is metabolized and reduces its elimination half-time, sleeping times are not prolonged. Thus metabolic inactivation of ketamine is probably not entirely responsible for the termination of ketamine's effect on the central nervous system. Alternatively, redistribution of ketamine (similar to thiopental and fentanyl) from the brain to inactive sites in other tissues probably contributes greatly to waning effects of ketamine.

Clinical Uses

Ketamine 1 to 2 mg/kg has a rapid onset of action (less than 60 seconds) when injected intravenously. Even an intramuscular injection of ketamine 4 to 6 mg/kg produces an effect in 2 to 4 minutes. The rapid onset of action plus the cardiovascular stimulating effects of ketamine make this an attractive drug to select for induction of anesthesia in patients who are considered to be hypovolemic or for whom anesthetic drugs with negative inotropic effects would be undesirable. As such, ketamine is often an alternative to thiopental for induction of anesthesia. Nevertheless, even ketamine may produce undesirable cardiovascular depression in hemorrhaged patients in whom catecholamine depletion has occurred.[17] Presumably, the absence of an adequate catecholamine-induced sympathetic nervous system response allows the direct cardiac depressant effects of ketamine to be unmasked. Furthermore, maintenance of blood pressure in hypovolemic patients by ketamine-induced vasoconstriction could jeopardize tissue perfusion. Indeed, in hemorrhaged animals, it was not possible to document an advantage of ketamine over thiopental when used in minimal dosages for induction of anesthesia.[18]

Ketamine can also be used for maintenance of anesthesia. For example, ketamine has been used extensively in patients for burn dressing changes and debridements.

Disadvantages of using ketamine for maintenance of anesthesia include accumulation of drug with delayed recovery after multiple doses. Furthermore, tolerance often accompanies repeated administrations of ketamine.

Postanesthesia Emergent Reactions. A major disadvantage associated with the clinical use of ketamine is emergent reactions characterized by unpleasant dreams and occasionally hallucinations. These emergent reactions are more likely to occur after rapid intravenous injections of ketamine or when atropine or droperidol are included in the preoperative medication. Conversely, benzodiazepines appear to be effective in attenuating postanesthesia emergent reactions. Specifically, diazepam, 0.15 to 0.3 mg/kg intravenously will greatly reduce the incidence of unpleasant dreams.

ETOMIDATE

Etomidate is a carboxylated imidazole derivative which, when administered intravenously, produces unconsciousness in less than 60 seconds with recovery in 4 to 10 minutes.[1] The distribution of etomidate is rapid because of its lipid solubility. When distribution of etomidate is complete, only 7 percent of the drug is in the central compartment and available for elimination at any one time. Eventually, about 90 percent of the drug appears in the urine, of which only about 2 percent is unchanged etomidate. This indicates that clearance of etomidate is primarily via liver metabolism.

Etomidate produces minimal changes in blood pressure and heart rate. Likewise, ventilation seems minimally altered. Evidence for drug-induced cerebral vasoconstriction is decreased cerebral blood flow. Disadvantages of etomidate include a high incidence of myoclonic movements (70 percent of patients) and pain associated with injection (50 percent). Myoclonic movements are not associated with epileptiform discharges on the electroencephalogram. Also, the prior administration of fentanyl or diazepam will reduce the incidence of myoclonic movements. Finally, etomidate produces transient depression of adrenocortical function manifesting as decreased serum cortisol concentrations.[19] During this drug-induced suppression the adrenal cortex is not responsive to adrenocorticotrophic hormone.

REFERENCES

1. Stanley TH. Pharmacology of intravenous non-narcotic anesthetics. In: Miller RD, ed., Anesthesia. New York, Churchill Livingstone 1981:451–85.
2. Eckstein JW, Hamilton WK, McCammond JM. The effect of thiopental on peripheral venous tone. Anesthesiology 1961;22:525–8.
3. Stanski RD, Watkins WD. Intravenous anesthetics. In: Stanski RD, Watkins WD, eds., Drug disposition in anesthesia. New York, Grune and Stratton, 1982:78–82.
4. Becker KE, Tonnesen AS. Cardiovascular effects of plasma levels of thiopental necessary for anesthesia. Anesthesiology 1978;49:197–200.
5. Maze M. Clinical implications of membrane receptor function in anesthesia. Anesthesiology 1981;55:160–71.
6. McCammon RL, Hilgenberg JC, Stoelting RK. Hemodynamic effects of diazepam and diazepam-nitrous oxide in patients with coronary artery disease. Anesth Analg 1980;59:438–41.
7. Reves JG, Samuelson PN, Vinik HR. Midazolam. In: Brown BR, ed., New Pharmacologic vistas in anesthesia. Philadelphia, FA Davis Company, 1983:147–62.
8. Stanley TH. Pharmacology of intravenous narcotic anesthetics. In: Miller RD, ed., Anesthesia. New York, Churchill Livingstone, 1981:425–38.
9. Lowenstein E, Philbin DM. Narcotic anaesthesia. In: Bullingham RES, ed., Clinics of Anesthesiology. London, WB Saunders Company, 1983:5–15.
10. Hameroff SR. Opiate receptor pharmacology. Mixed agonist: antagonist narcotics. In: Brown BR, ed., New pharmacologic vistas in anesthesia. Philadelphia, FA Davis Company, 1983:27–44.
11. Rosow CE, Moss J, Philbin DM, Savarese JJ. Histamine release during morphine and fentanyl anesthesia. Anesthesiology 1982;56:93–6.
12. Stoelting RK, Gibbs PS, Creasser CW, Peterson C. Hemodynamic and ventilatory responses to fentanyl, fentanyl-droperidol, and nitrous oxide in patients with acquired valvular heart disease. Anesthesiology 1975;42:319–24.
13. Tomicheck RC, Rosow CE, Philbin DM, Moss J, Teplick RS, Schneider RC. Diazepam-fentanyl interaction–hemodynamic and hormonal effects in coronary artery surgery. Anesth Analg 1983;62:881–4.
14. Stanski DR, Hug CC. Alfentanil—a kinetically predictable narcotic analgesic. Anesthesiology 1982;57:435–8.
15. Becker LD, Paulson BA, Miller RD, Severinghaus JW, Eger EI. Biphasic respiratory depression after fentanyl-droperidol or fentanyl alone used to supplement nitrous oxide anesthesia. Anesthesiology 1976;44:291–6.
16. White PF, Way WL, Trevor AJ. Ketamine—its pharmacology and therapeutic uses. Anesthesiology 1982;56:119–36.
17. Waxman K, Shoemaker WC, Lippmann M. Cardiovascular effects of anesthetic induction with ketamine. Anesth Analg 1980;59:35–8.
18. Weiskopf, RB, Bogetz MS, Roizen MF, Reid IA. Cardiovascular and metabolic sequelae of inducing anesthesia with ketamine or thiopental in hypovolemic swine. Anesthesiology 1984;60:214–9.
19. Wagner RL, White PF, Kan PB, Rosenthal MH, Feldman D. Inhibition of adrenal steroidogenesis by the anesthetic etomidate. N Engl J Med 1984;310:1415–21.

7

Local Anesthetics

Local anesthetics are drugs which, when applied in sufficient concentrations at the site of action, prevent conduction of electrical impulses by the membranes of nerve and muscle. This chapter is based on several more extensive reviews of local anesthetics.[1-3]

HISTORY

Since prehistoric times, the natives of Peru have chewed the leaves of the indigenous plant, erythroxylon coca, the source of cocaine, to obtain a feeling of well being and reduced fatigue. It was not until 1860, however, that cocaine was actually isolated by Nieman. In 1884 it was introduced into clinical medicine by Köller as a topical anesthetic for the cornea. Cocaine unfortunately was found to have strong addicting actions on the central nervous system, but nevertheless was used for 30 years because it was the only local anesthetic available. In 1905 Einhorn synthesized procaine, which became the dominant local anesthetic for many subsequent years. Since then, many local anesthetics have been synthesized. The overall goals in developing new local anesthetics were to reduce local irritation and tissue damage, minimize systemic toxicity, have a shorter onset of action, and have a longer duration of action. Lidocaine, synthesized in 1943 by Lofgren, is currently considered the prototype local anesthetic with which others are compared.

USES OF LOCAL ANESTHETICS

Topical Anesthesia

Topical or surface anesthesia is the application of local anesthetic to the skin or, more commonly, mucus membranes. For example, local anesthetics are commonly applied to the pharynx and trachea prior to induction of general anesthesia and intubation of the trachea. A local anesthetic is frequently inserted into the urethra prior to cystoscopic examinations. Local anesthetics used for these purposes are often ointments, which are water soluble and sterile. Spraying with a local anesthetic liquid is commonly employed but sometimes produces uneven anesthesia because the droplets may vary in size. One disadvantage is that topically applied local anesthetic to an area high in surface blood flow may result in the absorption of local anesthetic into the blood stream nearly as rapid as a direct intravenous injection. Therefore, the chances for a systemic reaction will be increased when the local anesthetic is applied to highly vascular areas.

Infiltration

Infiltration is the injection of a local anesthetic without respect to the specific neuroanatomy of the area. For example, with a lacerated hand or arm, a local anesthetic may be infiltrated around the laceration, rather than a specific nerve block. Likewise, a local anesthetic is often infiltrated (skin wheal) at the site where the skin will be punctured to place a catheter in a vein or artery.

Nerve Block

To block nerve conduction distal to its application, a local anesthetic can be injected near a specific peripheral nerve or placed in the subarachnoid or epidural space (see Chapters 13 and 14). This approach requires knowledge of the specific anatomy of the nerves to be blocked.

Treatment of Cardiac Dysrhythmias

Many cardiac antidysrhythmics, such as quinidine and propranolol, have local anesthetic effects. It is, therefore, not surprising that some local anesthetics have antidysrhythmic effects. Indeed, lidocaine is often the drug of choice for the treatment of cardiac ventricular dysrhythmias.

Supplementation of General Anesthesia

Procaine and lidocaine have been administered intravenously to supplement general anesthesia. More common is the administration of 1 to 1.5 mg/kg of lidocaine intravenously to attenuate the cardiovascular changes associated with intubation of the trachea. Similarly, lidocaine is sometimes given intravenously to minimize coughing during and following extubation of the trachea.

PHYSIOLOGY AND BIOCHEMISTRY OF LOCAL ANESTHETIC ACTION

Nerve Structure and Function

A typical peripheral nerve consists of several groups of axons. Each peripheral nerve axon possesses its own membrane called the axolemma. Nonmyelinated nerves are also surrounded by a Schwann

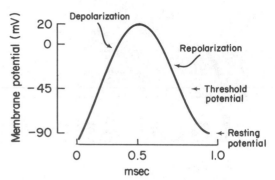

Figure 7-1. A membrane potential of approximately minus 90 mV is maintained by constant extrusion of sodium from the cell. In response to a stimulus, there is an increase in sodium permeability reflected by an increase in the membrane potential from minus 90 mV to minus 45 mV. An even further increase in sodium permeability occurs subsequently with a resultant membrane potential of approximately plus 20 mV. When the critical threshold potential is achieved, a propagated action potential occurs. Sodium permeability then rapidly diminishes and potassium permeability increases until the resting membrane potential is reestablished.

cell sheath. Most nerves, however, are insulated by a lipid-insulating membrane called myelin, which separates the axon from the Schwann cell sheath. Myelin greatly increases the speed of conduction by producing saltatory conduction via the nodes of Ranvier which are merely interruptions in the myelin sheath.

The nerve membrane maintains a voltage difference of about 90 mV between its inner and outer aspects. This membrane potential reflects the constant extrusion of sodium from within the cell by an energy-dependent sodium-potassium pump. In the absence of local anesthetics, stimulation of the nerve will cause the permeability of the nerve membrane to sodium to increase rapidly, decreasing the membrane potential from approximately minus 90 mV to minus 45 mV (Fig. 7-1). When this critical threshold potential is reached, the increase in sodium permeability is even more dramatic. The sudden inward rush of sodium ions reverses the membrane potential to approximately plus 20 mV (Fig. 7-1). When the critical threshold potential is achieved, a propagated action potential occurs along the entire length of the nerve membrane. Subsequently, the permeability of the membrane to sodium decreases and permeability to potassium increases until the resting membrane potential is re-established. The conduction of an impulse is an all-or-none phenomenon. If the critical threshold potential is not reached (e.g., a change in membrane potential from minus 90 mV to minus 45 mV), then propagation of the impulse will not occur (Fig. 7-1).

Mechanism of Local Anesthetic Action

Changes in membrane potential of nerve membranes, as described above, are probably due to the passage or conductance of sodium and potassium ions through protein-like channels. There are two receptors which are located on the external and internal aspects of the sodium channel.[1-3] The internal receptor site is probably the site where local anesthetics act to alter sodium permeability such that the rate of depolarization is reduced and critical threshold potential is not reached. When critical threshold potential is not reached, an action potential cannot occur, resulting in local anesthetic-induced block of nerve conduction.

The ability of most local anesthetics to block nerve conduction is partly dependent on the state of the channel. Channels in the rested state (which predominate at more negative membrane potentials) have a much lower affinity for local anesthetics than activated (open state) and inactivated channels (which predominate at more positive membrane potentials). Thus, the effect of a given local anesthetic concentration is more prominent in rapidly firing axons than in resting fibers.

Local Anesthetic Molecule

The basic structure of a local anesthetic molecule is a tertiary amine separated from an unsaturated benzene ring by an intermediate chain (Table 7-1). The intermediate chain contains either an ester or amide linkage; therefore, local anesthetics are classified as either ester or amide compounds. The ester or amide linkage contributes to the anesthetic potency. The benzene ring provides a lipophilic character to the local anesthetic, whereas the tertiary amine is relatively hydrophilic.

Kinetics of How a Local Anesthetic Penetrates the Nerve

Local anesthetics are marketed as hydrochloride salts, which are soluble in water but insoluble in organic solvents. The pKa of the local anesthetic and the tissue pH determine the amount of drug that exists in the un-ionized (free base) or ionized (positively charged cation) form when injected into living tissue.

$$pH = pKa - \log \frac{[base]}{[cation]} \text{ or}$$

$$R:N + HCl \rightleftarrows R:NH^+ + Cl$$

$$R:N = \text{uncharged tertiary amine}$$

$$R:NH^+ = \text{the charged}$$

quarternary amine

Both the un-ionized and ionized form of the local anesthetic are necessary to block nerve conduction. Apparently, the un-ionized form is necessary to traverse the lipophilic nerve sheath. Once this passage has occurred, however, the ionized form of the local anesthetic binds to the nerve membrane to actually block conduction.

FACTORS THAT ALTER LOCAL ANESTHETIC ACTION

Nerve Fiber Size and Myelin

The ability of a local anesthetic to block nerve conduction is indirectly related to the diameter of the nerve fiber. In other words, higher concentrations of local anesthetic are required to inhibit impulse conduction

Table 7-1. Structure and Properties of Several Ester and Amide Local Anesthetics

	Lipophilic Group	Intermediate Chain	Amine Substitutes	Maximum Dose/70 kg (mg)	Threshold[a] Dose (mg/kg)	Serum Level[b] Producing Convulsions (μg/ml)	Potency
Esters							
Procaine		C_6H_5—C(=O)—O—CH_2—CH_2—N(C_2H_5)$_2$		1000	19.2	—	1
Tetracaine		HN(C_4H_9)—C_6H_4—C(=O)—O—CH_2CH_2—N(CH_3)$_2$		200	2.5	—	16
Amides							
Lidocaine	2,6-(CH_3)$_2$$C_6H_3$—	NH—C(=O)—CH_2—N(C_2H_5)$_2$		500	6.4	18–26	4
Bupivacaine	2,6-(CH_3)$_2$ ring—	NH—C(=O)— ring—C_4H_9		200	1.6	4.5–5.5	16
Etidocaine	2,6-(CH_3)$_2$ ring—	NH—C(=O)—CH(C_2H_5)—N(C_2H_5)$_2$		300	3.4	4.3	16

[a] Dose producing CNS symptoms in man.
[b] Serum level producing convulsions in monkey.

in larger nerves than are required in smaller nerves. Also, the presence of myelin enhances the ability of a local anesthetic to block nerve conduction. For example, if two nerves exist with the same diameter, the one with myelin will be blocked by smaller concentrations of local anesthetic than will the one without myelin. Likewise, small diameter unmyelinated C fibers are blocked with about the same concentration of local anesthetic as large diameter myelinated delta fibers. Nerves can be classified according to fiber diameter, the presence of myelin, and function (Table 7-2).

Location of a Nerve in a Nerve Bundle

Despite the A alpha fiber being the largest diameter myelinated fiber, motor blockade frequently is observed to develop prior to sensory blockade, when performing a brachial plexus block. Winnie et al[4] explained this apparent paradox by pointing out that

Table 7-2. Relative Size and Susceptibility to Blockade by Local Anesthetics of Types of Nerve Fibers

Fiber Type	Myelin	Diameter (μ)	Sensitivity to Block	Function
Type A				
Alpha	Yes	12–20	+	Proprioception, motor
Beta	Yes	5–12	+ +	Proprioception, motor
Gamma	Yes	3–6	+ +	Muscle tone
Delta	Yes	2–5	+ + +	Pain, temperature, touch
Type B	Yes	<3	+ + + +	Preganglionic autonomic
Type C	No	0.3–1.2	+ + + +	Pain and postganglionic autonomic

Symbols: + + + + = extremely sensitive; + + + = very sensitive; + + = moderately sensitive; + = slightly sensitive.

the distribution of motor fibers in core bundles is peripheral to the distribution of sensory axons (Fig. 7-2).[3] Therefore, the local anesthetic reaches the larger diameter motor fibers of the core bundles first, thus explaining the observation that 1 percent solutions of lidocaine and mepivacaine

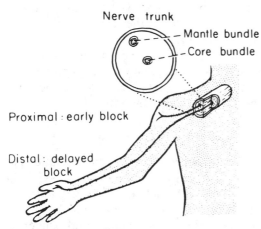

Figure 7-2. Relative locations of the mantle and core bundles in a nerve trunk. Proximal areas of the extremity are innervated by mantle bundles, while distal areas are served by core bundles. Within each bundle, motor fibers are distributed exterior to sensory fibers. Thus, sensory blockade proceeds from proximal to distal regions and motor blockade may become apparent before distal blockade. (deJong RH. Physiology and pharmacology of local anesthetics, Springfield, Illinois, Charles C Thomas, 1970, as modified in Savarese JJ, Covino BG, Pharmacology of local anesthetics. In: Miller RD, ed. Anesthesia, New York, Churchill Livingstone, 1981; 563–91.)

often produce motor blockade in advance of sensory blockade of the fingers. These concentrations of local anesthetic are sufficient to easily block conduction in the large motor A fibers. When a lower concentration of local anesthetic is used (e.g., 0.25 percent bupivacaine), which contains insufficient local anesthetic to produce significant motor blockade, sensory blockade then does precede motor blockade.

pH

A given concentration of local anesthetic is more potent in an alkaline pH than in an acidic pH. A high pH increases the fraction of local anesthetic existing in the un-ionized form, therefore providing greater transfer of drug across the lipophilic nerve sheath. Conversely, an acidic pH limits the fraction of drug which exists in the un-ionized form, explaining the observation that local anesthetics are relatively ineffective when injected into acidic infected tissues.

Vasoconstrictors

Vasoconstrictors, such as epinephrine and phenylephrine, reduce systemic absorption of local anesthetics by decreasing regional perfusion in the areas into which the local anesthetics have been injected. Vasoconstrictors are especially effective in enhancing the duration of action of otherwise intermediate and short-acting local anesthetics, such as lidocaine and procaine.

As a result, the blood levels of these local anesthetics are reduced by approximately 30 percent, which should reduce the chance of systemic toxicity from the local anesthetic. Vasoconstrictors are far less effective in prolonging the anesthetic properties of the long-acting local anesthetics, such as bupivacaine and etidocaine, probably because these local anesthetics are highly tissue bound, reflecting their greater lipid solubility.

Calcium

Elevated extracellular concentrations of calcium partially antagonize the action of local anesthetics. This reversal is caused by the calcium-induced increase of the surface potential on the membrane, which favors the low-affinity rested state.

Nerve Stimulation Rate

Local anesthetics have a higher potency with higher rates of stimulation. Even though this physiologic effect is well documented, its clinical importance, if any, has not been determined.

PHARMACOKINETICS

Systemic absorption of local anesthetics from the site of injection is dependent on dose, site of injection (blood flow and tissue binding), vasoconstrictors, physicochemical properties, and pharmacologic properties of the local anesthetics.[5]

Once the local anesthetic enters the blood stream, it is distributed widely with volumes of distribution at steady state ranging from 73 to 133 liters. By using a three-compartment distribution model, the elimination half-time of most local anesthetics ranges from 1.6 to 2.7 hours, which probably reflects hepatic metabolism. Indeed, renal excretion of unchanged drug accounts for less than 5 percent of the originally administered dose. Such pharmacokinetic values are unavailable for most ester-type agents because their plasma half-lives in vivo are extremely short due to rapid hydrolysis by pseudocholinesterase enzyme in the plasma. The amide local anesthetics are metabolized more slowly in the liver to water soluble inactive metabolites for excretion in the urine.

LOCAL ANESTHETIC TOXICITY

Toxicity of local anesthetics is usually directly related to the rate at which the local anesthetic diffuses from the tissue site of action to the systemic circulation and the resulting peak blood concentration. These two events dictate the total amount of local anesthetic that can be administered for a nerve block. Threshold doses of local anesthetic producing early symptoms and signs of central nervous system toxicity in humans and the associated plasma concentration vary with the drug administered (Table 7-1, Fig. 7-3).[1] These doses may be considered as maximum recommended quantities, particularly during intercostal, caudal, or paracervical blocks because these areas have a high blood flow.

Central Nervous System

Central nervous system manifestations of local anesthetic include sleepiness, light headedness, visual and auditory disturbances, and restlessness. With higher blood concentrations, nystagmus and shivering occur. Finally, with even higher blood concentrations, overt tonic-clonic seizures develop, followed by central nervous system depression and death. Local anesthetics apparently lead to depression of cortical inhibitory pathways, thereby allowing unopposed activity of excitatory components.

Prevention and Treatment

Over 90 percent of serious toxic reactions manifesting as seizures are due to excessive blood concentrations of local anesthetics. These toxic effects can be minimized by ad-

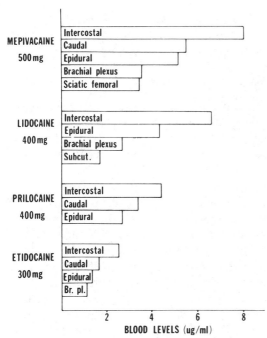

Figure 7-3. Peak plasma concentrations of local anesthetics resulting during performance of various types of regional anesthetic procedures. (Covino BG, Vassallo HG. Local anesthetics: Mechanisms of action and clinical use, New York, Grune & Stratton, 1976, by permission.)

ministering the smallest possible dose of local anesthetic needed to accomplish the desired clinical end point.

In animals, pretreatment with diazepam 0.25 mg/kg intramuscularly increases the dose of lidocaine required to produce seizures. Based on these data, preoperative medication with a benzodiazepine, such as diazepam, may be logical in an attempt to provide protection against systemic toxic effects of local anesthetics in patients.

If seizures do occur, arterial hypoxemia must be prevented. Although administration of oxygen is recommended in the treatment of seizures due to local anesthetics, oxygen inhalation itself does not prevent seizure activity. Hypercarbia and acidosis appear to promote the appearance of seizures. Thus, hyperventilation is recommended during treatment of seizures. Hyperventilation causes an alkalosis, which in turn lowers extracellular potassium. This decrease hyperpolarizes the transmembrane potential of the nerve membranes which then favors the rested or low-affinity state of the sodium channels, resulting in decreased local anesthetic activity.

Seizures induced by local anesthetics can also be treated with small intravenous doses of thiopental, 0.5 to 2.0 mg/kg. Alternatively, succinylcholine 0.5 to 1.0 mg/kg will stop peripheral manifestations of the seizure, but the brain will continue to exhibit hyperactivity. The proponents of administering succinylcholine point out, however, that postictal depression will be less if a muscle relaxant rather than a sedative-hypnotic is administered. Certainly, when seizures persist despite treatment with sedatives, it is necessary to administer a paralyzing dose of succinylcholine and intubate the trachea with a cuffed tube. Placement of a cuffed tube will reduce the likelihood of pulmonary aspiration of gastric contents and facilitate hyperventilation therapy.

Cardiovascular System

The cardiovascular effects of local anesthetics result partly from direct effects on cardiac and smooth muscle membranes and from indirect effects on autonomic nerves. Local anesthetics block cardiac sodium channels and thus depress cardiac pacemaker activity, excitability, and conduction. They also depress the strength of cardiac contraction and cause arteriolar dilatation. The only exception to this is cocaine.

With toxic doses, local anesthetics slow conduction in the heart, manifesting on the electrocardiogram as an increased P–R interval, and sinus bradycardia. These changes reflect a decrease in automaticity. Most local anesthetics seem to cause central nervous system irritability before myocardial depression. With adequate ventilation of the lungs during a seizure, evidence of cardiac toxicity is usually absent.

Cocaine. Among the local anesthetics, cocaine has unique cardiovascular effects. Blockade of uptake of norepinephrine back into the postganglionic nerve ending by cocaine manifests as vasoconstriction, hypertension, and cardiac dysrhythmias. This vasoconstricting property of cocaine can be used clinically to reduce the likelihood of bleeding from mucosal damage secondary to nasotracheal intubation (see Chapter 12).

Bupivacaine. The long-acting local anesthetics, bupivacaine and etidocaine, may have greater myocardial depressant effects than the other local anesthetics.[7] Specifically, several case reports suggest that simultaneous seizures and cardiovascular collapse occur without antecedent arterial hypoxemia from typical clinical doses of these local anesthetics that are inadvertently administered intravascularly. In awake sheep, equivalent doses of bupivacaine or lidocaine produced similar central nervous system toxicity when rapidly injected intravenously but serious cardiac dysrhythmias occurred only after bupivacaine.[8] Administration of bupivacaine concentrations above 0.5 percent to patients is not recommended so as to limit the dose administered should an inadvertent intravascular injection occur.

Methemoglobinemia. Administration of large doses (>10 mg/kg) of prilocaine may lead to accumulation of the metabolite o-toluidine, an oxidizing agent capable of converting hemoglobin to methemoglobin. When sufficient methemoglobin is present (3 to 5 mg/dl) the patient may appear cyanotic and the blood chocolate-colored. Such levels of methemoglobinemia are tolerated by healthy individuals, but may cause decompensation in patients with cardiac or pulmonary disease. Treatment with reducing agents such as methylene blue or, less satisfactorily, ascorbic acid may be given intravenously to rapidly convert methemoglobin to hemoglobin.

Local Tissue Toxicity

Local anesthetics are not neurotoxic when administered at recommended clinical concentrations. Yet, an accidental injection of large volumes of chloroprocaine into the subarachnoid space during the intended performance of an epidural block has been reported to result in sensory and motor deficits persisting for several weeks after the initial total spinal had subsided.[9,10] Sodium bisulfite, an antioxidant in chloroprocaine, produces similar neurologic deficits when placed in the subarachnoid space of rabbits.[11] Conversely, chloroprocaine without sodium bisulfite does not produce neurologic changes. Based on these data, it would seem that adverse effects that have followed inadvertent placement of chloroprocaine in the subarachnoid space are due to sodium bisulfite and not the local anesthetic or the low pH of the commercially available solution.

Allergic Reactions

Ester local anesthetics are metabolized to para-aminobenzoic acid derivatives. These metabolites can be responsible for allergic reactions in a small percentage of the population. Amides are not metabolized to para-aminobenzoic acid, and allergic reactions to local anesthetics in this group are extremely rare. Usually, patients are labelled as allergic to a local anesthetic when in fact they have experienced an adverse reaction due to excessive blood levels of drug or increased vagal activity. Thus, overall, the chances for having allergic reactions to local anesthetics are exceedingly rare. Furthermore, there is no cross-sensitivity between the ester and amide types of local anesthetics. Therefore, a patient known to be allergic to an ester could receive an amide local anesthetic without an increased risk of experiencing an allergic reaction.

SUMMARY

After years of experience, the commonly used ester and amide local anesthetics are well known in terms of their safety and relative nontoxic profiles. Even if a toxic effect does occur, it usually can be treated without prolonged adverse effect to the patient. Therefore, the versatility and safety of local anesthetics can be exceedingly useful to the anesthesiologist. The two most important controversies regarding local anesthetics are the possible myocardial toxicity of bupivacaine and neurotoxicity of chloroprocaine.

REFERENCES

1. Covino BG, Vassallo HG. Local anesthetics: Mechanisms of action in clinical use. New York, Grune & Stratton, 1976.
2. Savarese JJ, Covino BG. Pharmacology of local anesthetics. In: Miller RD, ed. Anesthesia, New York, Churchill Livingstone, 1981;563–91.
3. deJong RH. Physiology and pharmacology of local anesthetics. Springfield, Illinois, Charles C Thomas, 1970.
4. Winnie AP, LaVallee DA, PeSosa B, Masud KZ: Clinical pharmacokinetics of local anesthetics. Can Anaesth Soc J 1977;24:252–62.
5. Tucker GT, Mather LE. The clinical pharmacokinetics of local anesthetics. Clin Pharmacokinet 1979;4:241–78.
6. deJong RH, Heavner JE. Diazepam prevents local anesthetic seizures. Anesthesiology 1971;34:523–31.
7. Albright GA. Cardiac arrest following regional anesthesia with etidocaine or bupivacaine. Anesthesiology 1979;51:285–7.
8. Kotelko DM, Shnider SM, Dailey PA, Brizgys RV, Levinson G, Shapiro WA, Koike M, Rosen MA. Bupivacaine-induced cardiac arrhythmias in sheep. Anesthesiology 1984;60:10–8.
9. Ravindran RS, Bond VK, Tasch MD. Gupta CD, Luerssen TG. Prolonged neural blockade following regional analgesia with 2-chloroprocaine. Anesth Analg 1980;59:447–51.
10. Reisner LS, Hochman BN, Plumer MH. Persistent neurologic deficit and adhesive arachnoiditis following intrathecal 2-chloroprocaine injection. Anesth Analg 1980;59:452–4.
11. Wang BC, Hillman DE, Spielholz NI, Turndorf H. Chronic neurological deficits and Nesacaine-CE: An effect of the anesthetic 2-chloroprocaine, or the antioxidant, sodium bisulfite? Anesth Analg 1984;63:445–7.

8

Muscle Relaxants

Muscle relaxants are drugs which act at the neuromuscular junction to produce skeletal muscle paralysis. As such, these drugs are more accurately described as neuromuscular blockers. Nevertheless, the designation as muscle relaxants remains most commonly used. Skeletal muscle relaxation or paralysis can also be achieved by high doses of volatile anesthetics or regional anesthesia.

Several approaches are used when giving muscle relaxants during general anesthesia. One extreme has been the use of nitrous oxide, oxygen, and large doses of muscle relaxants. The philosophy of this approach is to administer sufficient anesthetic to provide amnesia and to prevent movement by administration of a muscle relaxant. Patients usually are amnesic, although awareness during anesthesia has been described.[1] In general, we believe that smaller doses of muscle relaxants should be used as adjuvants, and not substitutes, for anesthesia (see Chapter 9). By not administering muscle relaxants to patients who are showing signs of inadequate anesthesia (e.g., moving, hypertension, tachycardia) and monitoring neuromuscular function with a peripheral nerve stimulator, large doses of muscle relaxants can be avoided—which should decrease the incidence of prolonged paralysis and/or inadequate reversal of neuromuscular blockade.

NORMAL NEUROMUSCULAR FUNCTION

Neuromuscular transmission at the endplate is initiated by arrival of an impulse at the motor nerve terminal with an associated influx of calcium and a resultant release of acetylcholine (Fig. 8-1).[2] Acetylcholine then diffuses across the synaptic cleft to the nicotinic cholinergic receptor located on the motor endplate. When acetylcholine reacts with the receptor, permeability of the membrane in the endplate region increases to sodium primarily, but also to potassium. Sodium moves from outside to inside the membrane and the resting membrane potential depolarizes. This change in voltage is termed the *endplate potential*. The magnitude of the endplate potential is directly related to the amount of acetylcholine released. If the endplate potential is small, the permeability and the endplate potential return to normal without an impulse being propagated from the endplate region to the rest of the muscle membrane. If the endplate potential is large, the muscle membrane is depolarized and an impulse will be propagated alone the entire muscle fiber. Muscle contraction is then initiated by a process known as *excitation-contraction coupling*. The released acetylcholine is removed from the endplate region by diffusion and rapid hydrolysis by the enzyme

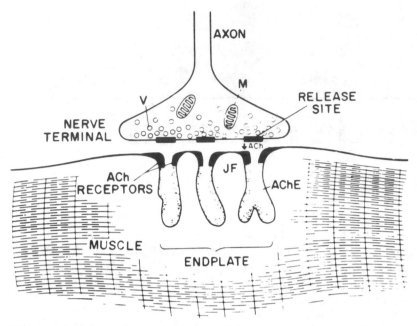

Figure 8-1. Schematic representation of the neuromuscular junction. V = transmitter vesicle, M = mitochondria, ACh = acetylcholine, AChE = acetylcholinesterase, JF = junctional folds. (Drachman DB. Myasthenia gravis. N Engl J Med 1978;298:136–42.)

acetylcholinesterase (true cholinesterase). Acetylcholinesterase is primarily located in the folds of the endplate region (Fig. 8-1).[2]

Skeletal muscle relaxation and paralysis can occur from interruption of function at several sites, including the central nervous system, myelinated somatic nerves, un- myelinated motor nerve terminals, and cholinergic receptors. Although muscle re- laxants and their antagonists have several sites of action, the primary blocking effect occurs at the cholinergic receptor. The cholinergic receptor itself, however, can be blocked by a variety of mechanisms (Fig.

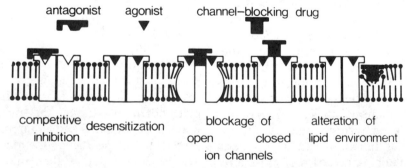

Figure 8-2. Possible modes of action of muscle relaxants on acetylcholine receptors hindering the flow of ions through channels. Agonist might be either acetylcholine or succinylcholine, whereas antagonist might be d-tub- ocurarine. (Dreyer F. Acetylcholine receptor. Br J Anaesth 1982;54:115– 30.)

8-2).[3] First, the receptor can be blocked by binding with a competitive inhibitor, preventing receptor activation by acetylcholine. This is the primary mechanism by which nondepolarizing muscle relaxants act. Secondly, desensitization produced by prolonged exposure of an agonist (e.g., succinylcholine) to the receptor can cause blockade. Conceptually, some channels enter a prolonged closed state, which cannot be opened by acetylcholine. They recover slowly to the resting state upon removal of the agonist molecules. Thirdly, drug-induced blockade of open ion channels will prevent not only closing of the channels, but also the flow of ions. This is probably what happens with huge overdoses of nondepolarizing muscle relaxants. Unfortunately, this type of blockade cannot be reversed by neostigmine. Fourthly, drug molecules may be bound to the ion channel in its shut formation preventing the opening of the channels. Lastly, the lipid environment around the acetylcholine receptor can be altered, thereby changing the channel properties. It is probable that the inhaled anesthetics, particularly enflurane, partly act by this mechanism.

PHARMACOLOGY OF MUSCLE RELAXANTS

Muscle relaxants are divided into two categories. One category is the nondepolarizing muscle relaxants, which includes d-tubocurarine, metocurine, gallamine, pancuronium, atracurium, and vecuronium. The other category of muscle relaxants is the depolarizing type. Succinylcholine is the only muscle relaxant in this group that is used clinically.

Nondepolarizing Muscle Relaxants

Mechanism of Action. Nondepolarizing muscle relaxants combine with the cholinergic receptors but do not activate them as does acetylcholine. This type of postsynaptic blockade is illustrated in the first panel of Figure 8-2.[3] If sufficient receptors are occupied by a nondepolarizing muscle relaxant, and therefore are unavailable to acetylcholine, neuromuscular transmission will fail. This is the main mechanism by which these muscle relaxants act, but they may also have presynaptic effects, such as decreasing the amount of acetylcholine released in response to an impulse. Because this is a competitive neuromuscular blockade, neuromuscular transmission can be reestablished by increasing the amount of acetylcholine at the neuromuscular junction and displacing the muscle relaxant from the receptor. This mechanism is achieved clinically by administration of an anticholinesterase (neostigmine, pyridostigmine, or edrophonium) which inhibits acetylcholinesterase, thereby allowing acetylcholine to accumulate at the neuromuscular junction. Anticholinesterases may also stimulate the presynaptic release of acetylcholine. The general characteristics of a nondepolarizing neuromuscular blockade are summarized in Table 8-1.

Duration of Action. Muscle relaxants can be categorized according to their duration of action (Table 8-2). There are no currently administered nondepolarizing muscle relaxants which are ultra short-acting. Vecuronium and atracurium are of short or intermediate duration of action, whereas d-tubocurarine, metocurine, pancuronium, and gallamine have a long duration of action. The duration of action of any nondepolarizing muscle relaxant is dependent on the dose administered. For example, with a large overdose, even a short-acting muscle relaxant can be made to be long-acting. With usual clinical doses, however, the duration of a long-acting muscle relaxant is about 60 minutes. In contrast, the duration of action of vecuronium or atracurium is about 30 minutes. A rule of thumb is that the duration of action of vecuronium and atracurium is about one-half

Table 8-1. Comparison of a Typical Nondepolarizing Muscle Relaxant (Pancuronium) and Depolarizing Muscle Relaxant (Succinylcholine)

	Pancuronium	Succinylcholine	
		Phase I	Phase II
Administrtion of pancuronium	Augment	Antagonize	Augment
Administration of succinylcholine	Antagonize	Augment	Augment
Administration of neostigmine	Antagonize	Augment	Antagonize
Initial excitatory effect on skeletal muscle	None	Fasciculation	None
Train-of-four ratio	<0.7	>0.7	<0.4
Response to tetanic stimulus	Unsustained	Sustained	Unsustained
Posttetanic facilitation	Yes	No	Yes
Rate of recovery[a]	30–60 min	4–8 min	>20 min

[a] Rate of recovery depends on dose. Larger doses cause a longer duration of blockade.

to one-third that of the long-acting muscle relaxants, such as pancuronium.

Pharmacokinetics. The rate of disappearance of a nondepolarizing muscle relaxant from blood is characterized by a rapid initial disappearance followed by a slower decay (Fig. 8-3).[4] Distribution to tissues is a major cause of the initial decrease, whereas the slower decay is due to excretion, usually via the kidney and/or bile. Because muscle relaxants are highly ionized, they do not cross lipid membranes easily and have a limited volume of distribution

(80 to 140 ml/kg) which is not much larger than the blood volume.

Table 8-3 summarizes the various muscle relaxants by their dependence on the kidney for their elimination. d-Tubocurarine, metocurine, and gallamine are not metabolized. Gallamine is essentially entirely dependent on the kidney for its elimination. In contrast, d-tubocurarine and metocurine are only partially dependent on the kidney for their elimination, while pancuronium is intermediate between these drugs and gallamine. Although the major route of excretion of pancuronium is via the kidney, it is

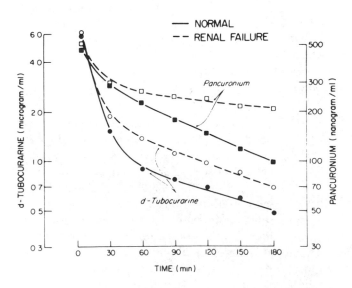

Figure 8-3. Rates at which the plasma concentrations of d-tubocurarine and pancuronium decrease in patients with and without renal failure. Note that the decay rates are about the same in patients with normal function. However, the decay rate is much slower in patients with renal failure receiving pancuronium than in those receiving d-tubocurarine. (Miller RD, Savarese JJ. Pharmacology of muscle relaxants, their antagonists and monitoring of neuromuscular function. In: Miller RD, ed. Anesthesia. New York, Churchill Livingstone, 1981;487–538, pancuronium data from Br J Anaesth 1976;48:341, and *d*-tubocurarine data from J Pharmacol Exp Ther 1977;202:1)

Table 8-2. Classification of Muscle Relaxants According to Duration of Action

Ultra-short
 Succinylcholine
Short
 Atracurium
 Decamethonium
 Vecuronium
Long
 d-Tubocurarine
 Gallamine
 Pancuronium
 Metocurine

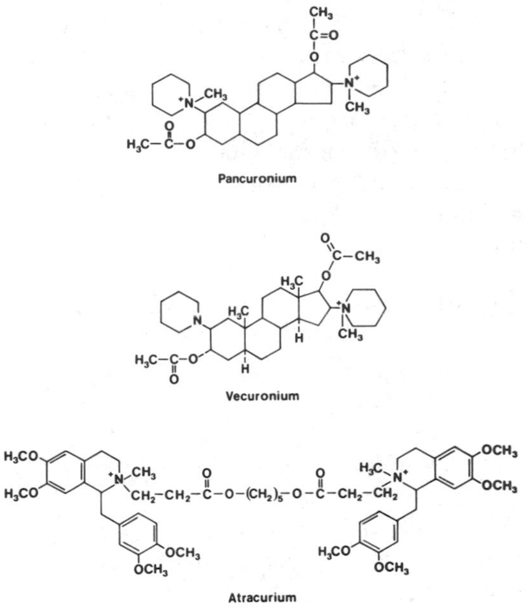

Figure 8-4. The chemical formula of pancuronium, vecuronium, and atracurium.

also metabolized (approximately 15 to 25 per cent of an injected dose) to 3-hydroxy, 17-hydroxy, and 3, 17-dihydroxy pancuronium. 3-Hydroxy pancuronium is about one-half as potent as its parent drug, pancuronium. Although the remaining metabolites also have neuromuscular blocking properties, they are very weak. The route of excretion for that muscle relaxant still remaining in the body that is not eliminated by the kidneys is unclear, although presumably biliary excretion accounts for most of it. A substantial amount of these muscle relaxants may remain in mucopolysaccharides of connective tissues for prolonged periods of time.

Vecuronium is a short-acting muscle relaxant which has a steroid nucleus and is a close analogue of pancuronium. Vecuronium differs from pancuronium only in that the nitrogen at position 2 is tertiary instead of quaternary, so that only the acetylcholine moiety associated with ring D remains (Fig. 8-4). Despite the apparent triviality in the structural difference, vecuronium has pharmacologic properties that are markedly different from those of pancuronium. Of prime importance is that, unlike pancuronium, vecuronium is not heavily dependent on the kidney for its elimination (Table 8-3). Animal studies indicate that most of the vecuronium (greater than 50 percent) is excreted unchanged into the bile. Vecuronium undoubtedly is metabolized via the same pathways as pancuronium, although the specific extent of metabolism has not been determined.

Atracurium is another short-acting muscle relaxant with a duration of action similar to that of vecuronium. This muscle relaxant is structurally related to some of the curare alkaloids (Fig. 8-4). Unlike other curare alkaloids, however, atracurium appears to be completely metabolized and, therefore, is not dependent on the kidney for its removal

Table 8-3. Classification of Muscle Relaxants According to Dependence on Renal Excretion for Their Elimination

Greater than 90 percent[a]
 Gallamine
 Decamethonium
60–80 percent
 Pancuronium
40–60 percent
 d-Tubocurarine
 Metocurine
Less than 20 percent
 Atracurium
 Succinylcholine
 Vecuronium

[a] Percent of injected dose dependent on the kidney for its elimination.

from blood. The main method by which atracurium is metabolized is probably by Hoffman elimination. Also, atracurium undergoes hydrolysis in the plasma. The main breakdown products are laudanosine and a related quaternary acid, neither of which exerts a neuromuscular blocking action.

Cardiovascular Effects. With the probable exception of vecuronium, all nondepolarizing muscle relaxants produce cardiovascular effects. Many of these effects are mediated by the autonomic nervous system and histamine receptors (Table 8-4).[4] d-Tubocurarine and, to a much lesser extent, metocurine and atracurium produce hypotension, probably as a result of liberation of histamine. With very large doses of d-tubocurarine, ganglionic blockade may also be a factor.

Pancuronium causes a modest increase in heart rate and blood pressure and to a lesser extent cardiac output, with little or no change in systemic vascular resistance. Although the tachycardia is primarily due to a vagolytic action, release of norepinephrine from adrenergic nerve endings and blockade of neuronal uptake of norepinephrine have been suggested as secondary mechanisms.

Depolarizing Muscle Relaxants

Mechanism of Action. Although decamethonium is still available, succinylcholine is the only depolarizing muscle relaxant commonly used clinically. Structurally, succinylcholine is two molecules of acetylcholine. Indeed, its neuromuscular effects can be conveniently characterized as almost identical to those of acetylcholine, except that succinylcholine produces a prolonged rather than brief depolarization of the neuromuscular junction. Succinylcholine reacts with the receptor to cause depolarization at the endplate and this, in turn, spreads to and depolarizes adjacent membranes, causing generalized disorganized contraction of motor units. Since succincylcholine is not metabolized as rapidly as acetylcholine, the membranes remain depolarized and unresponsive to additional impulses. Because excitation-contraction coupling requires repolarization and repetitive firing to maintain muscle tension, a flaccid paralysis results. The characteristics of a depolarizing (phase I) neuromuscular blockade are summarized in Table 8-1.

With continued exposure to succinylcholine, the initial depolarization decreases and the membrane becomes repolarized. Despite this repolarization, the membrane sometimes cannot be depolarized again by acetylcholine as long as succinylcholine is present. The mechanism for this response is not known, but one hypothesis is that a nonexcitable area develops in the investing muscle membrane immediately surrounding the endplate, which becomes repolarized shortly after the arrival of succinylcholine. This area presumably impedes centrifugal spread of impulses initiated by action of

Table 8-4. Autonomic Effects of Muscle Relaxants

Drug	Autonomic Ganglia	Muscarinic Receptors	Histamine Release
Succinylcholine	Stimulates	Stimulates	Slight
d-Tubocurarine	Blocks[a]	None	Moderate
Metocurine	Blocks weakly	None	Slight
Gallamine	None	Blocks strongly	None
Pancuronium	None	Blocks moderately	None
Vecuronium	None	None	None
Atracurium	None	None	Slight

[a] Only with high doses.
(Modified from Miller RD, Savarese JJ. Pharmacology of muscle relaxants, their antagonists and monitoring of neuromuscular function. In: Miller RD, ed. Anesthesia. New York, Churchill Livingstone, 1981;487–538.)

acetylcholine on the receptor. Because the endplate is partially repolarized and still does not respond to acetylcholine, some investigators have stated that the membrane is in a desensitized state to the effects of acetylcholine and the block is described as a desensitization (Phase II) block. This terminology is not entirely accurate, however, in that neostigmine or edrophonium can antagonize a phase II block (Table 8-1). Another possibility is that with prolonged exposure to acetylcholine, some channels enter a prolonged closed state, which cannot be opened by acetylcholine (Fig. 8-2).[3] This explanation still does not provide an answer as to why neostigmine or edrophonium can antagonize this type of blockade. The characteristics of a phase II block are nearly identical to those of a nondepolarizing blockade (Table 8-1).

Duration of Action and Pharmacokinetics. Succinylcholine is rapidly hydrolyzed by pseudocholinesterase (plasma cholinesterase), an enzyme in the liver and plasma. The initial metabolite, succinylmonocholine, is a much weaker neuromuscular blocker. It, in turn, is metabolized to succinic acid and choline. Pseudocholinesterase has an incredible capacity to hydrolyze succinylcholine at a very rapid rate. Consequently, only a small fraction of the originally administered intravenous dose of succinylcholine reaches the neuromuscular junction. Since there is little or no pseudocholinesterase at the motor endplate, the neuromuscular blockade of succinylcholine is terminated by diffusion away from the endplate into extracellular fluid. Pseudocholinesterase, therefore, influences the duration of action of succinylcholine by controlling the rate at which the latter is hydrolyzed before it reaches the endplate. Thus metabolism by pseudocholinesterase and diffusion away from the endplate account for succinylcholine's initial brief duration of action (Table 8-1).

Neuromuscular blockade by succinylcholine may be prolonged in patients with an atypical variant of pseudocholinesterase of genetic origin. The "dibucaine number" is a test to determine whether atypical or normal pseudocholinesterase is present in the plasma. Under standardized test conditions, dibucaine inhibits normal pseudocholinesterase activity by about 80 percent (dibucaine number 80), whereas dibucaine only inhibits atypical pseudocholinesterase activity by about 20 percent (dibucaine number 20). Although many genetic variations of pseudocholinesterase have been identified, the dibucaine-related variances are the most important. It is important to recognize that the dibucaine number does not indicate how much (quantity) pseudocholinesterase is present but rather indicates what type (normal or atypical) of pseudocholinesterase is available. When atypical pseudocholinesterase is present, the duration of action of a clinical dose of succinylcholine (1 to 2 mg/kg) is increased from usually less than 15 minutes to several hours.

Cardiovascular Effects. Succinylcholine-induced cardiac dysrhythmias are many and varied. Succinylcholine stimulates all autonomic and nicotinic receptors in both sympathetic and parasympathetic ganglia and muscarinic receptors in the sinus node of the heart (Table 8-4).[4] In low doses, both negative inotropic and chronotropic responses occur that can attenuated by administration of atropine. With large doses, positive inotropic and chronotropic effects may result. Bradycardia has been most often observed following the first dose of succinylcholine administered to children and following the second dose administered to adults, especially when the interval between doses is about 5 minutes. This bradycardia can be attenuated or prevented by the intravenous administration of atropine or a nonparalyzing dose of nondepolarizing muscle relaxant 1 to 3 minutes before injection of succinylcholine. Atropine administered intramuscularly with the preoperative medication does not protect against succinylcholine-induced bradycardia. Direct myocardial effects, increased muscarinic stimulation, and ganglionic stimulation may all be involved in the bradycardic response.

Complications of Succinylcholine. Several complications have been associated with the administration of succinylcholine. By far, the most important one is a massive hyperkalemic response to succinylcholine, although increases in intraocular pressure, intragastric pressure, and muscle pains have also been associated with succinylcholine administration.

Massive hyperkalemia can occur following administration of succinylcholine to patients with extensive burns, trauma (particularly crush injuries), nerve damage (spinal cord transection), or neuromuscular disease.[5] Conceptually, it is felt these events result in proliferation of sites on the postjunctional membrane where changes in permeability during depolarization can occur. As a result, depolarization produced by succinylcholine can result in permeability changes to potassium along the entire membrane, manifesting as hyperkalemia and cardiac arrest. In normal patients, succinylcholine increases the serum potassium concentration less than 0.5 mEq/L.

Although hyperkalemia has been associated with closed head injury, cerebral vascular accidents and intra-abdominal infections, these increases in serum potassium levels have not usually produced catastrophic results as have been reported with burns, trauma, or nerve damage. It also has been proposed that succinylcholine should not be given to patients in renal failure. Several studies, however, have failed to document that patients with renal failure are uniquely susceptible to a massive hyperkalemic response from succinylcholine.[6]

Because succinylcholine is not dependent on the kidney for its elimination, it has been our muscle relaxant of choice in patients undergoing renal transplantation. With the introduction of vecuronium and atracurium, reliance on succinylcholine for patients with renal failure may ultimately be less important.

The susceptibility to succinylcholine-induced hyperkalemia exists probably only between about 5 to 60 days post-injury. Pretreatment with a nonparalyzing dose of nondepolarizing muscle relaxant (e.g., 3 mg/70 kg of d-tubocurarine 3 minutes before injection of succinylcholine) is not effective in preventing this potassium release. Because this massive hyperkalemic response is so catastrophic, it is recommended that a patient who has had a burn or trauma longer than 5 days should not be given succinylcholine. The rule of thumb that succinylcholine may be given 60 days following injury is only valid if the burn or trauma heals without infection. If infection is present, tissues are probably continuing to degenerate and, therefore, the 60-day rule should be extended. In terms of neurological disease and the unpredictability with which patients will be susceptible to a massive hyperkalemic response from succinylcholine, it is probably prudent not to administer succinylcholine to any patient who has nerve damage or neuromuscular disease, especially those with hemiplegia or paraplegia secondary to upper motor neuron lesions.

Increased intraocular pressure. Succinylcholine causes an increase in intraocular pressure which is manifested 1 minute after injection, is maximum at 2 to 4 minutes, and subsides after 5 to 7 minutes. The mechanism for this effect has not been clearly defined but may involve contraction of myofibrils or transient dilation of choroidal blood vessels. Despite the increase in pressure, the use of succinylcholine for ophthalmologic surgery is not contraindicated unless the anterior chamber is to be opened (see Chapter 25). It is debatable as to whether prior administration of a nonparalyzing dose of a nondepolarizing muscle relaxant will prevent the increase in intraocular pressure associated with succinylcholine administration (see Chapter 25).

Increased intragastric pressure. In some patients, especially muscular males, fasiculations associated with succinylcholine will cause an increase in intragastric pressure, ranging from 5 to 40 cm/H_2O.[7] This may make regurgitation and pulmonary aspiration of gastric contents more likely, although this conclusion is purely speculative. The increase in intragastric pressure produced by succinylcholine can be prevented by pretreatment with a nondepolarizing dose of a nondepolarizing muscle relaxant.

Muscle pain. The incidence of muscle pain following succinylcholine administration varies from 0.2 to 89 percent. Muscle pain occurs more frequently in ambulatory patients than in those who are bedridden. The pain is probably secondary to damage produced in the muscle by the unsynchronized contraction of adjacent muscle fibers just before the onset of paralysis. Muscle damage has been verified by the appearance of myoglobinuria following the use of succinylcholine. Muscle pain can probably be attenuated, but not eliminated, by prior administration of a nondepolarizing muscle relaxant (see Chapter 29).

Interaction with Other Drugs

There are many drugs with which muscle relaxants interact. Inhaled anesthetics, antibiotics, and local anesthetics probably represent the most important ones. In addition, magnesium as used to treat toxemia of pregnancy and lithium as administered to treat manic depressive psychoses can potentiate the effects of muscle relaxants.

Inhaled anesthetics augment neuromuscular blockade produced by nondepolarizing muscle relaxants in a dose-dependent fashion. Of the drugs that have been studied, inhaled anesthetics augment the effects of muscle relaxants in the following order: isoflurane and enflurane augment more than halothane, which, in turn, augments more than nitrous oxide-barbiturate-narcotic anesthesia. For example, the dose of d-tubocurarine necessary to depress twitch 95 percent in adults is about 0.08 mg/kg during 1.25 MAC enflurane, 0.18 mg/kg during 1.25 MAC halothane and 0.31 mg/kg during a nitrous oxide-barbiturate-narcotic anesthetic. The most important factors involved in this augmentation are depression of sites proximal to the neuromuscular junction such as the central nervous system, and decreased sensitivity of the postjunctional membrane to depolarization by acetylcholine. Augmentation of succinylcholine neuromuscular blockade by inhaled anesthetics, with the possible exception of isoflurane, is not prominent.

Antibiotics. There have been over 100 clinical reports of enhancement of neuromuscular blockade by antibiotics, especially the aminoglycosides, which include neomycin, streptomycin, kanamycin, and polymixin B. Many of the antibiotics depress release of acetylcholine similar to that caused by magnesium. For this reason, some of the antibiotic-induced neuromuscular blockades can be antagonized by calcium. Furthermore, several antibiotics have postjunctional activity. Because the clinician is usually confronted with a combined nondepolarizing muscle relaxant-antibiotic neuromuscular blockade, it is our policy to administer the usual reversal dose of anticholinesterase intravenously. If that dose is unsuccessful in antagonizing the neuromuscular blockade, then ventilation of the lungs should be continued until the blockade dissipates spontaneously. Further attempts at antagonism with an anticholinesterase may actually augment the neuromuscular blockade. We do not administer calcium because antagonism is usually transient, and theoretically, calcium could antagonize the antibacterial effect of the antibiotics. Antibiotics that do not enhance neuromuscular blockade include the penicillins and cephalosporins.

Local anesthetics and antidysrhythmics, which are involved with channel blockade and/or membrane stabilization, enhance the neuromuscular blockade from both nondepolarizing and depolarizing muscle relaxants. In low doses, local anesthetics depress posttetanic potentiation, which is thought to be a neural prejunctional effect. With higher doses, local anesthetics block acetylcholine-induced muscle contractions. This stabilizing effect is the result of blockade of the ionic channels linked to the nicotinic receptor. Calcium channel blockers probably potentiate neuromuscular blockade by muscle relaxants.

MONITORING AND ITS INFLUENCE ON MUSCLE RELAXANT ADMINISTRATION

Monitoring of neuromuscular function in the perioperative period serves two useful functions.[8-10] First, monitoring serves as a guide to muscle relaxant administration intraoperatively. Monitoring allows the clinician to answer the question as to whether sufficient muscle relaxant has been administered or, more importantly, whether too much muscle relaxant has been given. Secondly, monitoring can be utilized to determine whether a neuromuscular blockade has been adequately antagonized either intraoperatively or postoperatively. Although muscle relaxants can be administered without monitoring of neuromuscular function, surveys have been performed which indicate that patients are frequently returned to the recovery room partially paralyzed when intraoperative monitoring is not employed. Despite a normal tidal volume these patients may not have the strength necessary to overcome airway obstruction. For example, Viby-Mogensen et al.[11] found that 24 percent of patients were unable to sustain head lift for 5 seconds in the recovery room and 42 percent had a train-of-four ratio less than 0.7. None of these 72 patients had been monitored with a peripheral nerve stimulator in the operating room. The implication is that more patients would arrive in the recovery room with neuromuscular blockade adequately antagonized if monitoring had been performed by use of a peripheral nerve stimulator.

Patients also vary in their responses to muscle relaxants. Therefore, whenever possible, a muscle relaxant should be titrated to a given end-point rather than arbitrarily administered in large bolus doses. Routine monitoring with a peripheral nerve stimulator makes it possible to achieve precise individual dosing of both muscle relaxants and their antagonists. Those patients in whom the response to muscle relaxants is especially unpredictable and therefore monitoring with a peripheral nerve stimulator imperative include (1) patients with reduced ability to excrete muscle relaxants (e.g., kidney and liver disease), (2) patients in poor general health, (3) patients with severe pulmonary disease, (4) patients with neuromuscular disease, (5) morbidly obese patients, and, (6) patients having to undergo prolonged surgery (e.g., greater than 4 hours).

Methods of Monitoring

Although the clinical assessment of the adequacy of muscle relaxation intraoperatively and various tests of ventilation postoperatively can be performed, use of a peripheral nerve stimulator is probably the most consistent and reliable method of monitoring neuromuscular function. Several peripheral nerve stimulators are available. Whatever stimulator is utilized, the ability to administer a single twitch (e.g., 0.1 Hz at 0.1–0.2 msec), tetanic stimulus of 50 or 100 Hz, and train-of-four stimulation should be available. Train-of-four stimulation is application of four supramaximal stimuli (2 Hz) at intervals of 0.5 seconds over a period of 2 seconds. Single twitch reflects predominately postsynaptic respones, while the tetanic stimulus and the train-of-four stimulation mirror predominately presynaptic events at the neuromuscular junction. Stimulation of the ulnar nerve, either with surface electrodes or needle electrodes, is frequently utilized (Fig. 8-5).[10]

Interpretation of Monitoring

Either a combination of a single twitch and tetanic stimulus or train-of-four stimulation will allow one to distinguish between a nondepolarizing and depolarizing neuromuscular blockade (Figs. 8-6, 8-7).[10] Using a peripheral nerve stimulator, a phase II desensitization neuromuscular blockade due to succinylcholine is indistinguishable from a nondepolarizing neuromuscular blockade. In an adequately anesthetized patient, a twitch height of less than 10 percent or a train-of-four ratio of less than 0.2 should provide adequate surgical relaxation. In essence, this means that if a patient is paralyzed with a nondepolarizing muscle relaxant, the response to a single twitch stimulus can be just barely felt or seen, and only the response to the first two of the four stimulations of the train-of-four can be seen or felt (Figs. 8-5, 8-6, 8-7).[10] If the twitch response is depressed greater than this level, difficulties with antagonism may develop.

ANTAGONISM OF NEUROMUSCULAR BLOCKADE

Reversal of a nondepolarizing neuromuscular blockade can be achieved by the intravenous administration of neostigmine, 40

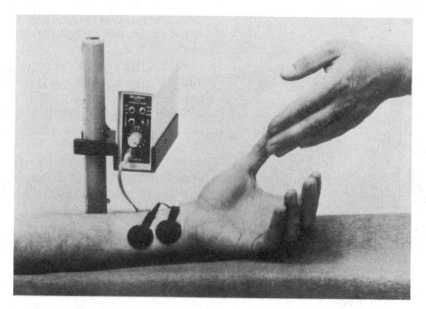

Figure 8-5. Monitoring of neuromuscular blockade without recording equipment. A peripheral nerve stimulator is utilized to provide stimuli via surface electrodes. The evoked response of the thumb or strength of contraction of the thumb is determined by tactile or visual evaluation. (Viby-Mogensen J. Clinical assessment of neuromuscular transmission. Br J Anaesth 1982;54:209–23.)

to 70 µg/kg (3 to 5 mg/70 kg), pyridostigmine 150 to 300 µg/kg (10 to 20 mg/70 kg) or edrophonium 0.5 to 1 mg/kg (35 to 70 mg/70 kg). The quaternary ammonium structure of these three drugs greatly limits their entrance into the central nervous system such that selective reversal of the effects of nondepolarizing muscle relaxants at the neuromuscular junction is possible. To prevent the peripheral cardiac muscarinic effects of neostigmine and pyridostigmine (e.g., bradycardia and hypotension), approximately 15 µg/kg of atropine must be given. The use of glycopyrrolate 7.5 µg/kg reduces the initial tachycardic response and probably the frequency of cardiac dysrhythmias when

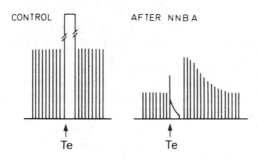

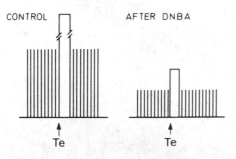

Figure 8-6. A diagramatic illsutration of the evoked response to tetanic and posttetanic stimulation following injection of a nondepolarizing (upper panel) and depolarizing (lower panel) muscle relaxant. Te = tetanic stimulus, NNBA = nondepolarizing muscle relaxant, DNBA = depolarizing muscle relaxant. (Viby-Mogensen J. Clinical assessment of neuromuscular tansmission. Br J Anesth 1982;54:209–23.)

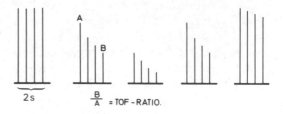

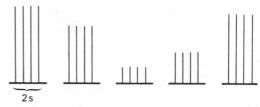

Figure 8-7. A diagramatic illustration of the evoked response to train-of-four (TOF) nerve stimulation following injection of nondepolarizing (upper panel) and depolarizing (lower panel) muscle relaxants. Note the "fade" in the train-of-four response during a nondepolarizing neuromuscular blockade. (Viby-Mogensen J. Clinical assessment of neuromuscular transmission. Br J Anaesth 1982;54:209–23.)

combined with neostigmine or pyridostigmine. If glycopyrrolate is given with edrophonium, however, an initial bradycardia will occur. This bradycardia reflects a more rapid onset of action of edrophonium than glycopyrrolate. Atropine with a more rapid onset of action should, therefore, be administered with edrophonium. The dose of atropine is 7 to 9 µg/kg, as edrophonium is

Table 8-5. Time to Onset of Action (min) of Edrophonium, Neostigmine, Pyridostigmine[a]

Response	Edrophonium (35 mg/70 kg)	Neostigmine (3 mg/70 kg)	Pyridostigmine (15 mg/70 kg)
50 percent	0.4	3.2	4.0
Peak effect	1.2	7.1	12.2

[a] Time from antagonist administration to 50 percent of peak effect and time to peak effect.
(Cronnelly R, Morris RB. Antagonism of neuromuscular blockade. Br J Anesth 1982;54:183–94.)

Table 8-6. Suggested Comparison, Advantages, and Disadvantages of Tests of Neuromuscular Transmission

Test	Estimated Receptors Occupied (Percent)	Disadvantages
Tidal volume	80	Insensitive
Twitch height	75–80	Insensitive, uncomfortable, need to know twitch before relaxant administration
Sustained tetanus at 30 Hz	75–80	Insensitive, uncomfortable
Vital capacity	70–75	Insensitive, need patient cooperation
Train-of-four	70–75	Not very sensitive
Sustained tetanus at 100 Hz	50	Very painful
Inspiratory force	50	Sometimes difficult to perform without endotracheal intubation
Head lift and hand grip	33	Need patient cooperation

(Miller RD, Savarese JJ. Pharmacology of muscle relaxants, their antagonists and monitoring of neuromuscular function. In: Miller RD, ed. Anesthesia. New York, Churchill Livingstone 1981;487–538.)

less likely than neostigmine or pyridostigmine to cause bradycardia.[12] Edrophonium may also have an advantage in that it has a quicker onset of action than does neostigmine or pyridostigmine (Table 8-5).[12]

Reversal of a nondepolarizing neuromuscular blockade by administration of an anticholinesterase should not be initiated before there is a response to a single stimulus or train-of-four. If an anticholinesterase is given when only the first response in the train-of-four is present or twitch height is less than 5 percent of control, 15 to 30 minutes will be required before twitch height reaches its normal height or the train-of-four ratio is greater than 0.7. If all four twitches from train-of-four stimulation can be felt, even though the ratio may be very low, reversal of neuromuscular blockade can be achieved in less than 10 minutes (Table 8-5).[12] In the postoperative period, a peripheral nerve stimulator can be used in the differential diagnosis of a patient who is having difficulty breathing. If the train-of-four ratio is greater than 0.7 and there is an absence of fade in response to a tetanic stimulus, or if the patient can lift his or her head for 5 seconds (Table 8-6),[4] it is highly unlikely that residual neuromuscular blockade is responsible for the patient's symptoms.

In view of the multiple factors involved with antagonism of neuromuscular blockade,[4,12] no more than 5 mg/70 kg of neostigmine, 20 mg/70 kg of pyridostigmine, or 70 mg/70 kg of edrophonium are recommended unless the following questions have been answered.

1. Has enough time been allowed for the anticholinesterase to antagonize the block (e.g., at least 15 to 30 minutes)?
2. Is the neuromuscular blockade too intense to be antagonized?
3. Is the acid-base and electrolyte status normal?
4. Is the temperature normal?
5. Is the patient receiving any drugs that may make antagonism difficult?
6. Has excretion of the muscle relaxant been reduced (e.g., reduced renal excretion)?

Answers to these questions often will provide the reason for failure of neostigmine, pyridostigmine, or edrophonium to antagonize a nondepolarizing neuromuscular blockade.

REFERENCES

1. Editorial. On being aware. Br J Anaesth 1979;51:711.
2. Drachmen DB. Myasthenia gravis. N Engl J Med 1978;298:136–42.

3. Dreyer F. Acetylcholine receptor. Br J Anaesth 1982;54:115–30.
4. Miller RD, Savarese JJ. Pharmacology of muscle relaxants, their antagonists and monitoring of neuromuscular function. In: Miller RD, ed., Anesthesia. New York, Churchill Livingstone 1981:487–538.
5. Gronert GA, Theye RA. Pathophysiology of hyperkalemia induced by succinylcholine. Anesthesiology 1975;43:89–99.
6. Miller RD, Way WL, Hamilton WK. Succinycholine-induced hyperkalemia in patients with renal failure? Anesthesiology 1972;36:138–41.
7. Miller RD, Way WL. Inhibition of succinylcholine-induced increased intragastric pressure by nondepolarizing muscle relaxants and lidocaine. Anesthesiology 1971;34:185–8.
8. Miller RD. Antagonism of neuromuscular blockade. Anesthesiology 1976;44:318–29.
9. Ali HH, Savarese JJ. Monitoring of neuromuscular function. Anesthesiology 1976;45:216–49.
10. Viby-Mogenson J. Clinical assessment of neuromuscular transmision. Br J Anaesth 1982;54:209–23.
11. Viby-Mogensen J, Chraemmer-Jorgensen B, Ording H. Residual curarization in the recovery room. Anesthesiology 1979;50:539–41.
12. Cronnelly R, Morris RB. Antagonism of neuromuscular blockade. Br J Anaesth 1982;54:183–94.

Section III
Preoperative Preparation and Intraoperative Management

9

Preoperative Evaluation and Choice of Technique of Anesthesia

Preoperative evaluation and preparation for anesthesia begins when the anesthesiologist reviews the patient's medical record and visits with the patient, ideally the day before elective surgery. Important aspects of the preoperative evaluation performed by the anesthesiologist include a history, review of current drug therapy, and a physical examination. Another important aspect of this preoperative visit is to inform the patient and other interested adults about events to expect on the day of surgery (Table 9-1). The planned management of anesthesia is discussed with the patient and informed consent obtained. Indeed, the patient or guardian must sign a consent statement authorizing the administration of anesthesia. Informed consent does not require that the anesthesiologist describe to the patient remote risks associated with the administration of anesthesia, as this would serve only to alarm a patient who is most likely already apprehensive. The anesthesiologist should describe, however, specific potential complications if an unusual technique or drug is to be employed or if the physical condition of the patient makes adverse responses likely, such as dislodgement of loose or diseased teeth during direct

laryngoscopy. Finally, the apprehension-allaying effect on the patient produced by the anesthesiologist's preoperative visit is an important aspect of preoperative medication (see Chapter 10).

Following the preoperative visit a summary of pertinent findings should be written in the patient's medical record. This summary includes details of the history, current drug therapy, physical examination, and laboratory data. In addition, a physical status classification is assigned and the technique of anesthesia that has been discussed with the patient is detailed. Specific potential complications associated with the administration of anesthesia that have been described to the patient should be noted. Finally, orders for the preoperative medication are written (see Chapter 10).

On occasion, it may be the anesthesiologist's opinion, based on the preoperative evaluation, that the patient is not in optimal medical condition prior to elective surgery. This judgment should be discussed with the patient's primary physician and, if necessary, elective surgery deferred until the patient's medical condition can be improved. When surgery is urgent, however, the benefits of immediate treatment offset the haz-

Table 9-1. Perioperative Events that Should be Discussed with the Patient Preoperatively

Preoperative insomnia and medication available for its treatment
Time, route of administration, and expected effects from the preoperative medication
Time of anticipated transport to operating room for surgery
Anticipated duration of surgery
Awakening after surgery in the recovery room
Likely presence of catheters on awakening (tracheal, gastric, bladder, venous, arterial)
Time of expected return to hospital room after surgery
Magnitude of postoperative discomfort and methods available for its treatment
Incidence of postoperative nausea and vomiting

ards introduced by less than optimal medical preparation, and the surgery is not delayed.

HISTORY

The history obtained preoperatively should seek details relating to previous anesthetics experienced by the patient or relatives as well as a careful review of organ system function as altered by co-existing diseases (Table 9-2). Co-existing diseases that influence the management of anesthesia may be related to the reason for surgery. Adverse events related to previous anesthetics should be specifically sought. Questions relating to major organ system function serve to elicit the presence and impact of co-existing diseases. The reader should consult specific sections of subsequent chapters for detailed discussions of the importance of co-existing diseases in the management of anesthesia.

CURRENT DRUG THERAPY

Current drug therapy must be carefully reviewed during the preoperative evaluation, since adverse interactions of these medications with drugs administered in the perioperative period must be considered. For example, current drug therapy can alter anesthetic requirements (MAC) for volatile drugs, potentiate muscle relaxants, exaggerate responses to sympathomimetics, re-

Table 9-2. Specific Areas to Investigate in Preoperative History

Previous adverse responses related to anesthesia
  Allergic reactions
  Prolonged skeletal muscle paralysis
  Delayed awakening
  Nausea and vomiting
  Hoarseness
  Myalgia
  Hemorrhage
  Jaundice
  Postspinal headache
  Adverse responses in relatives
Central nervous system
  Cerebrovascular insufficiency
  Seizures
Cardiovascular system
  Exercise tolerance
  Angina pectoris
  Prior myocardial infarction
  Hypertension
  Rheumatic fever
  Claudication
  Tachydysrhythmias
Lungs
  Exercise tolerance
  Dyspnea and orthopnea
  Cough and sputum production
  Bronchial asthma
  Cigarette consumption
  Pneumonia
  Recent upper respiratory tract infection
Liver
  Ethanol consumption
  Hepatitis
Kidneys
  Nocturia
  Pyuria
Skeletal and muscular systems
  Arthritis
  Osteoporosis
  Weakness
Endocrine system
  Diabetes mellitus
  Thyroid gland dysfunction
  Adrenal gland dysfunction
Coagulation
  Bleeding tendency
  Easy bruising
  Hereditary coagulopathies
Reproductive system
  Menstrual history
  Sexually transmitted diseases
Dentition
  Dentures
  Caps

Table 9-3. Current Drug Therapy and Potential Interactions with Drugs Administered in the Perioperative Period

Increase anesthetic requirements (MAC) for volatile drugs
  Monoamine oxidase inhibitors
  Tricyclic antidepressants (?)
  Chronic ethanol abuse
  Acute dextroamphetamine
  Acute cocaine
Decrease anesthetic requirements (MAC) for volatile drugs
  Acute ethanol intoxication
  Alpha methyldopa
  Clonidine
  Chronic amphetamine
  Verapamil
  Cimetidine (?)
Potentiate neuromuscular blockers
  Magnesium
  Aminoglycoside antibiotics
  Lidocaine
  Quinidine
  Lithium
Exaggerate response to sympathomimetics
  Monoamine oxidase inhibitors
  Tricyclic antidepressants
Reduce peripheral sympathetic nervous system activity
  Alpha methyldopa
  Guanethidine
  Clonidine
  Propranolol or other beta-adrenergic antagonists
Enhance metabolism
  Barbiturates
  Phenytoin
  Chronic ethanol abuse
  Corticosteroids
  Isoniazid
Impair metabolism
  Monoamine oxidase inhibitors
  Disulfiram
  Echothiophate
  Organophosphates (insecticides)

duce peripheral sympathetic nervous system activity, or enhance or impair the metabolism of drugs (Table 9-3).[1–7] The reader should consult Chapters 3, 5, and 8 for detailed discussions of these drug interactions. Potential drug interactions, however, do not dictate the need to discontinue preoperatively drugs that are producing desirable therapeutic responses. Indeed, with the exception of monoamine oxidase inhibitors and possibly anticoagulants, current drug therapy (antihypertensives, antianginal drugs, digitalis, diuretics, anticonvulsants, hormone replacement) should be continued throughout the perioperative period. Nevertheless, the safety of maintaining current drug therapy is based on the anesthesiologist's awareness of potential adverse drug interactions and appropriate modifications in perioperative selection of drugs and doses as well as techniques of monitoring.

PHYSICAL EXAMINATION

The physical examination performed by the anesthesiologist is primarily directed toward the cardiovascular system, lungs, and upper airway. Blood pressure obtained in the supine and standing position, heart rate and its regularity, and auscultation for cardiac murmurs, carotid artery bruits, and the presence of abnormal breath sounds such as rales or expiratory wheezing are part of the usual physical examination performed by the anesthesiologist. It is particularly important to listen for the murmur of aortic stenosis (systolic murmur at the right sternal border maximum in the second intercostal space), because patients with this valvular abnormality may be asymptomatic but vulnerable to unexpected cardiac dysrhythmias or adverse reductions in stroke volume should blood pressure, heart rate, or systemic vascular resistance change abruptly during anesthesia and surgery. The presence of orthostatic hypotension may reflect previously unrecognized hypovolemia or drug-induced impairment of peripheral sympathetic nervous system activity (see Chapters 3 and 18).

Physical characteristics of the patient that could make management of the airway difficult such as obesity, short neck, limited temporomandibular and/or cervical spine mobility, and prominent central incisors should be appreciated at this time (see Chapter 12). Availability of peripheral venous sites, including the external jugular veins, should be noted. The adequacy of collateral blood flow probably should be determined using the Allen's test if the plan is to insert an arterial catheter in the perioperative period (see Chapter 16). It may be important to evaluate the effect of the operative position on circulation. For example, extending or turning the head may not be tolerated in the presence of carotid or vertebral artery occlusive disease. Furthermore, patient immobility due to arthritis may limit positioning of the arms and/or legs during surgery. Finally, if regional anesthesia is planned, it is essential to inspect the likely site of local anesthetic injection for any anatomical abnormalities or signs of infection.

LABORATORY DATA

Many hospitals and departments of anesthesia have specific rules as to which tests should or must be performed on all patients prior to anesthesia for elective surgery. Ideally, however, only those laboratory tests indicated on the basis of positive findings elicited during the history and physical examination of the patient should be ordered.[8] Likewise, the age of the patient and complexity of the planned opreation should be considered in determining which laboratory tests need to be obtained preoperatively. Nevertheless, because patients frequently enter the hospital the evening before surgery, it has become common to order routine laboratory screening tests prior to the history and physical examination and regardless of the age of the patient or complexity of the planned surgery (Table 9-4).

Hemoglobin Concentration

Routine determination of the hemoglobin concentration (or hematocrit) is indicated prior to anesthesia for elective surgery. It is difficult to justify proceeding with an elective operation in the presence of anemia (hemoglobin less than 10 g/dl) due to an unknown cause that is discovered by the

Table 9-4. Examples of Laboratory Screening Tests Frequently Ordered Prior to Anesthesia for Elective Surgery

Hemoglobin concentration
Blood chemistries
Blood glucose
Blood urea nitrogen
Serum glutamic oxalacetic transaminase
Serum potassium
Coagulation studies
Prothrombin time
Plasma thromboplastin time
Urinalysis
Electrocardiogram
Radiograph of the chest
Pulmonary function studies
Arterial blood gases and pH
Forced exhaled volume in 1 second (FEV_1)
Vital capacity (VC)
FEV_1/VC
Maximum breathing capacity

measurement of the hemoglobin concentration preoperatively. Nevertheless, there are no data to confirm that treatment of moderate normovolemic anemia in the preoperative period leads to a decrease in perioperative morbidity or mortality.[8] Perhaps the duration of anemia is important also, as with time the cardiovascular system adjusts to the reduced concentration of hemoglobin by increasing the cardiac output so as to maintain tissue oxygen delivery despite reduced oxygen carrying capacity of the blood.

In contrast to anemia, there is evidence that the preoperative presence of polycythemia is associated with adverse perioperative events such as hemorrhage and/or thrombosis. Furthermore, the presence of unexpected polycythemia may be a clue preoperatively to the unexpected existence of chronic arterial hypoxemia or depletion of intravascular fluid volume related to diuretic therapy.

Blood Chemistries

Routine blood chemistry screening tests (SMA-12) in the absence of positive findings in the history or physical examination reveal unexpected abnormal findings in about 2.5 percent of patients under 40 years of age. This incidence of unexpected abnormal findings increases to about 7.5 percent in patients over 60 years of age. About 70 percent of the unexpected abnormal findings are related to measurement of the blood glucose concentration and blood urea nitrogen concentration. Based on these data, the recommendation is to measure the blood glucose concentration and blood urea concentration prior to anesthesia for elective surgery in all patients over 40 years of age even in the absence of positive findings in the history and physical examination.[8]

Determination of the serum glutamic oxalacetic transaminase concentration as a routine screening test for the detection of unexpected hepatocellular disease can be considered for adult patients. Indeed, about 1 in 750 otherwise healthy adults manifest unexpected abnormal liver function tests preoperatively and 1 in 3 of these patients will subsequently become jaundiced.

Serum potassium concentration should be measured routinely prior to anesthesia for elective surgery if the patient has been receiving chronic diuretic therapy.

Coagulation Studies

In the absence of positive findings in the history or physical examination suggesting the possibility of abnormal coagulation, the routine performance of prothrombin time and partial thromboplastin time prior to anesthesia for elective surgery is not necessary.

Urinalysis

Routine urinalysis as a screen before anesthesia for elective surgery offers little or no new information and in many respects only duplicates the blood chemistry measurements.

Electrocardiogram (ECG)

In the absence of positive findings in the history and physical examination, it is concluded that a routine resting ECG prior to

Table 9-5. Unexpected Abnormalities Detected on a Preoperative Electrocardiogram

Atrial fibrillation
Atrioventricular heart block
ST-T changes suggestive of myocardial ischemia
Atrial premature contractions
Ventricular premature beats
Left or right ventricular hypertrophy
Prolonged Q-T segment
Tall peaked T waves
Evidence of preexcitation syndrome
Evidence of a prior myocardial infarction

anesthesia for elective surgery is not necessary in patients less than 40 years of age.[8] This recommendation assumes that careful observation of the ECG will take place in the operating room prior to the induction of anesthesia. Indeed, most if not all the important abnormalities that might alter the management of anesthesia should be recognizable on a single lead ECG as routinely observed prior to the induction of anesthesia (Table 9-5). After 40 years of age, a routine ECG prior to anesthesia for elective surgery is recommended.

Radiograph of the Chest

A routine radiograph of the chest prior to anesthesia for elective surgery reveals unexpected abnormal findings in about 1.5 percent of patients under 40 years of age, in approximately 5 percent of patients 40 to 60 years of age, and in 6 to 30 percent of patients above 60 years of age (Table 9-6).[8] There is no logic, therefore, in obtaining a routine preoperative radiograph of the chest

Table 9-6. Unexpected Abnormalities Detected on a Preoperative Radiograph of the Chest

Tracheal deviation
Mediastinal masses
Pulmonary masses
Pulmonary blebs
Aortic aneurysm
Pulmonary edema
Pneumonia
Atelectasis
Fractures of the ribs or vertebrae
Cardiomegaly
Dextrocardia

in patients less than 40 years of age with no evidence of chest disease in the history and physical examination.

Pulmonary Function Tests

Pulmonary function tests are not necessary in the absence of positive findings in the history and physical examination of patients undergoing elective surgery that does not involve the chest. Conversely, pulmonary function tests are useful in the preoperative preparation and subsequent intraoperative and postoperative management of patients with evidence of pulmonary disease and undergoing upper abdominal or intrathoracic operations (see Chapter 20).

PHYSICAL STATUS CLASSIFICATION

Assignment of a physical status classification (Class 1 through 5) is based on the physical condition of the patient independent of the planned operation (Table 9-7).[9] It is important to recognize that the physical status classification is not intended to represent an estimate of anesthetic risk. Instead, the physical status classification serves as a "common language" between different institutions for subsequent examination of anesthetic morbidity and mortality. Not surprisingly, intraoperative cardiac arrest is more frequent in the poor physical status classification, particularly if emergency surgery is necessary.

TECHNIQUES OF ANESTHESIA

Following the preoperative evaluation, the anesthesiologist selects as the technique of anesthesia either a general anesthetic, regional anesthetic (see Chapter 13), or peripheral nerve block (see Chapter 14). The technique of anesthesia is determined by several considerations (Table 9-8). In many instances, more than one technique of anesthesia may be acceptable. It is the responsibility of the anesthesiologist to evaluate the medical condition and unique needs of

Table 9-7. Physical Status Classification of the American Society of Anesthesiologists (ASA)

Status	Disease State
ASA Class 1	No organic, physiologic, biochemical, or psychiatric disturbance
ASA Class 2	Mild to moderate systemic disturbance that may or may not be related to the reason for surgery
	Examples: Heart disease that only slightly limits physical activity, essential hypertension, diabetes mellitus, anemia, extremes of age, morbid obesity, chronic bronchitis
ASA Class 3	Severe systemic disturbance that may or may not be related to the reason for surgery
	Examples: Heart disease that limits activity, poorly controlled essential hypertension, diabetes mellitus with vascular complications, chronic pulmonary disease that limits activity, angina pectoris, history of prior myocardial infarction
ASA Class 4	Severe systemic disturbance that is life-threatening with or without surgery
	Examples: Congestive heart failure, persistent angina pectoris, advanced pulmonary, renal, or hepatic dysfunction
ASA Class 5	Moribund patient who has little chance of survival but is submitted to surgery as a last resort (resuscitative effort)
	Examples: Uncontrolled hemorrhage as from a ruptured abdominal aneurysm, cerebral trauma, pulmonary embolus
Emergency Operation (E)	Any patient in whom an emergency operation is required
	Example: An otherwise healthy 30-year-old female who requires a dilatation and curettage for moderate but persistent hemorrhage (ASA Class 1 E)

(From information in American Society of Anesthesiologists. New classification of physical status. Anesthesiology 1963; 24:111.)

Table 9-8. Considerations that Determine the
Technique of Anesthesia

Co-existing disease that may or may not be related
  to the reason for surgery
Site of surgery
Body position of patient during surgery
Elective or emergency surgery
Likelihood of the presence of increased amounts of
  gastric contents
Age of patient
Preference of patient

each patient and select the most appropriate
technique of anesthesia.

General Anesthetic

Induction of general anesthesia is most
often accomplished by the intravenous administration of a drug (ultrashort-acting barbiturate or benzodiazepine) that produces
the rapid onset of unconsciousness (see
Chapter 6). Commonly, succinylcholine is
also administered intravenously shortly
after the ultrashort-acting barbiturate or
benzodiazepine to produce skeletal muscle
relaxation so as to facilitate direct laryngoscopy for intubation of the trachea. The
injection of a drug to produce unconsciousness followed immediately by succinylcholine is referred to as a "rapid sequence induction." Frequently, the patient is
breathing oxygen via a mask (preoxygenation) prior to a rapid sequence induction. A
typical rapid sequence induction includes
preoxygenation, the intravenous administration of a defasiculating dose of a nondepolarizing neuromuscular blocker (d-tubocurarine 3 to 5 mg) followed 1 to 3 minutes
later by thiopental (3 to 5 mg/kg) and succinylcholine (1 to 2 mg/kg) intravenously.
Direct laryngoscopy for intubation of the
trachea may be initiated about 60 seconds
following administration of succinylcholine. Preoxygenation minimizes the likelihood of arterial hypoxemia developing during the period of apnea necessary for
insertion of the tracheal tube. Alternatively,
a nondepolarizing muscle relaxant can be
substituted for succinylcholine, realizing

that the onset of skeletal muscle paralysis
that is considered ideal for intubation of the
trachea may be delayed compared with the
rapid onset of relaxation produced by succinylcholine. Following intubation of the
trachea, it may be prudent to insert a gastric
tube through the mouth to decompress the
stomach and remove any easily accessible
fluid. This orogastric tube should be removed at the conclusion of anesthesia.
When gastric suction is needed postoperatively, the tube should be inserted through
the nares rather than the mouth.

An alternative to the rapid sequence induction of anesthesia is the inhalation of nitrous oxide plus a volatile anesthetic with
or without the prior intravenous administration of a "sleep dose" of an ultrashort-
acting barbiturate or benzodiazepine (see
Chapter 6). This is referred to as an "inhalation or mask induction." An inhalation
induction is often utilized in pediatric anesthesia, particularly when prior insertion of
a venous catheter is not practical. When an
inhalation induction of anesthesia is selected, a depolarizing or nondepolarizing
muscle relaxant is administered intravenously when it is deemed appropriate to intubate the trachea. Alternatively, skeletal
muscle relaxation produced by the volatile
anesthetic can be utilized to facilitate intubation of the trachea. Finally, it may be
the decision of the anesthesiologist not to
place a tube in the trachea, and anesthesia
is then maintained by inhalation via a mask.

The objectives of maintenance of general
anesthesia are analgesia, unconsciousness,
skeletal muscle relaxation, and control of
sympathetic nervous system responses to
noxious stimulation. These objectives are
achieved most often by the use of a combination of drugs that may include inhaled
and/or injected anesthetics with or without
muscle relaxants. Each drug selected
should be administered with a specific goal
to be achieved that is relevant to that drug's
known pharmacologic effects at therapeutic
doses. For example, it is not logical to ad-

minister high concentrations of a volatile anesthetic to produce skeletal muscle relaxation when muscle relaxants are specific for achieving this goal. Likewise, it is not acceptable to obscure skeletal muscle movement due to insufficient doses of anesthetics by administering excessive amounts of a muscle relaxant. The selective use of drugs for their specific effect permits the anesthesiologist to tailor the anesthetic to the medical condition of the patient and any unique needs introduced by the surgery.

Despite its lack of potency, nitrous oxide is the most frequently administered inhaled anesthetic. Typically, nitrous oxide (50 to 70 percent inhaled concentration) is administered in combination with a volatile anesthetic or a narcotic. It is important to remember that it is the partial pressure of an inhaled anesthetic (nitrous oxide, halothane, enflurane, isoflurane) that produces its pharmacologic effect. For example, 60 percent inhaled nitrous oxide administered at sea level exerts a partial pressure of 456 mmHg (60 percent of the total barometric pressure of 760 mmHg). The same inhaled concentration of nitrous oxide (or a volatile anesthetic) administered at altitude where the barometric pressure is less than 760 mmHg exerts a reduced pharmacologic effect because the partial pressure of the anesthetic that can be achieved in the brain is less.

Volatile anesthetics have the advantage of high potency and of being readily controlled in terms of the concentration delivered from the anesthetic machine, allowing titration of the dose so as to produce a desired response. Excessive sympathetic nervous system responses evoked by noxious stimulation are predictably attenuated by a volatile anesthetic. Dose-dependent cardiac depression is a major disadvantage of volatile anesthetics (see Chapter 4). Indeed, a volatile drug is seldom administered as the sole anesthetic, but instead these drugs are more often administered in combination with nitrous oxide. Substitution of nitrous oxide for a portion of the dose of the volatile anesthetic allows a reduction in the delivered concentration of the volatile drug, which results in less cardiac depression despite the same total dose of anesthetic drugs (see Chapter 4).

In certain instances, it is acceptable to administer a muscle relaxant to assure lack of patient movement and to permit a decrease in the delivered concentration of volatile anesthetic. This use of muscle relaxants, however, must not be interpreted as an endorsement for the administration of an inadequate dose of anesthetic that is obscured by skeletal muscle paralysis.

Narcotics which generally do not depress the cardiovascular system are combined most often with nitrous oxide (see Chapter 6). In patients with normal left ventricular function, however, the lack of narcotic-induced cardiovascular depression and absence of attenuation of sympathetic nervous system reflex may lead to elevated blood pressure. When this occurs, the addition of a low concentration of volatile anesthetic to the delivered gases is often effective in returning the elevated blood pressure to an acceptable level. Muscle relaxants are often necessary even in the absence of the need for skeletal muscle relaxation, since adequate doses of narcotic with nitrous oxide are unlikely to prevent patient movement in response to a painful stimulus. Another disadvantage of injected drugs compared with inhaled anesthetics is the inability to accurately titrate and maintain a therapeutic concentration of the injected drug. This disadvantage can be offset to some extent by continuous intravenous infusion of the injected anesthetic at a rate previously determined in other patients to be associated with a therapeutic concentration in the blood.

The methods and equipment necessary for accurate administration of inhaled gases and the vapors of volatile anesthetics are described in Chapter 11.

Regional Anesthetic

A regional anesthetic is selected when maintenance of consciousness during surgery is desirable. Skeletal muscle relaxation is also produced by a regional anesthetic. Patients may have preconceived and inaccurate conceptions about regional anesthesia that will require reassurance by the anesthesiologist as to the safety of this technique of anesthesia. A regional anesthetic should not be performed against the wishes of the patient. Disadvantages of this technique of anesthesia include the occasional failure to produce adequate anesthesia for the surgical stimulus and the reduction in blood pressure that accompanies the peripheral sympathetic nervous system block produced by the regional anesthetic, particularly in the presence of hypovolemia.

A regional anesthetic technique is most often selected for surgery that involves the lower abdomen or lower extremities in which the level of sensory anesthesia required is associated with minimal sympathetic nervous system block. This should not imply that a general anesthetic is an unacceptable technique for similar types of surgery.

Peripheral Nerve Blocks

Peripheral nerve blocks are most appropriate as a technique of anesthesia for superficial operations on the extremities (see Chapter 14). Advantages of a peripheral nerve block include maintenance of consciousness and continued presence of protective upper airway reflexes. The isolated anesthetic effect produced by a peripheral nerve block is particularly attractive in the patient with chronic pulmonary disease, severe cardiac impairment, or inadequate renal function. For example, insertion of a vascular shunt in the upper extremity for hemodialysis in a patient who often has associated pulmonary and cardiac disease is ideally accomplished with anesthesia provided by peripheral nerve block of the brachial plexus. Likewise, the avoidance of the need for muscle relaxants in this type of patient circumvents the possible prolonged effect produced by these drugs in the absence of renal excretion.

A disadvantage of peripheral nerve block as a technique of anesthesia is the unpredictable attainment of adequate sensory and motor anesthesia for performance of the surgery. The success rate of a peripheral nerve block is often inversely related to the frequency with which the anesthesiologist utilizes this technique of anesthesia. Finally, the patient must be cooperative for a peripheral nerve block to be effective. For example, the acutely intoxicated and agitated patient is not an ideal candidate for a peripheral nerve block.

PREPARATION FOR ANESTHESIA

Preparation for anesthesia after the preoperative medication has been administered and the patient is transported to the operating room is similar regardless of the technique of anesthesia that has been selected (Table 9-9). Upon arrival in the operating room, the patient is identified and the scheduled surgery reconfirmed. The nurse's notes are consulted by the anesthesiologist to learn of any unexpected changes in the patient's medical condition, vital signs, or body temperature and to determine that the preoperative medication has been administered. Likewise, any laboratory data that has become available since the anesthesiologist's prior visit should be reviewed.

Initial preparation for anesthesia, regardless of the technique of anesthesia selected, begins with insertion of a catheter in a peripheral vein and application of a blood pressure cuff. This initial preparation may be accomplished in a holding area or in the operating room. Use of separate rooms (induction rooms) distinct from the operating room for induction of anesthesia is not recommended because of the questionable

Table 9-9. Routine Preparation Prior to Induction of Anesthesia Regardless of Technique of Anesthesia Selected

---

Anesthetic machine
  Attach an anesthetic breathing system with a proper-sized face mask
  Occlude the patient end of the anesthetic breathing system and fill with oxygen from the anesthetic machine ("flush valve"). Applying manual pressure to the distended reservoir bag checks for leaks in the anesthetic breathing system and confirms the ability to provide positive pressure ventilation of the patient's lungs with oxygen.
  Check soda lime for color changes
  Check liquid level and content of vaporizers
  Confirm function of mechanical ventilator
  Confirm availability and function of wall suction
Drugs
  Local anesthetic for infiltration anesthesia (lidocaine)
  Ultrashort-acting barbiturate (thiopental, thiamylal, or methohexital)
  Anticholinergic (atropine)
  Sympathomimetic (ephedrine, phenylephrine)
  Depolarizing muscle relaxant (succinylcholine)
  Nondepolarizing muscle relaxants (d-tubocurarine, metocurine, pancuronium, atracurium, or vecuronium)
  Anticholinesterase (pyridostigmine, neostigmine, or edrophonium)
  Narcotic antagonist (naloxone)
  Catecholamine to treat an allergic reaction (epinephrine)
Equipment
  Intravenous solution and connecting tubing
  Intracath or extracath for vascular cannulation
  Suction catheter
  Oral and/or nasal airway
  Laryngoscope
  Tracheal tube
  Nasogastric tube

---

safety of routinely moving anesthetized patients with the necessary attached equipment from one area to another. Monitors such as the ECG, peripheral nerve stimulator, and chest stethoscope are also applied while the patient is still awake. Immediately prior to the induction of anesthesia base line vital signs (blood pressure, heart rate, cardiac rhythm, ventilation rate) are recorded.

Regardless of the technique of anesthesia selected, the anesthetic machine is present and functional and specific drugs and equipment are always immediately available (Table 9-9). If nothing else, it is mandatory to be able to suction the patient's pharynx followed by ventilation of the lungs with oxygen via a cuffed tube placed in the trachea.

PROFESSIONAL LIABILITY

The anesthesiologist is responsible for the management of and recovery from anesthesia. Physicians administering anesthetics are not expected to guarantee a favorable outcome to the patient but are required to exercise ordinary or reasonable care or skill compared with other anesthesiologists. That the anticipated result does not follow or that complications occur does not imply negligence. Furthermore, an anesthesiologist is not responsible for an error in judgment unless it is so gross as to be inconsistent with the skill expected of every physician. An anesthesiologist, however, as a specialist is responsible for making medical judgments that are consistent with national, not local, standards. Anesthesiologists carry professional liability (malpractice) insurance that provides financial protection should a court judgment against them occur.

A certified registered nurse anesthetist can be held legally responsible for the technical aspects of the administration of anesthesia. It is likely, however, that legal responsibilities for the actions of the nurse will be shared by the physician responsible for supervising the administration of anesthesia. If an anesthesiologist employs the nurse or advises the hospital as to the qualifications or conditions of employment, the anesthesiologist may be held responsible for the nurse's actions even though not directly concerned in supervision at the time of an alleged act of negligence.

Medical students and resident physicians are not immune to court action and should be protected by professional liability insurance in the same manner as the anesthesiologist or certified registered nurse anesthetist. Insurance coverage for the medical student or resident physician is most often provided by the institution that provides the course for credit for the medical student or who employs the resident physician.

It is inconceivable that anesthesia can always be administered without accident or complication. Nevertheless, mortality or irreversible morbidity related solely to the administration of anesthesia is extremely rare. When adverse events do occur, it is often difficult to establish the exact mechanism. In many instances, it is impossible to separate an adverse event due to an inappropriate action of the anesthesiologist from an unavoidable mishap despite optimal care.[10–12]

Most patients and/or families are understanding and satisfied by frank discussion of problems related to administration of anesthesia. In the event of an accident or complication related to the administration of anesthesia, the anesthesiologist should immediately document the facts on the patient's medical record. Treatment should be noted and consultation with other physicians sought when appropriate. The anesthesiologist should provide the hospital and the company that holds the physician's professional liability insurance with a complete account of the incident. Should a lawsuit be threatened or legal inquiry made concerning a patient, the anesthesiologist should immediately notify the insurance company and, when appropriate, seek legal assistance.

Malpractice is a theory arising from tort law. A tort is a civil (not criminal) wrong for which a patient can seek compensation through legal action for an alleged act of negligence of the anesthesiologist. The patient who claims injury obtains legal counsel and files a malpractice suit. Depositions are taken by attorneys for both sides to elicit plantiffs,' defendants,' and witnesses' opinions as to the facts of the event, a court hearing is arranged, usually with a jury present, and witnesses, including experts, for the defendant (physician) and plantiff (patient) give testimony. The judge explains the points of law to the jury, and the jury then makes a decision and recommendation of compensation for damages. This chain of events may be interrupted at any point. For example, the plantiff may drop the suit or the defendant may be advised by counsel to make a settlement. A settlement can be arranged with the aid of the judge at any time during the trial prior to the jury verdict. Indeed, about 80 percent of malpractice suits are settled out of court, and, of those that go to court trial, physicians win more than they lose.

The best protection for the anesthesiologist against medicolegal action lies in the thorough and up-to-date practice of anesthesia coupled with interest in the patient by virtue of preoperative and postoperative visits plus detailed records of the course of anesthesia.

REFERENCES

1. Tinker JH, Tarhan S. Discontinuing anticoagulant therapy in surgical patients with cardiac valve prosthesis. JAMA 1978;239: 138–9.
2. Miller RD, Way WL, Eger EI. The effects of alpha-methyldopa, reserpine, guanethidine, and iproniazid on minimum alveolar anesthetic requirement (MAC). Anesthesiology 1968;29:1153–8.
3. Ghoneim MM, Long JP. The interaction between magnesium and other neuromuscular blocking agents. Anesthesiology 1970;32: 23–7.
4. Sokoll MD, Gergis SD. Antibiotics and neuromuscular function. Anesthesiology 1981; 55:148–59.
5. Edwards RP, Miller RD, Roizen MF, Ham J, Way WL, Lake CR, Roderick L. Cardiac responses to imipramine and pancuronium during anesthesia with halothane or enflurane. Anesthesiology 1979;50:421–5.
6. Hilgenberg JC. Water and electrolyte disturbances. In: Stoelting RK, Dierdorf SF, eds. Anesthesia and Co-Existing Disease. New York. Churchill Livingstone 1983;411– 36.
7. Rao TLK, El-Etr AA. Anticoagulation following placement of epidural and subarach-

noid catheters. Anesthesiology 1981;55: 618–20.

8. Roizen MF. Routine preoperative evaluation. In: Miller RD, ed. Anesthesia. New York. Churchill Livingstone 1981:3–19.

9. American Society of Anesthesiologists. New classification of physical status. Anesthesiology 1963;24:111.

10. Hamilton WK. Unexpected deaths during anesthesia: Wherein lies the cause? Anesthesiology 1979;7:25–32.

11. Keats AS. What do we know about anesthetic mortality? Anesthesiology 1979;50: 387–92.

12. Engel HL. Deaths related to anesthesia (letter). Anesthesiology 1980;52:93–4.

10

Preoperative Medication

Management of anesthesia begins with the preoperative psychological preparation of the patient and administration of a drug or drugs selected to elicit specific pharmacologic responses. This initial psychological and pharmacologic component of anesthetic management is referred to as preoperative medication. Ideally, all patients should enter the preoperative period free from apprehension, sedated but easily arousable, and fully cooperative.

PSYCHOLOGICAL PREMEDICATION

Psychological premedication is provided by the anesthesiologist's preoperative visit and interview with the patient and family members (see Chapter 9). A thorough description of the planned anesthetic and events to anticipate in the perioperative period serves as a nonpharmacologic antidote to anxiety.[1] Indeed, the incidence of anxiety is reduced in patients visited by the anesthesiologist preoperatively compared with patients receiving only pharmacologic premedication and no visit (Table 10-1).[1] Nevertheless, a shortage of time and the fact that some patients' problems do not lend themselves to reassurance may limit the value of the preoperative interview.

PHARMACOLOGIC PREMEDICATION

Pharmacologic premedication is typically administered in the patient's hopsital room 1 to 2 hours before the anticipated induction of anesthesia. The goals for pharmacologic premedication are multiple (Table 10-2) and must be individualized to meet each patient's unique requirements. Some previously acceptable goals of pharmacologic premedication are either no longer valid or are better achieved by intravenous administration of the drug at a time more likely to correspond to the period when a pharmacologic effect is necessary (Table 10-3). The best drug or drug combination to achieve the desired goals of pharamcologic premedication is not known and oftcn is influenced by the individual physician's previous experience.

The appropriate drug or drugs and doses to be used for pharmacologic premedication can be selected only after the psychological and physiological condition of the patient have been evaluated. Drug choice and dose must take into account multiple factors (Table 10-4). There are certain types of patients who should not recieve depressant pharmacologic premedication, while others

Table 10-1. Value of Preoperative Interview Compared with Pentobarbital

	Percent of Patients			
	Interview Only	Pentobarbital[a] Only	Interview and Pentobarbital[a]	No Interview No Pentobarbital
Feel nervous	40	61	38	58
Feel drowsy	26	30	38	18
Judged adequately sedated by anesthesiologist	65	48	71	35

[a] 2 mg/kg intramuscularly 1 hour before surgery.

(Data from Egbert LD, Battit GE, Turndorf H, Beecher HK. The value of the preoperative visit by an anesthetist. JAMA 1963;185:553–5.)

Table 10-2. Primary Goals for Pharmacologic Premedication

Anxiety relief
Sedation
Analgesia
Amnesia
Antisialagogue effect
Elevation of gastric fluid pH
Reduction of gastric fluid volume
Prophylaxis against allergic reactions

Table 10-3. Secondary Goals for Pharmacologic Premedication

Reduction of cardiac vagal activity—better achieved with an intravenous injection just before the time of anticipated need
Facilitation of induction of anesthesia—not necessary in view of availability of potent intravenous induction drugs
Decreased anesthetic requirements—not of sufficient magnitude to be clinically significant
Postoperative analgesia—better achieved with the intravenous injection of an analgesic just before the time of anticipated need
Prevention of postoperative nausea and vomiting—better achieved with the intravenous injection of an antiemetic just before the time of anticipated need

Table 10-4. Determinants of Drug Choice and Dose

Patient age and weight
Physical status
Level of anxiety
Tolerance for depressant drugs
Previous adverse experiences with drugs used for preoperative medication
Elective or emergency surgery
Inpatient or outpatient surgery

deserve aggressive pharmacologic attempts to decrease preoperative anxiety and produce sedation (Table 10-5). Nevertheless, the patient who requests to be "asleep" before being transported to the operating room must be assured that this is neither a desired or safe goal of pharmacologic premedication.

DRUGS ADMINISTERED FOR PHARMACOLOGIC PREMEDICATION

Several classes of drugs are available to facilitate achievement of the desired goals for pharmacologic premedication in each individual patient (Table 10-6). These drugs are often administered intramuscularly, but, when possible, the oral route of administration should be considered to improve patient comfort. The small amount of water (30 to 60 ml) utilized to facilitate oral administration of drugs introduces no hazards related to gastric fluid volume. Ulti-

Table 10-5. Is Depressant Pharmacologic Premedication Indicated?

No	Yes
Less than 1 year of age	Cardiac surgery
Elderly	Cancer surgery
Outpatients	Inpatients
Decreased level of consciousness	Regional anesthesia
Intracranial pathology	
Severe chronic pulmonary disease	
Hypovolemia	

Table 10-6. Drugs and Doses Used for Pharmacologic Premedication

Classification	Drug	Typical Adult Dose (mg[a])	Route of Administration
Barbiturates	Secobarbital	50–150	Orally, IM
	Pentobarbital	50–150	Orally, IM
Narcotics	Morphine	5–15	IM
	Meperidine	50–100	IM
Benzodiazepines	Diazepam	5–10	Orally, IM
	Lorazepam	2–4	Orally, IM
Butyrophenones[b]	Droperidol	1.25	IV
Antihistamines	Diphenhydramine	25–75	Orally, IM
	Promethazine	25–50	IM
	Hydroxyzine	50–100	IM
Anticholinergics	Atropine	0.3–0.6	IM
	Scopolamine	0.3–0.6	IM
	Glycopyrrolate	0.2–0.3	IM
H_2-antagonists	Cimetidine	300	Orally, IM, IV
	Ranitidine	150	Orally
Antacids	Participate	15–30 ml	Orally
	Nonparticulate	15–30 ml	Orally
Stimulants of gastric motility	Metoclopramide	10–20	Orally, IM, IV

Abbreviations: IM, intramuscularly; IV, intravenously.
[a] Except for antacids.
[b] Recommended for use as an antiemetic to be administered near the conclusion or surgery.

mately, the specific drugs selected are based on a consideration of desirable goals to be achieved balanced against the potential undesirable effects these drugs may produce.

Barbiturates

Advantages of barbiturates as used for pharmacologic premedication include sedation, minimal ventilatory depressent effects, as evidenced by an unchanged response to carbon dioxide, minimal circulatory depression, rarity of nausea and vomiting, and effectiveness when administered orally. Disadvantages include lack of analgesia, disorientation, especially if administered to patients in pain, and absence of a specific pharmacologic antagonist. Stimulation of hepatic microsomal enzyme activity is not a consideration with a one-time administration of barbiturates for preoperative medication. A patient with porphyria, however, should not receive barbiturates as these drugs may precipitate an acute exacerbation of this disease (see Chapter 23).

Narcotics

Advantages of narcotics as used for pharmacologic premedication include the absence of direct myocardial depression and the production of analgesia in patients who are experiencing pain preoperatively or who will require insertion of invasive monitors before the induction of anesthesia. Discomfort associated with institution of a regional anesthetic is another indication for use of a narcotic as pharmacologic premedication. Pharmacologic premedication with an intramuscular narcotic may seem reasonable when a nitrous oxide-narcotic anesthetic is planned. The narcotic, however, may be just as logically given intravenously immediately before the induction of anesthesia.

Adverse effects of narcotics as used for pharmacologic premedication include depression of the medullary respiratory center, as evidenced by decreased responsiveness to carbon dioxide, and orthostatic hypotension due to relaxation of peripheral vascular smooth muscle. Orthostatic hypotension will be further exaggerated if a narcotic is administered to a patient with decreased intravascular fluid volume. The euphoric effect of narcotics in patients with pain may be dysphoria in the absence of pain. Nausea and vomiting most likely reflect narcotic stimulation of the chemoreceptor trigger zone in the medulla. Recumbency seems to minimize nausea and vomiting after administration of a narcotic, suggesting that stimulation of the vestibular apparatus may also be important in production of this undesirable effect. Narcotic-induced smooth muscle constriction may manifest as choledochoduodenal sphincter spasm, causing some to question the use of narcotics in patients with biliary tract disease (see Chapter 21).

Benzodiazepines

Diazepam and lorazepam act on specific brain receptors to produce selective antianxiety effects at doses that do not produce excessive sedation or cardiopulmonary depression (see Chapter 2). In addition, these drugs, particularly lorazepam, produce suppression of recall of events that occur in the period following (anterograde amnesia) their administration. Suppression of recall for preceding events (retrograde amnesia) is less predictable. In animals, diazepam increases the seizure threshold for lidocaine but there is no evidence in man that doses of benzodiazepines as used for pharmacologic premedication reduce the likelihood of local anesthetic toxicity.[2]

Disadvantages of benzodiazepines as used for pharmacologic premedication include excessive and prolonged sedation in occasional patients. This is particularly likely in patients who receive lorazepam in a dose that exceeds 50 μg/kg (total dose should not exceed 4 mg). Physostigmine,

and in the future specific antagonists may be effective in reversing sedation produced by benzodiazepines.

Cimetidine has been shown to delay the clearance of diazepam from the plasma, thus introducing the theoretical possibility of an adverse drug interaction when these drugs are administered together for preoperative medication. The clinical importance, if any, of the delayed clearance of diazepam when this drug is administered as preoperative medication in the presence of cimetidine is not known. Nevertheless, the same concern is not relevant for lorazepam, as this drug depends on glucuronidation in the liver which is not influenced by cimetidine. Furthermore, lorazepam metabolites are inactive, in contrast to the significant pharmacologic activity of the major metabolite of diazepam.

Butyrophenones

The use of droperidol for pharmacologic premedication is limited because of the occasional production of dysphoria following its administration. These patients express a fear of death and may refuse a previously agreed upon elective operative procedure. Another disadvantage of droperidol is production of dopaminergic receptor blockade, which may produce extrapyramidal symptoms in normal patients as well as those with co-existing paralysis agitans. Proponents of droperidol for use as preoperative medication cite its potential protection against epinephrine-induced cardiac dysrhythmias and production of a postoperative antiemetic effect.[3]

Antihistamines

Antihistamines are used for pharmacologic premedication because of their sedative and antiemetic properties. Promethazine combined with meperidine does not increase depression of ventilation produced by meperidine or alter the incidence of nausea and vomiting but does produce an additive sedative effect.

Prophylaxis Against Allergic Reactions. Diphenhydramine (0.5 to 1 mg/kg orally) has been recommended as pharmacologic premedication to provide prophylaxis against intraoperative allergic reactions in patients with a history of chronic atopy or undergoing procedures (radiographic dye studies, chemonucleolysis) known to be associated with allergic reactions.[4] Cimetidine (4 to 6 mg/kg orally) should also be administered with diphenhydramine (see the section *H_2-antagonist*). This combination of an H_1-antagonist (diphenhydramine) and H_2-antagonist (cimetidine) acts to occupy peripheral receptor sites normally responsive to histamine, thus reducing manifestations of any subsequent drug-induced release of histamine. Prednisone (50 mg every 6 hours for the 24 hours before surgery) may also be added to this prophylactic regimen.

Anticholinergics

Routine inclusion of an anticholinergic as part of the pharmacologic premedication is not necessary. The most frequent reasons for administering an anticholinergic are (1) production of an antisialagogue effect, (2) production of sedative and amnesic effects, and (3) prevention of reflex bradycardia.

Antisialagogue Effect. The need for including an anticholinergic in the preoperative medication to produce an antisialagogue effect has been questioned, since currently used inhaled anesthetics do not stimulate excessive upper airway secretions. Nevertheless, optimal conditions during general anesthesia, particularly when a tracheal tube is in place, are more likely when an anticholinergic is administered preoperatively.[5] An antisialagogue effect is particularly important for intraoral operations or when topical anesthesia is

necessary, as excessive secretions may interfere with the surgery or impair production of topical anesthesia by diluting the local anesthetic. Administration of an anticholinergic for an antisialagogue effect is not necessary when regional anesthesia is planned.

Glycopyrrolate and scopolamine are more potent antisialagogues than atropine. To avoid the discomfort of a dry mouth and throat, an anticholinergic can be given just before the patient leaves the ward for transportation to the operating room. Nevertheless, anxiety, fluid deprivation prior to elective surgery, and other drugs used for pharmacologic premedication may produce a dry mouth and throat even in the absence of an anticholinergic.

Sedative and Amnesic Effects. Atropine and scopolamine are tertiary amines that can cross lipid barriers, including the blood brain barrier. Resulting sedative and amnesic effects reflect penetrance of these drugs into the central nervous system. Scopolamine, more than atropine, produces useful sedative effects particularly in combination with barbiturates, narcotics, or benzodiazepines as used for pharmacologic premedication.

Prevention of Reflex Bradycardia. Use of an anticholinergic in the pharmacologic premedication for prevention of reflex bradycardia is a questionable objective, since the dose and timing of intramuscular administration is not appropriate. The most logical approach, particularly in children with increased vagal activity, is to administer atropine or glycopyrrolate intravenously shortly before the anticipated need.

Undesirable side effects of anticholinergics are multiple and must be considered in the decision to use these drugs for pharmacologic premedication (Table 10-7).

Table 10-7. Undesirable Side Effects of Anticholinergic Drugs

Central nervous system toxicity
Tachycardia
Relaxation of lower esophageal sphincter
Mydriasis and cycloplegia
Elevation of body temperature
Drying of airway secretions
Increased physiologic dead space

Central nervous system toxicity (central anticholinergic syndrome) produced by an anticholinergic manifests as delerium or prolonged somnolence after anesthesia. This undesirable response is more likely to follow administration of scopolamine than atropine, but the incidence should be low with the doses used for pharmacologic premedication. Nevertheless, elderly patients may be uniquely susceptible to central nervous system toxicity secondary to atropine or scopolamine[6] (see Chapter 30). Central nervous system toxicity is unlikely after the administration of glycopyrrolate, since this drug cannot easily cross the blood brain barrier. Finally, it must be remembered that toxicity attributed to the anticholinergic may also represent an uninhibited response to pain as the depressant effects of the anesthetic dissipate.

Tachycardia. Scopolamine or glycopyrrolate, which have minimal cardioaccelerator effects, are better selections than atropine for pharmacologic premedication when an increased heart rate would be undesirable—as in the patient with mitral stenosis and atrial fibrillation being treated with digitalis. Nevertheless, the most likely cardiac response after intramuscular atropine is heart rate slowing, presumably reflecting central vagal stimulation.

Relaxation of Lower Esophageal Sphincter. Intravenous administration of an anticholinergic results in relaxation of the lower esophageal sphincter. Intramuscular administration of these drugs should also lower esophageal sphincter pressure. When barrier pressure (lower esophageal sphincter pressure minus gastric pressure) is less than 13 cm H_2O, the patient becomes vulnerable to gastroesophageal reflux and the hazards of aspiration pneumonitis. At present, this remains a theoretical hazard of anticholinergics, as there is no evidence that the incidence of aspiration pneumonitis is increased in patients receiving these drugs as pharmacologic premedication.

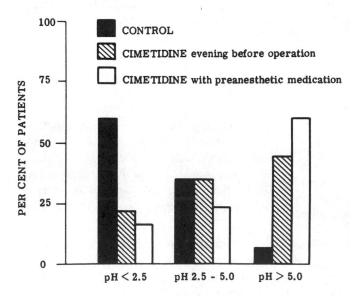

Figure 10-1. Compared with control patients, the percent of patients with a gastric fluid pH above 2.5 and 5 immediately following induction of anesthesia was significantly increased in those individuals receiving cimetidine 300 mg orally the evening before operation or with the preoperative (preanesthetic) medication. (Based on data in Stoelting RK. Gastric fluid pH in patients receiving cimetidine. Anesth Analg 1978;57:675–7.)

Mydriasis and Cycloplegia. Atropine and sopolamine may produce mydriasis and cycloplegia such that patients may experience visual impairment postoperatively. In this regard, scopolamine has a greater mydriatic effect than atropine. Conceivably, mydriasis could interfere with drainage of aqueous humor from the anterior chamber of the eye. There is no evidence, however, that inclusion of an anticholinergic in the pharmacologic premedication is contraindicated for the patient with glaucoma. Nevertheless, miotic eye drops should be continued throughout the perioperative period in those patients.

Elevation of Body Temperature. An anticholinergic may result in elevation of body temperature by suppressing sweat glands, which are innervated by cholinergic nerves via the sympathetic nervous system. Prevention of sweating by this mechanism may be undesirable in the presence of a co-existing increase in body temperature, particularly in children.

H$_2$-antagonists

H$_2$-antagonists (cimetidine, ranitidine) counter the ability of histamine to induce secretion of gastric fluid with a high hydrogen ion concentration. Therefore, these drugs offer a pharmacologic approach for increasing gastric fluid pH prior to the induction of anesthesia. Elevation of gastric fluid pH above 2.5 is desirable, since the severity of aspiration pneumonitis is accentuated by inhalation of fluid with a pH below 2.5.

Administration of cimetidine 300 mg orally 1 to 1.5 hours before induction of anesthesia increases gastric fluid pH above 2.5 in over 80 percent of patients (Fig. 10-1).[7] Conversely, gastric fluid pH is below 2.5 in about 60 percent of patients fasted overnight and receiving morphine with or without an anticholinergic as pharmacologic premedication (Fig. 10-2).[8]

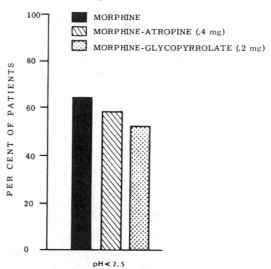

Figure 10-2. The percent of patients with a gastric fluid pH below 2.5 at the time of induction of anesthesia was not different (P>0.05) with or without the inclusion of an anticholinergic in the preoperative medication. All drugs were administered intramuscularly 1 to 1.5 hours before the induction of anesthesia. (Stoelting RK. Psychological preparation and preoperative medication. In Miller RD (ed): Anesthesia. New York, Churchill Livingstone, 1981, pp 95–105, based on data in ref. 8.)

Routine inclusion of an H$_2$-antagonist in the preoperative medication is appealing.[9] Certainly, use of an H$_2$-antagonist would be particularly attractive for inclusion in the pharmacologic premedication of (1) parturients, (2) patients with symptoms of gastroesophageal reflux, (3) obese patients who tend to have low gastric fluid pH values, (4) outpatients who may have unexpectedly low gastric fluid pH values, and (5) patients considered to be at risk for developing an allergic reaction. Intravenous administration of the H$_2$-antagonist is a consideration for patients requiring emergency surgery or those who cannot receive oral medications. An objection to routine inclusion of an H$_2$-antagonist in the preoperative medication is the concept that all therapies should be individualized to fit the patient, disease, and preoperative circumstances.[9]

Despite convincing evidence that H_2-antagonists increase gastric fluid pH, increased patient safety has not been shown to be present should inhalation of gastric fluid occur in those pretreated with cimetidine. Furthermore, these drugs are not 100 percent effective (e.g., an inherent failure rate) and they introduce potential adverse side effects (sedation, exacerbation of asthma). H_2-antagonists will not alter the pH of gastric fluid which is present before administration of the drug nor will they facilitate gastric emptying. Under no circumstances can preoperative medication with an H_2-antagonist be substituted for a technique of anesthesia (intubation of the trachea with a cuffed tube or maintenance of consciousness) known to protect the lungs from inhalation of gastric fluid (see Chapter 9). Aspiration is also a hazard at the conclusion of surgery when the trachea is extubated. In this regard, cimetidine administered as pharmacologic premedication is unlikely to offer protection at the conclusion of operations lasting more than 3 hours. Conversely, ranitidine may provide protection for up to 9 hours.

Antacids

Antacids administered 15 to 30 minutes before the induction of anesthesia are nearly 100 percent effective in elevating the gastric fluid pH above 2.5. Inhalation of gastric fluid containing particulate antacids, however, may be associated with severe and persistent pulmonary dysfunction despite a high pH of the aspirated material.[10] In contrast, a nonparticular antacid, sodium citrate, effectively raises gastric fluid pH above 2.5 and does not produce significant pulmonary dysfunction should inhalation of fluid containing this antacid occur (Fig. 10-3).[11]

Compared with H_2-antagonists, the administration of an antacid is effective in raising the pH of gastric fluid that is present in the stomach at the time of administration.

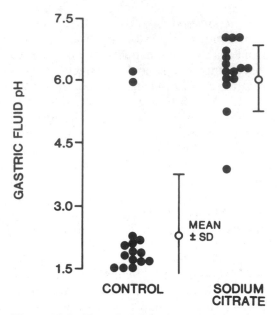

Figure 10-3. The administration of 15 ml of 0.3 molar sodium citrate 15 to 20 minutes before the induction of anesthesia raised the gastric fluid pH above 2.5 in every patient. The mean gastric fluid pH was 6.0 in patients treated with sodium citrate compared with 2.4 in the control patients (Based on data in Viegas OJ, Ravindran RS, Shumacker CA. Gastric fluid pH in patients receiving sodium citrate. Anesth Analg 1981; 60:521–3.)

This desirable effect, however, is predictably associated with an increased gastric fluid volume that does not occur with H_2-antagonists. Furthermore, antacids may slow the speed of gastric emptying. Since the severity of aspiration pneumonitis is likely to depend on both the volume (greater than 0.4 ml/kg) and pH (below 2.5) of the inhaled fluid, the increased gastric fluid volume produced by the administration of antacids must be considered. In addition, complete mixing of antacids with gastric fluid may not occur in patients who remain immobile.

Metoclopramide

Metoclopramide speeds gastric emptying by selectively increasing motility of the upper gastrointestinal tract and relaxing the

Table 10-8. Effects of Drugs Used for Pharmacologic Premedication

Effect	Effect for All Drugs Studied[a]
Decreased anxiety	None
Sedation	All to some degree except diazepam[b]
Dry mouth and throat	20 to 30 percent of patients (placebo groups similar)
Nausea	7 to 10 percent of patients (placebo groups similar)
Vomiting	None
Rating of premedication by anesthesiologist who was unaware of the drug administered	Satisfactory in 40 to 60 percent of patient (placebo groups similar)

[a] Drugs and doses (intramuscular) studied were pentobarbital (50 mg, 150 mg); secobarbital (50 mg, 150 mg); morphine (5 mg, 10 mg); meperidine (50 mg, 100 mg); diazepam (5 mg, 10 mg, 15 mg); hydroxyzine (50 mg, 100 mg, 150 mg).

[b] Absence of sedation in patients receiving diazepam was attributed to poor absorption after intramuscular injection of this drug.

(Data from Forrest WH, Brown CR, Brown BW. Subjective responses to six common preoperative medications. Anesthesiology 1977; 47:241–7.)

pyloric sphincter (Fig. 10-4).[12] The onset of metoclopramide's effect is 30 to 60 minutes after oral administration and 1 to 3 minutes following intravenous injection. Conceivably, this drug may find a place in preoperative medication for use in reducing gastric fluid volume, particularly in the patient with diabetes mellitus and associated gastroparesis, the parturient, and the patient who has recently ingested food and subsequently requires emergency surgery for disease unrelated to the gastrointestinal tract.

Side effects of metoclopramide are related to its passage into the central nervous system and production of dopaminergic receptor blockade manifesting as extrapyramidal symptoms. Metoclopramide, however, has no effect on the pH of gastric fluid. Finally, the increased speed of gastric emptying from metoclopramide may be offset by the opposite effects of a narcotic as often used for preoperative medication.

Table 10-9. Suggestions for Preoperative Medication for Adult Patients Prior to Elective Surgery[a]

1. Patient interview by anesthesiologist the day before surgery
2. Flurazepam (orally) to treat insomnia the night before surgery
3. Diazepam or lorazepam (orally) 1 to 2 hours before surgery
4. Substitute morphine (intramuscularly) for number 3 if analgesia is desired
5. Scopolamine (intramuscularly) 1 to 2 hours before induction of anesthesia if reliable sedation and amnesia are desired; otherwise, follow recommendation number 8 or do not administer an anticholinergic
6. Cimetidine or ranitidine (orally) 1 to 2 hours before induction of anesthesia
7. Metoclopramide (orally) 1 to 2 hours before induction of anesthesia—not routine at present
8. Glycopyrrolate (intramuscularly) when patient is ready to be transported to the operating room if an antisialogogue effect is desired

[a] See Table 10-6 for doses.

EVALUATION OF DEPRESSANT DRUGS USED FOR PHARMACOLOGIC PREMEDICATION

Precise methods to evaluate the value of depressant drugs as used for pharmacologic premedication are not available. For example, anxiety relief is a subjective response that may be influenced by differences in the emotional state of the patient as well as what the patient expects from the preoperative medication. Sedation is a more objective measurement, but drowsiness does not always parallel relief of anxiety. Comparison of studies on pharmacologic premedication is hampered by different drug doses, sites, and routes of administration and varying times for measuring responses. Despite these complexities, a well-controlled study suggested that desirable and undesirable effects of pharmacologic premedication were difficult to distinguish from placebo effects (Table 10-8).[13] This casts doubt on the ability to measure and confirm the value of drugs used to decrease anxiety and produce sedation, but

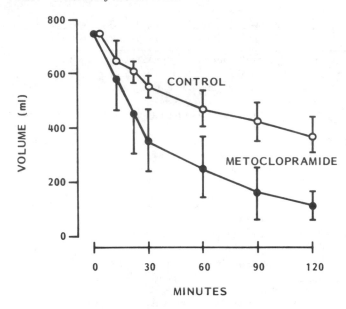

Figure 10-4. Gastric emptying time was measured in parturients during labor. Following administration of 750 ml of water via a nasogastric tube, the gastric fluid volume decreased at a faster rate in those patients treated with metoclopramide (10 mg intramuscularly) as compared with patients not receiving this drug (control) (Based on data in Howard FA, Sharp DS. Effect of metoclopramide on gastric emptying during labour. Br Med J 1973;1:446–8.)

the study's results should not be accepted as evidence that pharmacologic premedication fails to produce a more comfortable patient in the preoperative period.

RECOMMENDED PREOPERATIVE MEDICATION FOR ADULT PATIENTS PRIOR TO ELECTIVE SURGERY

Preoperative medication begins with the anesthesiologist's interview and subsequent decision as to the need for and type of pharmacologic premedication (Table 10-9). Timing of drug administration is as important as the drugs selected for pharmacologic premedication. Drugs administered to decrease anxiety and produce sedation are more appropriately administered 1 to 2 hours before induction of anesthesia. A benzodiazepine and/or an H_2-antagonist is also conveniently administered orally at this time. Metoclopramide is a logical consideration for inclusion in the pharmacologic premedication when a predictable reduction in gastric fluid volume is important. Emergency surgery requiring general anesthesia in a patient who has recently eaten would seem an appropriate situation for intravenous administration of cimetidine and metoclopramide. Intramuscular administration of morphine is an alternative to a benzodiazepine if analgesia is an important objective of preoperative medication. Intramuscular scopolamine administered at the same time as the drug selected to decrease anxiety is indicated when it is desirable to exploit the amnesic and sedative effects of this anticholinergic. For example, the combination of intramuscular morphine with or without an oral benzodiazepine plus intramuscular scopolamine is ideal for producing sedation in patients most deserving of aggressive pharmacologic premedication (Table 10-5).

An anticholinergic selected solely to produce an antisialagogue effect is most appropriately administered intramuscularly immediately before the patient is transported to the operating room. This timing minimizes the duration of the uncomfortable sensation of a dry mouth and throat experienced by the patient prior to the induction of anesthesia. Glycopyrrolate is the most logical drug to select if an antisialagogue response without central nervous system effects is desired.

Drugs to decrease vagal activity (atropine, glycopyrrolate), to protect against postoperative emesis (droperidol), or to provide postoperative analgesia are most logically administered intravenously at a time just preceding the desired effect. Finally, insomnia often occurs the night before elective surgery. Drugs such as flurazepam or temazepam are effective treatment for insomnia.

REFERENCES

1. Egbert LD, Battit GE, Turndorf H, Beecher HK. The value of the preoperative visit by an anesthetist. JAMA 1963;185:553–5.
2. Moore DC, Balfour RI Fitzgibbons D. Convulsive arterial plasma levels of bupivacaine and the response to diazepam therapy. Anesthesiology 1979;50:454–6.
3. Cohen SE. Antiemetic efficacy of droperidol and metoclopramide. Anesthesiology 1984; 60:67–9.
4. Stoelting RK. Allergic reactions during anesthesia. Anesth Analg 1983;62:341–56.
5. Falick YS, Smiler BG. Is anticholinergic premedication necessary? Anesthesiology 1975;43:472–3.
6. Smith DS, Orkin FK, Garnder SM, Zakeosian G. Prolonged sedation in the elderly after intraoperative atropine administration. Anesthesiology 1979;51:348–9.
7. Stoelting RK. Gastric fluid pH in patients receiving cimetidine. Anesth Analg 1978; 57:675–7.
8. Stoelting RK. Responses to atropine, glycopyrrolate, and Riopan of gastric fluid pH and volume in adult patients. Anesthesiology 1978;48:367–9.
9. Coombs DW. Aspiration pneumonia prophylaxis (Editorial). Anesth Analg 1983;62: 1055–8.
10. Gibbs CP, Schwartz DJ, Wynne JW, Hood CI, Kuck EJ. Antacid pulmonary aspiration in the dog. Anesthesiology 1979;51:380–5.
11. Viegas OJ, Ravindran RS, Shumacker CA. Gastric fluid pH in patients receiving sodium citrate. Anesth Analg 1981;60:521–3.
12. Howard FA, Sharp DS. Effect of metoclopramide on gastric emptying during labour. Br Med J 1973;1:446–8.
13. Forrest WH, Brown CR, Brown BW. Subjective responses to six common preoperative medications. Anesthesiology 1977;47: 241–7.

11

Anesthetic Equipment and Breathing Systems

Delivery of known concentrations of inhaled anesthetics and oxygen to the patient requires appropriate equipment including an anesthetic machine, vaporizer, and anesthetic breathing system. An understanding of the principles governing the performance of this anesthetic equipment is mandatory to assure maximal patient safety. Furthermore, the implications of bacterial contamination of anesthetic equipment and the role of anesthetic equipment in pollution of the atmosphere with anesthetic gases should be considered.

ANESTHETIC MACHINE

Anesthetic machines, regardless of their manufacturer, consist of the same basic components (Figs. 11-1 and 11-2.[1] These include (1) a source of compressed gases; (2) flowmeters to assure delivery of known flows and concentrations of these gases into an ancsthctic breathing system, and (3) means to vaporize and deliver known concentrations of the vapor of liquid anesthetics. The anesthetic machine may be equipped with a mechanical ventilator and devices to monitor the electrocardiogram, blood pressure, body temperature, and inhaled and exhaled concentrations of oxygen and carbon dioxide. Alarm systems to signal apnea or disconnection of the anesthetic

breathing system from the patient are also available. Many anesthetic machines are equipped with a fail-safe valve designed to prevent delivery of hypoxic gas mixtures from the machine due to failure of the oxygen supply. This valve shuts off the flow of all gases when the pressure in the oxygen delivery line decreases below about 30 psi. This will protect against an unrecognized exhaustion of oxygen delivery from a cylinder attached to the anesthetic machine or from a central source. This valvc, however, does not prevent the delivery of pure nitrous oxide when the oxygen flowmeter is turned off but pressure in the circuit of the anesthetic machine is maintained by an open oxygen cylinder or central supply source. In this situation, an oxygen analyzer would be necessary to detect the delivery of an hypoxic gas mixture. Far superior to the fail-safe valve or oxygen analyzer is a vigilant and alert anesthesiologist.

Compressed Gases

Gases used in the administration of anesthesia are available in cylinders attached to the anesthetic machine (Table 11-1). Compression of gas to a liquid offers the most economical and practical volume for storage. Oxygen stored in cylinders in the

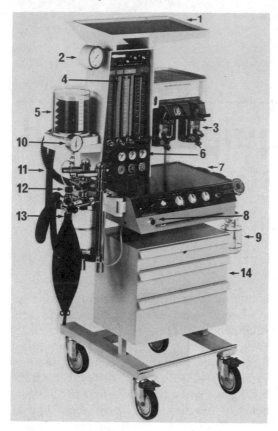

Figure 11-1. Anesthetic machine (1) shelf for monitors such as the electrocardiogram and oxygen analyzer; (2) blood pressure gauge; (3) agent specific vaporizers; (4) flowmeters; (5) ventilator; (6) pressure guages; (7) attachment for compressed gas cylinders; (8) oxygen flush; (9) suction; (10) airway pressure gauge; (11) circle anesthetic breathing system; (12) gas evacuation (scavenging system); (13) canister for carbon dioxide granules; and (14) drawers for storage.

operating room is a gas, since the temperature (critical temperature) at which oxygen exists as a liquid is far below room temperature. Nevertheless, liquid oxygen stored in large insulated containers (5 to 10 atm, minus 150 Celsius) can be vaporized for supply throughout the hospital. Unlike oxygen, nitrous oxide is compressible to a liquid at a temperature far above room temperature.

Oxygen and nitrous oxide may be piped to the operating room from a central source for delivery to the anesthetic machine via pressure tubing. Even with a central source, cylinders of oxygen and nitrous oxide should be attached to the anesthetic machine should the central supply fail. Gas cylinders are attached to yokes on the anesthetic machine. The position of two metal pins on the yoke corresponds to holes in the valve casing of the gas cylinder (pin-index) which makes it impossible to attach the gas cylinder to the wrong yoke. Otherwise, a cylinder containing nitrous oxide could be attached to the oxygen yoke, resulting in the delivery of nitrous oxide when the oxygen flowmeter was activated. Anesthetic machines usually have double yokes so that two cylinders of oxygen and nitrous oxide can be attached. Check valves prevent one gas cylinder from transfilling the other. This valve allows exchange of empty gas cylinders for full ones while the other tank is in use. Imprinted letters and numbers near the top of the gas cylinder refer to cylinder size (E,H), maximal permissable pressure in psi, manufacturer's serial number, and date of original and retest dates for pressure tolerance. The contents of the gas cylinder are not designated by any permanent notation on the tank. Instead, the contents of the gas cylinder are indicated only by a detachable label and the color of the cylinder (green for oxygen, blue for nitrous oxide).

Color-coded pressure gauges (green for oxygen, blue for nitrous oxide) on the anesthetic machine indicate the pressure of the gas in the corresponding gas cylinder. The pressure in an oxygen cylinder is directly proportional to the volume of oxygen in the cylinder. For example, a full oxygen cylinder (E size) contains 625 liters of oxygen at a pressure of 2000 psi and one-half this volume when the pressure is 1000 psi. Therefore, it is possible to calculate accurately how long a given flow rate of oxygen can be maintained before the cylinder is

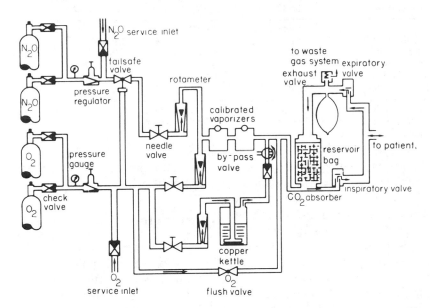

Figure 11-2. Schematic diagram of anesthetic machine and circle anesthetic breathing system. Oxygen and nitrous oxide enter the anesthetic machine from gas cylinders attached to yokes on the machine or from a central (service inlet) supply source. Check valves prevent transfilling of gas cylinders or flow of gas from the cylinders into the central supply source. Pressure regulators reduce pressure in the tubing from gas cylinders to about 50 psi. The failsafe valve prevents flow of nitrous oxide if the pressure in the oxygen supply circuit decreases below about 30 psi. Needle valves control gas flows to flowmeters (rotameters). Agent-specific vaporizers (calibrated vaporizers) provide a means to deliver a preselected concentration of volatile anesthetic. An interlock allows only one vaporizer to be on at a time. Gas flow to a Copper Kettle vaporizer is via a separate flowmeter and the effluent gas reenters the total gas flow to assure dilution of the saturated vapor concentration delivered by this type of vaporizer. A bypass valve must be in the ON position for effluent gas from the Copper Kettle to enter the total gas flow. Any flow metered to the Copper Kettle when the bypass valve is in the OFF position is vented to the atmosphere. After mixing in the manifold of the anesthetic machine, the total gas flow enters the circle anesthetic breathing system where unidirectional valves assure gas flow from the patient through the carbon dioxide absorber. Excess gases are vented through the overflow valve (exhaust valve) into the gas scavenging system (waste gas system). The gas reservoir bag compensates for variations in inspiratory flow rate. (Anesthesia equipment. In: Dripps RD, Eckenhoff JE, Vandam LD, eds. Introduction to Anesthesia. The principles of safe practice. Philadelphia, WB Saunders, 1982:45–68.)

Table 11-1. Characteristics of Compressed Gases Stored in E Size Cylinders that May Be Attached to the Anesthetic Machine

Characteristics	Oxygen	Nitrous Oxide	Carbon Dioxide	Air
Cylinder color	Green[a]	Blue	Gray	Yellow[a]
Physical state in cylinder	Gas	Liquid	Liquid	Gas
Cylinder contents (liters)	659	1590	1590	625
Cylinder weight empty (kg)	5.90	5.90	5.90	5.90
Cylinder weight full (kg)	6.76	8.80	8.90	
Cylinder pressure full (psi)	2200	745	838	1800

[a] The World Health Organization specifies that cylinders containing oxygen for medical use be painted white but U.S. manufacturers use green. Likewise, the international color code for air is white and black while cylinders in the U.S. are color coded as yellow.

empty. In contrast to oxygen, the pressure gauge for nitrous oxide does not indicate the amount of gas remaining in the cylinder. This occurs because the pressure in the gas cylinder remains at 750 psi as long as any liquid nitrous oxide is present. When nitrous oxide as a vapor leaves the cylinder, additional liquid is vaporized to maintain an unchanging pressure in the cylinder. When all the liquid nitrous oxide is vaporized, the pressure begins to decrease and it can be assumed that about 75 percent of the contents of the gas cylinder have been exhausted. Since a full nitrous oxide cylinder (E size) contains 1590 liters, approximately 400 liters remain when the pressure gauge begins to decrease from its previously constant value of 750 psi. Vaporization of a liquefied gas (nitrous oxide) as well as the expansion of a compressed gas (oxygen) absorbs heat, which is extracted from the metal cylinder and the surrounding atmosphere. For this reason, atmospheric water vapor often accumulates as frost on gas cylinders and in valves particularly during high flows. Internal icing does not occur because compressed gases are free of water vapor.

When gas leaves the cylinder, it enters metal tubing in the anesthetic machine and is directed through a pressure-reducing valve or regulator. This device lowers and maintains pressure constant at 50 psi before delivery of the gas to the flowmeters. If the gases are delivered from a central source, the reducing valve is usually located at this site and the line pressure maintained at about 50 psi.

Flowmeters

Flowmeters measure the flow of gases based on the principle that flow past a resistance is proportional to pressure. Typically, gas flow enters the bottom of a vertically positioned and tapered (cross-sectional area increases upward from site of gas entry) glass tube. Gas flow into the flowmeter raises a float that is shaped as a bobbin or ball. The float comes to rest when gravity is balanced by the fall in pressure caused by the float. The upper end of the bobbin or equator of the ball indicates the gas flow in milliliters or liters per minute. Proportionality between pressure and flow is determined by the shape of the tube (resistance) and physical properties (density and viscosity) of the gas. The flowmeters are initially calibrated for the indicated gas at the factory. Since few gases have the same density and viscosity, flowmeters are not interchangeable with other gases. The scale accompanying an oxygen flowmeter is green and the scale for the nitrous oxide flowmeter is blue.

Gas flow exits the flowmeters and passes into a manifold (mixing chamber) located at the top of the flowmeters (Fig. 11-2).[1] To ensure against accidental decreases in the delivered oxygen concentration, the oxygen flowmeter should be the last in the sequence of flowmeters and thus the last gas added to the manifold. This arrangement assures that leaks in the apparatus proximal to oxygen inflow cannot diminish the delivered oxygen concentration, while leaks distal to that point result in loss of volume without a qualitative change in the mixture. Gases mix in the manifold and flow to an outlet port on the anesthetic machine where they are directed into either a vaporizer or an anesthetic breathing system. For emergency puposes, provision is made for delivery to the outlet port of a large volume of oxygen through an oxygen flush valve that bypasses the flowmeters and manifold to deliver pure oxygen at 50 L/min.

VAPORIZERS

Potent inhaled anesthetics (halothane, enflurane, isoflurane) are liquids at room temperature and atmospheric pressure. Vaporization, which is the conversion of a liquid to a vapor, is accomplished in a closed container which is referred to as a vaporizer. The vapor concentration resulting from vaporization of a volatile liquid anesthetic must be delivered to the patient with the same accuracy and predictability as other gases (nitrous oxide, oxygen). The safe use of vaporizers for this purpose requires an understanding of the physics of vaporization.

Physics of Vaporization

Molecules comprising a liquid are in constant random motion. In a vaporizer containing a volatile liquid anesthetic, there is an asymmetrical arrangement of intermolecular forces applied to the molecules at the liquid-oxygen interface. The result of this assymetrical arrangement is a net attractive force pulling the surface molecules into the liquid phase. This force must be overcome if surface molecules are to enter the gas phase where their relatively sparse density constitutes a vapor. Energy necessary for molecules to escape from the liquid is supplied as heat. Heat of vaporization of a liquid is the number of calories required at a specific temperature to convert 1 gram of a liquid into a vapor. Heat of vaporization necessary for molecules to leave the liquid is greater when the temperature of the liquid decreases.

Vaporization in the closed confines of a vaporizer ceases when equilibrium is reached between the liquid and vapor phases such that the number of molecules leaving the liquid phase is the same as the number re-entering. The molecules in the vapor phase collide with each other and the walls of the container, creating a pressure. This pressure is termed vapor pressure. Vapor pressure is different and unique for each volatile anesthetic (see Chapter 2). Furthermore, vapor pressure is temperature dependent such that a reduction in temperature of the liquid is associated with a lower vapor pressure and fewer molecules in the vapor phase. Cooling of the liquid anesthetic reflects a loss of heat (heat of vaporization) necessary to provide energy for vaporization. This cooling is undesirable, as it lowers the vapor pressure and limits the attainable vapor concentration.

Vaporizer Design

Vaporizer design often includes an attempt to offset the loss of heat from the liquid that occurs during vaporization. In this regard, vaporizers may be constructed with copper (Copper Kettle) or bronze (Vernitrol), as these metals readily conduct heat from the surrounding parts of the anesthetic machine and the environment.[2] Conduction of heat from outside the vaporizer means less heat is lost from the liquid, providing a more constant temperature and thus level of vaporization. Other vaporizer designs include a temperature sensitive metallic strip that functions as "gate" to counter the impact of a decrease in liquid temperature on vaporization by allowing more carrier gas to flow through the vaporizing chamber. As such, these vaporizers are considered to be temperature-compensated. An important safety feature in vaporizer design is the location of the filling port in a relatively low position to prevent spillage of liquid anesthetic into the anesthetic breathing system. An indicator window is present on the vaporizer to facilitate visual verification of the amount of liquid anesthetic in the vaporizing chamber (Fig. 11-3).

Classification of Vaporizers

Vaporizers are classified as flow-over or bubble-through, depending on the method for saturating the carrier gas that flows through the vaporizing chamber (Table 11-2). Agent-specific vaporizers are examples of flow-over vaporizers, while the Copper Kettle and Vernitrol are examples of bubble-through vaporizers.

Agent-specific vaporizers accept the entire fresh gas flow from the anesthetic machine. The vapor concentration of the liquid anesthetic in the effluent gas from the vaporizer is determined by the setting of the concentration dial on the vaporizer (Fig. 11-3). This concentration dial setting determines the proportion of the total gas flow (carrier gas) that is diverted into the vaporizing chamber to pass near (flow-over) the anesthetic liquid (Fig. 11-4).[1] In addition to directing the carrier gas as close to the liquid as possible, vaporization may be enhanced by increasing the areas of contact between a carrier gas and liquid (gas-liquid interface) by placing a wick in the vaporizing chamber.

Agent-specific vaporizers are temperature-compensated by virtue of a heat-sensitive metallic strip which changes position with decreases in temperature of the liquid anesthetic so as to increase the carrier gas flow into the vaporizing chamber (Fig. 11-

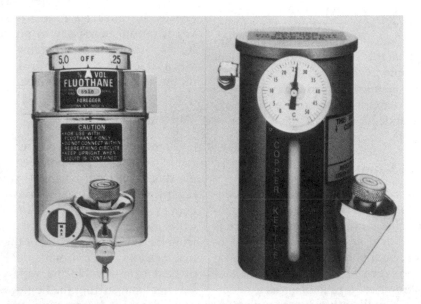

Figure 11-3. An agent-specific vaporizer for halothane (Fluothane) and a Copper Kettle. Note the position of the filling ports near the bottom of the vaporizers and a window to visualize the level of liquid in the vaporizing chamber. A temperature gauge on the Copper Kettle depicts the temperature of the liquid anesthetic in the vaporizing chamber.

Table 11-2. Classification of Vaporizers

Flow-over (Agent-specific)
  Fluotec (halothane)
  Fluomatic (halothane)
  Enfluromatic (enflurane)
  Ethrane (enflurane)
  Forane (isoflurane)
  Drager (halothane, enflurane, isoflurane)
Bubble through
  Copper Kettle
  Vernitrol

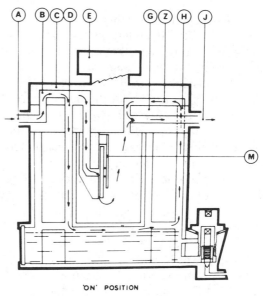

'ON' POSITION

Figure 11-4. Schematic diagram of an agent-specific (Fluotec Mark III) vaporizer. Counterclockwise rotation of the concentration dial (E) allows carrier gases (nitrous oxide and/or oxygen) to enter (A) and pass through channels (B,D) into the vaporizing chamber where wicks saturated with liquid anesthetic assure a large gas-liquid interface for efficient vaporization. Carrier gas also flows through an opening (M) the size of which is determined by a heat-sensitive metallic strip. All gases entering the vaporizing chamber exit at J. The position of the concentration dial determines the size of the opening of H and the flow through it. When the concentration dial is in the OFF position, carrier gases flow directly from A to J and ports D and H are closed. An indexed filling port and drain are pictured on the lower right. (Reproduced with permission of Cyprane North America Inc.)

4).[1] As a result, the vapor concentration is maintained constant within certain temperature and flow ranges. It must be appreciated, however, that these vaporizers are accurate only at the total gas flows specified by the manufacturer. For example, the vapor concentration in the effluent gas from these vaporizers may not be predictable at low (less than 2 L/min) total gas flows. This characteristic limits the usefulness of agent-specific vaporizers during low flow anesthesia (see the section *Closed System*). Concentration markings on the dial are determined by the manufacturer. The accuracy of these markings should be verified periodically according to recommendations of the manufacturer. A typical recommendation is to return the vaporizer at yearly intervals to the manufacturer for verification of continued accurate function. It must be appreciated that the vapor concentration delivered by the vaporizer when the dial setting is between "off" and the first concentration marking may not be linear.[3] This impairs the ability to reliably deliver a vapor concentration that is less than the lowest concentration marking on the dial.

Preservatives, such as thymol, present in halothane accumulate in the vaporizer because of their low volatility. These residues can lead to difficulty in turning the concentration dial, necessitating rinsing of the vaporizer with a solvent such as ether. This problem does not occur with enflurane or isoflurane, since these liquid anesthetics do not require the addition of preservatives to maintain stability during storage.

Placing of a liquid anesthetic in the vaporizer that is different from the drug for which the vaporizer was calibrated will result in the delivery of an unknown vapor concentration. The similar vapor pressures of halothane and isoflurane, however, mean the concentration dial settings on agent-specific vaporizers for either of these liquids would also be accurate with the other liquid. Nevertheless, interchanging these liquids is not encouraged, since this practice would condone deliberate filling of the vaporizer with the "wrong" anesthetic. Furthermore, an overdose of halothane (MAC 0.75 percent) is possible should the concentration dial settings be used as if the administered anesthetic is isoflurane (MAC 1.15 percent). Finally, the filling ports of some agent-specific vaporizers are constructed such that only the delivery system of a specially shaped bottle (keyed-vaporizer filling device) containing the correct liquid anesthetic will adapt to the filling port of the agent-specific vaporizer.

Copper Kettle. A Copper Kettle receives oxygen as the carrier gas from a separate dedicated flowmeter on the anesthetic machine. The efficiency of vaporization is maximized by passing this carrier gas through a sintered bronze disk at the bottom of the vaporizer (bubble-through) to form streams of fine bubbles (Fig. 11-5).[4] The bubbles produce maximal vaporization efficiency by providing a large surface for the liquid-gas interface. The scales of the oxygen flowmeters dedicated to these vaporizers are white, brown, or black to distinguish them from the green scales of flowmeters that deliver oxygen not passing through the vaporizer. Construction of the Copper Kettle with copper facilitates the transfer of heat from the surrounding metal parts of the anesthetic machine and environment.[1] This design characteristic offsets heat loss due to heat of vaporization and provides a more constant liquid temperature and level of vaporization. Neverthe-

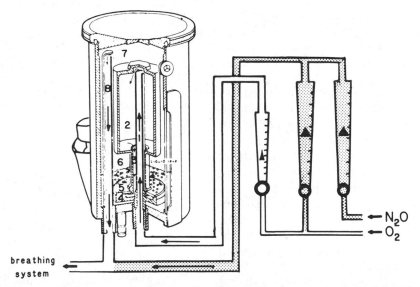

breathing
system

Figure 11-5. Schmatic diagram of a Copper Kettle vaporizer. A metered flow of oxygen enters the base of the vaporizer, travels up a center tube (1) and then turns downward (2–4) before passing through a sintered bronze disk (5) to form fine bubbles. The resultant bubbles rise through the liquid anesthetic (6) in the vaporizing chamber (7). The saturated vapor concentration exits through an outlet tube (8) where it is diluted by the total gas flow enroute to the anesthetic breathing system. (Reproduced by courtesy of Foregger Co. Reprinted by permission of the publisher from Hill DW. Physics applied to anesthesia. 4th edition. London: Butterworths (Publishers) Ltd. 1980, as modified in Orkin FK. Anesthetic systems. In: Miller RD, ed. Anesthesia. New York, Churchill Livingstone, 1981:117–56.)

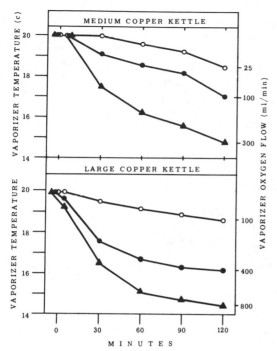

Figure 11-6. The temperature of the liquid anesthetic (vaporizer temperature) in medium and large sized Copper Kettle vaporizers decreases with time during continuous carrier gas flow (vaporizer oxygen flow) through the vaporizer. The magnitude of the temperature decrease is directly related to the total carrier gas flow. (Gartner J, Stoelting RK. A laboratory comparison of Copper Kettle, Fluotec Mark 2, and Pentec Vaporizers. Anesth Analg 1974;53:187–90.)

less, the temperature of the liquid anesthetic, as depicted by a temperature gauge mounted on the vaporizer, predictably decreases during prolonged use of the Copper Kettle particularly at high carrier gas flow rates (Fig. 11-6).[3] Furthermore, the traditional maintenance of operating room temperatures in a "cold" range limits the efficency of temperature compensation by conduction of heat from the environment. For these reasons, the Copper Kettle, unlike agent-specific vaporizers, is not considered to be a temperature compensated vaporizer.

Effluent gas from the Copper Kettle is maximally saturated with vapor, the concentration being equal to the vapor pressure

of the anesthetic at the temperature of the liquid in the vaporizer divided by barometric pressure (Table 11-3). This concentration must be diluted before delivery to the anesthetic breathing system, since the saturated vapor concentration would produce cardiovascular collapse within a few breaths. Indeed, the major hazard of the Copper Kettle is delivery of an excessive concentration of anesthetic vapor. This hazard is less with agent-specific vaporizers, since the maximum dial setting is far below the saturated vapor concentration of that agent. An advantage of the Copper Kettle compared with an agent-specific vaporizer is its interchangeability with all liquid anesthetics and predictable accuracy with low carrier gas flows as necessary during closed system anesthesia (Fig. 11-7).[3] Dilution of the vapor concentration delivered by a Copper Kettle is accomplished by mixing the effluent gas from tbe vaporizer with the separately metered flows of nitrous oxide and/or oxygen from the anesthetic machine. The resulting concentration of anesthetic vapor in the gases delivered to the breathing system must be calculated (Table 11-4). This contrasts with agent-specific vaporizers in which the delivered concentration is determined by the dial setting on the vaporizer.

A rapid means of calculating the delivered concentration of anesthetic vapor delivered to the patient using a Copper Kettle is based on the fraction of barometric pressure represented by the vapor pressure of the liquid being vaporized (Table 11-3). For example, the vapor pressures of halothane and isoflurane (244 and 240 mmHg respectively) are about one-third of an atmosphere at 20 Celsius. Therefore, one-third of the effluent gas from a Copper Kettle will be anesthetic vapor. When 100 ml/min of oxygen is metered into a Copper Kettle, the effluent gas will be 100 ml of oxygen plus about 50 ml of halothane or isoflurane vapor. This 50 ml of anesthetic vapor diluted in a total gas flow of 5 L/min is roughly

Table 11-3. Calculation of Vapor Concentration and Output
Using a Bubble-Through Vaporizer

$$\begin{array}{l}\text{Vapor concentration (percent)} \\ \text{in effluent gas from vaporizer}\end{array} = \frac{\begin{array}{c}\text{vapor pressure of anesthetic at the}\\\text{temperature of the liquid (VPanes), mmHg}\end{array}}{\text{barometric pressure (}P_B\text{), mmHg}}$$

Example calculations—assuming a liquid anesthetic temperature of 20 Celsius and sea level

$$\text{Halothane} = 244/760 = 32 \text{ percent}$$

$$\text{Enflurane} = 172/760 = 23 \text{ percent}$$

$$\text{Isoflurane} = 240/760 = 31 \text{ percent}$$

$$\begin{array}{l}\text{Vapor output (ml)}\\\text{in effluent gas from vaporizer}\end{array} = \frac{\begin{array}{c}\text{carrier gas flow of oxygen into the}\\\text{vaporizer (CG), ml/min} \times \text{VPanes}\end{array}}{P_B - \text{VPanes}}$$

Example calculations—assuming a CG flow of 100 ml/min and liquid anesthetic temperature of 20 Celsius

$$\text{Halothane} = \frac{100 \times 244}{760 - 244} = 47 \text{ ml}$$

$$\text{Enflurane} = \frac{100 \times 172}{760 - 172} = 30 \text{ ml}$$

$$\text{Isoflurane} = \frac{100 \times 240}{760 - 240} = 46 \text{ ml}$$

Clinical example

Anesthetic machine flowmeters are set to deliver nitrous oxide 3 L/min, oxygen 2 L/min, and 100 ml/min of oxygen as carrier gas through a Copper Kettle containing isoflurane. The 46 ml of isoflurane vapor (see above calculations) in the effluent gas from the vaporizer will be diluted in a total gas flow of 5146 ml. Ignoring the 146 ml effluent gas flow from the vaporizer (46 ml isoflurane vapor and 100 ml oxygen carrier gas), the estimated delivered isoflurane concentration is 1%. The ease of estimating the delivered concentration of isoflurane (or halothane) when diluted in a total gas flow of about 5 L is one of the reasons for the popularity of 5 L flows in clinical practice.

1 percent, ignoring the 100 ml/min of oxygen from the vaporizer. This is the reason total gas flows of 5 L/min are frequently selected during administration of halothane or isoflurane. Reducing the total gas flow below 5 L/min without changing the carrier gas flow through the Copper Kettle increases the anesthetic concentration. Likewise, an increase in total gas flow results in greater dilution of the vaporizer output and a decreased anesthetic concentration. Enflurane has a vapor pressure (172 mmHg at 20 Celsius) such that 100 ml/min of oxygen entering the Copper Kettle will exit with about 30 ml of enflurane vapor. Dilution of this 30 ml in a total gas flow of 3 L/min is about 1 percent or 0.5 percent if total gas flow is 6 L/min.

A switch on the table top of the anesthetic machine must be in the "on" position for the effluent gas from the Copper Kettle to enter the total gas flow. When carrier gas flow is zero but the switch is in the "on" position, surges of anesthetic-containing gas may enter the anesthetic breathing system during positive pressure ventilation of the lungs. This reflects a back-flushing of gases from the anesthetic breathing system into the vaporizer. Prevention of back-flushing of gases into the vaporizer is provided by inserting a unidirectional valve in the effluent circuit from the vaporizer or by

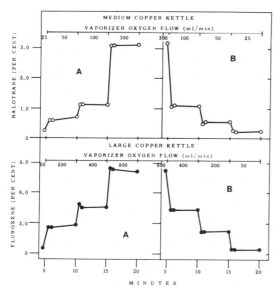

Figure 11-7. The average anesthetic concentration provided by three Copper Kettle vaporizers at 20 Celsius was measured after 5 minutes of continuous carrier gas flow (vaporizer oxygen flow) through the vaporizer. Diluent oxygen flow was 5 L/min. The carrier gas flow was then increased (A) or decreased (B) and the delivered anesthetic concentration was measured after 30 seconds, 1 minute, and 5 minutes. This sequence was then repeated at the next indicated carrier gas flow. The change in delivered anesthetic concentration following an alteration in carrier gas flow through the Copper Kettle was detectable within 30 seconds. Furthermore, the measured anesthetic concentration agreed with the predicted concentration based on the vapor pressure of the liquid anesthetic at 20 Celsius and diluent oxygen flow of 5 L/min. (Gartner J, Stoelting RK. A laboratory comparison of Copper Kettle, Fluotec Mark 2, and Pentec Vaporizers. Anesth Analg 1974;53:187–90.)

placing the switch on the table top of the anesthetic machine in the "off" position when the vaporizer is not in use. If the switch is in the "off" position, any carrier gas flow metered to the vaporizer is vented to the atmosphere. On many anesthetic machines, this switch when turned to the side directly opposite the "on" position for vaporizer flow turns "on" the emergency oxygen flush system.

The Vernitrol is identical to the Copper Kettle except that bronze (thermal conductivity similar to copper) rather than copper is used for its construction.

ANESTHETIC BREATHING SYSTEMS

Anesthetic breathing systems consist of the components necessary to deliver anesthetic gases and oxygen from the anesthetic machine to the patient.[4] Conceptually, the anesthetic breathing system is a tubular extension of the patient's upper airway. Because peak inspiratory flows as high as 60 L/min are reached during spontaneous inspiration, anesthetic breathing systems can add considerable resistance to inhalation. The resistance imparted by an anesthetic breathing system is influenced by unidirectional valves and connectors. Minimizing resistance to breathing requires that components of the anesthetic breathing system, particularly the tracheal tube connector, have the largest possible lumen. Increased airway resistance due to sharp bends produced by right-angle connectors is minimized by replacing these devices with curved connectors. Finally, increased resistance to breathing due to the anesthetic breathing system can be offset by substituting controlled ventilation of the lungs for spontaneous breathing.

Anesthetic breathing systems are classified as open, semiopen, semiclosed, and closed, according to the presence or absence of (1) a gas reservoir bag in the system, (2) rebreathing of exhaled gases, (3) means to chemically neutralize exhaled carbon dioxide, and (4) unidirectional valves (Table 11-4).[5] In addition, the composition and flow rate of the inflow gases should be stated when describing an anesthetic breathing system.

Open Anesthetic Breathing System

An open anesthetic breathing system is characterized by the absence of a gas reservoir bag and the absence of rebreathing

Table 11-4. Classification of Anesthetic Breathing Systems

System	Gas Reservoir Bag	Rebreathing of Exhaled Gases	Chemical Neutralization of Carbon Dioxide	Unidirectional Valves	Fresh Gas Inflow Rate[b]
Open					
Insufflation	No	No	No	None	Unknown
Open drop	No	No	No	None	Unknown
Semiopen					
Mapleson A, B, C, D	Yes	No[a]	No	One	High
Bain	Yes	No[a]	No	One	High
Mapleson E	No	No[a]	No	None	High
Jackson-Rees	Yes	No[a]	No	One	High
Semiclosed					
Circle	Yes	Partial	Yes	Three	Moderate
Closed	Yes	Total	Yes	Three	Low

[a] No rebreathing of exhaled gases only when fresh gas inflow is adequate.
[b] High = greater than 6 L/min; moderate = 3 to 6 L/min; low = 0.3 to 0.5 L/min.

of exhaled gases (Table 11-4). The absence of a physical connection of this anesthetic breathing system to the patient results in spillage of anesthetic gases into the atmosphere (see the section *Pollution of the Atmosphere with Anesthetic Gases*) and an inability to assist or control ventilation of the lungs. The depth of anesthesia provided by an open anesthetic breathing system is unstable. For example, light anesthesia and the associated increase in ventilation results in increased dilution of the inhaled gases with room air such that even lighter levels of anesthesia result. Conversely, as the level of anesthesia deepens, the patient's tidal volume decreases and less dilution with room air occurs, resulting in deeper anesthesia.

Examples of open anesthetic breathing systems are insufflation and open drop administration of anesthetic gases.

Insufflation is the delivery of gases from the anesthetic machine via a delivery tube or mask held above the patient's face. During inspiration, the inhaled mixture is composed of gases delivered from the anesthetic machine plus room air. This is a useful technique for the induction of anesthesia in the pediatric patient. During maintenance of anesthesia, as during bronchoscopy or laryngoscopy, insufflation of anesthetic gases and oxygen into the pharynx is facilitated by the use of a delivery device that fits on the corner of the mouth (insufflation hook) so as to direct gases into the pharynx.

Open drop administration of an anesthetic (most often ether but possible with all volatile anesthetics) is achieved by dripping the anesthetic liquid onto layers of gauze stretched over a wire frame in the shape of a face mask. Placement of this mask firmly on the face may introduce some degree of rebreathing of exhaled gases. The carbon dioxide trapped under the mask also dilutes the inhaled concentration of oxygen. The decrease in oxygen concentration is offset by flowing oxygen under the mask (250 to 500 ml/min), but it must be appreciated that this flow reduces the inhaled concentration of anesthetic. The inhaled gases are cold, reflecting cooling of the gauze consequent to heat of vaporization. Open drop administration of anesthetic gases is rarely used, but its portability and simplicity favors its use in disaster situations.

Semiopen Anesthetic Breathing System

A semiopen anesthetic breathing system includes a gas reservoir bag and utilization of a unidirectional valve and/or high fresh gas inflow rates to prevent rebreathing of exhaled gases (Table 11-4).[5] These systems are lightweight, portable, easy to clean, and offer low resistance to breathing. Their principal advantage, however, is that the absence of rebreathing of exhaled gases results in a composition of the inspired gas that approximates that delivered by the anesthetic machine. As a result, an accurate estimate of the concentration of anesthetic gases and oxygen being delivered to the patient is possible. The presence of a gas reservoir bag enables assisted or controlled ventilation of the lungs. Like the open anesthetic breathing system, there is no conservation of respiratory moisture and body heat and the operating room atmosphere is contaminated with anesthetic gases (see the section *Pollution of the Atmosphere with Anesthetic Gases*).

Unidirectional Valve. The presence of a unidirectional valve in the semiopen anesthetic breathing system functions to direct fresh gases into the patient and exhaled gases out of the system. As a result, the total fresh gas inflow can be reduced often to a flow that equals the patient's minute ventilation. Disadvantages of a unidirectional valve include increased resistance to breathing and valve malfunction due to condensation of moisture. In addition, respiratory obstruction with a subsequent pneumothorax can occur in the presence of a unidirectional valve when the patient's minute ventilation exceeds fresh gas inflow into the anesthetic breathing system. Construction of the unidirectional valve to allow room air to enter when the patient's minute ventilation exceeds fresh gas inflow (Steen valve) prevents this adverse effect but re-

sults in dilution of the concentration of anesthetic gases and oxygen. Semiopen anesthetic breathing systems employing a unidirectional valve are frequently utilized in equipment designed for cardiopulmonary resuscitation (see Chapter 34).

High Fresh Gas Inflow. Semiopen anesthetic breathing systems that lack a unidirectional valve to prevent rebreathing of exhaled gases require high fresh gas inflow rates. These systems are classified as Mapleson A through E, depending on the location of the fresh gas inflow relative to the patient or overflow valve (Fig. 11-8).[4] The arrangement of these components influences the efficiency of the elimination of carbon dioxide. Mapleson systems are most often used in pediatric patients up to about 10 kg body weight. The limiting factor in the use of these systems is the fresh gas inflow rate (often based on ml/kg or a multiple of the patient's minute ventilation) required to prevent rebreathing of exhaled gases. The high fresh gas inflow rates reduce the usefulness of these systems as body weight increases.

Mapleson A System. The Mapleson A system (Magill attachment) is characterized by placement of the overflow valve near the patient and separation of the gas reservoir bag from this valve by a corrugated tube (Fig. 11-8).[4] Fresh gas inflow is into the gas reservoir bag. This placement of the overflow valve and fresh gas inflow is the most efficient for elimination of carbon dioxide during spontaneous ventilation.[4] Elimination of carbon dioxide reflects the preferential spillage of alveolar gas that contains carbon dioxide through the overflow valve during exhalation (Fig. 11-9).[4] For example, during exhalation, physiologic dead space gas followed by alveolar gas flows back into the corrugated tube. Pressure increases in the corrugated tube as exhaled gases meet fresh gas inflow. When the pressure is suf-

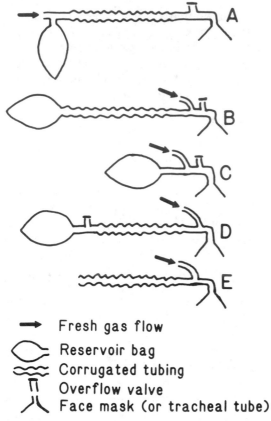

→ Fresh gas flow

Reservoir bag

Corrugated tubing

Overflow valve

Face mask (or tracheal tube)

Figure 11-8. Anesthetic breathing systems categorized as semiopen Mapleson A through E. (Mapleson WW: The elimination of rebreathing in various semiclosed anesthetic systems. Br J Anaesth 1954; 26: 323, as redrawn in Orkin FK. Anesthetic systems. In: Miller RD, ed. Anesthesia. New York, Churchill Livingstone, 1981:117–56.)

ficiently elevated, the overflow valve opens and the last gas to be exhaled (alveolar gas containing carbon dioxide) is preferentially vented to the atmosphere. Indeed, rebreathing of exhaled gases containing carbon dioxide does not occur using this system until fresh gas inflow decreases to a value equal to the patient's alveolar ventilation. Conservation of physiologic dead space gas is desirable, since this gas resembles fresh gas inflow in that carbon dioxide has not been added and anesthetic gases and oxygen have not been removed.

Compared with spontaneous ventilation, the Mapleson A system is less efficient during assisted or controlled ventilation of the lungs. This reflects the need to tighten the overflow valve to permit production of positive airway pressure when the gas reservoir bag is manually compressed. As a result, gases exit from the system during manually produced inspiration rather than during exhalation, leading to rebreathing of exhaled alveolar gas. The fresh gas inflow required to prevent rebreathing during assisted or controlled ventilation of the lungs using this system is difficult to estimate. Therefore, the Mapleson A system is best used in the presence of spontaneous ventilation.

Mapleson B System. The Mapleson B system is characterized by placement of the fresh gas inflow just distal to the overflow valve which is located near the patient (Fig. 11-8).[4] This location of the fresh gas inflow results in a system that is less efficient than the Mapleson A system during spontaneous ventilation. In contrast to the Mapleson A system, however, the Mapleson B system behaves in a similar manner during spontaneous, assisted, or controlled ventilation of the lungs. (Fig. 11-9).[4] A fresh gas inflow equal to at least twice the patient's minute ventilation is recommended to prevent rebreathing of exhaled gases.

Mapleson C System. The Mapleson C system is a Mapleson B system in which the expiratory limb has been shortened (Fig. 11-8).[4] As a result, the inhaled gases contain more alveolar gas (Fig. 11-9).[4] Therefore, the fresh gas inflow rate should be at least twice the patient's minute ventilation to prevent rebreathing of exhaled gases. The Mapleson C system may be used with any mode of ventilation.

Mapleson D System. The Mapleson D system resembles the Mapleson A system except that the locations of the fresh gas inflow and the overflow valve are reversed

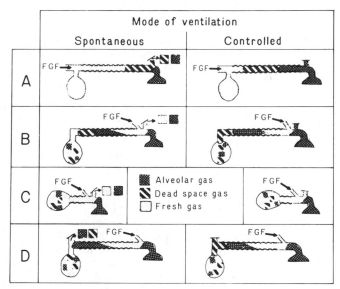

Figure 11-9. Gas disposition at end-exhalation during spontaneous or controlled ventilation of the lungs using Mapleson A–D anesthetic breathing systems. (Sykes MK: Rebreathing circuits: A review. Br J Anesth 1968;40:666, as redrawn in Orkin FK. Anesthetic systems. In: Miller RD, ed. Anesthesia. New York, Churchill Livingstone, 1981:117–56.)

(Fig. 11-8).[4] Placement of the fresh gas inflow near the patient produces efficient elimination of carbon dioxide regardless of the mode of ventilation (Fig. 11-9).[4] When the fresh gas inflow rate is equal to twice the patient's minute ventilation, the amount of rebreathing of exhaled gases is negligible.

Bain System. The Bain system is a co-axial version of a Mapleson D system in which the fresh gas inflow enters through a narrow tube within the corrugated expiratory limb (Fig. 11-10).[4] Advantages claimed for the Bain system include (1) warming of the fresh gas inflow by the surrounding exhaled gases in the expiratory limb, (2) improved humidification as a result of partial rebreathing, and (3) ease of scavenging waste anesthetic gases from an overflow valve. Availability of this system as a disposable item facilitates sterility and its light weight is particularly important when anesthetic equipment must be far-removed from the airway, as during head and neck surgery.

During controlled ventilation of the lungs using a Bain system, a fresh gas inflow rate equal to about 70 ml/kg will maintain normocarbia.[6] Similar fresh gas inflow rates during spontaneous ventilation of the lungs

may result in hypercarbia, since the patient may not be able to sufficiently increase alveolar ventilation in the presence of anesthetic-induced depression of ventilation. Therefore, fresh gas inflow rates of 200 to 300 ml/kg have been recommended when the Bain system is utilized during spontaneous ventilation.[6] In addition to hypercarbia, other complications associated with the use of the Bain system include increased resistance to breathing, rebreathing of exhaled gases due to unrecognized disconnection of the inner tube, and absence of fresh gas inflow due to unrecognized kinking of the inner tube.

Mapleson E System. The Mapleson E system consists of an expiratory limb connected to an Ayre's T piece (Fig. 11-8).[4] The Ayre's T piece is a metal tube with an internal diameter of 1 cm that receives fresh gas inflow via a side arm. During exhalation both exhaled and fresh gases flow down the open expiratory limb. During inspiration, varying ratios of fresh and exhaled gases can be inhaled, depending upon the fresh gas inflow rate and the volume of the expiratory limb. For example, a fresh gas inflow rate equal to three times the patient's minute ventilation avoids rebreathing of ex-

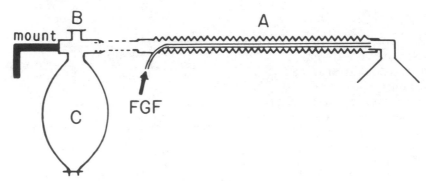

Figure 11-10. Schematic diagram of the Bain system showing fresh gas flow (FGF) into a narrow tube within the corrugated expiratory limb (A). The only valve in this system is an overflow valve (B) located near the gas reservoir bag (C). (Bain JA, Spoerel WE: A streamlined anesthetic system. Can Anaesth Soc J 1972;19:426, as relabelled in Orkin FK. Anesthetic systems. In: Miller RD, ed. Anesthesia. New York, Churchill Livingstone, 1981:117–56.)

haled gases during spontaneous ventilation when the volume of the expiratory limb is one-third the patient's tidal volume. Although there is no gas reservoir bag, ventilation of the lungs can be controlled by intermittent manual occlusion of the expiratory limb which forces gas into the trachea.

Jackson-Rees Modification of the Ayre's T Piece. The addition of a gas reservoir bag with an adjustable overflow valve to the expiratory limb of a Mapleson E system is designated the Jackson-Rees modification of the Ayre's T piece (Fig. 11-11).[7] The advantage of this arrangement is ease of instituting assisted or controlled ventilation of the lungs as well as monitoring ventilation by movement of the gas reservoir bag during spontaneous breathing. This system is particularly popular for pediatric patients because of its minimal dead space and low

resistance to breathing. Furthermore, this system can be used with a mask or a tracheal tube. Scavenging systems can be adapted to this system so as to reduce pollution of the atmosphere with anesthetic gases. The major disadvantage of this system is the need to deliver a fresh gas inflow rate equal to at least twice the patient's minute ventilation so as to assure the absence of rebreathing of exhaled gases.

Semiclosed Anesthetic Breathing System

A semiclosed anesthetic breathing system is the most commonly used system for delivery of anesthetic gases and oxygen to children and adults. This system has a gas reservoir bag and provides for partial rebreathing of exhaled gases (Table 11-4).[5] Rebreathing of exhaled gases is acceptable because of the use of chemical neutraliza-

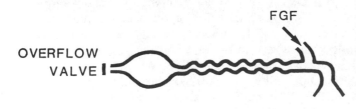

Figure 11-11. Schematic diagram of the Jackson-Rees modification of the Ayre's T piece showing fresh gas flow (FGF) entering near the patient and an adjustable overflow valve in the distal end of the gas reservoir bag.

tion of carbon dioxide. As a result of partial rebreathing of exhaled gases, there is some conservation of airway moisture and body heat. Furthermore, the fresh gas inflow rate can be less than the patient's minute ventilation, which diminishes pollution of the surrounding atmosphere with anesthetic gases. The price paid for these desirable characteristics includes increased resistance to breathing, bulkiness with loss of portability, and enhanced opportunity for malfunction of a more complex apparatus.

Circle System. The circle system is the most commonly used semiclosed anesthetic breathing system (Fig. 11-12).[4] The circle system is a true breathing circuit, as anesthetic gases and oxygen circulate in one direction entirely within the confines of the

components of the system. The essential components of this system are (1) a gas reservoir bag, (2) two corrugated tubes ("elephant tubes"), (3) two unidirectional valves, (4) a canister containing a carbon dioxide absorbent, and (5) an overflow valve to permit escape of excess gases. The gas reservoir bag maintains an available reserve volume to satisfy inspiratory flow rates (up to 60 L/min) which greatly exceed conventional fresh gas inflows (3 to 6 L/min) from the anesthetic machine. The two corrugated tubes serve as the conduits to deliver anesthetic gases and oxygen to the patient. These large lumen tubes (22 mm) provide minimal resistance to breathing and are corrugated to prevent kinking. Two unidirectional valves are situated so that one tube is for inhalation and the other for ex-

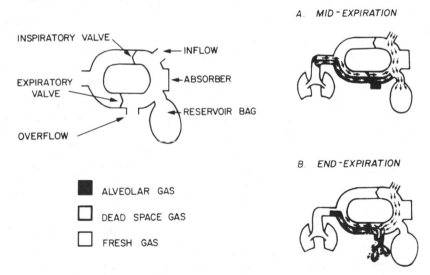

Figure 11-12. Circle anesthetic breathing system showing placement of valves relative to fresh gas inflow, carbon dioxide absorber and gas reservoir bag. Alveolar and dead space gas undergo complete mixing during mid-exhalation (A) and end-exhalation (B). Placement of the inspiratory and exhalation valves near the patient with the overflow valve immediately distal to the exhalation valve results in preferential elimination of alveolar gas. This arrangement, however, is bulky and clumsy such that placement of the valves more distal to the patient as pictured in the schematic diagram is the most frequently used system. (Eger EI II: Anesthetic uptake and action. Baltimore, Williams & Wilkins, 1974. © 1974 EI Eger II, MD as redrawn in Orkin FK. Anesthetic systems. In: Miller RD, ed. Anesthesia. New York, Churchill Livingstone, 1981:117–56.)

halation. This arrangement eliminates the inhalation of exhaled gases until they have passed through the carbon dioxide absorber (see the section *Elimination of Carbon Dioxide*) and have had their oxygen content replenished. Incompetence or absence of a unidirectional valve permits breathing back and forth in one tube, resulting in rebreathing of exhaled gases and the development of hypercarbia.

Prevention of rebreathing of exhaled gases using a circle system mandates that a unidirectional valve be placed between the patient and gas reservoir bag on both the inspiratory and expiratory limbs of the circuit.[8] The most efficient arrangement of components for both spontaneous and controlled ventilation of the lungs is placement of the (1) unidirectional valves near the patient, (2) overflow valve near the patient just distal to the exhalation valve, and (3) fresh gas inflow entering between the carbon dioxide absorber and inhalation valve. In this arrangement, fresh gas inflow preferentially expels ("flushes") alveolar gas (as in th Mapleson A system) while physiologic dead space gas is conserved. Nevertheless, this optimal arrangement is impractical, as the bulky unidirectional valves and overflow valve are located near the patient. A more practical but less efficient arrangement is placement of the unidirectional valves and overflow valve more distal to the patient (Fig. 11-12).[4]

Rebreathing of exhaled gases using a semiclosed anesthetic breathing system influences the inhaled anesthetic concentrations of these gases. For example, when uptake of an anestheic gas is high, as during induction of anesthesia, rebreathing of exhaled gases depleted of anesthetic greatly dilutes the concentration of anesthetic in the fresh gas inflow. This dilutional effect of uptake is offset clinically by increasing the delivered concentration of anesthetic. As uptake of anesthetic diminishes, the impact of dilution on the inspired concentra-

tion produced by rebreathing of exhaled gases is lessened.

Closed Anesthetic Breathing System

A closed anesthetic breathing system is present when the fresh gas inflow into a circle system is decreased sufficiently to permit closure of the overflow valve, and all the exhaled carbon dioxide is neutralized in the carbon dioxide absorber. The fresh gas inflow for a closed system (150 to 500 ml/min) satisfies the patient's metabolic oxygen requirements (150 to 250 ml/min during anesthesia) and replaces anesthetic gases lost by virtue of tissue uptake.

Advantages of the closed anesthetic breathing system compared with the semiclosed anesthetic breathing system include (1) maximal humidification and warming of inhaled gases, (2) less pollution of the surrounding atmosphere with anesthetic gases, and (3) economy in the use of anesthetics. A disadvantage of the closed anesthetic breathing system is the inability to rapidly change the delivered concentration of anesthetic gases and oxygen due to the low fresh gas inflow. The principal dangers of a closed anesthetic breathing system are delivery of (1) unpredictable and possibly insufficient amounts of oxygen, and (2) unknown and possibly excessive concentrations of potent anesthetic gases.

Unpredictable Amounts of Oxygen. Unpredictable and possibly insufficient concentrations of oxygen using a closed anesthetic breathing system are particularly likely when nitrous oxide is included in the fresh gas inflow. For example, decreased tissue uptake of nitrous oxide with time in the presence of continued and unchanged uptake of oxygen can result in a decreased concentration of oxygen in the alveoli (Table 11-5). Therefore, the use of an oxygen analyzer placed on the inspiratory or expiratory limb of the circle system is man-

Table 11-5. Alveolar Gas Concentration Using a Closed Anesthetic Breathing System

Example 1

Gas inflow is nitrous oxide 300 ml/min and oxygen 300 ml/min maintained for 15 minutes. Nitrous oxide uptake by tissues at this time is 200 ml/min and oxygen consumption is 250 ml/min.

Alveolar gas after tissue uptake consists of 100 ml nitrous oxide and 50 ml oxygen. The alveolar concentration of oxygen (F_AO_2) is:

$$F_AO_2 = \frac{50 \text{ ml oxygen}}{100 \text{ ml nitrous oxide} \atop \text{plus } 50 \text{ ml oxygen}} \times 100 = 33 \text{ percent}$$

Example 2

Gas inflow is as in example 1, but duration of administration is 1 hour. At this time, tissue uptake of nitrous oxide has decreased to 100 ml/min but oxygen consumption remains unchanged at 250 ml/min.

Alveolar gas after tissue uptake consists of 200 ml nitrous oxide and 50 ml oxygen. The alveolar concentration of oxygen (F_AO_2) is:

$$F_AO_2 = \frac{50 \text{ ml oxygen}}{200 \text{ ml nitrous oxide} \atop \text{plus } 50 \text{ ml oxygen}} \times 100 = 20 \text{ percent}$$

datory when nitrous oxide is delivered using a closed anesthetic breathing system.

Unknown Concentrations of Potent Anesthetic. Exhaled gases, freed of carbon dioxide, form a major part of the inhaled gases when a closed anesthetic breathing system is used. This means the composition of the inhaled gases is influenced by the concentration present in the exhaled gases. The concentration of anesthetic in exhaled gases reflects tissue uptake of the anesthetic. Initially, tissue uptake is maximal and the concentration of anesthetic in the exhaled gases is reduced. Subsequent rebreathing of these exhaled gases dilutes the inhaled concentration of anesthetic delivered to the patient. Therefore, high inflow concentrations of anesthetic are necessary to offset maximal tissue uptake. Conversely, little or no anesthetic needs to be added to the inflow gases when tissue uptake is reduced. The unknown impact of tissue uptake on the concentration of anesthetic in the exhaled gases makes it difficult to estimate the inhaled concentration delivered to the patient using a closed anesthetic breathing system. This disadvantage can be partially offset by administering higher fresh gas inflows (3 L/min) for about 15 minutes before instituting use of a closed anesthetic breathing system. This approach permits elimination of nitrogen from the lungs and corresponds to the time of greatest tissue uptake of anesthetic.

ELIMINATION OF CARBON DIOXIDE

Elimination of carbon dioxide from an anesthetic breathing system can be achieved by venting all exhaled gases to the atmosphere, as occurs during the use of an open or semiopen anesthetic breathing system. More often, however, partial (semiclosed anesthetic breathing system) or total (closed anesthetic breathing system) rebreathing of exhaled gases is permitted and carbon dioxide is eliminated by chemical neutralization. Chemical neutralization of carbon dioxide is achieved by directing exhaled gases through a container (canister) containing a carbon dioxide absorbent such as soda lime or baralyme.

Table 11-6. Composition of Carbon Dioxide Absorbents

Soda Lime (percent of wet weight)	Baralyme (percent of wet weight)
Sodium hydroxide = 4 percent	Barium hydroxide = 20 percent
Potassium hydroxide = 1 percent	Calcium hydroxide = 80 percent
Water = 14–19 percent	Water = bound water of crystallization in the octahydrate salt of barium hydroxide
Silica = 0.2 percent	Silica = none
Calcium hydroxide = balance	

Soda Lime

Soda lime granules consist of calcium hydroxide plus smaller amounts of sodium hydroxide and potassium hydroxide that are present as activators (Table 11-6). A specific water content of soda lime granules is necessary to assure optimal activity. Silica is added to the granules to give hardness and thus minimize the formation of alkaline dust. Formation of this alkaline dust must be prevented, since its inhalation can produce irritation of the airways manifesting as bronchospasm.[9]

Neutralization of carbon dioxide begins with the reaction of this gas with the water present in soda lime granules and exhaled gases to form carbonic acid (Table 11-7). Carbonic acid then reacts with the hydroxides present in soda lime granules to form carbonates, water, and heat. The water formed by the neutralization of carbon dioxide is useful for humidifying the inhaled gases and for dissipating some of the heat generated in the exothermic neutralization reaction. Accumulation of this highly alkaline water in the bottom of the canister can produce burns on contact with the skin. The heat generated during neutralization of carbon dioxide can be detected by warmness of the canister. Failure of the canister to become warm to touch should alert the anesthesiologist to the possibility that chemical neutralization of carbon dioxide is not taking place.

Baralyme

Baralyme granules consist of barium hydroxide and calcium hydroxide (Table 11-6). Unlike soda lime, the addition of silica to baralyme granules is not necessary to assure hardness. This inherent hardness of baralyme granules reflects the presence of bound water of crystallization in the octahydrate salt of barium hydroxide. This bound water also accounts for the more reliable performance of baralyme than soda lime in dry environments. As with soda lime, the neutralization of carbon dioxide by baralyme results in the formation of carbonates, water, and heat (Table 11-7).

Table 11-7. Chemical Neutralization of Carbon Dioxide

Soda lime

$$CO_2 + H_2O \rightarrow H_2CO_3$$

$$H_2CO_3 + NaOH \rightarrow Na_2CO_3 \text{ (rapid)} + 2H_2O + Heat$$

$$H_2CO_3 + Ca(OH)_2 \rightarrow CaCO_3 \text{ (slow)} + 2H_2O + Heat$$

Baralyme

$$CO_2 + H_2O \rightarrow H_2CO_3$$

$$H_2CO_3 + Ba(OH)_2 \rightarrow BaCO_3 \text{ (rapid)} + 2H_2O + Heat$$

$$H_2CO_3 + Ca(OH)_2 \rightarrow CaCO_3 \text{ (slow)} + 2H_2O + Heat$$

Efficiency of Carbon Dioxide Neutralization

Efficiency of carbon dioxide neutralization is influenced by the size of the carbon dioxide absorbent granules and presence or absence of channeling in the canister containing the carbon dioxide absorbent. In addition, optimal absorptive conditions provide that the equivalent of the patient's tidal volume be accommodated entirely within the void space of the canister. Therefore, about one-half the volume of a properly packed canister should consist of intergranular spaces.

A pH sensitive dye is added to soda lime or baralyme by the manufacturer. A change in color of the absorbent granules is produced when this dye is activated by carbonic acid that accumulates due to exhaustion of the activity of absorbent granules. If the exhaused absorbent granules are not replaced with fresh granules, the color change often disappears during disuse. Minimal regeneration of absorbent granule activity, however, will have occurred and, upon reuse, the dye quickly produces the color change again.

The maximum volume of carbon dioxide that can be absorbed is approximately 26 liters of carbon dioxide per 100 grams of absorbent granules. Usually, considerably less carbon dioxide is absorbed due to factors such as canister design and the specific end-point used to detect exhaustion of absorbent granule activity. For example, only 10 to 15 liters of carbon dioxide per 100 grams of absorbent are neutralized in a single-chambered canister, whereas 18 to 20 liters are absorbed in a dual-chambered (jumbo) canister. In the jumbo canister, the chamber through which the exhaled gases flow first is replaced with new absorbent granules when the indicator dye changes color and at the same time the canister is inverted so the second chamber is moved to the position formerly occupied by the first canister. This sequence is intended to maximally utilize the activity of the absorbent granules in both canisters.

Absorbent granule size is designated as mesh size. For example, an absorbent granule size of 8 mesh (2.5 mm) will pass through a screen having 8 or fewer wires per 2.5 cm. Empirically, the optimal absorbent granule size of soda lime or baralyme has been found to be 4 to 8 mesh. This absorbent granule size represents a compromise between absorptive activity and resistance to air flow through the canister. Absorptive activity increases as absorbent granule size decreases because total surface area increases. The smaller the absorbent granules, however, the smaller the interstices through which gases must flow, resulting in increased resistance to flow.

Channeling is the preferential passage of exhaled gases through the canister via pathways of low resistance such that the bulk of the carbon dioxide absorbent granules are bypassed. Loose packing of the absorbent granules in the canister is the most frequent cause of channeling. Shaking the canister gently prior to use to assure firm packing of the absorbent granules reduces the likelihood of channeling without substantially increasing resistance to flow of gases. In addition, the absorbent granules are held in place with screens and baffles to facilitate uniform dispersion of gas flow.

HUMIDIFICATION

Humidification is a form of vaporization in which water vapor (moisture) is added to the gases delivered by the anesthetic breathing system. Normally, air passing through the nose is warmed to body temperature and saturated with water vapor before reaching the carina. Administration of dry anesthetic gases and oxygen at room temperature via an anesthetic breathing system that bypasses the nose leads to cytologic damage to the respiratory epithelium within 1 hour.[10] Breathing of dry gases for several hours can result in drying of secretions and, when a tracheal tube is used, airway obstruction from inspissated secretions in the tube. In addition, breathing dry and unwarmed gases is associated with water and heat loss from the patient (see Chapter 31). More important than water loss, however, is the heat loss which may lead to adverse reductions in body temperature, particularly in infants and children who are rendered poikilothermic by general anesthesia. Indeed, the most important reason to provide heated humidification during general anesthesia is to reduce heat loss and associated decreases in body temperature (Fig. 11-13).[11]

The simplest method for raising the water content of inhaled gases is passing these gases through the canister used for carbon dioxide absorption. Heating due to the exothermic reaction produced by the neutralization of carbon dioxide enables the inhaled gases to hold more water. The most reliable way to warm and humidify anesthetic gases and oxygen is to use specially designed humidifiers (see Chapter 31).

BACTERIAL CONTAMINATION OF ANESTHETIC EQUIPMENT

The role of bacterial contamination of the anesthetic machine and equipment and the subsequent development of pulmonary infection and cross-infection between patients is controversial.[12] Nevertheless, it is assumed that equipment used to deliver anesthesia is a potential source of bacterial contamination to patients. Based on this assumption, the use of disposable anesthetic breathing systems has become popular. The incidence, however, of postoperative pulmonary infection is not altered by the use of a sterile disposable anesthetic breathing system as compared with the use of a reusable system that is cleaned with basic hygenic techniques but not sterilized between uses. Likewise, the incidence of postoperative pulmonary infection is not altered by inclusion of a bacterial filter in the anesthetic breathing system.

The reason anesthetic equipment has not been implicated as a cause of infection, in

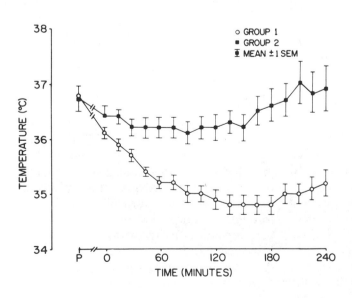

Figure 11-13. Nasopharyngeal temperature was measured in 10 patients breathing gases that were heated to 37 Celsius and 100 percent humidified (Group 1) and 10 patients breathing gases delivered at room temperature (Group 2). Preoperative oral temperatures (P) and nasopharyngeal temperatures immediately following induction of anesthesia (0 time) were similar in both groups of patients. Subsequently, nasopharyngeal temperature decreased only in patients not receiving warmed and humidified gases. (Stone DR, Downs JB, Paul WL, Perkins HM. Adult body temperature and heated humidification of anesthetic gases during general anesthesia. Anesth Analg 1981;60:736–41.)

contrast to the undeniable role of respiratory therapy equipment (particularly nebulizers), involves the low likelihood of airborne transmission of bacteria from the host. Furthermore, the environment presented to organisms that may be present in the anesthetic machine and breathing system is not conducive to bacterial survival.

Airborne Transmission

During anesthesia and quiet breathing only a small number of bacteria are likely to be liberated from the host. Indeed, the administration of anesthesia to patients with known colonization of gram-negative bacteria does not result in contamination of the anesthetic breathing system. Bacteria that are released from the airway during violent forms of exhalation originate almost exclusively from the anterior portion of the oropharynx and rarely the nose or pharynx which harbors respiratory pathogens. Furthermore, even low concentrations of oxygen are lethal to airborne bacteria.

Environment Presented to Bacteria

Airborne bacteria released into a circle anesthetic breathing system are exposed to shifts in humidity and temperature. Bacteria, particularly gram-negative organisms, are sensitive to both these changes. In fact, shifts in humidity and temperature are probably the most important factors responsible for bacterial killing that occurs within the anesthetic breathing system.

Most studies have shown that clinical concentrations of general anesthetics have little influence on the survival of bacteria in the anesthetic breathing system. However, bacteria placed in vaporizers containing liquid anesthetics do not survive. The role of anesthetic equipment in transmitting viral illnesses is not known.

Metallic ions of metals (copper, zinc, chromium, brass) present in the anesthetic machine and other equipment have a highly lethal effect on bacteria. A practical use for this effect has been the insertion of copper mesh or sponges into the expiratory limb of ventilators to prevent infection from contaminated respiratory therapy equipment.

Transmission of Tuberculosis

There has been no documented transmission of tuberculosis from a contaminated anesthetic machine or anesthetic breathing system to a patient.[12] Nevertheless, of all bacterial forms, acid-fast bacilli are the most adaptable and resistant to destruction. Therefore, a greater degree of vigilance should be observed in dealing with patients with pulmonary disease conceivably due to tuberculosis. This vigilance should include use of a disposable anesthetic breathing system and disinfection of nondisposable equipment with an appropriate chemical such as glutaraldehyde (Cidex). Finally, the anesthesiologist should be gloved and should keep intraoral manipulation to a minimum.

POLLUTION OF THE ATMOSPHERE WITH ANESTHETIC GASES

Chronic exposure to low concentrations of anesthetics that result from spillage of these gases into the atmosphere from the anesthetic machine and anesthetic breathing system constitutes a health hazard to operating room personnel[13,14] (see Chapter 5). For this reason removal (scavenging) of trace concentrations of anesthetic gases present in the atmosphere of the operating rooms is recommended. In addition, dental and veterinary settings should be provided with gas scavenging capabilities. The National Institute of Occupational Safety and Health (NIOSH) has proposed that nitrous oxide concentrations in the atmosphere should be less than 25 ppm (parts per million) and less than 5 ppm for volatile anesthetics. It must be recognized, however, that there is no evidence these proposed levels are either desirable or less hazardous than higher concentrations. Nevertheless, nitrous oxide concentrations in excess of 200 ppm as determined by gas chromatogrphy or infrared analysis should alert personnel to search for leaks and/or consider alterations in anesthetic techniques.

Source of Anesthetic Gases in the Environment

High pressure system leakage of anesthetic gases into the atmosphere occurs when a gas such as nitrous oxide escapes from tanks attached to the anesthetic machine (faulty yokes) or from tubing or connectors necessary for the delivery of nitrous oxide to the anesthetic machine from a central gas supply (faulty quick-coupler connector). Low pressure leakage is characterized by escape of anesthetic gases from sites located between the flow meters of the anesthetic machine and the patient, including spillage from the anesthetic breathing system.

Control of Gas Leakage

Control of gas spillage into the environment requires (1) periodic maintenance of anesthetic equipment, (2) removal of excess gases vented from the anesthetic breathing system by the process known as scavenging, (3) attention to technique of anesthesia, and (4) adequate ventilation of the operating rooms.[14]

Periodic maintenance of the anesthetic machine by a qualified service representative is the best protection against persistence of leaks in the high or low pressure system of the anesthetic machine and anesthetic breathing system. Spillage from high or low pressure system components can be detected by applying a soap solution to suspected areas of spillage. The presence and amount of leakage using a circle anesthetic breathing system can be determined by closing the overflow valve, occluding the patient end of the system, and noting the oxygen inflow required to maintain a pressure of 30 cm H_2O. Leakage varies linearly with pressure such that a 150 ml/min leakage rate at 30 cm H_2O will manifest as 50 ml/min spillage at 10 cm H_2O which is the typical average pressure in a circle anesthetic breathing system during controlled ventilation of the lungs. Leakage of 50 ml/min contributes less than 5 ppm to the average operating room concentration of anesthetic gases. Correction of leakage often involves simple steps such as replacing a worn canister gasket or removing a deformed washer on a yoke.

Scavenging is the term applied to collection and removal of excess gases that normally exit via the overflow valve of the anesthetic breathing system. Removal of these excess gases is accomplished by attaching a gas capturing device that includes suction to the anesthetic breathing system. Captured gases are most often delivered to the central vacuum system of the hospital for disposal. Attachment of this device to the anesthetic breathing system introduces the risk of removal of excessive volumes of gas from the system unless the fresh gas inflow is greater than the suction rate. The presence of an excessive rate of suction most often manifests as collapse of the gas reservoir bag. Conversely, occlusion of the gas disposal route may allow excessive pressure increases to occur in the anesthetic breathing system and lead to barotrauma. For these reasons, a pressure-balancing capability is included in the gas capturing device so as to prevent the development of negative or positive pressure in the anesthetic breathing system.

Technique of Anesthesia. Poor fit of the face mask, as well as allowing anesthetic gases to flow prior to placement of the mask on the patient's face or during intubation of the trachea, result in spillage of anesthetic gases into the atmosphere. Administration of oxygen at the conclusion of anesthesia serves to eliminate anesthetic gases from the patient and anesthetic breathing system and thus reduce spillage into the atmosphere. The use of low flow or closed system techniques diminishes but does not eliminate operating room pollution with waste anesthetic gases. Care should be exercised in filling vaporizers, as spillage of liquid anesthetic results in substantial pollution. For example, if halothane spillage is detectable by smell, the level of contamination is likely to exceed 30 ppm.

Room Ventilation. The efficiency of operating room ventilation in terms of room air turnovers per hour should be determined and ventilation filters checked at periodic intervals by the hospital engineer.

REFERENCES

1. Anesthesia Equipment. In: Dripps RD, Eckenhoff JE, Vandam LD, eds. Introduction to anesthesia. The principles of safe practice. Philadelphia, WB Saunders 1982:54–68.
2. Morris LE. New vaporizer for liquid anesthetic agents. Anesthesiology 1952;13:587–93.
3. Gartner J, Stoelting RK. A laboratory comparison of Copper Kettle, Fluotec Mark 2, and Pentec vaporizers. Anesth Analg 1974;53:187–90.
4. Orkin FK. Anesthetic systems. In: Miller RD, ed. Anesthesia. New York, Churchill Livingstone 1981:117–56.
5. Hamilton WK. Nomenclature of inhalation anesthetic systems. Anesthesiology 1964; 25:3–5.
6. Rose DK, Byrick RJ, Froese AB. Carbon dioxide elimination during spontaneous ventilation with a modified Mapleson D system: studies in a lung model. Can Anaesth Soc J 1978;25:353–65.
7. Jackson-Rees G. Anaesthesia in the newborn. Br Med J 1950;2:1419–22.
8. Eger EI II. Anesthetic systems: Construction and function, Anesthetic Uptake and Action. Baltimore, Williams & Wilkins Company, 1974, pp 206–207.
9. Lauria JI. Soda-lime dust contamination of breathing circuits. Anesthesiology 1975;42: 628–9.
10. Chalon J, Loew DAY, Malebranche J. Effect of dry anesthetic gases on tracheobronchial ciliated epithelium. Anesthesiology 1972;37:338–43.
11. Stone DR, Downs JB, Paul WL, Perkins HM. Adult body temperature and heated humidification of anesthetic gases during general anesthesia. Anesth Analg 1981; 60:736–41.
12. duMoulin GC, Hedley-Whyte J. Bacterial interactions between anesthesiologists, their patients, and equipment. Anesthesiology 1982;57:37–41.
13. Vessey MP. Epidemiological studies of the occupational hazards of anaesthesia—a review. Anaesthesia 1978;33:430–8.
14. Lecky JH. Anesthetic pollution in the operating room. A notice to operating room personnel. Anesthesiology 1980;52:157–9.

12

Airway Management

Intubation of the tracheal (translaryngeal intubation) is a safe and common practice in the patient undergoing general anesthesia.[1] Atraumatic intubation of the trachea requires a knowledge of the anatomy of the upper airway and appropriate use of equipment and drugs, particularly muscle relaxants.

PREOPERATIVE EVALUATION

Preoperative evaluation of the patient determines the route (oral or nasal) and method (awake or anesthetized) for intubation of the trachea. This evaluation includes an assessment of anatomic characteristics which may make intubation of the trachea difficult, a thorough dental examination, and an evaluation of temporomandibular joint and cervical spine mobility.

Anatomic Characteristics

Anatomic characteristics that impair alignment of oral, pharyngeal, and laryngeal axes (Fig. 12-1)[1] and make visualization of the glottic opening difficult by direct laryngoscopy include (1) a short muscular neck and a full set of teeth, (2) a receding mandible, (3) protruding maxillary incisors, (4) poor mandibular mobility, and (5) a long high arched palate associated with a long narrow mouth. If nasotracheal intubation is planned, the patency of the nares can be evaluated by asking the patient to breath through each naris while the examiner occludes the other. This is supplemented by direct questioning about previous nasal trauma or difficulty breathing through the nose.

Dental Examination

Teeth and dental prostheses are vulnerable to damage or dislodgment by the laryngoscope blade during direct laryngoscopy. Therefore, the preoperative dental examination should ascertain the presence of (1) loose teeth, (2) dental prostheses, and (3) co-existing dental abnormalities.[2]

Loose Teeth. Newly erupted deciduous or permanent teeth initially have little support because the roots are only partially formed. Deciduous teeth begin to erupt at about 6 months of age and permanent teeth start to appear at about 6 years of age. As a permanent tooth erupts, the root portion of the overlying deciduous tooth undergoes resolution such that just before exfoliation it may be held in place only by fibrous tissue. Children 6 to 12 years of age are considered to be in the mixed dentition stage. In adults, loosening of teeth most often reflects peridontal disease and loss of bony support.

Dental Prostheses. The position of fixed or removable dental prostheses should be determined preoperatively. An individual

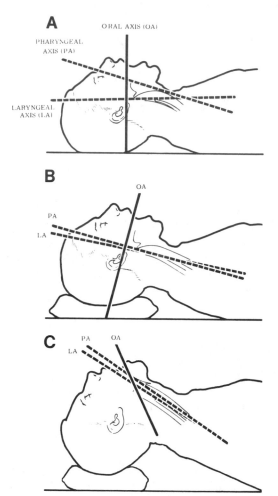

Figure 12-1. Schematic diagram demonstrating head position for intubation of the trachea. (A) Successful exposure of the glottic opening using direct laryngoscopy requires alignment of the oral, pharyngeal, and laryngeal axes. (B) Elevation of the head with pads under the occiput with the shoulders remaining on the table aligns the pharyngeal and laryngeal axes. (C) Subsequent head extension at the atlanto-occipital joint serves to create the shortest distance and most nearly straight line from the incisor teeth to glottic opening. (Stoelting RK. Endotracheal intubation. In: Miller RD, ed. Anesthesia. New York, Churchill Livingstone, 1981, 233–55.)

crown (cap) is affixed to an underlying natural tooth and is difficult to detect, particularly if it is porcelain. A permanent (non-removable) bridge fills a gap between one or more missing permanent teeth and prosthetic appliances are attached to the bridge. Nonpermanent bridges or dentures may be removed preoperatively or left in place until after induction of anesthesia so as to facilitate a mask fit to the face.

Co-Existing Dental Abnormalities. The position of missing teeth and chips or fractures (especially on maxillary incisors) is important to detect preoperatively. Otherwise, subsequent discovery of these abnormalities may be incorrectly attributed to damage produced by the laryngoscope blade. It must be appreciated that protruding maxillary incisors are particularly vulnerable to damage from levering effects exerted by the laryngoscope blade.

Temporomandibular Joint Mobility

Temporomandibular joint mobility can be evaluated by having the patient open his mouth as widely as possible. Normal mandibular opening in an adult is in the range of 40 mm or at least two finger breadths.[3] Limitation of mandibular mobility is most often due to involvement of the temporomandibular joint by arthritis. As a result, difficulty may be experienced in opening the mouth wide enough to permit direct laryngoscopy for intubation of the trachea.

Cervical Spine Mobility

Cervical spine mobility as demonstrated by flexion and extension of the head is essential for proper positioning in preparation for direct laryngoscopy (Fig. 12-1).[1] The normal range of flexion-extension of the head decreases approximately 20 percent by 75 years of age.[4]

Table 12-1. Indications for Orotracheal Intubation

Provide patent airway
Prevent inhalation (aspiration) of gastric contents
Need for frequent suctioning
Facilitate positive pressure ventilation of the lungs
Operative position other than supine
Operative site near or involving the upper airway
Airway maintenance by mask difficult
Disease involving upper airway

INDICATIONS FOR OROTRACHEAL INTUBATION

Orotracheal intubation may be considered for every patient receiving general anesthesia. There are also specific indications for intubation of the trachea in the surgical patient (Table 12-1). Specific indications for placement of a cuffed tracheal tube include provision of a patent airway and prevention of the inhalation (aspiration) of gastric contents, blood, or secretions into the lungs. Intubation of the trachea is mandatory in patients who have recently ingested food or in whom intestinal obstruction is present. Any patient requiring frequent tracheal suctioning is best managed with a tracheal tube in place. Operations in which positive pressure ventilation of the lungs is required (thoracotomy, presence of neuromuscular blockade) or in which prolonged controlled ventilation of the lungs is necessary are most reliably managed in the presence of a tracheal tube. Maintenance of a patent upper airway or controlled ventilation of the lungs is not reliable in the absence of a tracheal tube when operations are performed in other than the supine position (e.g., sitting, prone, lateral, lithotomy, or head-down position). Operations about the head, neck, or upper airway require a tracheal tube for both airway maintenance and/or removal of anesthetic equipment from the operative site. Difficult maintenance of a patent airway by mask may be an indication for tracheal intubation. For example, the upper airway of an edentulous patient is difficult to maintain

using a face mask, but intubation of the trachea is technically easy. Finally, disease involving the upper airway mandates placement of a tracheal tube when unconsciousness is to be produced with anesthetic drugs.

TECHNIQUE FOR OROTRACHEAL INTUBATION

Orotracheal intubation using direct laryngoscopy in an anesthetized patient is routinely chosen unless specific circumstances dictate a different approach. Equipment and drugs utilized in accomplishing intubation of the trachea include a proper sized tracheal tube, laryngoscope, functioning suction catheter, appropriate anesthetic drugs, and facilities to provide positive pressure ventilation of the lungs with oxygen. If a cuffed tracheal tube is chosen, the cuff should be checked for air-tightness. Techniques for induction of anesthesia prior to intubation of the trachea are describe in Chapter 9.

Head Position for Orotracheal Intubation

Elevating the head about 10 cm with pads under the occiput (shoulders remaining on the table) and extension of the head at the atlanto-occipital joint serves to align the oral, pharyngeal, and laryngeal axes such that the passage from the lips to glottic opening is most nearly a straight line (Fig. 21-1).[1] This posture is described as the "sniffing position." Extension of the head, without elevation of the occiput, increases the distance from the lips to glottic opening, rotates the larynx anteriorly, and may necessitate leverage on the maxillary teeth or gums with the laryngoscope blade in order to expose the glottic opening. The height of the operating table should be adjusted such that the patient's face is at the level of the standing anesthesiologist's xiphoid cartilage. If not opened by extension of the head, the patient's mouth may be manually opened by depressing the mandible with the right thumb. Simultaneously, the patient's lower lip can be rolled away with the right index finger to prevent its bruising by the laryngoscope blade.

Use of the Laryngoscope

The laryngoscope consists of a battery-containing handle to which blades with a light source may be attached and removed interchangeably (Fig. 12-2).[1] The laryngoscope is held in the left hand near the junction between the handle and blade of the laryngoscope. The blade is then inserted on the right side of the patient's mouth so as to avoid the incisor teeth and deflect the tongue to the left away from the lumen of the blade. Pressure on the teeth or gums must be avoided as the blade is advanced forward and centrally toward the epiglottis. The wrist is held rigid to prevent using the upper teeth or gums as a fulcrum with the

blade of the laryngoscope as a lever. When the epiglottis is visualized, the next step depends on the type of laryngoscope blade being used.

Curved (MacIntosh) Blade. The tip of the curved blade is advanced into the space between the base of the tongue and the pharyngeal surface of the epiglottis (Fig. 12-3A).[1] Forward and upward movement of the blade exerted along the axis of the laryngoscope handle while avoiding any temptation to lever the blade on the teeth or gums by pulling back on the handle serves to stretch the hypoepiglottic ligament, which elevates the epiglottis and exposes the glottic opening.

Straight (Jackson-Wisconsin) or Straight with Curved Tip (Miller) Blade. The tip of the straight blade is passed beneath the laryngeal surface of the epiglottis (Fig. 12-3B).[1] Forward and upward movement of the blade exerted along the axis of the laryn-

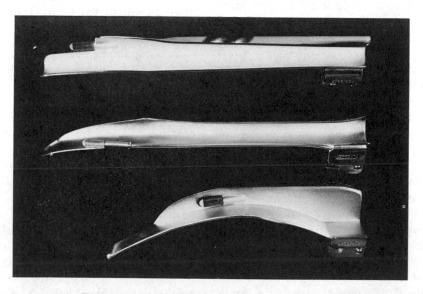

Figure 12-2. Examples of detachable laryngoscope blades which can be used interchangeably on the same handle include the straight blade (uppermost), straight blade with a curved distal tip (middle), and curved blade (lowermost). (Stoelting RK. Endotracheal intubation. In: Miller RD, ed. Anesthesia. New York, Churchill Livingstone, 1981, 233–55.)

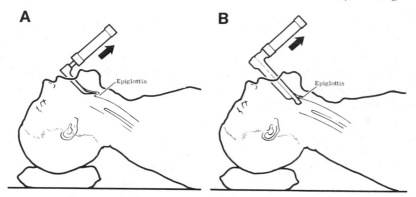

Figure 12-3. Schematic diagram depicting proper position of the laryngoscope blade for exposure of the glottic opening. (A) The distal end of the curved blade is advanced into the space between the base of the tongue and the pharyngeal surface of the epiglottis. (B) The distal end of the straight blade is advanced beneath the laryngeal surface of the epiglottis. Regardless of blade design, forward, and upward movement exerted along the axis of the laryngoscope handle as denoted by the arrows, serves to elevate the epiglottis and expose the glottic opening. (Stoelting RK. Endotracheal intubation. In: Miller RD, ed. Anesthesia. New York, Churchill Livingstone, 1981, 233–55.)

goscope handle while avoiding any temptation to lever the blade on the teeth or gums by pulling back on the handle serves to directly elevate the epiglottis and expose the glottic opening. Depression or lateral movement of the patient's thyroid cartilage externally on the neck with the anesthesiologist's right hand may facilitate exposure of the glottic opening.

Choice of Laryngoscope Blade. The choice of laryngoscope blade is often based on personal preference. Advantages cited for the curved blade include less trauma to teeth with more room for passage of the tube and less bruising of the epiglottis because the tip of the blade should not touch this structure. Advantages cited for the straight blade include better exposure of the glottic opening and less need for a stylet to direct a tube into an anterior glottic opening.

Tracheal Tube Size and Length

Tracheal tube sizes are specified according to internal diameter (ID) which is marked on each tube (Table 12-2) (Fig. 12-

4).[1] Tracheal tubes are available in 0.5 mm internal diameter increments. Most adult tracheas (after 14 years of age) readily accept a cuffed 8.0 to 9.0 mm internal diameter tracheal tube. The tracheal tube also has lengthwise cm markings starting at the distal trachael end to permit accurate determination of the tube length inserted past

Table 12-2. Size and Length of Tracheal Tubes

Age	Internal Diameter (mm)	Distance Inserted from Lips to Place Distal End in the Midtrachea (cm[a])
Premature	2.5	10
Full term	3.0	11
1–6 months	3.5	11
6–12 months	4.0	12
2 years	4.5	13
4 years	5.0	14
6 years	5.5	15–16
8 years	6.5	16–17
10 years	7.0	17–18
12 years	7.5	18–20
14 years and over	8.0–9.0	20–22

[a] Add 2 to 3 cm for nasal tubes.

the lips. The letters I.T. (implantation tested) or Z-79 indicate that the tracheal tube material has been determined to be free of any tissue irritant or toxic properties. Tracheal tube material should also be radiopaque to facilitate demonstration of tube position relative to the carina and transparent to permit visualization of secretions or cessation of air flow as evidenced by disappearance of breath fogging.

Tracheal Tube Cuff

Inflatable cuffs are built into the distal end of tracheal tubes (Fig. 12-4).[1] The cuff is inflated with air to create a seal against the underlying tracheal mucosa. This seal facilitates positive pressure ventilation of the lungs and reduces the likelihood of aspiration of pharyngeal or gastric secretions. Cuffs are classified as high pressure or low pressure.[5]

High pressure cuffs must be inflated to high intraluminal cuff pressures (180 to 250 mmHg) before they expand sufficiently to create a seal between the tube and tracheal mucosa. This high cuff pressure is partially transmitted to the underlying tracheal mucosa. Ischemia of the tracheal mucosa may occur whenever the pressure on the tracheal wall exceeds capillary arteriolar pres-

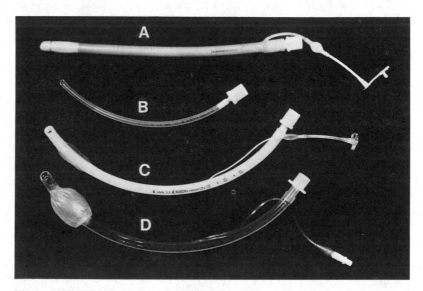

Figure 12-4. Various types of tracheal tubes and cuffs. Tube A is an armored or anode tube with built-in spiral wire to minimize the opportunity of collapse or kinking. Tubes B, C, and D are made of smooth plastic and are recommended for single use. Tube B is uncuffed and is a size appropriate for a child. Tubes C and D are appropriate for adults. Tubes A and C are equipped with built-in high pressure cuffs. Tube D is constructed to include a low pressure cuff. These cuffs are inflated by attaching an air-filled syringe to the small diameter tube that leads to the cuff. Distension of the small balloon near the attachment for the syringe confirms inflation of the cuff. Numbers and letters visible on tubes B, C, and D denote the internal diameter, length from the distal tracheal end, and confirmation the tubes have been tested for tissue compatibility. (Stoelting RK. Endotracheal intubation. In: Miller RD, ed. Anesthesia. New York, Churchill Livingstone, 1981, 233–55.)

sure (about 32 mmHg). Persistent ischemia of the tracheal mucosa may cause damage which in extreme cases manifests as destruction of cartilaginous tracheal rings. High pressure cuffs also tend to inflate asymmetrically, deforming the trachea and ultimately producing tracheal dilatation.

Low pressure cuffs inflate symmetrically, adapting to the contour of the tracheal wall and producing a seal with the tracheal mucosa at low intraluminal cuff pressures. The resulting tracheal wall pressure has been found to equal peak airway pressure (15 to 30 mmHg) during positive pressure ventilation of the lungs. These characteristics make tracheal mucosa ischemia and tracheal dilatation less likely than with high pressure cuffs. Indeed, low pressure cuffs decrease the severity of tracheal injury observed at the cuff site.[6] Tracheal tubes with low pressure cuffs are often recommended when intubation of the trachea is anticipated to be required for longer than 48 hours. Nevertheless, there is probably no period of tracheal intubation that does not produce some laryngotracheal damage. For example, ciliary denudation has been found to occur predominantly over the tracheal rings and underlying cuff site with only 2 hours of intubation and tracheal wall pressures less than 25 mmHg.[6]

Placement of a Tracheal Tube

The glottic opening is recognized by its triangular shape and pale white vocal cords (Fig. 12-5). The tracheal tube is held in the anesthesiologist's right hand like a pencil and introduced on the right side of the patient's mouth with the built in curve directed anteriorly. Attempts to insert the tube in the midline of the mouth and then down the lumen of the laryngoscope blade usually obscure vision of the glottic opening. The tube is advanced past the vocal cords until the cuff just disappears, which should correspond to the distance predicted to place the distal end of the tube midway between the vocal cords and carina (Table 12-1).[1] At this point, the laryngoscope blade is removed from the mouth. The tracheal tube cuff is next inflated with air to just a no leak volume during positive pressure ventilation of the lungs. Distension of the small pilot balloon attached to the inflation tube leading to the cuff confirms cuff inflation. Confirmation of placement of the tube in the trachea is evidenced by bilateral chest movement and air entry movement. Noting the depth of insertion as determined by the cm markings on the tracheal tube at the lips helps predict a midtrachea position of the distal end of the tube. For example, insertion of a tracheal tube 20 to 22 cm beyond the lips of an adult should reliably place the distal end of the tube in the midtrachea. Furthermore, if a cuffed tube is properly placed in the midtrachea, the anesthesiologist can easily detect, by external palpation, cuff distension in the suprasternal notch during rapid inflation of the cuff. Finally, the tube is secured in position with tape placed around the tube and applied above and below the lips, extending over the cheeks.

ALTERNATIVES TO OROTRACHEAL INTUBATION DURING GENERAL ANESTHESIA

Alternatives to orotracheal intubation during general anesthesia include awake orotracheal intubation, nasotracheal intubation, and intubation using a fiberoptic laryngoscope. These alternatives are considered when orotracheal intubation during general anesthesia might be unsafe (recent food ingestion, bowel obstruction, upper airway disease) or impossible because of altered anatomy (see the section *Anatomic Characteristics*).

Awake Orotracheal Intubation

Local anesthesia for awake orotracheal intubation utilizing direct laryngoscopy may include (1) topical spray of the lips,

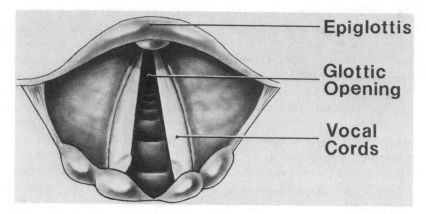

Figure 12-5. Schematic view of glottic opening as seen during direct laryngoscopy when the epiglottis is elevated with a curved or straight laryngoscope blade. The glottic opening is recognized by its triangular shape bordered by the pale white vocal cords.

tongue, palate and pharynx; (2) superior laryngeal nerve block; and (3) transtracheal injection of a local anesthetic, most often lidocaine. It is helpful to reduce oropharyngeal secretions with an anticholinergic. When vomiting is a hazard, only topical spray is recommended, thus avoiding anesthesia of areas necessary to protect against pulmonary aspiration.

Nasotracheal Intubation

Nasotracheal intubation may be performed electively for intraoral operations, when anatomic abnormalities or disease of the upper airway make direct laryngoscopy difficult or impossible and when long term intubation of the trachea is anticipated. Advantages cited for nasotracheal intubation include (1) more stable tube fixation, (2) less change for tube kinking, (3) greater comfort in an awake patient, and (4) fewer oropharyngeal secretions.

Awake blind nasotracheal intubation is usually reserved for situations in which direct laryngoscopy or ventilation of the lungs would be impossible or induction of anesthesia before intubation of the trachea would be hazardous. To insure maximum patient comfort and nasal patency and to minimize the chance of epistaxis, the nasal mucosa should be anesthetized and constricted with topical cocaine. If cocaine is not available, constriction but not anesthesia of the nasal mucosa can be produced with topical phenylephrine. Either naris may be chosen, depending on the history and physical examination, but the right naris is preferable because the bevel of most tracheal tubes when introduced through the right naris will face the flat nasal septum, reducing damage to the turbinates. Tracheal tubes can be used interchangeably for nasal or oral intubation of the trachea (Table 12-2).[1] In an adult, a 7.0 to 7.5 mm internal diameter tube is usually adequate. After passage through the naris into the oropharynx, the tracheal tube is advanced toward the glottic opening as long as breath sounds are maximal as determined by listening to exhaled air passing from the proximal end of the tube. Ideally, the tracheal tube is swiftly passed through the glottic opening just before inspiration, because the vocal cords are most open during this time and the risk of vocal cord trauma is thus minimized. Successful placement of the tube in the trachea is confirmed by continued breathing through the tube.

Nasotracheal intubation during general anesthesia is acceptable when vomiting is not a hazard and ventilation of the lungs can be maintained by a mask. General anesthesia is produced following vasoconstriction of the nasal mucosa with topical cocaine or phenylephrine. If blind nasotracheal intubation is to be performed, it is mandatory to maintain spontaneous ventilation in the patient so as to permit identification of the glottic opening as evidenced by exhaled air passing from the proximal end of the tube. Alternatively, nasotracheal intubation may be accomplished utilizing direct laryngoscopy to expose the glottic opening. When this approach is selected, succinylcholine is administered to produce skeletal muscle relaxation and the tracheal tube is placed through the right naris into the oropharynx. The glottic opening is then visualized using direct laryngoscopy and the tracheal tube guided through the glottic opening under vision by manually advancing it at the proximal end. Alternatively, the tracheal tube may be grasped in the oropharynx with intubating forceps (Magill forceps) and directed so that pressure on the proximal end causes the tube to pass between the vocal cords. The right naris is preferred because a left nasotracheal tube is clumsy to advance under direct vision with the anesthesiologist's left hand holding the laryngoscope.

Complications unique to nasotracheal intubation include (1) epistaxis, (2) dislodgement of pharyngeal tonsils (adenoids), (3) eustachian tube obstruction, (4) maxillary sinusitis, and (5) bacteremia.[7] Epistaxis most likely reflects avulsion of nasal mucosa covering the turbinates. Shrinkage of nasal mucosa with cocaine or phenylephrine and use of small and generously lubricated tracheal tubes should minimize this complication. When pharyngeal tonsils are prominent, as in children, it is preferable to perform all nasotracheal intubations utilizing direct laryngoscopy to expose the glottic opening so as to prevent unrecognized delivery into the trachea of a dislodged piece of tonsil. Bacteremia following nasotracheal intubation most likely reflects entrance of upper airway flora into the circulation via traumatized nasal mucosa. Therefore, prophylactic antibiotics are indicated when nasotracheal intubation is planned in patients with heart disease.

Intubation Using a Fiberoptic Laryngoscope

Intubation of the trachea using a flexible fiberoptic laryngoscope is ideal for the patient in whom the glottic opening cannot be visualized because of anatomic abnormalities (Fig. 12-6).[8] After topical anesthesia as described for awake blind nasotracheal intubation, the tracheal tube is passed through the naris into the oropharynx. The lubricated fiberoptic laryngoscope is then passed through the tracheal tube (tube must be about 8 mm internal diameter to allow easy passage of the fiberscope) until the epiglottis and glottic opening are visualized. The pediatric fiberoptic bronchoscope, however, will pass through a 5 mm internal diameter tracheal tube. The fiberoptic laryngoscope is passed between the vocal cords and the tracheal tube is advanced into the trachea using the fiberoptic laryngoscope as a guide. Orotracheal intubation using the fiberoptic laryngoscope is technically more difficult than the nasal approach.

OROTRACHEAL INTUBATION IN CHILDREN

Orotracheal intubation in children differs from adults because of anatomic differences in pediatric patients as well as the need to more carefully select the size and length of tracheal tube inserted in these young individuals (see Chapter 27).

Anatomic Differences from Adults

The newborn head and tongue are large and the neck is short. The larynx is more cephalad than in the adult. For example, the

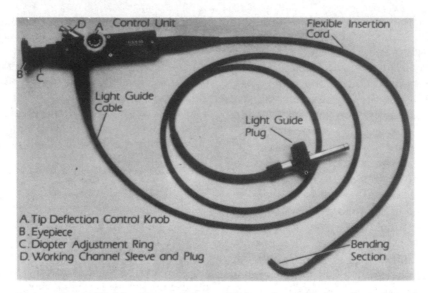

Figure 12-6. Flexible fiberoptic laryngoscope that will pass through an 8 mm internal diameter tracheal tube. (Intubation of the trachea. In: Dripps RD, Eckenhoff JE, Vandam LD, eds. Introduction to Anesthesia. The principles of safe practice. Philadelphia, WB Saunders, 1982:180–95.)

lower border of the cricoid cartilage is opposite the 4th cervical vertebra at birth and opposite the 5th cervical vertebra at age 6. The epiglottis is U-shaped and stiff. These anatomic differences result in difficulty aligning the oral, pharyngeal, and tracheal axes and elevating the epiglottis to expose the glottic opening (Fig. 12-1).[1] As such, the glottic opening of the newborn tends to be anterior compared with the adult. It must be remembered that the cricoid cartilage is the narrowest point in the larynx of children such that a tube that passes through the glottic opening may subsequently resist advancement at this site.

Tracheal Tube Size and Length

Selection of the appropriate tracheal tube size and length is critical in children, as the margin for error is small (Table 12-2).[1] Excessive tube size is responsible for unnecessary laryngotracheal trauma which may manifest as laryngeal edema when the tube is removed from the trachea. Likewise, the short glottis to carina distance in children necessitates careful calculation of correct tube length to assure a midtrachea position of the distal end of the tube (Table 12-2).[1] One must be aware that head flexion or change from the supine to head-down position may shift the carina upward, converting a midtrachea tube placement to an endobronchial intubation while head extension may place the distal end of the tube in the pharynx.

A tracheal tube one size above and below the calculated size should be available with the final choice made when the glottic opening is visualized and the tube is inserted into the trachea. Cuffed tubes are probably not necessary before 5 years of age because the narrow subglottic tracheal diameter insures an adequate seal between the tube and tracheal mucosa. Resistance to breathing is a consideration for the small lumen tracheal tubes and connectors necessary in children. When increased airway resistance is a concern, the best approach is placement of a proper (not the largest possible) sized tube in the trachea and controlled ventilation of the lungs to prevent excessive work of breathing.

Technique for Tracheal Intubation

Orotracheal intubation is routinely chosen for short-term intubation in children. Awake orotracheal intubation of the newborn is preferable. After about 2 weeks of age, infants are sufficiently strong to resist awake intubation of the trachea and anesthesia may be produced before direct laryngoscopy. A straight laryngoscope blade often provides better exposure of the glottic opening than the curved blade, especially in children less than 3 years of age.

EXTUBATION OF THE TRACHEA

Extubation of the trachea following general anesthesia is ideally accomplished while the patient is still adequately anesthetized so as to diminish the likelihood of coughing or laryngospasm (reflex closure of the vocal cords). This assumes that adequate ventilation of the lungs is present or can be maintained without the tracheal tube in place and that the presence of gastric contents is not a likely hazard. Suctioning of the pharynx should be performed prior to extubation of the trachea so that secretions proximal to the tube cuff do not drain into the trachea when the cuff is deflated. After the cuff is deflated, the tube is removed often with simultaneous pressure on the reservoir bag so the lungs are inflated and the initial gas flow is outward. This maneuver may facilitate a cough and expulsion of any aspirated material. When the presence of gastric contents is predictable at the conclusion of anesthesia, the trachea should not be extubated until protective laryngeal reflexes have returned. Vigorous reaction to the tracheal tube (''bucking'') signals the return of the protective cough reflex and at this point the trachea must be extubated or further sedation instituted to permit tolerance of the tube.

Laryngospasm and vomiting are the most serious immediate hazards following extubation of the trachea. Therefore, oxygen, succinylcholine, equipment for reintubation of the trachea, and suction must be immediately available.

COMPLICATIONS OF TRACHEAL INTUBATION

Complications of tracheal intubation are rare and should not influence the decision to place a tracheal tube. Certainly, the benefits of a properly placed and patent tracheal tube far exceed the risks of intubation of the trachea. Complications of tracheal intubation may be categorized as those occurring (1) during direct laryngoscopy and intubation of the trachea, (2) while the tracheal tube is in place, and (3) following extubation of the trachea either immediately or after a delay (Table 12-3).[7]

Complications During Direct Laryngoscopy and Intubation of the Trachea

Dental trauma is the most serious and frequent type of damage related to direct laryngoscopy. Avoidance of using the laryngoscope blade as a lever on the teeth will minimize the hazard of dental trauma. Should injury occur, immediate consultation with a dentist is indicated. A dislodged tooth must be recovered, but, if the search is unsuccessful, appropriate radiographs of the chest and abdomen taken to assure the tooth has not passed through the glottic opening.

Hypertension and tachycardia frequently accompany direct laryngoscopy (regardless of type of laryngoscope blade used) and intubation of the trachea.[9] These responses are usually transient and innocuous. In patients with coexisting hypertension or those

Table 12-3. Complications of Tracheal Intubation

During direct laryngoscopy and intubation of the
   trachea
      Dental and oral soft tissue trauma
      Hypertension and tachycardia
      Cardiac dysrhythmias
      Inhalation (aspiration) of gastric contents
While tracheal tube is in place
      Tracheal tube obstruction
      Endobronchial intubation
      Esophageal intubation
      Accidental extubation
      Increased resistance to breathing
      Tracheal mucosa ischemia
Immediate and delayed complications after
   extubation of the trachea
      Laryngospasm
      Inhalation (aspiration) of gastric contents
      Pharyngitis (sore throat)
      Laryngitis
      Laryngeal or subglottic edema
      Laryngeal ulceration with or without granuloma
        formation
      Tracheitis
      Tracheal stenosis
      Vocal cord paralysis
      Arytenoid cartilage dislocation

with coronary artery disease, however, these changes may be exaggerated or jeopardize the balance between myocardial oxygen requirements and delivery. In these types of patients, it is particularly important to minimize the circulatory responses by limiting the duration of direct laryngoscopy to less than 15 seconds. Serious or persistent cardiac dysrhythmias during intubation of the trachea are unlikely, particularly if adequate oxygenation during the period of apnea associated with direct laryngoscopy is assured by prior inflation of the lungs with oxygen.

Complications While the Tracheal Tube is in Place

Obstruction of the tracheal tube may occur due to the accumulation of secretions in the tube and kinking of the tube. Inadvertent endobronchial intubation is minimized by calculating the proper tracheal tube length for every patient and then noting the cm marking on the tube at the point of fixation at the lips. Flexion of the head may advance the tube up to 1.9 cm converting a tracheal placement into an endobronchial intubation. Conversely, extension of the head can withdraw the tube up to 1.9 cm and result in a pharyngeal intubation.

Immediate and Delayed Complications Following Extubation of the Trachea

Laryngospasm and/or inhalation of gastric contents are the two most serious potential immediate complications following extubation of the trachea. Laryngospasm is unlikely if the depth of anesthesia is sufficient during extubation of the trachea or the patient is allowed to awaken before extubation. It is the patient who is lightly anesthetized at the time of extubation of the trachea who is most at risk. If laryngospasm occurs, oxygen under positive pressure via a face mask and forward displacement of the mandible using the index fingers to apply pressure at the temporomandibular joints may be sufficient treatment. Administration of intravenous (alternatively intramuscular) succinylcholine is indicated if laryngospasm persists. Inhalation of gastric contents is most likely to occur in the debilitated patient or in the presence of recent food ingestion or gastrointestinal obstruction. Pharyngitis (sore throat) is a frequent complaint after extubation of the trachea, particularly in females presumably because of the thinner mucosal covering over the posterior vocal cords compared with males.[7] Skeletal muscle myalgia associated with administration of succinylcholine may manifest in the peripharyngeal muscles as postoperative sore throat which is incorrectly attributed to prior intubation of the trachea. Regardless of the mechanism, sore throat usually disappears spontaneously in 48 to 72 hours without any treatment. Symptomatic laryngeal or subglottic edema is most likely in children because a small amount of swelling greatly reduces the lumen of the larynx. The likely causes of laryngeal edema in children include traumatic intubation of the trachea, use of an oversized tracheal tube, or the presence of an upper respiratory tract infection. Even with ideal conditions, however, laryngeal edema may still occur. Laryngeal incompetence may be present in some patients in the first 4 to 8 hours following extubation of the trachea leading to an increased risk of pulmonary aspiration.[10]

The major complication of prolonged intubation of the trachea (greater than 48 hours) is damage to the tracheal mucosa which may progress to destruction of cartilaginous rings and subsequent circumferential cicatricial scar formation and tracheal stenosis. Stenosis becomes symptomatic when the adult tracheal lumen is reduced to less than 5 mm.

REFERENCES

1. Stoelting RK. Endotracheal intubation. In: Miller RD, ed. Anesthesia. New York, Churchill Livingstone 1981;233–55.
2. Wright RB, Manfield FFV. Damage to teeth during the administration of general anesthesia. Anesth Analg 1974;53:405–8.
3. Block C, Brechner VL. Unusual problems in airway management II: The influence of the temporomandibular joint, the mandible, and associated structures on endotracheal intubation. Anesth Analg 1971;50:114–23.
4. Brechner VL. Unusual problems in the management of airways: I. Flexion-extension mobility of the cervical vertebrae. Anesth Analg 1968;47:363–73.
5. Carroll R, Hedden M, Safar P. Intratracheal cuffs: Performance characteristics. Anesthesiology 1969;31:275–81.
6. Klainer AS, Turndorf H. Wen-Hsien WU, Maewal H, Allender P. Surface alterations due to endotracheal intubation. Am J Med 1975;58:674–83.
7. Blanc VF, Tremblay NAG. The complications of tracheal intubation. A new classification with a review of the literature. Anesth Analg 1974;53:202–13.
8. Intubation of the trachea. In: Dripps RD, Eckenhoff JE, Vandam LD, eds. Introduction to Anesthesia. The principles of safe practice. Philadelphia, WB Saunders 1982:180–95.
9. Stoelting RK. Blood pressure and heart rate changes during short duration laryngoscopy for tracheal intubation. Influence of viscous or intravenous lidocaine. Anesth Analg 1978;57:197–9.
10. Bishop MJ, Weymuller EA, Fink RB. Laryngeal effects of prolonged intubation Anesth Analg 1984;63:335–42.

13

Spinal, Epidural, and Caudal Blocks

Spinal, epidural, and caudal block are commonly referred to as regional or conduction block anesthesia. Spinal anesthesia is produced by administration of a local anesthetic into the lumbar intrathecal space. The local anesthetic blocks conduction in the spinal nerve roots, dorsal root ganglia, and probably the periphery of the spinal cord. Epidural anesthesia is accomplished by injecting the local anesthetic into the extradural space. The epidural space is usually identified by using a lumbar approach. Caudal anesthesia refers to identification and deposition of local anesthetic into the epidural space when the needle is introduced into the sacral hiatus. The epidural space is that compartment between the dura mater and the boney and ligamentus walls of the spinal canal. It is a potential space filled with fat and the internal vertebral plexus of veins.

Either spinal or epidural anesthesia has the advantage of providing anesthesia more selectively, in regard to the surgical site, than anesthesia of the total body as is produced by general anesthesia. The patient may be awake or sedated. Furthermore, profound skeletal muscle relaxation can be produced, which has the advantage of not requiring muscle relaxants. The gastrointestinal tract is usually contracted, which

facilitates exposure within the abdominal cavity for the surgeon. Despite these advantages, patients and/or surgeons may be biased against the use of spinal or epidural anesthesia. Most often these biases are based on the patient's fear of being awake during the surgery and the surgeon's concern that the block may be inadequate, resulting in a delay in starting the operation while the anesthesiologist induces general anesthesia.

SPINAL ANESTHESIA

Anatomy

The spinal canal extends from the foramen magnum to the sacral hiatus and is formed anteriorly by the bodies of the vertebra, laterally by the pedicles, and posteriorly by the lamina. The only openings into the canal are the intervertebral foramina, through which segmental nerves and blood vessels pass. The spinal dura mater is a continuation of the dura mater from the skull and extends from the foramen magnum to the second sacral segment. The spinal cord, however, is terminated at the L1-L2 junction. The subarachnoid space surrounds the spinal cord between the pia and arachnoid membranes and extends to the second sacral vertebra. Spinal anesthesia involves the introduction of local anesthetic into this space at the level of the lumbar vertebra.

To interpret the effects and complications of spinal and epidural anesthesia, knowledge of the sensory, motor, and autonomic distribution of spinal nerves is essential. A dermatome is that area of the skin supplied by a single spinal nerve. Other than the face, which is supplied by trigeminal dermatomes, the remainder of the body skin is supplied in sequence by dermatomes C2 through S5 (Fig. 13-1).

Before every anesthetic, especially a spinal or epidural block, a history, particularly as related to the blood volume and the potential to compensate for hypotension, should be elicited. Also, a careful neurologic history and examination should be performed to provide a baseline for monitoring recovery from regional anesthesia.

When discussing a spinal anesthetic with the patient, three common objections can arise. First, patients are fearful of being awake during a surgical procedure. Secondly, there is often a fear of having a needle in the back. Lastly, there is a fear of becoming paralyzed because of some unsubstantiated report of paralysis from another patient. Quite often, communication between a patient and his or her anesthesiologist is inadequate because of the definition of ''sleep.'' To an anesthesiologist, a patient's request to be asleep often refers to general anesthesia. To the patient, moderate sedation, being only partially aware of intraoperative events rather than overt general anesthesia, is often what is meant by wanting to be ''asleep.'' Our approach is to instruct patients that they will be sedated and asleep, although we may intermittently allow them to awaken. If, at any time, the patient feels that the sedation is inadequate, all he or she has to do is to request additional sedation, which will be given. In our experience, patients who are moderately sedated usually are quite pleased. The fear of having a needle in the back or possibly having paralysis can be minimized by outlining the sequence of events that will lead to the operative procedure.

Preoperative Medication

To alleviate apprehension associated with an unknown venture, such as spinal anesthesia and a surgical procedure, ad-

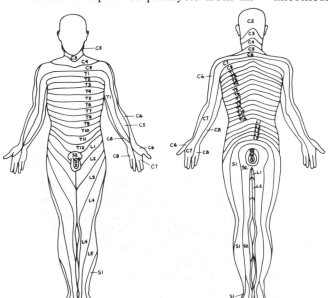

Figure 13-1. The dermatomes of the body shown in an orderly progression from the cranial to the caudal aspects of the body.

ministration of a drug which will produce sedation is often desirable in the immediate preoperative period. Furthermore, administration of a narcotic is helpful to alleviate some of the pain associated with institution of a spinal anesthetic. Although many preoperative medication schemes have been described and can be used (see Chapter 10), one approach is to combine the use of a narcotic, such as morphine 10 mg/70 kg intramuscularly, with a drug, such as diazepam 10 mg/70 kg orally. Anticholinergics are usually not required nor, in fact, desirable because of discomfort produced in an awake patient due to a dry mouth.

Technique for Institution of a Spinal Anesthetic

Equipment. Although reusable spinal anesthetic trays can be employed, use of a disposable commercially prepared tray is preferred (Fig. 13-2). Manufacturers of disposable trays have been able to duplicate almost completely those essential aspects of a reusable tray and provide more predictable sterilization procedures. A tray should include syringes for the intradermal injection of local anesthetic, a 5 ml glass or well functioning plastic syringe, 5 ml of 10 percent dextrose, 20 mg of tetracaine, 1 mg of epinephrine, and a 2.5 to 3.75 cm thin-walled 18 gauge introducer needle. Also, appropriate needles should be included such as a 25-gauge needle and an optional 22-gauge needle.

Most spinal anesthetics are performed with either a 22- or 25-gauge, 8.75 cm needle. For obese patients, a 12.5 cm needle is sometimes needed. The advantage of the 22-gauge needle is that it provides better proprioceptive information from the needle tip to the clinician, with regard to the tissues through which the needle is passing. Also, the 22-gauge needle is more rigid than the 25-gauge needle. Unfortunately, a 22-gauge needle has a significantly higher incidence of postspinal headache than does a 25-gauge needle, especially when used in younger pa-

tients. The disadvantage of a 25-gauge needle is that it can be easily distorted or bent with inappropriate usage. Some clinicians minimize this problem by utilization of an introducer needle placed into the interspinous ligament through which the 25-gauge needle is inserted with the introducer needle acting as a splint. Another disadvantage of the 25-gauge needle is the longer time it takes for the cerebrospinal fluid (CSF) to spontaneously track back through the needle and appear at the hub. Alternatively, CSF can be aspirated using a syringe attached to the needle.

Approaches to the Subarachnoid Space. There are three approaches that can be utilized for a lumbar dural puncture to produce spinal anesthesia. The most common one used is the midline approach.

Midline. The lateral or sitting position can be utilized. The lateral position is usually more satisfactory for patients who are ill or heavily sedated. The sitting position can be used when there is difficulty separating the lumbar spinous processes or a low level of spinal anesthesia is desired. In the lateral position, the patient should have his neck and legs flexed, but not into an uncomfortable or painful posture. The midline of the lumbar spinous processes are then identified, which may not necessarily be the midline of the skin of the back. When a well defined lumbar interspace is located, usually at L2-3, L3-4, or L4-5, the needle is introduced at right angles to the transverse plane of the back and directed somewhat cephalad (Fig. 13-3).[1] The needle should be introduced slowly through the thick and resistant ligamentum flavum until the point of the needle is free of the ligament. Then, the needle is advanced until the sensation of the needle going through the dura into the subarachnoid space is felt. An unsuccessful spinal puncture is almost always due to improper direction of the needle. Once the needle has traversed the dura and certainty exists that the bevel is entirely inside the

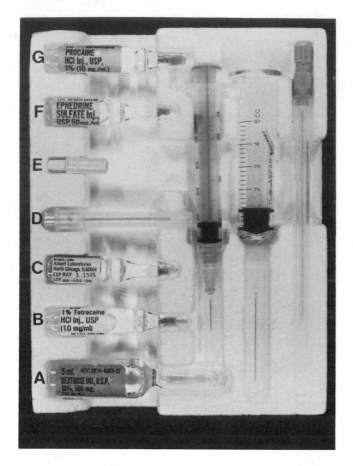

Figure 13-2. An illustration of a typical disposable tray used for spinal anesthesia. The contents of the vials are (A) 5 ml of 10 percent dextrose; (B) 2 ml of 1 percent tetracaine; (C) one ampule of epinephrine 1:1,000 (1 mg/ml); (D) a thin-walled introducer needle, (E) a 5 micron filter; (F) one ampule of ephedrine (50 mg/ml); and (G) 2 ml of 1 percent procaine.

subarachnoid space, the needle can be stabilized by grasping the hub of the needle between the thumb and forefinger of one hand and by resting the hand against the patient's back. If this is not done during the removal of CSF and injection of solution, the needle is apt to be displaced by traction or pressure on the syringe attached to the needle.

Paramedian. The paramedian approach has the advantage of not being so dependent on the patient properly flexing and is useful in obese patients. This approach is performed by introducing the needle 1 to 2 cm from the midline opposite the selected lumbar spinous process. The needle should be

directed slightly cephalad at an angle of 15 to 20 degrees. At the appropriate depth, the needle will pass through the ligamentum flavum, the epidural space, and then into the subarachnoid space.

Lumbosacral (Taylor). The largest interspace in the vertebral column is the L5-S1 interspace. To enter this interspace the needle should be introduced through the skin wheal approximately 1 cm medial and 1 cm cephalad to the posterior superior iliac spine (Fig. 13-3). The needle is then directed cephalad and medially. If the sacrum is contacted, the needle should be walked cephalad until it slips off the surface of the

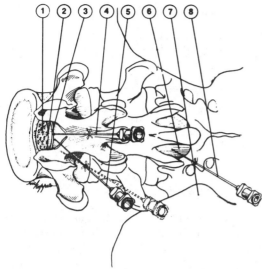

Figure 13-3. A dorsal view of the fourth and fifth lumbar vertebrae and their relation to the sacrum and iliac bones. (1) The cauda equina; (2) the dura mater; (3) the ligamentum flavum at the L3 to L4 interspace; (4) the midline approach for spinal and epidural techniques; (5) the paramedian approach when the needle puncture site is 1 to 2 cm lateral to the above midline approach; (6) a larger interspace between S5 and L1, which is situated 2 cm medial and cephalad from the (7) posterior superior iliac spine; (8) the needle can be introduced at this site in the "Taylor" approach to either the subarachnoid or epidural space. (Murphy TM. Spinal, epidural and caudal anesthesia. In: Miller RD, ed. Anesthesia. New York, Churchill Livingstone, 1981; 635–78.)

sacrum, pierces the ligamentum flavum, and enters the subarachnoid space.

Drugs and Factors Which Influence the Level of Anesthesia

Local Anesthetics and Vasoconstrictors. Although several local anesthetics are available for producing spinal anesthesia, procaine, lidocaine, and tetracaine are the most commonly used and provide a broad spectrum of durations of action (Table 13-1). The duration of spinal anesthesia can be increased by approximately 50 percent if a vasoconstrictor, such as epinephrine, is added to the solution injected into the CSF.

Either 0.1 mg or 0.2 mg of epinephrine (e.g., 0.1 or 0.2 ml of a 1:1,000 solution) is the most common vasoconstrictor used. Phenylephrine can also be injected in doses ranging from 1 to 4 mg. Phenylephrine appears to be more potent than epinephrine and can produce an even longer duration of spinal anesthesia. It should be emphasized that although certain doses of local anesthetic are required to achieve a given level of anesthesia, other factors such as baricity of the injected solution and position of the patient are the primary determinants of the level of anesthesia.

Baricity and Position of the Patient. CSF has a specific gravity of 1.003 to 1.009. A primary determinant as to what level of spinal anesthesia will be achieved is the specific gravity of the local anesthetic solution being injected relative to that of CSF. When the local anesthetic solution is heavier or has a higher specific gravity than CSF, it is termed a hyperbaric solution. Conversely, when the local anesthetic solution has a lower specific gravity than that of CSF, it is called a hypobaric solution. When the local anesthetic solution has a specific gravity equal to that of CSF, it is called an isobaric solution. The hyperbaric solution is most popular and is achieved by mixing the local anesthetic with a 10 percent dextrose solution. Being heavier than CSF, this solution will settle to the most dependent aspect of the subarachnoid space which is determined by the position of the patient. For example, if one wishes the level of spinal anesthesia to be high (e.g., T4), then putting the patient in the head-down position will enhance the cephalad spread of the local anesthetic. A common hyperbaric solution to inject is 10 to 12 mg of tetracaine (1.0 to 1.2 ml), 0.2 mg of 1:1000 epinephrine (0.2 ml), and 1.5 ml of 10 percent dextrose.

Hypobaric solutions are less frequently used, but at times can be very helpful, especially for perineal or rectal procedures, such as a hemorrhoidectomy, where the

Table 3-1. The Dose and Duration of Action of Drugs Used for Spinal Anesthesia

| Drug | Dose (mg)[a] | | | Duration (min) | |
	L1	T10	T4	Plain	Epinephrine 0.2 mg
Procaine	50	100	150	30–45	60–75
Lidocaine	50	75	100	45–60	60–90
Tetracaine	6	9	12	60–90	120–180

[a] Dose when diluted as described in text.

surgical approach requires the patient to be in the jack-knife prone position. Therefore, the highest part of the subarachnoid space is the sacral area. Hypobaric solutions introduced into the subarachnoid space will float to the caudal end of the subarachnoid space and produce effective analgesia of the sacral dermatomes. Also, with a total hip arthroplasty, the patient can be put into the lateral position for surgery before the local anesthetic is injected. Because it is hypobaric, the anesthetic solution will tend to rise to the nondependent side, which is the side upon which surgery will be performed. To achieve a hypobaric solution, the local anesthetic is usually mixed with sterile water. A common mixture is 8 to 10 mg of tetracaine (0.8 to 1.0 ml), 0.2 mg of 1 : 1000 epinephrine (0.2 ml), and 6 to 8 ml of sterile water.

Isobaric solutions are not widely used, but can be employed when anesthesia is required at a specific level, such as for lower extremity surgery or surgery for a fractured hip. The solution can be made by diluting the local anesthetic mixture with CSF.

Although several factors, such as intra-abdominal pressure and patient straining, can be influential, there is no doubt that the baricity of the solution to be injected into the subarachnoid space and the position of the patient at the time of the injection are the two most important criteria in determining the level of spinal anesthesia that is achieved, assuming an adequate dose of drug has been administered.

Problems with Technique

Paresthesias. A paresthesia which radiates to one of the legs during insertion of the needle presumably reflects contact of the needle with a nerve. Theoretically, it is important not to inject the local anesthetic during a paresthesia, as an intraneural injection might enhance the chances of a neurological complication postoperatively. Nevertheless, this supposition has not been proven. If, during the beginning of an injection, a paresthesia is elicited, the needle should be redirected and the injection then continued without paresthesia.

Failure to achieve spinal anesthesia can most often be attributed to failure to introduce all of the local anesthetic solution into the subarachnoid space. The needle has either been dislodged or the bevel was not totally within the subarachnoid space. When there is a failure to achieve spinal anesthesia, it is permissable to reintroduce the needle and reinject the same or a lesser amount of local anesthetic. A sufficient length of time should be taken, however, to be assured that lack of anesthesia is not merely due to a delay in onset (e.g., at least 20 minutes). In some patients, the needle may be introduced and a flow of CSF appears, but the anesthesiologist cannot aspirate fluid into the syringe. When this occurs, it may be helpful to rotate the needle, as the flow of CSF is probably obstructed by a segment of the pia mater or ligament.

Table 13-2. Level of Spinal Anesthesia Necessary for Certain Surgical Procedures

Level	Type of Surgery
S2–S5	Rectal surgery
L2–L3	Foot surgery
L1	Lower extremity
T10 (umbilicus)	Hip and transurethral surgery, resection of the prostate
T6 (xiphoid process)	Lower abdominal surgery
T4 (nipple)	Upper abdominal surgery

If CSF cannot be aspirated, it is prudent to remove and then reinsert the needle in the midline. Failure to aspirate CSF is often associated with a partial or complete failure to achieve spinal anesthesia.

Bloody Tap. Occasionally, blood-tinged CSF will flow from the needle. Frequently, the CSF will be clear of blood after several drops. If clear CSF can then be aspirated, the injection may proceed. If blood-tinged CSF continues to flow from the needle, the local anesthetic should not be injected.

Documentation of the Block

Within 30 to 60 seconds after injecting the local anesthetic, an attempt should be made to determine the developing level of spinal anesthesia. The desired level of anesthesia is dependent on the type of surgery that is being performed (Table 13-2). Because the sympathetic nerves are usually the first ones to be blocked, an early indication of the level of spinal anesthesia can be achieved by testing the patient with an alcohol sponge. In the area that is blocked by the spinal anesthetic, the alcohol sponge should produce a neutral or warm sensation, rather than the cold sensation that will be felt in the unblocked areas. Therefore, the response to temperature provides an early indication as to the developing level of spinal anesthesia. Classically, sympathetic nervous system blockade produced by spinal anesthesia is two dermatomes above the level of sensory blockade (e.g., zone of differential blockade). Motor blockade typically is two dermatomes below the level of sensory blockade. If an appropriate level of spinal anesthesia is not being achieved, as indicated by the response to the alcohol sponge, the patient can be repositioned in an attempt to alter the level of anesthesia. Soon thereafter, the level of sensory blockade can be tested by a pin prick. If one is performing many spinal anesthetics, perhaps a stamp could be made in which the anesthesiologist fills in the blanks as to which level of anesthesia had been achieved and what drugs had been administered, along with the other important details (Table 13-3).

Physiology of Spinal Anesthesia

Circulation. Peripheral sympathetic nervous system blockade is the major determinant of circulatory responses produced by spinal anesthesia. Since the level of sympathetic blockade is about two dermatomes higher than that of sensory blockade, it is predictable that a sensory level of T3 will result in total sympathetic blockade (remembering that the highest preganglionic sympathetic fibers arise from the spinal cord at T1). With a high spinal anesthetic, decreases in blood pressure and central venous pressure can be expected.[2] The magnitude of reduction in blood pressure parallels the level of sympathetic blockade produced by spinal anesthesia. The decrease in blood pressure is primarily due to a decrease in cardiac output secondary to pooling of blood in denervated veins. Arterial vasodilation with a decrease in calculated systemic vascular resistance contributes minimally to the decrease in blood pressure during spinal anesthesia. Bradycardia is common during spinal anesthesia, reflecting block of sympathetic cardiac nerves.

Treatment of hypotension during spinal anesthesia is to increase venous return

Table 13-3. Basic Documentation on the Anesthetic Record of a Spinal Anesthetic

Position _____	Paresthesias _____
Prep solution _____	Drugs injected _____
Needle size _____	Quality of CSF[a] _____
Level of injection _____	Level of anesthesia _____
Number of attempts _____	

[a] CSF, cerebrospinal fluid.

which facilitates cardiac output. This objective is best achieved by placing the patient in a modest head-down position and administering intravenous crystalloid solution. Excess fluid administration, however, may produce undesirable degrees of hemodilution. In some instances, a sympathomimetic, such as ephedrine 10 to 25 mg/70 mg intravenously, may be necessary to promptly increase blood pressure. Bradycardia that is associated with hypotension is treated with intravenous atropine 0.2 to 0.4 mg.

Respiration. Respiratory function is usually unimpaired with low levels of spinal anesthesia. For example, high sensory levels (T1) of spinal anesthesia are associated with an unchanged resting minute ventilation and arterial blood gases. Conversely, inspiratory capacity is minimally decreased and expiratory reserve volume is markedly decreased.[3] It is probable that the reduced expiratory reserve volume impairs the patient's ability to cough.

Gastrointestinal Tract. The preganglionic sympathetic fibers from T5 to L1 are inhibitory to the gastrointestinal tract. Therefore, during spinal anesthesia, the small intestine is contracted due to unopposed activity of the vagus nerve. In contrast, the sphincters are relaxed and peristalsis is active.

Complications

Headache. A headache is the most frequent complication following spinal anesthesia. Young parturients are most likely to develop this complication but the incidence of postspinal headache, even in this group, is only about 1 percent when a 25-gauge needle is used to perform the block. A postspinal headache is most likely due to a persistent leak of CSF through the needle hole in the dura mater with resultant intracranial tension on meningeal vessels and nerves. A true postspinal headache is characterized by its dependence on posture. Usually, the headache is not present in the supine position, but occurs when the patient attempts to assume the upright position. Typically, a postspinal headache is occipital in location. Transient diplopia associated with a postspinal headache most likely reflects stretch of the abducens nerve. It is important to establish whether the headache is due to the spinal anesthetic or to other causes. Careful assessment of the dependence of the headache on posture will markedly aid in the differential diagnosis.

Milder forms of the postspinal headache can be treated conservatively by enforcing bed rest for 24 to 48 hours. Symptomatic treatment can be achieved with analgesics and/or sedatives. Various approaches have been utilized to restore the pressure relationship between the epidural and subarachnoid spaces. These measures include use of abdominal binders forcing more venous blood through the epidural plexuses and aggressive hydration of the patient, either through administration of intravenous fluids or by forcing oral fluid intake of 3 liters or more daily.

For many years, the epidural administration of saline has been observed to frequently alleviate a postspinal headache, usually on a transient basis. For those patients who do not respond to conservative measures during the first 24 hours, administration of the patient's own blood, rather than saline, into the epidural space, usually results in permanent relief of the headache.[4] This is commonly called a "blood-patch epidural." Specifically, administration of 5 to 10 ml of the patient's own (aseptically drawn) blood into the epidural space at the site of the previous lumbar puncture results in prompt and persistent relief of the postspinal headache. Presumably a blood patch epidural is effective by stopping the leak of CSF such that normal pressures in the subarachnoid space are restored. This procedure may be repeated 24 hours later if the headache is not completely relieved. Complications from a blood patch epidural are few and minor. The most common one is a backache, which dissipates within 24 to 48 hours. Clearly, the blood patch epidural for treatment of a postspinal headache is a very effective approach with few known risks.

Urinary Retention. Because a spinal anesthetic blocks the nerve supply to the bladder, administration of large amounts of fluids intravenously can cause bladder distention, which may require catheter drainage. This often is a problem with patients who are having relatively minor surgery (e.g., inguinal hernia repair) and in whom it would be undesirable to catheterize the bladder. This problem can be minimized by being prudent with the amount of crystalloid solution administered intravenously.

Nausea and vomiting occasionally occur at the beginning of a spinal anesthetic, especially if hypotension is present. Treatment of the hypotension will sometimes be effective treatment for the nausea and vomiting. If the nausea and vomiting persist despite treatment of hypotension, administration of oxygen via a mask, or atropine, 0.2 to 0.4 mg/70 kg intravenously, if bradycardia is present, is often helpful. If the nausea and vomiting still persist, administration of diazepam or droperidol may be effective.

Neurologic Sequelae. Although neurologic sequelae to spinal anesthetics are feared and often the subject of conversation by lay persons, they are in fact extremely rare. In an analysis of 582,190 cases of spinal anesthesia, there was a zero incidence of permanent motor paralysis.[5] In another evaluation of 10,000 cases of spinal anesthesia, there was only one neurologic complication which could be attributed to the spinal anesthetic.[6] It is important that the anesthesiologist ascertain whether any neurological deficits exist preoperatively so as to assure that a postoperative neurological complication was not actually present preoperatively. Secondly, if a neurological complication does occur, it may be due to other causes. For example, is a subdural hematoma forming, which could be relieved surgically with no permanent neurological difficulties? Also, neurological injuries should be carefully evaluated as to their site (e.g., peripheral nerve vs. spinal cord). This classification will help identify whether the neurologic problem was secondary to positioning or operative trauma, rather than due to the spinal anesthesia.

EPIDURAL ANESTHESIA

Comparison of Epidural and Spinal Anesthesia

In most respects, epidural anesthesia is similar to spinal anesthesia. The major site of action of the local anesthetic placed in

Table 13-4. Dose and Duration of Anesthesia of Different Drugs Used for Epidural Anesthesia

Drug	Percentage	mg/Segment[a]	Duration (min)
Chloroprocaine	3.0	45	60
Lidocaine	1.5	23	50
Bupivacaine	0.5	7	120
Etidocaine	1.0	15	170
Mepivacaine	1.5	23	60

[a] Although this is stated in mg/segment, volume of the solution injected is very important. Generally, 1 to 1.5 ml of local anesthetic per segment are required.

the epidural space is probably at the nerve roots and dorsal root ganglia beyond the point of the meningeal covering. To a lesser extent, local anesthetics can be found to diffuse into the subarachnoid space itself.

At a given sensory level, the responses to epidural and spinal anesthesia are quantitatively different. The onset of peripheral sympathetic nervous system blockade and development of hypotension is slower with epidural anesthesia. In contrast to spinal anesthesia, the levels of sensory and sympathetic blockade produced by epidural anesthesia are similar while the zone of differential blockade for motor blockade is greater, being up to five dermatomes lower than the level of sensory anesthesia. A disadvantage of epidural anesthesia compared to spinal anesthesia is that much larger doses of local anesthetic are required, which enhances the chance of having a systemic reaction to the local anesthetic. Conversely, the incidence of a "postspinal" headache following an epidural anesthetic should be zero since the dura is not punctured. Lastly, insertion of a catheter into the epidural space permits repeated injection of local anesthetic or narcotic which can provide analgesia for many hours in the postoperative period.

Technique for Institution of an Epidural Anesthetic

Equipment. Usually, a 16- or 18-gauge Tuohy needle with a Huber point is utilized. The Tuohy needle is constructed so that the blunt leading edge of the needle has a lateral opening at the tip. This type of construction should reduce the incidence of dural puncture, because the blunt leading end will be less likely to puncture the dura than a sharp, pointed needle. Sometimes, the Crawford needle is utilized in which the orifice is at the distal end of the needle. With this needle, the risk of dural puncture can be reduced by injecting a bolus of saline or air as the epidural space is entered.

In general, the equipment necessary for an epidural injection is similar to that required for a spinal anesthetic, with two exceptions (Fig. 13-4). First, a different type of needle is utilized, as described above. Secondly, a well-functioning glass syringe which has no resistance upon moving the plunger is required when the loss of resistance technique is used for identifying the epidural space.

Location of Epidural Space. The position of the patient should be identical to that required for a dural puncture for spinal anesthesia. At the appropriate interspace, a 16- to 18-gauge needle can be introduced in the same manner as a spinal needle would be introduced. Because pressure in the epidural space is lower than atmospheric, the "loss of resistance" technique can be utilized. After inserting the needle until the intraspinous ligament or ligamentum flavum has been located, the stylet should be removed and a glass syringe attached to the needle. The needle is then advanced slowly until one feels a sudden loss of resistance to gentle compression of the plunger in the syringe.

Drugs. Although the number of mg per segment of anesthesia desired is often expressed, the volume of local anesthetic is of prime importance. In general, it takes about 1 to 1.5 ml of local anesthetic per segment to produce adequate anesthesia.

After the needle has been introduced into the epidural space, a 2 to 3 ml test dose

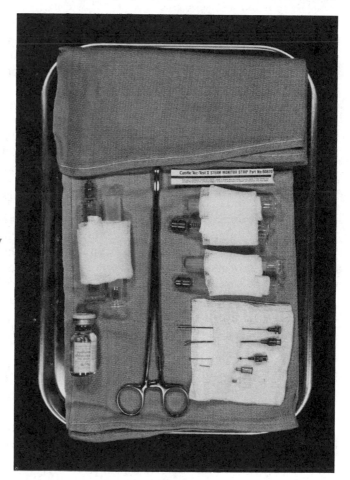

Figure 13-4. A typical epidural tray used for epidural anesthesia.

should be injected, usually with epinephrine, to ascertain whether the needle is subarachnoid or in a blood vessel. If the needle is intravascular, a tachycardia should result from injection of the local anesthetic with epinephrine. Absence of sensory analgesia or motor paralysis in the lower extremities or saddle area during a 3 to 5 minute period confirms that the needle is not subarachnoid and the remainder of local anesthetic can then be injected. The baricity of the local anesthetic solution does not influence the height of epidural anesthesia. If prolonged anesthesia is required, a plastic epidural catheter can be inserted through the needle approximately 2 to 3 cm beyond the tip. When the local anesthetic is introduced

through this catheter, an additional test dose should be injected because these catheters can migrate into the subarachnoid space or into a blood vessel even though the needle appears not to be in that location.

Factors Which Influence Level of Anesthesia

Weight and Height. Weight has little to do with the dose of local anesthetic required to produce epidural anesthesia. Extremes in height, however, will alter the dose. A rule of thumb is to use 1.0 ml of local anesthetic per segment for a person who is 150 cm tall, and then add 0.1 ml per segment for each 5 cm above 150 cm in height.

Age. The dose of local anesthetic required for epidural anesthesia decreases with increasing age. A rule of thumb is that 1.0 to 1.5 ml of local anesthetic per segment is required for a patient who is 20 to 40 years of age. For a patient who is 40 to 60 years of age, 0.5 to 1.0 ml per segment is required and 0.3 to 0.5 ml per segment for patients over 60 years of age.

Position. Although position is clearly important for a spinal anesthetic, it is of less importance for an epidural anesthetic. Still, there is no doubt that in the lateral position, the dependent part of the body will have a slightly more profound block than the non-dependent side.

Physiology of Epidural Anesthesia

Cardiovascular. Conceptually, an epidural anesthetic should produce hypotension similar to that of a spinal anesthetic. Although the degree of hypotension is probably similar, the onset time is delayed with an epidural anesthetic, reflecting a slower onset of peripheral sympathetic nervous system blockade. Furthermore, the presence of epinephrine in the local anesthetic mixture injected into the epidural space is associated with a larger decrease in blood pressure than when the local anesthetic is used without epinephrine.[7] Cardiac output, however, is increased when epinephrine is used. Therefore, the beta effect of epinephrine is predominant with the low circulating levels of epinephrine achieved from systemic absorption of an epinephrine-containing local anesthetic solution placed in the epidural space. When epinephrine is not included with the local anesthetic, the reductions in blood pressure and calculated systemic vascular resistance are minimal.

Respiration. The respiratory effects of epidural anesthesia are essentially the same as with spinal anesthesia. The loss of proprioception due to blockade of the thoracic sensory nerves leads to a reduction of sensory input to the respiratory motor nuclei and a subsequent reduced, but adequate, motor output carried via the phrenic nerves. Usually, normal respiratory gas exchange is achieved even with upper abdominal surgery. The only danger may be that the ability to cough is compromised because of the intercostal and abdominal wall skeletal muscle paralysis.

Complications

Accidental Dural Puncture. After apparent insertion of the needle into the epidural space, clear fluid may either spontaneously flow from the needle or be aspirated. This fluid may be CSF, saline that was injected during determination of the loss of resistance, or the local anesthetic. There are several techniques utilized to determine whether the fluid is CSF. If the drops of fluid are allowed to fall on the forearm of the anesthesiologist, the temperature of local anesthetic or saline will be cold compared to CSF. Also, if the fluid is allowed to drip onto a fresh test strip for glucose, the presence of glucose would indicate CSF.

Hopefully, administration of a test dose of local anesthetic would ascertain whether the needle was in the subarachnoid space. If a large dose of local anesthetic is inadvertently injected into the subarachnoid space, however, a total spinal anesthetic probably will result. The main danger of a total spinal anesthetic is the potential for profound hypotension and respiratory paralysis. The adverse effects of a total spinal anesthetic are easily managed, however, with prompt attention to ventilation of the lungs, head-down tilt, intravenous fluid infusion and, on occasion, the administration of a sympathomimetic to maintain perfusion pressure.

Intravascular Injection. Because the epidural space is highly vascular, and a large volume of local anesthetic is frequently required to achieve adequate anesthesia, a large dose of local anesthetic can be inadvertently injected intravascularly and produce systemic toxicity, mainly in the form of seizures (see Chapter 7).

Backache. Because larger needles are utilized, the incidence and severity of backache probably are more pronounced after epidural anesthesia than after spinal anesthesia. There are no data, however, to support this claim. If a backache does occur, it will usually disappear within 48 to 72 hours.

Epidural hematoma is an almost unheard complication of epidural anesthesia in patients who do not have a pre-existing coagulation defect. In all cases, however, there is a rapid onset of neurological deficit and/or severe back pain. When these signs occur, the presence of an epidural hematoma should be investigated, including consideration of myelography. A laminectomy should be performed if an epidural hematoma is present as recovery of neurologic function is likely if surgical decompression is performed promptly.

A prolonged bleeding time due to platelet dysfunction from aspirin therapy represents a dilemma if regional anesthesia is planned. Theoretically, the risk of formation of an epidural hematoma is increased. Nevertheless, there is no evidence that epidural block should be avoided in patients with prolonged bleeding time due to aspirin therapy.

CAUDAL ANESTHESIA

The epidural space can be located via the caudal (sacral) canal. Caudal anesthesia lends itself well to surgical procedures of the lower extremities, perineum, and lower abdomen. Most anesthesiologists, however, find the lumbar rather than sacral approach to the epidural space to be a more predictable and easier technique to utilize. Frequently, in obese patients, the land-

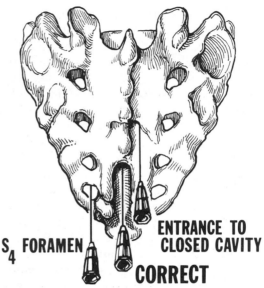

Figure 13-5. The correct placement for insertion of a needle for caudal anesthesia. Needles can be inadvertently inserted into a closed cavity, or into the fourth sacral foramen, as indicated above.

marks for insertion of the caudal anesthetic are obscure. Even with experienced anesthesiologists, there are occasional failures to achieve anesthesia because of abnormalities in the anatomy of the caudal canal.

Anatomy

The caudal canal is the distal continuation of the epidural space and is contained within the sacrum. The crucial landmark for identification of the caudal canal is the sacral hiatus which varies considerably between individuals. Typically, the sacral hiatus is about 5 cm from the tip of the coccyx in the midline. In some patients, however, the sacral hiatus can be in a more rostral position.

Technique for Institution of a Caudal Anesthetic

With the patient in the prone position, preferably with a pillow under the pubis, the sacral cornu are identified (Fig. 13-5). These are defined by palpating the tip of the coccyx and working the fingers cephalad until the tip of the finger identifies the depression into the sacral hiatus. Then, by moving the finger laterally, the sacral cornu on both sides can be identified. At the most cephalad point of the sacral hiatus, the needle should be introduced perpendicular to the skin until the sacrum is contacted. The needle is then slightly withdrawn and the angle reduced before advancing it through the sacrococcygeal membrane and into the caudal canal. The bevel of the needle is often turned downward to facilitate its passage through the caudal canal for a distance of approximately 3 to 3.5 cm. Confirmation that the needle is actually in the caudal canal can be made by injecting 4 to 5 ml of air through the needle and palpating the skin for a crepitant feeling. If no such feeling occurs, the needle is probably in the caudal canal. If a crepitant feeling is detected, however, the needle is probably posterior to the caudal canal and should be removed and reinserted.

Complications

Many of the complications associated with caudal anesthesia are the same as those for lumbar epidural anesthesia. Infection, however, is a more likely complication considering the close proximity of the caudal canal to the rectum Nevertheless, infection is extremely rare, particularly with a single shot injection. Continuous techniques which utilize a catheter are more likely to be associated with infection.

Another complication is the possibility of an intraosseous injection. Because the sacral bone is thin, the cortex can be easily penetrated. An intraosseous injection may manifest itself by the appearance of a gritty aspirate of a small volume of apparently pure blood following the test injection of local anesthetic solution. Lastly, a subarachnoid injection is possible with any epidural anesthetic technique. Because the dural sac ends at the lower level of S2, which is equivalent to a line joining the two posterior superior iliac spines, a dural puncture can be avoided by keeping the caudal needle distal to this site.

SUMMARY

Of the three anesthetic techniques described in this chapter, a spinal anesthetic is technically easiest to perform and, therefore, probably has more widespread use. An epidural anesthetic has the advantage of evoking cardiovascular effects which occur at a slower rate than with a spinal block. Furthermore, the avoidance of a postspinal headache is an advantage for epidural anesthesia. Overall, the use of spinal, epidural, or caudal anesthesia provides advantages over general anesthesia.[8–10] These techniques add to the flexibility of the various anesthetic options available to the surgical patient, especially with the opportunity to provide analgesia in the immediate postoperative period without the use of intravascularly or intramuscularly administered narcotics.

REFERENCES

1. Murphy TM. Spinal, epidural and caudal anesthesia. In: Miller RD, ed. New York, Churchill Livingstone, 1981:635–78.
2. Kennedy WF Jr. The effects of spinal and peridural blocks on renal and hepatic functions. In: Bonica JJ, ed. Regional anesthesia: recent advances and current status. Clinical Anesthesia Series II. Philadelphia, F. A. Davis, 1969:110–21.
3. Freund FG, Bonica JJ, Ward RJ, Akamatsu TJ, Kennedy WF Jr. Ventilatory reserve and level of motor block during high spinal and epidural anesthesia. Anesthesiology 1967;28:834–7.
4. Abouleish E. Epidural blood patch for treatment of chronic postlumbar puncture cephalgia. Anesthesiology 1978;49:291–2.
5. Lund PC. Principles and practice of spinal anesthesia. Springfield, Charles C Thomas, 1971.
6. Nolte H. Current and future status of spinal anesthesia for surgery. Regional Anesthesia, 1979;4:10.

7. Ward RJ, Bonica JJ, Freund FG. Epidural and subarachnoid anesthesia. JAMA 1965;191:275–8.

8. Bridenbaugh PO, Kennedy WF Jr. Spinal, subarachnoid neural blockade. In: Cousins MJ, Bridenbaugh PO, eds. Neural Blockade. Philadelphia, J. B. Lippincott Company, 1980;146–75.

9. Cousins MJ. Epidural neural blockade. In: Cousins MJ, Bridenbaugh PO, eds. Neural Blockade. Philadelphia, J. B. Lippincott Company, 1980;176–274.

10. McCaul K. Caudal blockade. In: Cousins MJ, Bridenbaugh PO, eds. Neural Blockade. Philadelphia, J. B. Lippincott Company, 1980;275–94.

14

Peripheral Nerve Blocks

Peripheral nerve blocks are used for (1) intraoperative anesthesia, (2) postoperative analgesia, and (3) diagnosis and/or therapy for chronic pain syndromes (see Chapter 33).[1,2] This type of anesthesia can offer significant advantages over other anesthetic techniques. For example, intraoperatively, if only that area upon which the surgical procedure is to be conducted is anesthetized, the cardiovascular and respiratory effects of inhaled anesthetics can be avoided. In other situations, complete relaxation of skeletal muscles can be achieved without the use of muscle relaxants. There are, however, disadvantages of peripheral nerve blocks, with the most important being the significant incidence of failure. This is in contrast to general anesthesia, which can permit successful surgery to be completed virtually 100 percent of the time. Obviously, success with a peripheral nerve block depends on placing the needle as close to the target nerve as possible. This requires a working knowledge of the surface landmarks and overall anatomy.

PREPARATION PRIOR TO THE BLOCK

Preoperative Visit

The main purpose of the preoperative visit is to discuss the choice of anesthetic and to ensure that the physical condition of the patient is appropriate for performing a peripheral nerve block to provide anesthesia for the planned surgical procedure. The first step is to inform and prepare the patient for a peripheral nerve block. As with regional anesthesia, patients often state that they would "rather be asleep" during the surgical procedure which may be misinterpreted as a desire to "be asleep" with general anesthesia. Quite often, this request to "be asleep" can be achieved by administration of small doses of a sedative-hypnotic and/or narcotic to produce light sleep or amnesic tranquilization. Patients can be reassured by the anesthesiologist that additional "sleep medication" can be given if, at any time during the surgical procedure, they feel uncomfortable. Reassurance that sleep medication will be given will often alleviate these fears and increase the acceptance of peripheral nerve block anesthesia by patients.

In addition to the usual preoperative evaluation, the landmarks needed for a particular peripheral nerve block should be examined to confirm that there are no impediments to performing a successful nerve block. Such impediments might include cutaneous infections, old operative scars, and osseous fusions. Lastly, patients should be questioned as to whether they have a bleeding tendency. If such a history is positive, confirmation of a normal clotting mechanism should be obtained. If abnormal, this would speak against not only peripheral nerve block anesthesia, but even perhaps the surgical procedure itself.

Preoperative Medication

Preoperative medication prior to anticipated peripheral nerve block should be given in sufficient amounts to minimize apprehension upon arrival in the operating room or holding area and to provide analgesia during insertion of the needles while performing the block. Yet, performing a successful peripheral nerve block often requires communication with the patient regarding paresthesias. Although there are many preoperative medication schemes, frequently the combination of a narcotic and a sedative-hypnotic will suffice (see Chapter 10). For example, morphine 10 to 15 mg/70 kg intramuscularly or diazepam 10 mg/70 kg orally is usually sufficient. The rationale for including a benzodiazepine in the preoperative medication is animal data demonstrating intramuscular diazepam is effective in elevating the seizure threshold for lidocaine.[1] For procedures that do not require patient cooperation to report paresthesias (e.g., intercostal nerve blocks), larger doses of premedication drugs can be considered. The administration of an anticholinergic is not necessary prior to a peripheral nerve block and in fact can lead to an uncomfortable awake patient because of a dry mouth.

Optimal Site in Operating Room Area to Perform Block

Although peripheral nerve blocks certainly can be performed in the operating room, performing them in another location has the advantage of avoiding the noise and pressure from an anxious surgical audience. Such areas might be a holding area adjacent to the operating room or the recovery room. This allows the peripheral nerve block to be performed either at the end of the previous surgical procedure or while the operating room is being prepared for the next pro-

cedure. Furthermore, the onset of anesthesia with a peripheral nerve block is often not rapid. If, for example, the nerve block is performed in the recovery room, the patient has to then be transported to the operating room, positioned, and prepped before the incision can be made. This process often provides time sufficient for a nerve block to take effect before the surgeons are ready to make the incision.

Equipment. The room in which the peripheral nerve block is to be performed should contain monitoring equipment and drugs for the diagnosis and treatment of toxic reactions to the local anesthetic.[2–4] Disposable peripheral nerve block trays are becoming increasingly available (Fig. 14-1). There is a wide spectrum of opinion as to what equipment should be on a basic nerve block tray. Most peripheral nerve blocks can be performed with standard needles and Luer-Lok syringes. Syringes that do not have a locking device may be associated with frustrating experiences of leaks of local anesthetic when the syringe detaches itself from the needle and sprays the solution widely. Some clinicians recommend that a control syringe with a ring holder should be available because it permits one-handed aspiration during the block (Fig. 14-2).[3] This is important for ascertaining whether the needle has entered a blood vessel or is in the subarachnoid space. By permitting one-handed operation of the syringe and drug administration, the anesthesiologist's other hand is free to stabilize the relationship of the needle.

Needles. It is desirable to have a variety of needle sizes that will attach to a Luer-Lok syringe. A 22-gauge needle is probably the most satisfactory for performance of the majority of peripheral nerve blocks. The tip of the needle should be blunt, rather than having a long, sharp taper. Long, thin-tapered needles have a tendency to pierce nerves, whereas blunt needles tend to push

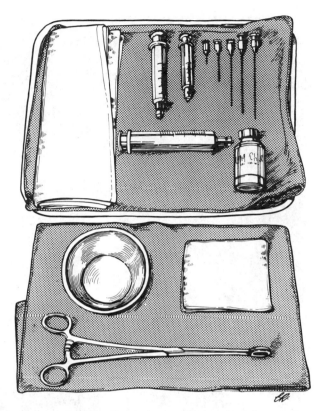

Figure 14-1. An illustration of a nerve block tray containing the essential ingredients necessary for performing a peripheral nerve block.

the nerve ahead of them which theoretically will reduce the risk of neural damage (Fig. 14-3).[3,5] Also, a blunt needle transmits changes of resistance more readily than a needle with a sharp point. Changes of resistance are important in certain nerve blocks as anatomic guides.

Safety. Whenever large doses of local anesthetic have been administered, certain resuscitative equipment should be available. An inadvertent intravascular injection of local anesthetic can result in seizures and myocardial depression (see Chapter 7). Therefore, an intravenous catheter should usually be present through which resuscitative drugs, such as diazepam, thiopental, or sympathomimetics, can be given. Equipment to maintain the airway includes a bag and mask apparatus (Ambu bag) plus a source of supplemental oxygen. Also, a laryngoscope and endotracheal tubes should be available in case intubation of the trachea is necessary.

INTRAOPERATIVE MANAGEMENT

Because there is a significant failure rate with peripheral nerve block anesthesia, and the pressures of the operating room team sometimes may dictate proceeding with surgery before the nerve block is 100 percent effective, equipment must be available to administer anesthesia, ranging from light sedation to a general anesthetic. In the presence of a successfully performed peripheral nerve block, however, adequate sedation and reassurance may be the difference between a failed and acceptable anesthetic. Small intravenous doses of a benzodiazepine, such as diazepam (2 to 5 mg/70 kg) are often useful in attenuating apprehension. Obviously, adequate monitoring of airway and cardiovascular functions are as essential during peripheral nerve block anesthesia as during other types of anesthesia. Also, the spoken word may be as effective as drugs in reassuring some patients. Anes-

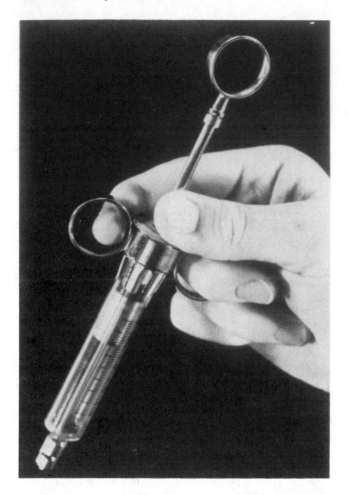

Figure 14-2. To grip the syringe, the index and middle fingers hold the syringe barrel via control rings; the thumb can be used to secure the metal piston and prevent drug leakage from the syringe during transfer. During injection, the thumb is inserted in the ring on the piston and pressure on this ring enables detection of "loss of resistance" to injection as the syringe and needle are advanced. (Murphy TM. Nerve blocks. In: Miller RD, ed. Anesthesia. New York, Churchill Livingstone, 1981;593–634.)

thesiologists use hypnosis, both knowingly and unknowingly, in reassuring and acquiring the cooperation of patients during the intraoperative period. Sedation can also be provided by allowing the patient to inhale 50 to 75 percent nitrous oxide. This approach permits the termination of sedation within minutes following surgery.

AIDS IN HELPING TO POSITION THE NEEDLE

Paresthesias

When the needle comes in contact with the desired nerve, the patient will experience paresthesias in the peripheral distribution of that nerve. Although this technique of needle positioning is advantageous in that it precisely identifies the nerve to be blocked, it is an uncomfortable sensation for the patient. If elicitation of paresthesias are essential, a moderately sedated patient may be more cooperative and experience less intraoperative apprehension.

Paresthesias elicited during performance of axillary blocks have been associated with an increased incidence of post-block nerve deficits.[6] Symptoms of such a lesion vary from mild paresthesia lasting a few weeks to severe paresthesia, ache, and paresis lasting more than a year. The absence of paresthesia is associated with fewer post-block lesions. Since paresthesias are essential, however, to successfully performing certain peripheral nerve blocks, it may be important to know whether the needle is in-

Figure 14-3. Note the shallow bevel of the needle on the left, which is the optimal type of point for performance of peripheral nerve blocks because it is less likely to traumatize nerves than the sharper needle. A 22-gauge needle is optimal for performance of most peripheral nerve blocks. (Murphy TM. Nerve blocks. In: Miller RD, ed. Anesthesia. New York, Churchill Livingstone, 1981; 593–634.)

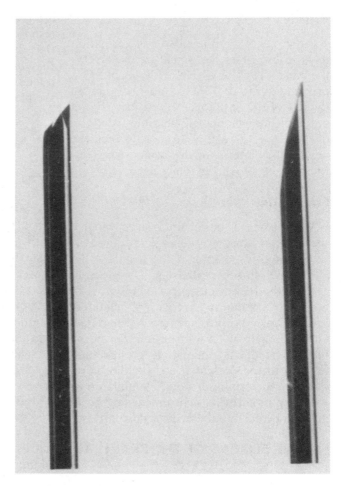

traneural. The rapid administration of 0.3 to 0.5 ml of local anesthetic produces a sudden and severe paresthesia if the needle is intraneural. The needle should then be moved a few millimeters before the full volume of local anesthetic is administered. Although not proven, intraneural injections probably are associated with post-block lesions.

Boney Landmarks

The close association of some nerves with boney prominences allows the use of boney landmarks to guide the direction in which the needle is inserted. For example, the ulnar nerve runs posteriorly to the medial epicondyle of the humerus where it is subcutaneous and readily palpable. Therefore, this boney landmark can be utilized to better locate the ulnar nerve.

Loss of Resistance

Some nerves lie in a compartment that is surrounded by a fascial sheath (neurovascular bundle). The axillary sheath surrounding the brachial plexus is an example of such a fascial sheath. In this situation, increased resistance is felt as the needle first meets the fascial sheath, presses against it, and then a sudden loss of resistance occurs when the sheath is penetrated. This often is confirmation that the needle is in the correct anatomic position. Sometimes the loss of resistance is described as a "popping" sensation.

Arteries

Some nerves run in close approximation to arteries. Thus, by palpating the artery, the nerve can be assumed to be in close proximation to it. Two examples of this are the use of the axillary artery to identify the cords of the brachial plexus, and palpation of the femoral artery to help direct the needle just lateral to the artery when attempting to block the femoral nerve.

Stimulating Needles

With several peripheral nerve blocks, there is only one way to ascertain the correct anatomic position of the needle—that is, elicitation of paresthesias. The most direct method of eliciting paresthesias is to utilize a "stimulating needle." A relatively low frequency, pulse-generated electrical current that can be transmitted via an exploring needle is optimal. A ground connection to the patient at a distal site is required. A peripheral nerve stimulator as used for monitoring neuromuscular blockade can be easily modified for this purpose.

NERVE BLOCKS OF THE BRACHIAL PLEXUS

The upper extremity can be completely or partially anesthetized by injecting local anesthetic around the brachial plexus.[2,4] The brachial plexus is derived from the anterior rami of C5-8 and T1. These nerves converge toward the upper surface of the first rib where they emerge between the anterior scalene and medial scalene muscles. The brachial plexus then passes under the midpoint of the clavicle to the apex of the axilla. Approaches to the brachial plexus for performance of a nerve block are designated as interscalene, axillary, and supraclavicular (Table 14-1).

Interscalene Approach

The interscalene approach makes use of the fact that nerves of the brachial plexus are grouped with major vessels going to the arm in a fascial sheath.[7] This technique has the advantage over the axillary approach in that the local anesthetic solution is introduced closer to the origin of the nerves of the plexus, including the musculocutaneous and axillary nerves. Furthermore, the site of needle insertion is high enough to avoid puncturing the pleura of the lung and, therefore, the chances of a pneumothorax should be minimized.

An interscalene block is usually carried out at the level of the sixth cervical vertebra. This vertebral level can be identified with a perpendicular line drawn posterior from the cricoid cartilage to intersect the posterior border of the sternomastoid muscle at or close to the interscalene groove. The external jugular vein is a fairly constant landmark, as it often crosses the sternomastoid muscles at the same site as the interscalene groove (Fig. 14-4). When the groove between the anterior and medial scalene muscles is identified, the needle is inserted in a caudal and medial direction. The needle need be only inserted between 1 to 4 cm before paresthesias of the C5 and C6 dermatomes are elicited to the radial border of the forearm, thumb, or index finger. Such a paresthesia is evidence that the needle is in close proximity to the upper roots of the brachial plexus and is an indication to proceed with the injection. After aspiration tests are satisfactory, 30 to 40 ml of local anesthetic are injected. Any "ballooning" of the subcutaneous tissue in the neck is an indication that the local anesthetic is probably being deposited outside the fascial sheath and an unsatisfactory block will result. In contrast to more peripheral blocks of the brachial plexus, the onset of an interscalene block follows a dermatomal and myotomal pattern, as occurs with an epidural block; that is, the anesthetic spreads from C5 distally down to T1. Therefore, the last myotome to be anesthetized in an interscalene block is T1, which involves the small muscles of the hand. Because the

Table 14-1. Advantages to Various Approaches to the Brachial Plexus

Location	Nerve Roots					
	C5	C6	C7	C8	T1	T2
Shoulder						
Interscalene	+++	+++	+++	+++	+	---
Supraclavicular	++	++	++	++	+	---
Axillary	---	---	---	---	---	---
Elbow						
Interscalene	+++	+++	+++	+++	++	---
Supraclavicular	++	++	++	++	++	---
Axillary	+	+	++	++	++	---
Wrist & Hand						
Interscalene	+++	+++	++	+	+	---
Supraclavicular	++	+++	+++	+++	++	---
Axillary	+	+	++	++	++	

Symbols: + + + = marked blockade; + + = moderate blockade; + = slight blockade; - - - = no blockade.

ulnar nerve is usually one of the last nerves to be anesthetized, blocking the ulnar nerve at the elbow will speed the onset of anesthesia. Finally, in contrast to more peripheral nerve blocks of the brachial plexus, the interscalene approach is suitable for surgical procedures on the acromioclavicular joint and the clavicle (Table 14-1).

Axillary Approach

The axillary approach is an excellent technique for surgical procedures distal to the elbow (Table 14-1). The main disadvantage of this approach is the difficulty in ensuring anesthesia of the musculocutaneous nerve. Furthermore, an axillary block of the

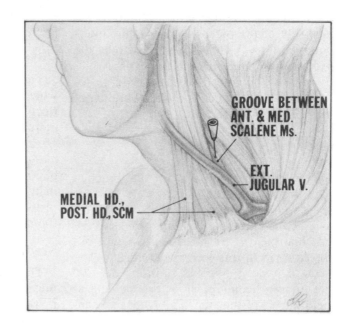

Figure 14-4. Outlined are the landmarks for performance of an interscalene approach for blocking the brachial plexus. Median lines depict medial and lateral aspects of the sternomastoid muscle (SCM). The apex of the V often is at the junction of the posterior border of the sternomastoid muscle and external jugular vein. Broad marks just medial to the needle indicate space between anterior and medial scalene muscles. The needle should be advanced in a plane about 45 degrees to the plane of the neck with the head turned to the opposite side.

brachial plexus usually is not suitable for surgical procedures of the proximal arm or shoulder.[8]

In the supine position, the arm should be abducted 90 degrees. In the axilla, the brachial artery can be palpated proximal to the insertion of the pectoralis major muscle anteriorly and the latissimus dorsi posteriorly. As the finger of one hand palpates the artery, the needle is inserted just anterior to the vessel but through the axillary sheath (Fig. 14-5). As the needle penetrates the sheath a sudden release or "popping" sensation is felt. The needle will then pulsate with the brachial artery. Approximately 15 to 20 ml of local anesthetic solution can be deposited and the needle moved to a position posterior to the artery where a similar amount is injected. Paresthesias are useful, but not essential, for confirming correct placement of the needle.

Application of pressure to the axillary sheath, either with a tourniquet or the anesthesiologist's hand, is often recommended in an attempt to ensure that the anesthetic moves proximal to the site in the sheath where the musculocutaneous nerve exits. The musculocutaneous nerve may also be blocked separately by injecting local anesthetic deep to the fascia just lateral to the insertion of the biceps tendon at the intercondylar line. A cuff of anesthesia over the proximal medial aspect of the axilla is recommended to anesthetize the intercostobrachial nerve, which is a lateral branch of the T2 intercostal nerve.

Supraclavicular Approach

The classic approach to the brachial plexus has been supraclavicular. The supraclavicular approach utilizes the first rib as its boney landmark and the trunks of the brachial plexus are blocked as they cross the first rib in the posterior triangle of the neck. The needle should be inserted 1 to 2 cm above the midpoint of the clavicle at right angles to the skin in all planes and advanced until the upper aspect of the first rib is contacted. The needle is then "walked" along the first rib in an anterior or posterior direction until paresthesias are obtained. This is an excellent approach to blocking the brachial plexus because the plexus is most compact at this point. Unfortunately, the supraclavicular approach is associated with about a 1 percent incidence of pneumothorax, even when experienced anesthesiologists are performing the block.

NERVE BLOCKS AT THE ELBOW

Radial Nerve Block

The landmarks for block of the radial nerve at the elbow can be determined by measuring four finger breadths above the lateral epicondyle of the humerus. The nerve can be palpated at this site in some individuals, where it emerges from its course in the spiral groove of the humerus. The needle should be inserted down to the humerus and local anesthetic deposited in a fan-like fashion along the lateral border of the humerus at the junction of its middle and lower third. A radial nerve paresthesia to the dorsal aspect of the thumb or first finger is confirmatory evidence of correct needle position. A total of 5 to 20 ml of local anesthetic is usually needed.

Ulnar Nerve Block

The ulnar nerve is identified at the elbow where it runs subcutaneously and posteriorly to the medial epicondyle of the humerus. Analgesia may be produced by infiltration of local anesthetic proximal to the medial epicondyle, as the nerve is more mobile at this site and is less likely to be traumatized by the needle. A total of 5 to 10 ml of local anesthetic is required for block of the nerve at this site.

Median Nerve Block

The median nerve is the most medial content of the antecubital fossa, and the landmark for localization is the brachial artery.

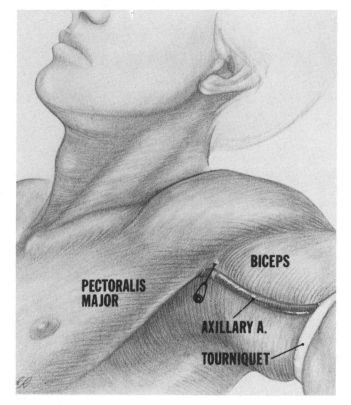

Figure 14-5. The axillary approach to blocking the brachial plexus. With the arm extended 90 degrees from the body, the axillary artery should be palpated. For convenience of injection, and to minimize displacement of the needle from the point at which the paresthesias are elicited, the needle can be connected by tubing to a syringe containing local anesthetic.

The brachial artery is immediately medial to the biceps tendon at the level of the flexion crease of the elbow and medial to it is the median nerve. Approximately 5 ml of local anesthetic injected at this site will effect analgesia of the peripheral distribution of the median nerve.

NERVE BLOCKS AT THE WRIST
(Fig. 14-6)

Radial Nerve Block

The radial nerve is found at the level of the proximal flexor crease on the lateral side of the radial artery. The radial artery is palpated and 3 ml of local anesthetic is infiltrated lateral to the artery. In addition, a subcutaneous cuff of anesthesia is produced on the lateral and dorsal aspects of the radial side of the wrist to anesthetize those branches of the radial nerve that have

left the parent trunk in the lower third of the forearm.

Ulnar Nerve Block

The ulnar nerve lies on the medial side of the ulnar artery and is blocked at this site at the level of the proximal flexor crease. Usually 3 ml of local anesthetic injected at this site will result in analgesia of the palmar and dorsal surfaces of the fifth digit and lateral half of the fourth digit.

Median Nerve Block

The median nerve is located at the level of the proximal flexor crease between the palmaris longus and the flexor carpi radialis tendons. The main body of the nerve passes deep to the flexor retinaculum. The needle should be advanced through the felxor retinaculum until loss of resistance is appre-

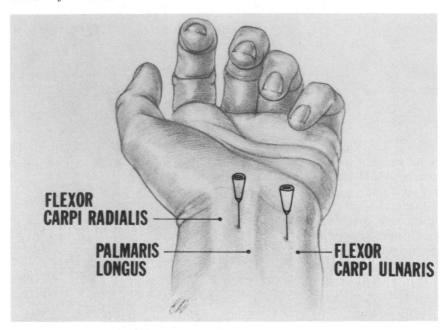

FLEXOR
CARPI RADIALIS

PALMARIS
LONGUS

FLEXOR
CARPI ULNARIS

Figure 14-6. An illustration of the approach to blocking the radial, ulnar, and median nerves at the wrist.

ciated and then 3 ml of local anesthetic injected to block the median nerve.

NERVE BLOCKS OF THE LOWER EXTREMITY

Unlike the compactness of the brachial plexus, the lower extremity is supplied by nerves which are widely separated from each other as they enter the thigh. The lumbar plexus is formed by the anterior primary rami of nerves T12 to L4. The lower components, including L2 to L4 are destined for the skin and musculature of the anterior and medial aspects of the thigh. These components eventually divide into an anterior and posterior division within the substance of the psoas major muscle. The anterior division forms the obturator nerve and the posterior division the femoral nerve.

Sciatic Nerve Block

The L4 to L5 and S1 to S3 nerves comprise the sacral plexus which results in the formation of the sciatic nerve. The sciatic nerve is the largest nerve in the body and can be blocked from several approaches. The traditional method is the posterior approach in the buttocks (Fig. 14-7). A line is drawn from the posterior superior iliac spine and the greater trochanter. A point about 5 cm caudad from the midsection of this line is the site for needle insertion. The needle is directed perpendicular to the skin for about 6 to 8 cm. The first paresthesia obtained is usually down the posterior aspect of the thigh due to the needle contacting the posterior cutaneous nerve of the thigh which lies just superficial to the sciatic nerve. Usually 10 to 25 ml of local anesthetic is needed to anesthetize the sciatic nerve.

Femoral Nerve Block

The femoral nerve is located immediately lateral to the femoral artery. Therefore, the needle is introduced lateral to the femoral artery just below the midpoint of the inguinal ligament. A loss of resistance is ob-

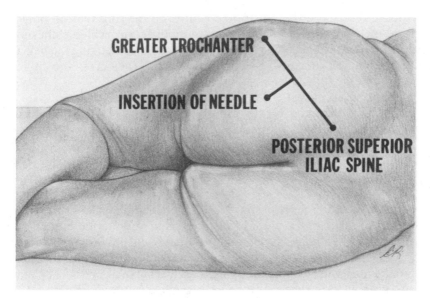

Figure 14-7. The traditional approach to blocking the sciatic nerve. The sciatic nerve may be blocked by identifying the midpoint of a line joining the posterior iliac spine to the greater trochanter. Needle insertion should be about 5 cm caudal to this midpoint.

tained as the needle "pops" through the fascia lata. A paresthesia may be sought, although injection of 10 to 15 ml of local anesthetic at this site is usually effective in blocking the femoral nerve.

Obturator Nerve Block

The obturator nerve enters the thigh through the obturator foramen and thus is located much deeper than the femoral and lateral femoral cutaneous nerves. The needle should be inserted 2 cm medial and 2 cm caudad to the pubic tubercle. A 10 cm needle will suffice in all but the most obese patients. The needle is introduced at right angles to the skin and advanced until it locates the inferior pubic ramus. At this point, the needle is walked medially and cephalad until it slips off the bone and lies at the obturator foramen. A paresthesia may be sought by adjusting the needle position at this site. This is a particularly difficult block to perform. It is stated that this block is necessary in order for surgery to be conducted

on the knee joint. Our experience, however, is that blocking the sciatic, femoral, and lateral femoral cutaneous nerves of the thigh is often sufficient anesthesia for surgery on the knee joint.

Lateral Femoral Cutaneous Nerve Block

The lateral femoral cutaneous nerve can be blocked immediately below its site of emergence through the inguinal ligament, 1 to 2 cm medial to the anterior superior iliac spine. The needle is inserted 2 cm medial and 2 cm below the anterior superior iliac spine. Infiltration with 5 to 8 ml of local anesthetic will usually be sufficient to block this nerve.

Psoas Compartment Block

As the lumbar plexus emerges from the psoas major muscle, it is wedged between this muscle anteriomedially and the quadratus lumborum and iliacus muscles posteriorly and laterally. All these muscles lie deep to the dense fascia over the posterior abdominal and pelvic walls. Local anesthetic injected into this fascial compartment between the two muscle masses will distribute itself around the lumbar plexus and will provide appropriate anesthesia. The two main routes to the lumbar plexus are the posterior approach and the perivascular or inguinal approach.[3,9]

Nerve Block at the Ankle

The nerve supply of the foot is primarily derived from the sciatic nerve and its branches, including the tibial, sural, and peroneal nerves. The femoral nerve also contributes to the innervation of the foot via its saphenous branch. For surgical proce-dures on the foot that do not require a leg tourniquet, surgical anesthesia can be provided by anesthetizing the nerves supplying the foot as they cross the ankle joint (Figs. 14-8, 14-9).

PARAVERTEBRAL BLOCK

Cervical Plexus Block

Upon leaving the intervertebral foramina, the cervical nerves pass behind the vertebral artery and lie with their anterior branches in the sulci of the transverse processes. The anterior branches of the first four cervical nerves join together just lateral to the transverse processes to form the cervical plexus. A cervical plexus block can provide anesthesia for thyroid surgery, car-

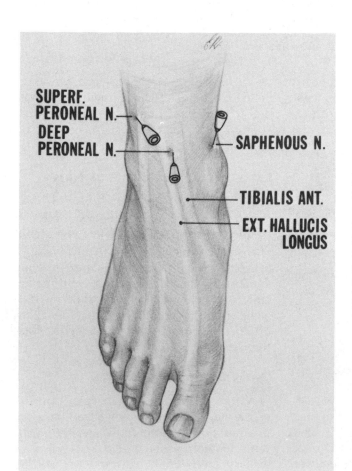

Figure 14-8. Nerve distribution for innervation of the foot. Block of the saphenous nerve, superficial peroneal nerve, and deep peroneal nerves are illustrated. (Modified from Bridenbaugh PO. The lower extremity: somatic blockade. In: Cousins MJ, Bridenbaugh PO, eds. Neural blockade. Philadelphia, JB Lippincott, 1980; 320–42.)

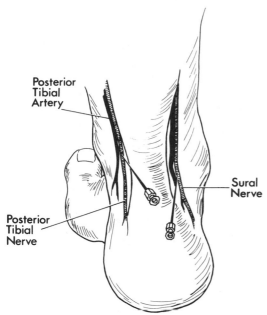

Figure 14-9. The approach to blocking the nerves that innervate the foot at the level of the ankle.

otid endarterectomy, and for the differential diagnosis of pain, such as cervical disc syndromes.

The intersection of a line drawn from the mastoid process to Chassiagnac's tubercle of the sixth cervical vertebra with a line drawn through the lower border of the ramus of the mandible is C4 (Fig. 14-10). A 22-gauge 5 cm needle should be inserted perpendicular to the skin and directed toward the transverse process. Once the transverse process is located, and hopefully a paresthesia obtained, anesthesia usually can be obtained with 3 to 5 ml of local anesthetic.

Lumbar Somatic Block

The paravertebral segmental nerves can be blocked in the paravertebral space from C1 to L5. Basically, the technique is the same for all levels, which involves location of the transverse process and then walking the needle off the transverse process into the paravertebral space. This block is used primarily for aiding in the diagnosis of chronic pain states, although it is quite feasible to produce operative anesthesia by a combination of paravertebral blocks.

An 8 cm needle is introduced at the rostral end of the spinous process of the vertebra to be blocked and advanced until the transverse process is located. The needle then should be walked posteriorly off the transverse process and advanced an additional 1 to 2 cm where 5 ml of local anesthetic should be injected.

Intercostal Nerve Block

Intercostal nerve blocks have a variety of uses, which include surgical anesthesia and providing analgesia postoperatively for patients who have undergone thoracotomy or upper abdominal surgery. Intercostal nerve blocks can also be used to provide relief of pain for patients who have rib fractures.

Intercostal nerves pursue a circumferential course along the inferior border of the ribs supplying the skin and abdominal wall muscles. To effectively produce anesthesia of the anterior and lateral thoracic and abdominal walls, intercostal nerves must be blocked before the lateral cutaneous branches arise at the midaxillary line. Therefore, the needle is usually inserted about 8 cm from the midline posteriorly where the rib can be palpated. The needle is advanced until the periosteum of the rib is located. At this point, the needle is directed caudad until it slips off the lower border of the rib. The patient is asked to hold his or her breath to reduce movement and possible needle displacement. An aspiration test is performed and approximately 5 ml of local anesthetic injected to block each intercostal nerve (Fig. 14-11).[3]

SYMPATHETIC NERVE BLOCKS

Stellate Ganglion

The cervical part of the sympathetic trunk contains three ganglia, a superior, middle, and lower. The latter is usually

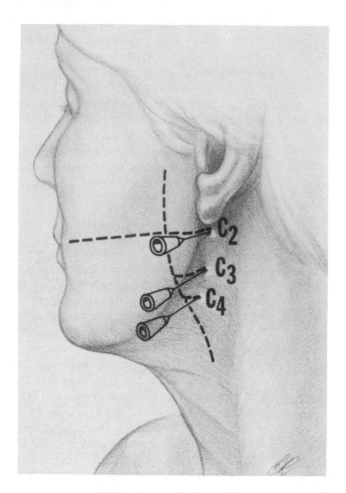

Figure 14-10. Superficial landmarks necessary for block of the cervical plexus.

fused with the first thoracic ganglia to form the stellate ganglion. Stellate ganglion block is useful in the diagnosis and treatment of abnormalities in the sympathetic nervous system distribution of the arm, which are commonly designated reflex sympathetic dystrophies (see Chapter 33).

With the patient in the supine position, and the head extended backwards on a pillow, the anesthesiologist's finger is inserted between the sternomastoid muscle and the trachea. The most easily palpated transverse process is sought, which is usually the sixth cervical transverse process (Chassiagnac's tubercle). The needle should be inserted through the skin over this transverse process and advanced until it makes contact with that transverse process. The point of the needle is then withdrawn a few millimeters and 15 to 20 ml of local anesthetic injected. A successful stellate ganglion block will be evident by the occurrence of a Horner's syndrome (ptosis, myosis, enophthalmos, and anhydrosis). Successful block of the sympathetic nervous system innervation of the arm is evidenced by a 3 to 5 Celsius increase in skin temperature.

Lumbar Sympathetic Block

The sympathetic chain is located on the anterolateral aspect of the vertebral bodies in a fascial compartment limited by the vertebral column, the psoas sheath, and the retroperitoneal fascia. Block of this chain re-

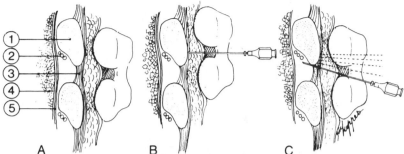

Figure 14-11. Intercostal nerve block. (A) The intercostal space is identified by the index and middle fingers of the anesthesiologist's nondominant hand. Numbers point to the (1) rib; (2) intercostal neurovascular bundle containing intercostal vein, artery, and nerve from within out; (3) intercostal muscles both internal and external; (4) lung; and (5) visceral and parietal pleural layers. (B) The anesthesiologist's fingers move the skin wheal cephalad over the rib above the intercostal space. The needle is now inserted at this site so that the rib acts as a bony end-point to prevent accidental excessive advancement with possible pleural puncture. (C) The needle is walked caudad as the skin wheal is allowed to retract in a similar direction. As the needle slips off the lower end of the rib, it pierces the intercostal muscles and enters the potential space between these muscles and the parietal pleura. A subtle loss of resistance is often appreciated at this stage and an injection is made into this space without any attempts to seek paresthesia. (Murphy TM. Nerve blocks. In: Miller RD, ed. Anesthesia. New York, Churchill Livingstone, 1981;593–634.)

quires the tip of the needle to be inserted from the patient's back into this space. This block can be used for conditions in which hyperactivity of the sympathetic nervous system exists. Furthermore, it can be used to provide increased blood flow in conditions such as incipient gangrene and vascular disease.

With the patient in the lateral position, and the waist supported by a pillow so that the vertebral column is curved in a lateral plane, needles should be inserted opposite the spinus process of L2 and L4, about 7 to 10 cm lateral to the midline. Each needle is advanced until the transverse process of the vertebra lying above it is contacted (Fig. 14-12).[10] The needle should then be redirected and advanced an additional 5 cm. The subsequent administration of 10 to 15 ml of local anesthetic at each needle site produces a complete sympathetic block.

Celiac Plexus Block

Celiac plexus block is one of the more useful techniques utilized by the anesthesiologist in control of chronic pain syndromes (see Chapter 33).[2,3] It is specifically useful in the treatment of intractable pain that is associated with carcinoma of the pancreas. A celiac plexus block denervates the nerve supply of the foregut and therefore can successfully interrupt stimuli from the pancreas, stomach, and liver. Generally, an anesthesiologist should not perform this block unless he or she has had considerable experience. This means that a celiac plexus block is usually utilized only by anesthesiologists who are actively engaged in the treatment of patients with chronic pain. Many favor performing this block with fluroscopy to assure proper placement of the needle.

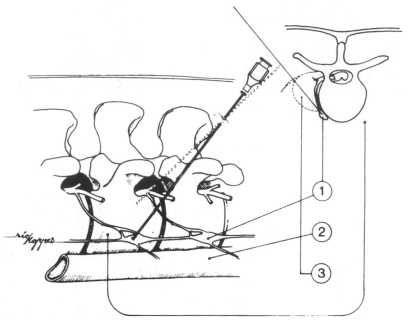

Figure 14-12. Lumbar sympathetic block. This figure shows the relationships of the lumbar sympathetic chain on the anterolateral aspect of the lumbar vertebral bodies to the large vessels and somatic nerves. Insert diagram shows how the needle must transverse and in its final position be anterior to the psoas major muscle and its sheath so as to block the sympathetic chain. If injections are made within the psoas major muscle, its sheath will prevent the drug from diffusing to the sympathetic chain. (1) Lumbar sympathetic chain, (2) abdominal aorta, (3) psoas major muscle. (Murphy TM. Treatment of chronic pain. In: Miller RD, ed. Anesthesia. New York, Churchill Livingstone, 1981;1459–91.)

INTRAVENOUS REGIONAL ANESTHESIA

Intravenous regional anesthesia is a simple method of producing analgesia of the arm or leg by injection of the local anesthetic intravenously while the circulation to that extremity is occluded. This method was first described by August Bier in 1908. As a result, this form of anesthesia is frequently called the "Bier Block." Advantages of this technique include ease of performance, relative safety, rapid onset and recovery, controllable duration of action, and excellent muscle relaxation.

A venous catheter is placed in a distal portion of the extremity and a blood pressure cuff or some other type of tourniquet applied to the limb proximal to the site of surgery. Some anesthesiologists believe that exsanguination of the limb assists in the production of complete analgesia. The usual method is to wrap an Esmarch bandage up the arm starting proximal to the catheter in the vein. When this is completed, the tourniquet should be inflated to a pressure above the patient's systolic arterial blood pressure. A tourniquet pressure of 200 to 250 mmHg should be adequate. Alternatively and probably preferably to eliminate tourniquet pain, the double tourniquet technique can be utilized. The proximal tourniquet can be initially inflated and the Esmarch bandage removed. The local anesthetic is then injected (25 to 50 ml for upper extremity and 100 to 200 ml for lower extremity). The onset of anesthesia is rapid, usually within 5 to 10 minutes. Local anesthetics which can be utilized for this block include 0.5 percent lidocaine, 0.5 percent procaine, 0.5 percent mepivacaine, or 0.5 percent prilocaine. Chloroprocaine is not recommended because of previous observations of venous irritation when this drug is used for this purpose. Although bupivacaine may be a suitable local anesthetic for intravenous regional anesthesia, it presently is not approved for this use.

After the initial injection, analgesia is produced up to, but not including, the limb under the proximal tourniquet. When the patient complains of tourniquet discomfort, the distal tourniquet is inflated over what will be analgetic skin. When continued occlusion is assured, the proximal tourniquet can be deflated. Approximately 45 to 60 minutes of satisfactory analgesia can be produced with this technique. If surgery is going to be longer than this, then deflation of the tourniquet with subsequent reexsanguination and reinjection of local anesthetic will probably be necessary or prospective selection of an alternative anesthetic technique will be needed. With deflation of the tourniquet, local anesthetic is flushed into the circulation providing the potential for a systemic toxic reaction (see Chapter 7). In fact, this is a rare event. Still, respiratory and cardiovascular monitoring is essential to detect any local anesthetic toxic effect.

SUMMARY

There are often advantages to avoiding general anesthesia in preference to the use of peripheral nerve block. Nevertheless, cooperation is required between the anesthesiologist, patient, and surgeon for this approach to succeed. Preoperatively, a detailed discussion with the patient and adequate preoperative medication is essential. In addition, a detailed knowledge of the anatomy is required with use of a technique that is as gentle as possible. Furthermore, psychological support must be provided during surgery and appropriate drugs given for sedation. A gentle surgeon may be the difference between a successful and unsuccessful peripheral nerve block. Lastly, the characteristics and pharmacology of local anesthetics must be understood so that appropriate treatment can be given in case a toxic reaction occurs (see Chapter 6). If the anesthesiologist and surgical team are willing to accept these qualifications, then peripheral nerve block anesthesia often provides a suitable and sometimes better alternative to general anesthesia.

REFERENCES

1. deJong RH, Heavner JE. Diazepam prevents local anesthetic seizures. Anesthesiology 1971;34:523–31.
2. Moore DC. Regional block. Springfield, Charles C Thomas Co., 1975.
3. Murphy TM. Nerve blocks. In: Miller RD, ed. Anesthesia. New York, Churchill Livingstone, 1981;593–634.
4. Kennedy WF Jr. Preparation for neural blockade: The patient, block equipment, resuscitation and supplementation. In: Cousins MJ, Bridenbaugh PO eds., Neural Blockade. Philadelphia, J. B. Lippincott, 1980;135–45.
5. Selander D, Dhuner KG, Lundborg G. Peripheral nerve injury due to injection needles used for regional anesthesia. Acta Anaesthesiol Scand 1977;21:182–8.
6. Selander I, Edshage S, Wolff T. Paresthesia or no paresthesia? Nerve lesions after axillary blocks. Acta Anaesthesiol Scand 1979;23:27–33.
7. Winnie AP. Interscalene brachial plexus block. Anesth Analg 1970;49:455–66.
8. deJong RH. Axillary block of the brachial plexus. Anesthesiology 1961;22:215–25.
9. Chayden D, Nathan H, Chayden M. The psoas compartment block. Anesthesiology 1976;45:95–9.
10. Murphy TM. Treatment of chronic pain. In: Miller RD, ed. Anesthesia. New York, Churchill Livingstone, 1981;1459–91.

15

Positioning

During surgery and anesthesia, the patient is usually positioned to offer optimal surgical conditions. Many surgical positions, however, have the danger of imposing limitations on physical and physiologic tolerances of the patient. If these tolerances are exceeded, either immediate (e.g., decreased cardiac output) or long-term (e.g., peripheral neuropathy), complications may result.

An inappropriate surgical position may lead to several adverse effects. First, nerve damage or a peripheral neuropathy may result from placing the patient in a position which stretches or applies pressure to the nerve. Secondly, the patient may undergo undue pressure in a vulnerable area, which may manifest itself as pressure necrosis of the skin, leading to ulceration, and even sometimes requiring skin grafting. Thirdly, damage to fingers or toes can occur when equipment, such as an operating room table, is positioned to achieve a certain position. Fourthly, alterations in position may cause cardiovascular changes because anesthetics blunt normal compensatory mechanisms. For example, suddenly changing a patient from the supine to sitting position may result in hypotension and decreased blood flow to the brain. Lastly, respiratory changes may occur. For example, the head-down position may compress the abdominal contents against the diaphragm, decreasing lung volumes. Furthermore, the lateral decubitus position may alter adversely the distribution between ventilation and circulation.

Despite the multiple complications that may occur, most of them are preventable with careful positioning of the patient and proper utilization of equipment.

COMMONLY TRAUMATIZED NERVES

Various areas of the body, especially the eyes, skin, fingers, and toes, can be damaged and undergo pressure necrosis from undue prolonged pressure. Nerves may be damaged because they are excessively stretched or compressed, leading to ischemia. If this ischemia is maintained for a sufficient period of time, necrosis of the nerve occurs in addition to stretching of the nerve bundle. If the hematoma is small the surrounding nerve fibers are merely compressed and may later recover. Conversely, a large hematoma may compress nerve fibers and result in necrosis. Finally, a tourniquet as used for surgical procedures on the upper extremity may exert excessive pressure on underlying nerves. This is the reason for limiting the duration of tourniquet inflation usually to less than 3 hours.

Excessive stretching and compression may occur in an anesthetized patient because muscle tone is reduced, especially when muscle relaxants are administered, thus allowing a patient to be placed in an unphysiologic position. Also, the anesthetized patient cannot complain of pain, and therefore may be placed in a position that he or she would normally not tolerate. Other factors that may contribute to peripheral nerve injuries include congenital anomalies, pre-existing diseases (e.g., diabetic neuropathy), hypothermia, hypotension, and application of a tourniquet.[1]

Brachial Plexus

Of the possible postoperative peripheral nerve complications, injury to the brachial plexus is the most common.[2] Because of being in close proximity to several freely moving structures, the brachial plexus can easily be compressed. Furthermore, malpositioning allows the brachial plexus to be easily stretched. For example, by dorsal extension and lateral flexion of the head to the opposite side in the supine position, the angle between the head and shoulder tip in-

creases and, therefore, stretches the brachial plexus.

Although the entire brachial plexus may be involved, usually only parts of the plexus are damaged such as one of the three cords. Britt et al[1] recommend that the easiest way to determine posterior cord damage is by seeking evidence in the dorsum of the first web space for the presence of sensation. A lateral cord palsy can be tested by determining whether sensation of the palmar pad of the distal phalanx of the index finger exists, whereas the palmar pad of the distal phalanx of the little finger can be tested for medial cord damage. Overall, damage to the brachial plexus can be minimized by avoiding excessive stretching of the plexus and assurance of proper shoulder rest placement when a patient is in the head-down position. The shoulder rest is properly placed over the acromioclavicular joint. Medial placement of the shoulder rest can pinch the brachial plexus between the clavicle and first rib. Lateral placement of the

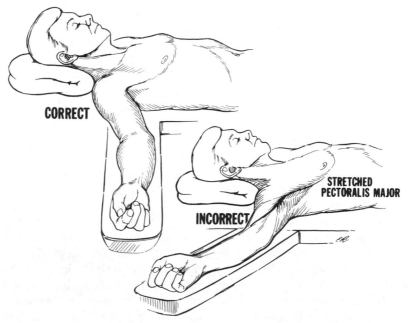

Figure 15-1. When the arm is extended more than 90 degrees, the brachial plexus may be injured. This possibility can be detected by palpation of the pectoralis major muscle. If the muscle is tense, it is likely that the brachial plexus is being unduly stretched.

shoulder rest can depress the head of the humerus and stretch the brachial plexus.

By palpating the pectoralis major muscle, one can indirectly assess the presence of pressure on the brachial plexus. If the pectoralis major muscle is not tense, then it is reasonable to assume that the brachial plexus is not being excessively stretched (Fig. 15-1). Turning the head toward the extended and internally rotated arm also minimizes stretch on the brachial plexus.

Radial Nerve

The radial nerve may be injured if the arm slips off the side of the operating room table or if pressure is applied to the nerve as it traverses the spiral groove of the humerus (Fig. 15-2). Damage to this nerve is manifested by the characteristic "wrist drop."

Median Nerve

If there is an inability to oppose the thumb and little finger, then damage to the median nerve should be suspected. Usually, this nerve is not damaged by malpositioning, but

by trauma during an intravenous injection of a drug, such as thiopental.

Ulnar Nerve

The ulnar nerve is the most common nerve to be injured because of its superficial path along the medial aspects of the elbow.[3] This injury is manifested by weakness and sensory loss on the ulnar side of the hand. The most common cause of ulnar nerve damage is inadvertently allowing the elbow to hang over the edge of the table leading to compression of the nerve between the medial epicondyle of the humerus and sharp edge of the table (Fig. 15-3).

Sciatic Nerve

In a patient who is lying on an improperly padded table, the sciatic nerve may be compressed as it exits from under the piriformis muscle when the opposite buttock is elevated, such as in a total hip arthroplasty. Also, in the lithotomy position, the sciatic nerve can be damaged if the thighs and legs are externally rotated, or if the knees are extended. To minimize this from happen-

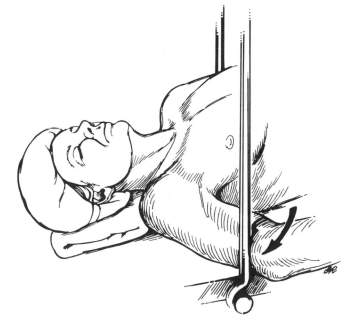

Figure 15-2. Compression of the arm against a frame for surgical drapes (ether screen) either in the supine or head-down position can cause compression and a resultant neuropathy of the radial nerve.

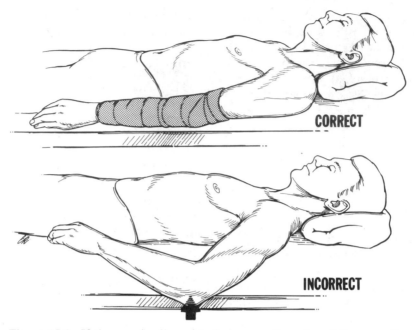

Figure 15-3. If the arm is allowed to hang over the edge of the operating table in the supine position, an ulnar nerve neuropathy may result.

ing, external rotation of the thighs and knees must be minimal and the knee should be flexed. The sciatic nerve may also be traumatized by an intramuscular injection into the buttock. Injury to the sciatic nerve manifests as paralysis of all muscles below the knee as well as numbness of the lateral half of the calf and almost all of the foot with the exception of the inner border of the arch.

Common Peroneal Nerve

The common peroneal nerve, which is a branch of the sciatic nerve, is the most frequently damaged nerve in the lower extremity. This nerve courses around the head of the fibula at the tibial condyles. Typically, the common peroneal nerve is compressed between the fibula and the metal brace utilized for the lithotomy position. Obviously, proper padding can minimize this complication from occurring. The physical findings of damage to the common peroneal nerve are foot drop, loss of dorsal extension of the toes, and inability to evert the foot.

Deep Peroneal Nerve

Foot drop may manifest postoperatively if the feet are plantar-flexed for extended periods during anesthesia. Patients in the sitting position should have a foot support under their feet, while patients in the prone position should have a roll placed under the anterior aspect of the ankle to maintain the extended position (Fig. 15-4).

Femoral Nerve

The femoral nerve may be compressed at the pelvic brim by the blade of a self-retaining retractor as used during a laparotomy or excessive angulation of the thigh when the patient is placed in the lithotomy position. On examination, there is loss of flexion of the hip and extension of the knee due to quadriceps femoris palsy. Sensation is absent over the superior aspect of the thigh and medial and anteromedial side of the calf. The possibility of femoral nerve injury due to the above mechanism must be remembered when neurologic deficits in the

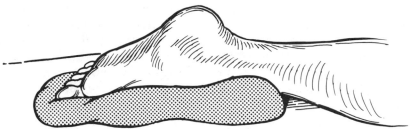

Figure 15-4. Injury to the foot can be minimized by proper padding in the prone position.

postoperative period are erroneously attributed to a prior regional block.

Saphenous Nerve

The saphenous nerve is a branch of the femoral nerve and can be damaged by compression against the medial tibial condyle if the foot is suspended lateral to a vertical brace (Fig. 15-5). Obviously, in the lithotomy position, there should be ample padding between the legs and these braces.

Obturator Nerve

Damage to the obturator nerve manifests as inability to abduct the leg and numbness of the medial side of the thigh. This nerve

may be damaged during difficult forceps delivery or by excessive flexion of the thigh to the groin.

COMMONLY TRAUMATIZED AREAS

Eye

Corneal abrasions can occur during general anesthesia from pressure of the anesthetic mask, surgical drapes, or operating room table. A rule of thumb is that if the orbit of the eye can be felt in its entirety, then pressure on the eye is unlikely. The eye must be protected during surgery to prevent the occurrence of a corneal abrasion (see Chapter 25).

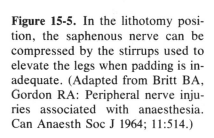

Figure 15-5. In the lithotomy position, the saphenous nerve can be compressed by the stirrups used to elevate the legs when padding is inadequate. (Adapted from Britt BA, Gordon RA: Peripheral nerve injuries associated with anaesthesia. Can Anaesth Soc J 1964; 11:514.)

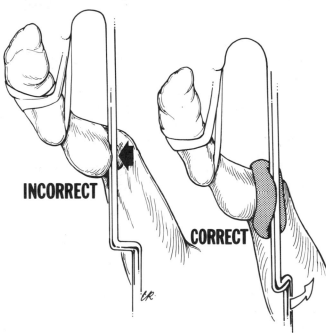

INCORRECT

CORRECT

Prolonged and excessive pressure on the eye, especially during hypotension, can cause thrombosis of the central retinal artery, with blindness upon waking from anesthesia. Such pressure is likely to occur in the prone position. Again, the patient should be systematically examined to ensure that pressure does not occur on the eye.

Skin

Excessive pressure over an area of skin may result in ischemia and localized ulceration. In severe cases, a skin graft may even be required. For example, taping of an endotracheal tube may cause ulceration of facial skin. Care must be taken to ensure that bolster-type orthopaedic frames to support patients during spinal column surgery are well padded to prevent pressure necrosis of the skin of the groin. The knees also must be padded. In essence, any area that has excessive pressure on it, particularly skin over a boney surface, is subject to the possibility of undergoing pressure necrosis.

Fingers or Toes

Whenever parts of a table are being moved, the possibility of a finger or toe being damaged in a progressively narrowing gap between the main portion and the part of the table being moved must be appreciated. Probably the most likely problem is having fingers traumatized when the foot of the operating table is returned from the lithotomy to horizontal position.

PROBLEMS FROM AN ANESTHETIC MASK

Several complications can occur from the improper application of an anesthetic mask, mask strap, or tracheal tube connector (Figs. 15-6 and 15-7). The most common complication is necrosis of the bridge of the nose from excessive pressure by the anesthetic mask. One approach to minimize the

chances of this happening is to remove the anesthetic mask every 5 minutes and massage the bridge of the nose with a piece of gauze to restore circulation to the compressed area. Another complication is loss of hair of the outer third of the eyebrow. Unfortunately, this hair often does not grow back. This complication can be minimized by putting a pad underneath the mask strap and avoiding pressure on the outer third of the eyebrow. Another complication from the mask strap is excessive pressure on the buccal branch of the facial nerve, causing loss of function of the orbicularis oris muscle. Also, excessive pressure on the ear by the mask strap can result in pressure necrosis. Both of these complications can be prevented by inserting a gauze between the skin and the mask and alleviating the associated pressure. On rare occasions, loss of hair has occurred from the back of the head from the mask strap. It is not clear what should be done to minimize this complication. Obviously, the less the duration of constant pressure, the less likely this complication will occur.

Compression of the supraorbital nerve by tracheal tube connector manifests as numbness of the forehead and pain in the eye. The facial nerve may be damaged by compression between the anesthesiologist's fingers and the ascending ramus of the patient's mandible if extreme and prolonged manual forward pressure is required to maintain a patent upper airway.

COMMONLY USED SURGICAL POSITIONS

Supine

Parks[2] evaluated 72 postoperative peripheral nerve complications and found that 33 of them occurred in the supine position. Fourteen of these involved the brachial plexus, with the ulnar nerve being most common. Therefore, care must be taken in protecting the brachial plexus and its branches from damage during anesthesia.

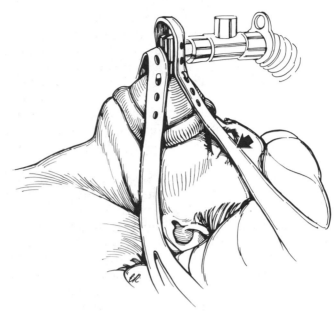

Figure 15-6. Several complications can occur from excessive pressure with application of an anesthetic mask and mask strap. The outer third of the eyebrow can disappear with excessive compression from the strap. The buccal branch of the facial nerve can be injured from the mask strap, and also necrosis of the bridge of the nose can occur from excessive pressure by the anesthetic mask.

Although there are several alterations in ventilation when changing from the standing to the supine position, they are less dramatic than with other position changes.[4] Froese and Bryan[5] studied diaphragmatic movement in patients who were awake and in those who were anesthetized either with spontaneous ventilation or during controlled ventilation of the lungs in the presence of skeletal muscle paralysis. In the anesthetized state, the diaphragm was displaced somewhat cephalad. Skeletal muscle paralysis caused a further cephalad shift in the end-expiratory position of the diaphragm, with the shift being especially large in the dependent region of the lungs. Obviously, during positive pressure ventilation of the lungs, the passive diaphragm is displaced in the most nondependent regions of the lung where abdominal pressure is the

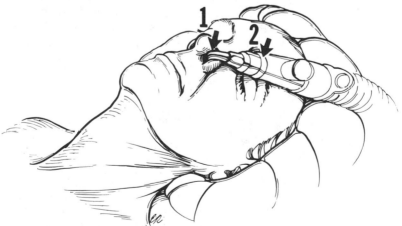

Figure 15-7. The supraorbital nerve can be compressed by a tracheal tube connector especially when padding is insufficient. Pressure on the nasal opening by the connector can result in tissue ischemia and damage.

least. This indicates that regional restriction of movement of the dependent diaphragm will decrease compliance, even in the absence of a change in functional residual capacity and the amount of airway closure. This implies that even though not totally effective, positive pressure ventilation of the lungs should be utilized in especially prolonged cases to minimize regional and peripheral atelectasis.

In general, the supine position has the fewest adverse effects on the circulation, unless there is a large abdominal mass, such as a tumor, acites, or a gravid uterus which can compress the inferior vena cava sufficiently to impede venous return, resulting in hypotension and a decreased cardiac output. During labor, such hypotension can be minimized by elevating the right hip, which tilts the uterus to the left and away from the inferior vena cava (see Chapter 26).

Prone

The prone position can result in several complications, mainly from pressure. The eye may be damaged by pressure with the face down. To ensure that pressure is not being applied to the eye, the boney orbit should be easily and entirely palpated. The brachial plexus can be injured if it is stretched, or by pressure from improperly placed supports (Fig. 15-8). Many of these injuries can be prevented by proper placement of pads and blankets (Fig. 15-9).

Any position that compresses the abdomen may cause a cephalad shift of the diaphragm, resulting in reduced lung volumes. Thus, rolls and/or bolsters should be inserted along the sides of the patient's abdomen and thorax to ensure freedom from pressure and to allow adequate expansion of the lungs. Another reason for avoiding compression of the abdomen is to avoid obstruction of the inferior vena cava. When flexion is added to the prone position, as during laminectomy, it is likely that blood will pool in dependent parts of the body. Thus, movement into this position should be done at a slow rate to ensure sufficient time for activation of compensatory mechanisms to prevent excessive pooling in the arms and legs.

Lateral Decubitus

Improper support of the head in the lateral decubitus position can result in stretch of the brachial plexus (Fig. 15-10). A pillow between the knees and under the elbows will help to distribute the weight of the upper extremity to the dependent extremity. Lastly, a small roll under the upper chest, but not the axilla, will take the weight off the dependent arm (Fig. 15-11).

In the lateral decubitus position, the dependent lung tends to be underventilated because it is compressed by the pressure of the abdominal contents and the weight of

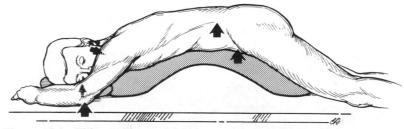

Figure 15-8. This position indicates the multiple problems that can occur with an improperly positioned patient in the flexed prone position. If excessively stretched, the brachial plexus can be damaged. The ulnar nerve can be damaged by inadequate padding of the elbow. Inadequate padding under the head can cause eye damage, or undue pressure to the face or lower eyelid. Excessive compression to the inferior vena cava can be minimized by padding under the inferior iliac spine.

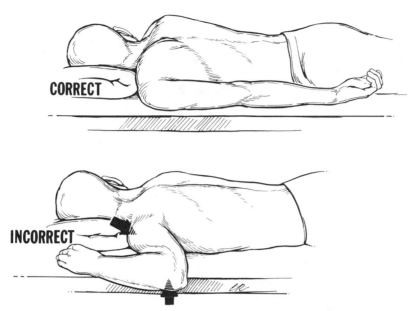

Figure 15-9. Proper padding in the prone position can minimize damage to the brachial plexus, especially the ulnar nerve.

the mediastinum. The nondependent lung is relatively overventilated because the compliance of this lung is increased particularly when the corresponding hemithorax is opened. At the same time, gravity favors distribution of pulmonary blood flow to the underventilated dependent lung. This accentuated mismatching of ventilation to perfusion introduced by the lateral decubitus position may manifest as unexpected arterial hypoxemia emphasizing the importance of monitoring PaO_2 of patients in this position.

From a circulatory point of view, there is the risk of compression of the inferior vena cava. Furthermore, raising the kidney rest

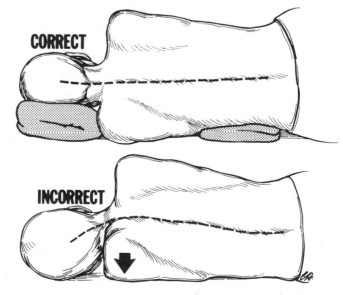

Figure 15-10. Injury to the nondependent brachial plexus can be minimized by proper padding underneath the head.

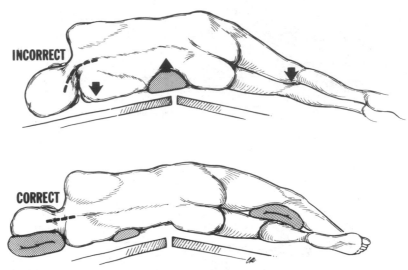

Figure 15-11. In the lateral decubitus position, pillows between the legs and elbows help distribute the weight of the upper extremity to that of the lower extremity.

can lead to marked reductions in venous return and subsequent hypotension.

Sitting

The sitting position is usually employed for posterior fossa and cervical spinal cord surgery. There are few neurological complications associated with this position, assuming that the knees are bent slightly and padded appropriately to avoid excessive pressure. The legs should be as high as possible to promote venous return. Also, the legs probably should be wrapped with elastic bandages to minimize pooling of blood and the development of thrombophlebitis. Venous air embolism is a major hazard associated with operative procedures performed with the patient in the sitting position (see Chapter 24).

Lithotomy

The main neurological problems associated with the lithotomy position are related to positioning of the legs (Fig. 15-5). These problems can be avoided by minimizing pressure from the stirrups that are utilized to elevate the legs. The four nerves most likely to be damaged are the common per-

ioneal, femoral, saphenous and obturator (see the section *Commonly Traumatized Nerves*). Trauma of these nerves can be prevented by cushioning the ankle and the knee against pressure from the metal stirrup. Wrapping a towel around the knee and ankle is effective in attenuating pressure. When positioning the patient, both legs should be elevated and flexed simultaneously. The thigh should be flexed at no more than 90 degrees before rotating the stirrups laterally.

An abdominal mass may obstruct the inferior vena cava, especially when the patient is in the lithotomy position (see Chapter 26).

SUMMARY

A patient ideally should be placed in the position of surgery before anesthesia is induced to identify abnormal physiologic consequences and undue pressure. Sometimes, however, the patient can only be positioned after anesthesia has been induced. The anesthesiologist must be aware of those areas that are especially vulnerable to injury. Also, whenever, an anesthetized patient is moved to a different position, it should be done slowly, with full recognition that compensatory mechanisms, such as baroreceptor activity, are often depressed by general anesthesia. Careful attention to the above details should minimize the adverse effects of various surgical positions.

REFERENCES

1. Britt BA, Joy N, Mackay MB. Positioning trauma. In: Orkin FK, Cooperman LH, eds., Complications of anesthesia. Philadelphia, J.B. Lippincott Company, 1983:646–70.

2. Parks BJ. Postoperative peripheral neuropathies. Surgery 1973;74:384–57.

3. Miller RG, Camp PE. Postoperative ulnar neuropathy. JAMA 1979;242:1636–9.

4. Smith BL. Physiological changes in the normal conscious human subject on changing from the erect to the supine position. In: Martin JT, ed., Positioning in anesthesia and surgery. Philadelphia, W.B. Saunders Company, 1978:10–31.

5. Froese AB, Bryan AC. Effects of anesthesia and paralysis on diaphragmatic mechanics in man. Anesthesiology 1974;41:242–7.

16

Monitoring

Monitoring involves the observation and collection of data which are evaluated and interpreted in order to provide the patient with the safest anesthetic possible. Therefore, monitoring includes evaluating the influence of surgery (e.g., blood loss), drug effects (e.g., circulatory effects of anesthetics), and of vital functions (e.g., adequate perfusion of the heart, brain, liver, and kidney). Monitoring should be sufficient to allow prompt recognition of a problem or deleterious trend, to estimate the severity of the problem, and to evaluate the response to therapy. Conversely, adequacy of monitoring must be weighed against the complications associated with monitoring, especially when utilizing invasive approaches (e.g., pulmonary artery catheter). For these reasons, not only the benefits but also the complications of the more specialized and intensive monitoring approaches must be understood.

ROUTINE MONITORING FOR ALL ANESTHETIZED PATIENTS

Routine monitoring of the anesthetized patient is an extension of the basic elements of physical diagnosis, which include inspection, palpation, percussion, and auscultation.[1] With the increased emphasis on gadgets and sophisticated electrical monitoring, these routine noninvasive and nonharmful methods of monitoring must not be forgotten (Table 16-1).

Routine monitoring includes use of a sphygmomanometer to measure blood pressure, and either a precordial or esophageal stethoscope to monitor heart and breath sounds (Fig. 16-1). The electrocardiogram (ECG), body temperature, and peripheral nerve stimulator are increasingly becoming mandatory monitoring for all anesthetized patients. Also, various disconnect alarm systems are routinely available on anesthetic machines. Lastly, the inspired oxygen concentration is monitored to avoid the rare accidental case of a low inspired concentration of oxygen.

Noninvasive Blood Pressure Monitoring

Sphygmomanometry. A sphygmomanometer measures the pressure required to occlude a major artery in an extremity. A cuff, located in a pneumatic bladder positioned over the artery, is inflated to a pressure greater than systolic blood pressure. While releasing the air from the bladder, sphygmomanometry techniques used to detect the systolic, and possibly the diastolic blood pressure include the following:

1. Oscillation of the cuff pressure
2. Auscultation of Korotkoff sounds
3. Ultrasonic detection of arterial wall motion under the cuff

213

Table 16-1. Monitoring That Requires No Instrumentation

Inspection
    Skin—color, capillary refill, rash, edema
    Nail beds—color, capillary refill
    Mucous membranes—color, moisture, edema
    Surgical field—color of tissues and blood, rate of blood loss, skeletal muscle relaxation
    Movement—purposeful or reflex
    Eyes—Conjunctiva (color and edema), pupils (size, reactivity)

Palpation
    Skin—temperature and texture
    Pulse—fullness, rate, and regularity
    Muscle—tone

Percussion
    Gastric—distention
    Chest—pneumothorax

Auscultation
    Chest—ventilation and cardiac sounds
    Blood pressure—sphygmomanometry

Location of gastric tube

(Adapted from Hug CC. Monitoring. In: Miller RD, Anesthesia. New York, Churchill Livingstone, 1981:157–201.)

4. Detection of blood flow distal to the sphygmomanometer cuff by palpation of an arterial pulse

Auscultation of Korotkoff sounds is probably the most frequently used method to measure blood pressure. The most common problems are the inaccuracy of the aneroid manometers and the size and positioning of the blood pressure cuff. Aneroid manometers should regularly be calibrated against a mercury manometer. The width of the blood pressure cuff should be greater than one-third of the circumference of the limb.

The bladder should cover at least one-half of the circumference of the arm with the middle of the bladder positioned directly over the artery. Even when these details are followed, discrepancies have been noted, especially in patients who have hypertension, obesity, hypothermia, and/or shock. When these problems are anticipated, perhaps other methods of monitoring blood pressure should be utilized during extensive surgery.

Automated Blood Pressure Recorders. Utilizing a Doppler ultrasound transducer or oscillometric approach, automatic devices are available which periodically measure blood pressure and heart rate as often as every 60 seconds (Fig. 16-2). Alarm systems are present to alert the anesthesiologist when pressure either above or below predetermined limits is exceeded. The Doppler detects sudden vibrations in the arterial wall when the cuff pressure falls slightly below systolic blood pressure and distal arterial blood flow occurs. This arterial blood flow produces an audible sound that varies rhythmically with the heart beat. At this point, systolic blood pressure is noted on the manometer. An oscillometric device, such as the Dinamap, measures blood pressure and heart rate via a cuff that inflates automatically. Once the artery is occluded, the cuff will begin to deflate in average increments of about 8 mmHg. At each step, the monitor will measure the amplitude of the oscillations introduced into the cuff by

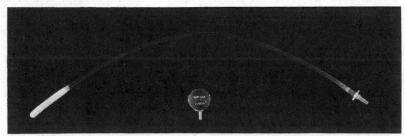

Figure 16-1. A typical weighted, precordial stethoscope and esophageal stethoscope.

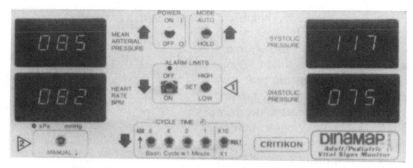

Figure 16-2. An example of a digital display of an automatic monitoring device.

the movement of the arterial wall. During deflation, the microcomputer will process and store two consecutive pressure pulsations of equal amplitude and frequency. At each pressure level, the microcomputer stores the cuff's pressure, the pulsation amplitude, and the time between sucessive heart beats. By analyzing these variables, the monitor determines the point in the cuff pressure where pulsations increase, peak, and decrease. This process of stepped deflation continues until the microcomputer has found the desired variables, or until the cuff pressure decreases to near 0 mmHg. The resultant determinants are systolic blood pressure, mean arterial blood pressure, diastolic blood pressure, and heart rate.

Advantages of an oscillometric device are that the cuff is both an actuator and a transducer. No separate transducer is needed and cuff application is simple, with no accurate transducer positioning required. Furthermore, the system is not sensitive to electrosurgical interference. The accuracy of the oscillometric technique has been evaluated in critically ill newborn infants. Kimble et al.[2] compared arterial blood pressure obtained with the automatic oscillometric technique with intra-arterial measurements and found a close correlation between the two methods. They concluded that this is a satisfactory, noninvasive method with which to measure blood pressure in critically ill infants.

When monitoring patients with extremely low blood pressures, the oscillometric device may display mean arterial blood pressure and not systolic and diastolic blood pressures. This is because of the low level pressure fluctuations or deflections in the cuff due to very low amplitudes in the systolic/diastolic wave form. The mean arterial pressure, however, probably is accurate. Determination of the blood pressure with the oscillometric device takes longer than other methods. For example, the germination period normally is 20 to 45 seconds. Finally, if the cuff is inflated too often (e.g., every 60 seconds), the possibility exists of edema and other ischemic changes occurring in the arm distal to where the blood pressure is being monitored. Indeed, when using a Dinamap in a 3 month old, 6 kg infant, in which blood pressures were measured at 60 second intervals, the arm distal to the blood pressure cuff became edematous, cyanotic, and with petechiae 90 minutes later.[3] This problem can be minimized by not measuring the blood pressure every 60 seconds and/or close observation of the arm to detect any ischemic changes.

Precordial and Esophageal Stethoscope

One of the most valuable noninvasive monitoring devices is a stethoscope. A well functioning stethoscope can provide continuous information regarding cardiac and respiratory function in an anesthetized patient. For example, ventricular and most atrial dysrhythmias can be detected by listening through a stethoscope and, in fact, diagnosed without an ECG. Also, the rate and character of the heart sounds can be detected. Subtle changes in heart tone may reflect a change in cardiac contractility. From a respiratory point of view, the quality and intensity of respiratory sounds can be valuable in diagnosing airway obstruction, and alterations in airway resistance. Also, a sudden change in the pattern of breathing may reflect depth of anesthesia.

There are two types of stethoscopes used during anesthesia. The first one is a chest wall stethoscope, either in a bell-shape or diaphragm (Fig. 16-1). The bell-shaped stethoscope is probably preferred, since an airtight seal on the chest wall is more easily obtained than with a diaphragm design. The bell-shaped stethoscope is frequently used during induction of anesthesia.

The second type of stethoscope is an esophageal tube monitor, which is often employed when anesthesia is administered via a tracheal tube (Fig. 16-1). It has the advantage of being so close to the heart that sounds are enhanced in intensity. An esophageal stethoscope also cannot be displaced with position changes of the patient or by movement of the drapes. This type of monitor should be used whenever possible to continuously monitor heart sounds and breath sounds.

For both types of stethoscopes, a major cause of inadequate intensity response is related to the poor fitting of the ear piece. Most anesthesiologists prefer using one ear, so that the other is available for operating room communication. As a result, a well fitting ear piece is essential. Acrylic ear pieces fit snugly, cause no discomfort, and are quite durable. These can be purchased commercially or can be custom made by a hearing aid company or a dental appliance laboratory. Rubber molded ear plugs may be fixed to the stethoscope, but do not fit as well as the acrylic ear pieces.

Body Temperature

To ensure that patients do not become unduly hypothermic and to be able to detect the rare case of malignant hyperthermia, the standard of practice is to monitor body temperature in all patients undergoing general anesthesia, except for those who have extremely brief, minor surgical procedures. Body temperature commonly decreases 1 to 4 Celsius during anesthesia and surgery performed in a cold operating room.[4] Although this type of decrease in body temperature is usually not serious, postoperative shivering may increase oxygen demand by as much as 400 percent.

There are several sites which can be utilized to monitor body temperature. The rectum is a common site, but the accuracy of the measured temperature as a reflection of core temperature depends on rectal blood flow. Indeed, rectal temperatures often do not reflect core body temperature accurately. Probably the most accurate site would be to insert a temperature probe into the lower one-third of the esophagus. This temperature would reflect the actual core temperature. Other sites for monitoring temperature include the skin, axilla, nasopharynx, and tympanic membrane. The skin and axilla have the disadvantages that their temperature varies with subcutaneous blood flow, sweating, radiation, and conduction of heat to and from other objects. Nasopharyngeal and upper esophageal temperature recordings can reflect the temperature of the inhaled gases. Insertion of the temperature probe into the nares has the propensity to cause epistaxis. A tympanic membrane probe can be valuable in that it approximates the temperature of the blood perfusing the brain when the probe is close to the tympanic membrane. Cerumen, however, can act as an insulator. Also, tympanic membrane measurement of temperature can be associated with external auditory canal bleeding, particularly in patients who are anticoagulated. When placing the tympanic membrane probes in an awake patient, there is a tendency to leave the device too distal in the canal so that adequate probe contact is lacking and temperature values may not reflect the body temperature. Lastly, there is a risk of perforation of the tympanic membrane.

Electrocardiogram (ECG)

The ECG has become a standard monitor in all anesthetized patients being useful intraoperatively for detection of (1) cardiac dysrhythmias, (2) myocardial ischemia, and (3) electrolyte changes, particularly potassium. The ECG needs to be displayed on an oscilloscope. In patients who are at high risk for having cardiac problems intraoperatively, it may be desirable to have a unit that allows freezing and holding of a set of complexes. Also, hard-copy recordings probably should be available in high-risk patients in order to better analyze the ECG changes. For example, a 1 mm or greater ST segment depression from base line may be a sign of myocardial ischemia. Lastly, an audible indicator of the QRS complex is frequently employed, which allows the anesthesiologist to carry on other activities, while listening to a possible change in cardiac rate of rhythm.

Although any lead in routine ECG monitoring can be used to detect cardiac dysrhythmias, a modified, bipolar chest lead is most commonly used. The positive electrode is placed in the usual V_1 position, and the negative electrode is placed near the shoulder. A third electrode is placed in a more remote area of the chest and serves as a ground (Fig. 16-3). This lead is of major value in cardiac rhythm evaluation. Lead II can also be used for detection of cardiac dysrhythmias as this lead parallels the P wave vector, resulting in maximum amplitude of the P wave on the ECG. For example, identification of the P wave can facilitate differentiation of supraventricular from ventricular dysrhythmias. Inferior wall myocardial ischemia may also be reflected by ST segment depression in lead II. More common sites of myocardial ischemia, however, are the anterior and lateral walls, which are best monitored by a precordial lead in the V_5 position (5th intercostal space along the anterior axillary line). For this reason, a V_5 lead is used when the goal is to monitor the ECG for the detection of myocardial ischemia. The equivalent of a V_5 lead can be obtained using three electrodes by placing the left arm electrode in the V_5 position and selecting lead aVL on the monitor.

It should be remembered that the ECG reflects only the electrical activities occurring in the heart and in no way is a measure of heart function. For example, it has been demonstrated that a normal ECG complex can be observed on the oscilloscope in the absence of an effective cardiac output (electromechanical dissociation). Although this latter example is extreme, it should be clearly understood that the ECG is not a measure of functional activity of the heart.

Ventilation

Clinical Assessment. The pattern of ventilation (rate, depth, and regularity) should be continuously monitored by the anesthesiologist. This is accomplished by visual and tactile (hand on the bag) monitoring of the movements of the reservoir bag on the anesthetic breathing system, by observing chest movement, and by auscultation of the chest via either a precordial or an esophageal stethoscope. The character of respiratory movements is helpful in assessing both depth of anesthesia and the extent to which air is moving. During general anesthesia with an inhaled anesthetic, ventilation is typically shallow with a rapid rate, whereas narcotics usually decrease the rate of respiration while tidal volume may actually increase. Also, by correlating chest movements to movements of the reservoir bag, a judgment can be made regarding the na-

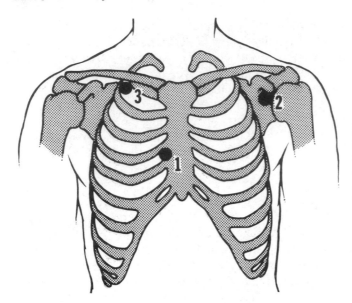

Figure 16-3. A modified CL_1 lead system for monitoring; (1) positive electrode in V_1 position; (2) negative electrode near the left shoulder; and (3) ground electrode.

ture and degree of possible respiratory obstruction. Unfortunately, the anesthesiologist frequently limits his or her observations to the rebreathing bag, and thus fails to obtain valuable information by not correlating this with movement of the chest.

Volume Measurement. To provide a more quantitative assessment of ventilation, a ventimeter or respirometer can be utilized. These devices measure tidal volume and provide a visual clue as to the nature and extent of respiratory movements. Measurement of tidal volume can be used to calculate minute ventilation (tidal volume times respiratory rate). All leaks in the anesthetic breathing system must be eliminated for accurate measurement of tidal volume.

Respiratory Gas Exchange. The adequacy of respiratory gas exchange is best determined by analysis of arterial blood gases and pH (see Chapter 17). Exhaled carbon dioxide concentrations can be measured by infrared analysis. Increased exhaled concentrations of carbon dioxide occur in the presence of hypoventilation, and increased carbon dioxide production.

Sudden decreases in the exhaled concentration of carbon dioxide may reflect esophageal intubation, venous air embolism, or disconnection of the tracheal tube from the anesthetic breathing system.

Exhaled physiologic and anesthetic gases can also be monitored by mass spectrometry. These devices allow monitoring of inspired and expired concentrations of oxygen, carbon dioxide, and inhaled anesthetics.[5]

Transcutaneous measurement of oxygen tension can be used to estimate the partial pressure of oxygen in arterial blood (PaO_2). The accuracy of this measurement is dependent on skin perfusion. With improved technology, measuring the oxygen tension transcutaneously is increasingly becoming a more accurate indicator of PaO_2.

Oxygen analyzers should be routinely utilized in all anesthetic machines to ensure that the inhaled concentration of oxygen is adequate. Oxygen analyzers are relatively inexpensive and provide a means for quantifying the oxygen content to the inhaled or exhaled gases. An oxygen analyzer is mandatory for low-flow or closed circuit administration of anesthetic mixtures containing nitrous oxide (see Chapter 11). The sensor for the oxygen analyzer may be placed on the inspiratory or expiratory side of the anesthetic breathing circuit.

SPECIALIZED AND INTENSIVE MONITORING

Urinary Output

In more complex cases, determination of urinary output can be a valuable guide to the adequacy of intravascular fluid volume and dynamics. When urinary output decreases below about 0.5 ml/kg/hr, oliguria exists (see Chapter 22). Correlation of the central venous pressure and urinary output is frequently a valuable guide in assessing the degree to which renal failure and intravascular fluid volume are interrelated. Lastly, monitoring urinary output permits early detection of hemoglobinuria, which is one of the initial signs of a hemolytic transfusion reaction.

Invasive Blood Pressure Monitoring

Although several arteries are accessible for percutaneous cannulation and direct measurement of arterial blood pressure, the radial artery is the most frequently used. Information derived from this kind of monitoring includes continuous blood pressure analysis on a beat-to-beat basis. Also, cannulation of a radial artery allows analysis of pulse wave form and facilitates collection of arterial blood for analysis of blood gases, pH, and electrolytes. The catheters to be used for cannulation of the radial artery should be small in diameter (such as a 20- or 22-gauge non-tapered Teflon catheter). A small catheter is important in minimizing thrombosis and occlusion of the artery because of the relationship between diameter of the catheter and the artery. For example, Bedford[6] found an 8 percent incidence of radial artery occlusion following cannulation with a 20-gauge catheter as compared to a 34 percent incidence of occlusion with

an 18-gauge catheter. In addition, Bedford[6] found that small radial arteries (less than 2 mm in diameter) are more likely to occlude and remain thrombosed than are larger radial arteries. Patients who have small wrists (circumference less than 18 cm) tend to have small arteries and may be at a greater risk for developing occlusive lesions than are patients with larger wrists.

Allen's test is utilized to determine the adequacy of collateral flow from the ulnar artery prior to cannulation of the radial artery. The Allen's test can be performed by occluding both the radial and ulnar arteries and asking the patient to make a tight fist. This maneuver forces blood from the hand such that the palmar surface becomes blanched and appears pale. Pressure over only the ulnar artery is then released and the patient instructed to open his or her hand avoiding hyperextension of the digits. If collateral circulation via the ulnar artery is adequate, color will return to the palmar surface of the hand within 5 to 15 seconds. Collateral flow is considered inadequate if color does not return to the hand in this period of time. Traditionally, inadequate collateral ulnar artery blood flow has been considered a relative contraindication to the insertion of a catheter into the radial artery. Slogoff et al.,[7] however, cannulated the radial arteries of 16 patients whose Allen's test results were abnormal and found no adverse results. In 22 patients, the ulnar artery was cannulated after multiple punctures of the ipsilateral radial artery and no ischemic changes occurred. They concluded that in the absence of peripheral vascular disease, Allen's test is not a predictor of ischemia of the hand during or following radial artery cannulation. They also concluded that when decreased or absent radial artery flow followed cannulation, it is of little or no clinical consequence and that radial artery cannulation is a low risk, high benefit monitoring technique that deserves wide clinical use, particularly during the intraoperative period.

Cannulation of the radial artery should be performed with the hand supinated, the forearm immobilized on an arm board, and the wrist dorsiflexed approximately 40 to 60 degrees over a towel or gauze sponges (Fig. 16-4). The skin is prepared with 1 percent iodine or 70 percent alcohol and, if the patient is awake, the anticipated entry site infiltrated with a small amount of local anesthetic. Sometimes it is helpful to make a small superficial incision to avoid damaging the tip of the plastic catheter as it is introduced through the skin. The needle is inserted at a 15 to 30 degree angle and advanced until the lumen of the artery is entered. While the catheter is advanced into the lumen of the artery, free blood must be continuously seen at the hub. After successful placement the catheter should be flushed continuously with a solution containing 1 to 2 units of heparin in saline at a rate of 1.5 to 3.0 ml/hr. This continuous flush is important in minimizing thrombus formation and maintaining an adequate blood pressure wave form.

Central Venous Pressure

Catheterization of the central veins has become an important maneuver both for measuring central venous pressure and pro-viding long term intravenous feedings, especially hyperalimentation. Furthermore, in an emergency, such as after acute hemorrhage with peripheral vasoconstriction, it may be impossible to catheterize a peripheral vein percutaneously and only a central vein may be available to infuse fluids for rapid restoration of blood volume. The four veins commonly utilized for catheterization are the brachial, subclavian, external jugular, and internal jugular. The relative advantages and disadvantages of utilizing each vein are summarized on Table 16-2.

Cannulation of the brachial vein is associated with a low complication rate, but advancement of a catheter centrally via this route can be time consuming and often unsuccessful. For example, it is often difficult to entice the catheter to turn the corner around the shoulder and enter the superior vena cava. The subclavian vein is a continuation of the axillary vein beginning at the outer border of the first rib. It may be cannulated by utilizing either a supraclavicular or infraclavicular approach. The subclavian vein has a wide caliber, is held open by surrounding tissue even in severe circulatory collapse, and is easily accessible to the anesthesiologist during a surgical procedure. The use of the subclavian vein allows the catheter to be securely fixed on the

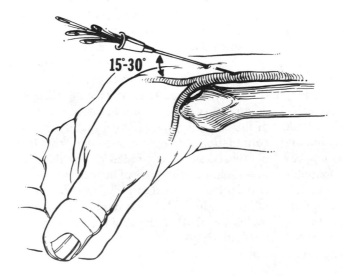

15°-30°

Figure 16-4. A diagramatic illustration of an approach to cannulating the radial artery.

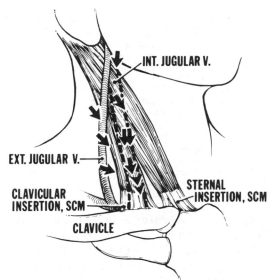

Figure 16-5. The arrows indicate the various approaches utilized to cannulate the internal jugular vein. The position of the internal jugular vein is indicated by the dashed lines.

chest wall. Most clinicians report a high success rate for central placement, but serious complications occur much more frequently with cannulation of the subclavian vein than with other routes. Pneumothorax is the most common complication, so the technique should be used with caution, if at all, in patients with severe lung disease. Attempts to cannulate both subclavian veins are best avoided because of the risk of producing bilateral pneumothorax.

The external jugular vein in usually visible and easy to cannulate. It is therefore a

useful alternative to the arm veins. Blitt et al.[8] used a modified Seldinger technique with a flexible J-shaped wire, which can be threaded through the external jugular vein and manipulated into the superior vena cava, enabling the central venous catheter to be inserted into a peripheral vein over the J-shaped wire. Successful central venous placement has been reported to be over 90 percent.

The internal jugular vein is probably preferred to the subclavian vein since there is a lower incidence of major complications. The nursing management of neck catheters, however, may be difficult. The right internal jugular vein is ideal as it forms a shorter, straighter line than the left internal jugular vein to the superior vena cava. Techniques in which the needle is inserted well above the clavicle are less likely to cause major complications and, therefore, are most often selected. Although various approaches can be utilized to locate the internal jugular vein, there are several points of management common to all techniques (Fig. 16-5). To avoid unnecessary trauma, the vein can be first located with a small (23-gauge) "seeker" needle. The small needle is then removed and a larger needle introduced along the side, using the small needle as a guide. Saline should be injected through the larger needle after puncturing the skin to clear the needle of any tissue. The primary complication of this approach is puncture of the carotid artery and he-

Table 16-2. Advantages of Different Approaches to Central Vein Catheterization

	Vein			
	Brachial	Subclavian	External Jugular	Internal Jugular
Ease of insertion	+	+	+ +	+ +
Success rate	+	+ +	+ + +	+ +
Complications	+ + +	+	+ +	+
Ability to insert pulmonary artery catheter	−	−	+	+ +

Symbols: + + + = marked advantage; + + = moderate advantage; + = minimal advantage; − = no advantage.

matoma formation. Although other complications are rare, thrombophlebitis, infection, pneumothorax, nerve damage, thoracic duct injury (left internal jugular vein cannulation), hematoma, neck tenderness, tracheal tube cuff puncture, venous air embolism, vocal cord paralysis, mediastinal infiltration, and cardiac tamponade have been reported.

From a clinical point of view, the central venous pressure or right atrial pressure is influenced by the right ventricular volume. If the right ventricle fails to empty because of pulmonary hypertension or, more often, left heart failure, the central venous pressure will be elevated and may draw the incorrect inference that the patient's blood volume is expanded. If left heart failure is suspected, additional monitoring, such as a pulmonary artery catheter, is needed.

Pulmonary Artery Catheter

A flow-directed, balloon-tipped pulmonary artery catheter (Swan-Ganz) enables catheterization of the right heart for measurement of pressures without requiring the manipulative and radiologic control demanded by other methods of cardiac catheterization.[1] The flow-directed pulmonary artery catheter has been further developed for measuring cardiac output by the thermodilution technique and for cardiac pacing. This catheter is most frequently inserted percutaneously via the right internal jugular vein.

Indications for use of a flow-directed pulmonary artery catheter are constantly evolving (Table 16-3). For example, the need for intravascular fluid volume replacement as well as the response to intravenous fluid infusion is commonly monitored with a pulmonary artery catheter. Measurement of cardiac output and calculation of systemic and pulmonary vascular resistance are essential information for evaluating the response to inotropes and/or vasodilators in patients with valvular heart disease or cor-

Table 16-3. Some Indications for Insertion of a Flow-Directed Pulmonary Artery Catheter (Swan Ganz) in Noncardiac Surgery Cases

Evaluation of response to fluid administration, inotropes, or vasodilators
Impaired left ventricular function
Severe, uncontrolled arterial hypertension
Pericardial disease with tamponade
Massive trauma
Sepsis
Pulmonary emboli
Aortic surgery with cross-clamping
Portal systemic shunt surgery
Severe respiratory failure

onary artery disease. Subendocardial myocardial ischemia may manifest as a V wave on the tracing of the pulmonary artery occlusion pressure even before changes on the ECG suggest myocardial ischemia. Normal pressures in various sites of the cardiovascular system are summarized in Table 16-4, while the interpretation of various disease states are summarized in Table 16-5.

Neuromuscular

A peripheral nerve stimulator should be utilized to monitor the degree of neuromuscular blockade produced by muscle relaxants (see Chapter 8).

Central Nervous System

The electroencephalogram (EEG) can be monitored during anesthesia for procedures in which localized brain ischemia may occur

Table 16-4. Normal Pressures of Various Cardiovascular Sites

Location	Abbreviation	Pressure (mmHg)
Central venous	CVP	6
Right atrial	RAP	4
Right ventricular		
Systolic	—	24
Diastolic	RVEDP	4
Pulmonary artery		
Systolic	PAsP	24
Diastolic	PAdP	10
Mean	PAP	16
Pulmonary artery occlusion	PAo	9
Left atrial	LAP	7
Left ventricular		
Systolic	—	130
Diastolic	LVEDP	7

Table 16-5. Use of a Flow-Directed Pulmonary Artery Catheter (Swan Ganz) in the Interpretation of Various Low Cardiac Output States

Cause of Low Cardiac Output	CVP	PAo	PAdP vs PAo Pressure
Hypovolemia	Decreased	Decresed	PAdP = PAo
Left ventricular failure	Increased	Increased	PAdP = PAo
Right ventricular failure	Increased	No change	PAdP = PAo
Pulmonary embolism	Increased	No change	PAdP > PAo
Cardiac tamponade	Increased	Increased	PAdP = PAo

Abbreviations: CVP, central venous pressure; PAo, pulmonary artery occlusion pressure; PAdP, pulmonary artery diastolic pressure.

(see Chapter 24). For example, it has been recommended that an EEG be utilized in carotid endarterectomy surgery. Traditionally, the EEG has proven to be of little value in monitoring depth of anesthesia because of a variable response and alterations in such factors as $PaCO_2$. Recently, however, more sophisticated EEG monitoring has provided some promise in regard to accurate monitoring of anesthetic depth.

RECORDING OF INTRAOPERATIVE DATA (ANESTHESIA RECORD)

The anesthesia record is a required and indispensable part of anesthetic care (Fig. 16-6). As in all aspects of medicine, the anesthetic and surgical events need to be documented for medical and legal purposes. The anesthesia record is the only continuous record which provides a detailed account of the intraoperative course of a patient. The intraoperative record provides documentation of drugs and fluids that have been given. This information, for example, correlated with urinary output, can aid in predicting future drug and fluid needs. Also, a recording of the vital signs and analgesic responses to narcotics will aid the ward physicians in estimating narcotic tolerance. In essence, the anesthesia record provides a mechanism by which patient responses can be analyzed and appropriate action taken. Furthermore, this record can provide a reminder to the anesthesiologist of observations other than cardiopulmonary variables that need to be made. For ex-

ample, the anesthesia record may provide spaces to record fluid and blood replacement, estimated blood loss, urinary output, temperature, ECG findings, end-tidal PCO_2, and central venous pressure. Also, if the anesthesiologist becomes distracted, a record exists as to when the last vital signs were determined.

Although patient care should take priority over making a neat and current anesthesia record, every effort should be made to keep the anesthesia record as current as possible. There can be no doubt that information recorded based on someone's memory will be highly suspect in its accuracy.

Retrospective review of anesthesia records can provide valuable information. For example, the effect, hazards, and disadvantages of a particular anesthetic technique can be assessed. Questions such as the magnitude of hypotension after a spinal anesthetic and how many of these patients required vasopressor therapy can be quantitated. An overall assessment of anesthetic techniques and drugs used in a particular hospital can be determined. Also, a particular problem can be assessed by analyzing multiple anesthesia records. As an example, the question may be raised as to the adequacy of monitoring for a particular procedure. By analysis of all past anesthesia records, the current practice can be established.

When litigation becomes a factor in assessing an anesthetic, it is essential that the anesthesia record be as complete as possible. A random observation of anesthesia

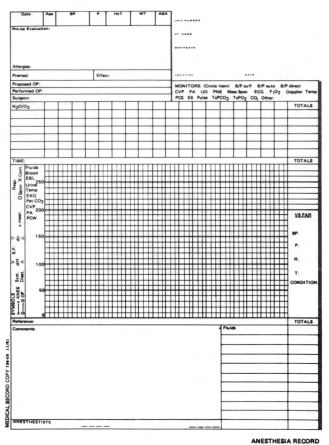

Figure 16-6. A typical anesthesia record form.

records in the author's hospitals, and several other hospitals, indicates that these records are rarely complete. An incomplete anesthesia record makes it difficult for attorneys to ascertain an accurate course of perioperative events. The anesthesiologist needs to develop work habits consistent with providing complete anesthesia records, which are properly dated, timed, and signed. It is further recommended that the anesthesiologist make postanesthesia rounds and record on the patient's chart findings relevant to the prior anesthetic.

PATIENT SAFETY

In the anesthetized state, the patient is totally dependent on the anesthesiologist for safety and comfort (see Chapter 15).

This requires a keen awareness for potential harm to the patient. Protection of the patient from accidental electrocution or burns due to malfunctioning monitoring equipment is essential. Isolation transformers limit the hazard of macroshock but not microshock to the patient. Isolated patient inputs on monitoring equipment limit the current that could actually pass to the patient. Battery powered monitors present little chance of electrocution to the patient or anesthesiologist since leakage current does not exist.

The electrosurgical unit can result in high frequency current burns when the return plate ("ground") malfunctions. If disconnection of the return plate occurs, all the high frequency current generated by the electrosurgical unit will seek a return via alternate pathways such as electrodes for the ECG or internal temperature probes. Burns occur reflecting the high current density at these sites.

REFERENCES

1. Hug CC. Monitoring. In: Miller RD, ed, Anesthesia. New York, Churchill Livingstone, 1981:157–201.
2. Kimble KJ, Darnall RA, Yelderman M, Ariagno RL, Ream AK. An automated oscillometric technique for estimating mean arterial pressure in critically ill newborns. Anesthesiology 1981;54:423–5.
3. Showman A. Hazards of automatic noninvasive blood pressure monitoring. Anesthesiology 1981;55:717–8.
4. Morris RH. Operating room temperature and the anesthetized, paralyzed patient. Arch Surg 1971;102:95–7.
5. Ozanne GM, Young WG, Mazzel WS, Severinghaus JW. Multipatient anesthetic mass spectrometry. Anesthesiology 1981;56:62–70.
6. Bedford RF. Radial arterial function following percutaneous canulation with 18- and 20-gauge catheters. Anesthesiology 1977;47:37–9.
7. Slogoff S, Keats AS, Arlund C. On the safety of radial artery cannulation. Anesthesiology 1983;59:42–7.
8. Blitt CD, Wright WA, Petty WC, Webster TA. Central venous catheterization via the external jugular vein. A technique employing the J-wire. JAMA 1974;229:817–8.

17

Acid-Base Balance and Blood Gas Analysis

All living organisms depend on maintenance of acid-base equilibrium and oxygenation for survival.[1,2] Regulation of acid-base balance is actually regulation of the hydrogen ion (H^+) and bicarbonate ion (HCO_3^-) concentration in body fluids. Maintenance of the H^+ concentration over a narrow range is necessary to (1) insure the optimal function of enzymes, (2) maintain the proper distribution of electrolytes, (3) optimize myocardial contractility, and (4) maintain an optimal saturation of hemoglobin. The normal H^+ concentration in the arterial blood and extracellular fluid is 36 to 44 nanomoles/L which is equivalent to an arterial pH (pHa) of 7.44 to 7.36, respectively. The normal concentration of HCO_3^- is 24 ± 2 mEq/L.

MAINTENANCE OF THE HYDROGEN ION CONCENTRATION

All body fluids are provided with buffer systems which represent the first line of defense against excessive changes in pHa produced by excess acid or alkali. The bicarbonate buffer system is the most important and readily available buffer system, representing over 50 percent of the total buffering capacity of the body. The most important nonbicarbonate buffer system is hemoglobin, which is responsible for about 35 percent of the buffering capacity in blood. The remainder of buffering capacity is provided by phosphates and plasma proteins.

The bicarbonate buffer system is dependent on the hydration of carbon dioxide to carbonic acid (H_2CO_3) in the plasma and erythrocytes (Fig. 17-1). Hydration of carbon dioxide in the plasma is a slow process, but in erythrocytes this reaction is greatly accelerated by the presence of the enzyme carbonic anhydrase. The H^+ formed by dissociation of H_2CO_3 in the erythrocytes and plasma is buffered by reduced hemoglobin. Hemoglobin can also transport carbon dioxide as carbaminohemoglobin. The HCO_3^- formed by dissociation of H_2CO_3 in erythrocytes enters the plasma where it functions as a buffer. At the same time, chloride ions enter the erythrocytes (chloride shift) to maintain electrical neutrality.

In addition to buffers, other compensatory mechanisms necessary for maintenance of an appropriate pHa include (1) alterations in the alveolar ventilation, (2) reabsorption of HCO_3^- by renal tubule cells, and (3) secretion of H^+ by renal tubule cells (Figs. 17-2 and 17-3).[1,2] Ultimately, the kidneys are the most powerful of the acid-base regulatory systems, but, in contrast to the instantaneous action of buffers and rapid adjustments in ventilation (1 to 3

$$CO_2 + H_2O \xrightleftharpoons[\text{anhydrase}]{\text{carbonic}} H_2CO_3 \rightleftharpoons H^+ + HCO_3^-$$

Figure 17-1. Carbon dioxide (CO_2) formed from aerobic metabolism undergoes hydration to form carbonic acid (H_2CO_3). Hydration of CO_2 in the plasma is a slow process, while in erythrocytes this reaction is greatly accelerated by the presence of the enzyme carbonic anhydrase. Dissociation of H_2CO_3 to hydrogen ion (H^+) and bicarbonate ion (HCO_3^-) is spontaneous.

minutes), the compensation via the kidneys requires 12 to 48 hours.

The Henderson-Hasselbach equation emphasizes that a normal pHa depends upon maintenance of an optimal 20 to 1 ratio of the concentration of HCO_3^- to carbon dioxide (Table 17-1). Acid-base disturbances characterized by changes in the plasma concentration of HCO_3^- are predictably accompanied by appropriate compensatory changes in the $PaCO_2$ secondary to alterations in alveolar ventilation. If changes in the plasma concentration of HCO_3^- and $PaCO_2$ are proportional such that a 20 to 1 ratio is maintained, the pHa will remain near or within the normal range despite disturbances of acid-base balance. For example, acid-base disturbances due to respiratory acidosis or alkalosis are compensated for by renal-induced changes in the plasma concentration of HCO_3^- such that the 20 to 1 ratio is maintained. As a result, the pHa in the presence of chronic respiratory acid-base disturbances is near normal despite persistent abnormalities of the $PaCO_2$. Likewise, acid-base disturbances due to metabolic abnormalities are compensated for by adjustments in alveolar ventilation in an effort to place the $PaCO_2$ in a range that preserves the 20 to 1 ratio.

DIFFERENTIAL DIAGNOSIS OF ACID-BASE DISTURBANCES

The differential diagnosis of acid-base disturbances (respiratory acidosis, respiratory alkalosis, metabolic acidosis, metabolic alkalosis) is based on the direct measurement of the pHa and $PaCO_2$ plus a derived estimate of the plasma concentration of HCO_3^- using a nomogram (Table 17-2, Fig. 17-4).[3] Acidemia is present when the pHa is less than 7.36; alkalemia is present when the pHa is greater than 7.44. A $PaCO_2$ greater than 44 mmHg is defined as hypoventilation; hyperventilation is present when the $PaCO_2$ is less than 36 mmHg. Hypoventilation is synonomous with respiratory acidosis, and hyperventilation is synonomous with respiratory alkalosis. Acidemia and alkalemia characterized by

Table 17-1. Henderson-Hasselbach Equation[a]

pHa	$= pK + \log \dfrac{HCO_3^-}{0.03 \times PaCO_2}$
pHa	= negative logarithm of the arterial concentration of hydrogen ions
pK	= 6.1 at 37 Celsius
HCO_3^-	= concentration of bicarbonate ions
0.03	= solubility coefficient for CO_2 in plasma
$PaCO_2$	= arterial partial pressure of CO_2

[a] Substitution of normal values for pHa (7.4) and $PaCO_2$ (40 mmHg) results in a calculated HCO_3^- concentration of 24 mEq/L. Maintenance of this concentration of HCO_3^- relative to the concentration of CO_2 (0.03 × 40) results in an optimal 20 to 1 ratio. Likewise, alterations in HCO_3^- or the concentration of CO_2 will not significantly change the pHa if the 20 to 1 ratio is preserved.

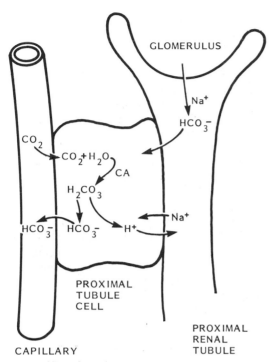

Figure 17-2. Proximal renal tubule cells can regulate acid-base equilibrium by acidifying or alkalizing the urine via reabsorption of bicarbonate ions (HCO_3^-) and/or secretion of hydrogen ions (H^+). In addition to reabsorption of HCO_3^-, proximal renal tubule cells are able to synthesize new HCO_3^- via hydration of CO_2 and subsequent dissociation of H_2CO_3. Hydration of CO_2 in these cells is accelerated by the presence of the enzyme carbonic anhydrase (CA). Reabsorbed and newly synthesized HCO_3^- can pass from renal tubule cells into capillaries to replenish that lost due to buffering. H^+ ions formed by dissociation of H_2CO_3 in proximal renal tubule cells are secreted into the urine in exchange for cations, usually sodium (Na^+) so as to maintain electrical neutrality.

deviations of the HCO_3^- concentration above or below 24 mEq/L are considered to be primary metabolic disturbances. Predictable adverse responses accompany acidemia and alkalemia (Table 17-3 and 17-4).

Interpretation of the plasma concentration of HCO_3^- as derived from the nomogram requires an adjustment for the impact of ventilation (Fig. 17-4). For example, an increased $PaCO_2$ leads to the hydration of

carbon dioxide with a subsequent increase in the plasma concentration of HCO_3^- (Fig. 17-1). Normalization of the HCO_3^- concentration above or below 24 mEq/L in the presence of an increased or decreased $PaCO_2$ is achieved by applying a correction factor that is dependent on the rapidity and direction of change in the $PaCO_2$ (Table 17-5).

In discussing abnormalities of acid-base balance, primary alterations should be distinguished from changes that reflect compensatory responses. Compensation is the restoration of pHa toward 7.4 despite the continued presence of the primary acid-base abnormality. Indeed, compensatory responses frequently result in mixed acid-base disturbances. Ultimately, differentiation between primary respiratory or metabolic causes of acid-base disturbances is necessary to assure proper treatment.

RESPIRATORY ACIDOSIS

Respiratory acidosis is present when the $PaCO_2$ exceeds 44 mmHg (Table 17-2). Measurement of the pHa or estimate of the plasma concentration of HCO_3^- provides evidence as to the chronicity of the acid-base disturbance and gives an indication as to the primary or compensatory nature of the respiratory change (Table 17-2). An increased $PaCO_2$ is due either to decreased elimination of carbon dioxide by the lungs (hypoventilation) or increased metabolic production of carbon dioxide (Table 17-6).

The initial effect of an increase in the $PaCO_2$ is a decreased pHa due to hydration of carbon dioxide (Fig. 17-1). The reduction in pH occurs to a similar extent in arterial blood and cerebrospinal fluid (CSF) since carbon dioxide rapidly crosses lipid barriers such as the blood brain barrier. The response to a reduction in pHa is stimulation of ventilation via the carotid bodies, while the decreased pH of the CSF stimulates medullary chemoreceptors located in the fourth cerebral ventricle.[4] With time, stim-

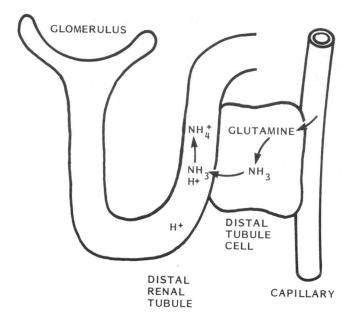

GLOMERULUS

NH$_4^+$

GLUTAMINE

NH$_3$
H+

NH$_3$

H+

DISTAL
TUBULE
CELL

DISTAL
RENAL
TUBULE

CAPILLARY

Figure 17-3. The formation of ammonia (NH_3) from glutamine in distal renal tubule cells facilitates the elimination of hydrogen ions (H^+) in the urine as ammonium (NH_4^+). Neutralization of H^+ in the urine by formation of NH_4^+ is essential, since secretion of H^+ by proximal renal tubule cells (see Fig. 17-3) ceases when the urine pH is less than 4.5. Renal disease may impair the ability of distal renal tubule cells to form NH_3, resulting in decreased secretion of H^+ by renal tubule cells as the urine pH decreases below 4.5.

ulation of ventilation via medullary chemoreceptors is eliminated as the CSF pH is restored to normal by the active transport of HCO_3^- into the CSF.[4] Therefore, the volume of ventilation after restoration of the CSF pH to normal is less than that present during the initial phase of respiratory acidosis. It should be appreciated that volatile anesthetics greatly reduce the carotid body mediated response to acidemia.

Compensatory Responses

The absolute reduction in pHa produced by respiratory acidosis depends on the degree of compensation provided by the secondary increase in the plasma concentration of HCO_3^-. It is estimated that the hydration of carbon dioxide increases the plasma concentration of HCO_3^- about a mEq/L for every 10 mmHg increase of the PaCO$_2$ above normal (Table 17-5). This compensatory increase in the plasma concentration of HCO_3^- occurs within seconds following the increase in PaCO$_2$. In addition, hydration of carbon dioxide in proximal renal tubule cells promotes secretion of H^+ into the urine (Fig. 17-2). At the same time, sodium is exchanged for H^+ which facilitates reabsorption of HCO_3^- (Fig. 17-2). Likewise, distal renal tubule cells secrete H^+ (Fig. 17-3). This renal compensation requires 12 to 48 hours but eventually increases the plasma HCO_3^- concentration by about 2 mEq/L for every 10 mmHg elevation in the PaCO$_2$ above normal (Table 17-5). Thus, the total increase in the plasma concentration of HCO_3^- produced by hydration of carbon dioxide and renal reabsorption of HCO_3^- is about 3 mEq/L for every 10 mmHg increase of the PaCO$_2$ above normal (Table 17-5). The net effect of this compensatory response is a return of the pHa to normal or near normal in patients with chronic elevations in the PaCO$_2$. Acute respiratory acidosis is recognized by a reduced pHa and less than the predicted increase in the plasma concentration of HCO_3^- (Table 17-2).

Treatment

Treatment of chronic respiratory acidosis is by correction of the disorder responsible for decreased elimination of carbon dioxide by the lungs or increased metabolic pro-

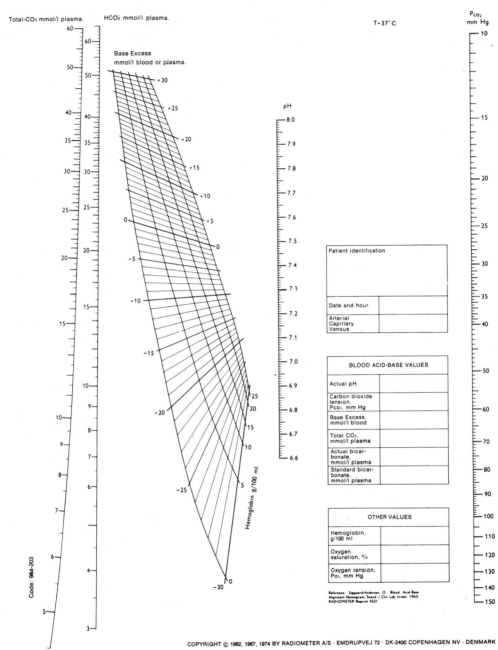

Figure 17-4. The Siggard-Andersen alignment nomogram is used to derive the estimated plasma concentration of bicarbonate ions (HCO_3^-) or, alternatively, determination of base excess. A line connecting the measured partial pressure of carbon dioxide (PCO_2) and pH will transect the vertical column representing the plasma concentration of HCO_3^- or base excess (Nomogram originally appeared in Siggard-Andersen O. Blood acid-base alignment nomogram. Scand J Clin Lab Invest 1963;15:211–7).

Table 17-2. Differential Diagnosis of Acid-Base Disturbances

Disturbance	pHa (7.36 to 7.44)	PaCO$_2$ (36 to 44 mmHg)	HCO$_3^-$ (24 mEq/L)
Respiratory acidosis			
Acute	Moderate decrease	Marked increase	Slight increase
Chronic	Slight decrease to no change	Marked increase	Moderate increase
Respiratory alkalosis			
Acute	Moderate increase	Marked decrease	Slight decrease
Chronic	Slight increase to no change	Marked decrease	Moderate decrease
Metabolic acidosis			
Acute	Moderate to marked decrease	Slight decrease	Marked decrease
Chronic	Slight decrease	Moderate decrease	Marked decrease
Metabolic alkalosis			
Acute	Marked increase	Moderate increase	Marked increase
Chronic	Marked increase	Moderate increase	Marked increase

duction of carbon dioxide (Table 17-6). Mechanical ventilation of the lungs will be necessary when acute or chronic elevation of the PaCO$_2$ is marked. Rapid lowering of a chronically elevated PaCO$_2$, however, can result in metabolic alkalosis and central nervous system irritability due to washout of total body carbon dioxide more rapidly than the kidneys can produce a corresponding reduction in the plasma concentration of HCO$_3^-$. Therefore, it is mandatory to slowly reduce a chronically elevated PaCO$_2$ so as to assure time for renal elimination of excess HCO$_3^-$. Hypochloremia due to augmentation of renal excretion of chloride in order to enhance proximal renal tubule cell reabsorption of HCO$_3^-$ may require treatment in some patients.

Table 17-3. Adverse Effects of Respiratory or Metabolic Acidosis

Increased serum potassium concentration
Central nervous system depression
Cardiovascular depression due to direct depressant effects on the vasomotor center, arteriolar smooth muscle and myocardial contractility (offset until severe acidosis by increased secretion of catecholamines and elevated plasma concentrations of ionized calcium)
Increased incidence of cardiac dysrhythmias
Decreased precapillary and increased postcapillary sphincter tone leading to hypovolemia

Mixed Acid-Base Disturbances

Respiratory acidosis complicated by metabolic acidosis is evidenced by an increase in the plasma concentration of HCO$_3^-$ which is less than 3 mEq/L for every 10 mmHg increase of the PaCO$_2$ above normal. This combination of acid-base disturbances may occur when cardiac output and renal blood flow are greatly reduced due to cor pulmonale in the presence of chronic obstructive pulmonary disease. An increase in the plasma concentration of HCO$_3^-$ that exceeds 3 mEq/L for every 10 mmHg elevation of the PaCO$_2$ above normal suggests

Table 17-4. Adverse Effects of Respiratory or Metabolic Alkalosis

Decreased serum potassium concentration
Decreased ionized calcium concentration (altered neuromuscular function manifesting as tetany, decreased myocardial contractility)
Central nervous system excitation
Decreased cerebral blood flow
Decreased availability of oxygen to tissues due to leftward shift of the oxyhemoglobin dissociation curve (Bohr effect)
Increased incidence of cardiac dysrhythmias
Increased airway resistance and right-to-left intrapulmonary shunting (respiratory alkalosis only)
Increased oxygen consumption
Increased cardiac output
Decreased cardiac output

Table 17-5. Normalization of Plasma Concentration of Bicarbonate for Alveolar Ventilation

Change in $PaCO_2$ from 40 mmHg	Change in HCO_3^- Concentration from 24 mEq/L
Acute 10 mmHg increase	Increase 1 mEq/L
Acute 10 mmHg decrease	Decrease 2 mEq/L
Chronic 10 mmHg increase	Increase 3 mEq/L
Chronic 10 mmHg decrease	Decrease 5 mEq/L

the presence of respiratory acidosis complicated by metabolic alkalosis. Metabolic alkalosis complicating respiratory acidosis is likely in the presence of hypochloremia and/or hypokalemia. Treatment of metabolic alkalosis associated with respiratory acidosis is with the intravenous administration of potassium chloride and avoidance of mechanical hyperventilation of the lungs.

RESPIRATORY ALKALOSIS

Respiratory alkalosis is present when the $PaCO_2$ is less than 36 mmHg (Table 17-2). Measurement of the pHa or estimate of the plasma concentration of HCO_3^- provides evidence as to the chronicity of the acid-base disturbance and gives an indication as to the primary or compensatory nature of the respiratory change (Table 17-2). A decreased $PaCO_2$ is due either to increased elimination of carbon dioxide by the lungs

Table 17-6. Causes of Respiratory Acidosis

Decreased eliminaton of carbon dioxide by the lungs (hypoventilation)
   Central nervous system depression due to drugs (anesthetics)
   Decreased skeletal muscle strength (diseases, skeletal muscle relaxants)
   Intrinsic pulmonary disease
   Rebreathing of exhaled gases (exhausted soda lime, incomplete one-way valve in anesthetic breathing system)
Increased metabolic production of carbon dioxide
   Hyperthermia
   Increased glucose load (hyperalimentation)

(hyperventilation) or decreased metabolic production of carbon dioxide (Table 17-7). The initial effect of a decrease in the $PaCO_2$ is an increased pHa due to decreased hydration of carbon dioxide (Fig. 17-1). The decreased $PaCO_2$ and increased pHa reduces the stimulus to breath normally mediated by the carotid bodies and medullary chemoreceptors. Active transport of HCO_3^- out of the CSF subsequently restores the CSF pH to normal.[4] As a result, the activity of the medullary chemoreceptors becomes normal and the volume of ventilation is increased, despite persistence of a decreased $PaCO_2$. By the same mechanism, mechanical hyperventilation of the lungs during anesthesia can result in the initiation of spontaneous ventilation at a lower $PaCO_2$ than present before hyperventilation (Fig. 17-5).[5] This initiation of ventilation reflects a normal CSF pH which maintains ventilation via stimulation from the medullary chemoreceptors. Likewise, continued hyperventilation upon returning to sea level from altitude reflects maintenance of ventilation by the medullary chemoreceptors exposed to a normal pH.

Compensatory Responses

Three events occur simultaneously to reduce the plasma concentration of HCO_3^- and thus offset the increase in pHa that accompanies respiratory alkalosis. There is an immediate response via the bicarbonate buffer system resulting in the production of carbon dioxide (Fig. 17-1). In addition, alkalosis stimulates the activity of phosphofructokinase enzyme, which results in glycolysis and generation of lactic acid. These two mechanisms operate rapidly to reduce the plasma concentration of HCO_3^- by about 2 mEq/L for every 10 mmHg decrease in the $PaCO_2$ below normal (Table 17-5). The third compensatory mechanism is decreased proximal renal tubule cell reabsorption of HCO_3^- which becomes maxi-

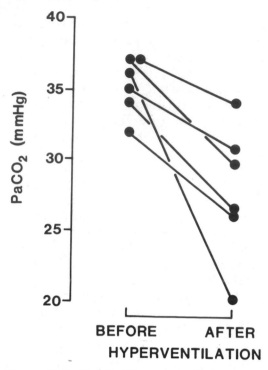

Figure 17-5. The $PaCO_2$ present during spontaneous ventilation before and after mechanical hyperventilation to a $PaCO_2$ of 20 mmHg for 2 hours was measured in six adult patients. The return of spontaneous ventilation at a lower $PaCO_2$ following mechanical hyperventilation reflects restoration of the cerebrospinal fluid pH to normal despite persistent reductions in the $PaCO_2$. This is equivalent to resetting the threshold of the medullary chemoreceptors for carbon dioxide. (Modified from Moorthy SS. Acid-base disturbances. In: Stoelting RK, Dierdorf SF, eds, Anesthesia and co-existing disease. New York Churchill Livingstone, 1983;227–37; and based on data in reference 5.)

mal by 12 to 48 hours (Fig. 17-2). The reduction in the plasma concentration of HCO_3^- produced by these three compensatory mechanisms is about 5 mEq/L for every 10 mmHg decrease in the $PaCO_2$ below normal (Table 17-5). This degree of metabolic compensation is sufficient to return the pHa to normal or near normal in patients with chronic reductions in the $PaCO_2$ (Table 17-2). Chronic respiratory alkalosis complicated by metabolic acidosis

Table 17-7. Causes of Respiratory Alkalosis

Increased elimination of carbon dioxide by the lungs (hyperventilation)
    Iatrogenic-mechanical or self-induced
    Pain
    Anxiety
    Decreased barometric pressure
    Central nervous system injury
    Arterial hypoxemia
    Pulmonary vascular disease
    Cirrhosis of the liver
    Sepsis
    Hyperthermia

Decreased metabolic production of carbon dioxide
    Hypothermia
    Skeletal muscle paralysis

is reflected by less than a 5 mEq/L increase in the plasma concentration of HCO_3^-.

Treatment

Treatment of chronic respiratory alkalosis is directed at correcting the underlying disorder responsible for the increased elimination of carbon dioxide by the lungs or decreased metabolic production of carbon dioxide (Table 17-7). During anesthesia, treatment of acute respiratory alkalosis is most often accomplished by adjustment of the mechanical ventilator to decrease the alveolar ventilation. In addition, rebreathing of exhaled gases that contain carbon dioxide can be provided by adding dead space to the anesthetic breathing system. Finally, carbon dioxide delivered from a metered source can be added to the inhaled gases in an attempt to reestablish a normal $PaCO_2$.

METABOLIC ACIDOSIS

Metabolic acidosis is present when the pHa is less than 7.36 and the plasma concentration of HCO_3^- is decreased below 24 mEq/L (Table 17-2). Measurement of the $PaCO_2$ supplies evidence as to the chronicity of the acid-base disturbance and gives an indication as to the primary or compensatory nature of the metabolic change (Table 17-2). A decreased pHa in associa-

Table 17-8. Causes of Metabolic Acidosis

Decreased renal tubule elimination of hydrogen ions
    Renal failure
    Cirrhosis of the liver with decreased conversion
      of lactate to glucose

Increased metabolic production of hydrogen ions
    Anaerobic glycolysis due to decreased delivery
      of oxygenated blood to tissues
    Diabetic ketoacidosis
    Metabolism of amino acids in hyperalimentation
      solutions
    Idiopathic
    Excessive loss of gastrointestinal fluids formed
      distal to the pylorus (diarrhea, ileostomy)
      leading to a relative excess of hydrogen ions
    Renal tubular acidosis (inability of kidneys to
      reabsorb bicarbonate ions present in the
      glomerular filtrate results in a relative excess
      of hydrogen ions)

tion with a reduced plasma concentration of HCO_3^- is due either to decreased renal tubule cell elimination of H^+ or increased metabolic production of H^+ relative to HCO_3^- (Table 17-8).

Compensatory Responses

Compensatory responses initiated by metabolic acidosis include proximal renal tubule cell secretion of H^+ with reabsorption of HCO_3^- (Figure 17-2), distal renal tubule cell secretion of H^+ (Fig. 17-3), and increased alveolar ventilation due to stimulation of the carotid bodies by H^+. The reduction in $PaCO_2$ produced by increased alveolar ventilation is rapidly reflected as a corresponding decrease in the $PaCO_2$ in the CSF. As a result, the CSF pH increases, leading to an inhibition of the activity of the medullary chemoreceptors and a blunting of the increase in ventilation produced by the carotid bodies.[4] With time, however, the CSF pH normalizes, reflecting the active transport of HCO_3^- into the CSF. Therefore, the inhibition of ventilation provided by the medullary chemoreceptors is removed and there is a further, although delayed, increase in alveolar ventilation. As with respiratory acidosis, volatile anesthetics blunt the carotid body mediated response to metabolic acidosis.[8] Another

compensatory mechanism is the use of buffers present in bone to neutralize the nonvolatile acids present in the circulation. Indeed, chronic metabolic acidosis is commonly associated with loss of bone mass.

A useful guideline is that a 1 mmHg change in $PaCO_2$ above or below 40 mmHg results in a 0.008 unit pH change in the opposite direction. Therefore, a patient with a $PaCO_2$ of 30 mmHg and a pHa of 7.38 has a "corrected" pHa of 7.30. Routine use of this rule in the initial interpretation of the $PaCO_2$ and pHa permits rapid recognition of an acid-base abnormality due to a metabolic disturbance. Another useful guideline is that $PaCO_2$ decreases about 1 mmHg for every mEq/L reduction in the plasma concentration of HCO_3^- below 24 mEq/L. When metabolic acidosis is complicated by respiratory acidosis, the magnitude of reduction in the $PaCO_2$ is less than 1 mmHg for each mEq/L reduction in the plasma concentration of HCO_3^-.

Treatment

Treatment of metabolic acidosis is with removal of the cause for the accumulation of nonvolatile acids in the circulation (Table 17-8). In addition, the intravenous administration of sodium bicarbonate is indicated if metabolic acidosis is associated with myocardial depression or cardiac dysrhythmias. Calculation of the dose of sodium bicarbonate (Table 17-9) requires use of a nomogram to determine the plasma concentration of HCO_3^- or, alternatively, the base excess (Fig. 17-4).[3] The best approach is to administer about one-half of the calculated dose of sodium bicarbonate followed by a repeat measurement of the pHa to evaluate the impact of therapy.

METABOLIC ALKALOSIS

Metabolic alkalosis is present when the pHa is greater than 7.44 and the plasma concentration of HCO_3^- is increased above 24

Table 17-9. Calculation of the Dose of Sodium Bicarbonate to Treat Metabolic Acidosis

Dose of sodium bicarbonate	=	Body weight (kg)	×	Deviation of HCO₃⁻ from 24 mEq/L[a]	×	Extracellular fluid volume as a fraction of body mass (0.2)

[a] The normal value for HCO_3^- (24 mEq/L) must be adjusted for deviations in the $PaCO_2$ from 40 mmHg (see Table 17-5).

mEq/L (Table 17-2). Measurement of the $PaCO_2$ supplies evidence as to the chronicity of the acid-base disturbance and gives an indication as to the primary or compensatory nature of the metabolic change (Table 17-2). An increased pHa due to metabolic alkalosis reflects events that result in an excess of HCO_3^- relative to H^+ (Table 17-10). An example of an event that results in a relative excess of HCO_3^- is conversion of citrate in the liver to HCO_3^-. Indeed, metabolic alkalosis is not an infrequent finding following administration of large amounts of stored whole blood containing citrate anticoagulant.[6] Clinically, metabolic alkalosis correlates with reductions in the total body concentrations of chloride and potassium. For example, diuretics which facilitate chloride loss via the renal tubules are associated with increased proximal renal tubule cell reabsorption of HCO_3^- to maintain electrical neutrality. Likewise, hypokalemia secondary to diuretic therapy is associated with similar renal changes that contribute to metabolic alkalosis (Table 17-11).

Compensatory Responses

Compensatory responses initiated by metabolic alkalosis include increased proximal renal tubule cell reabsorption of H^+ (Fig. 17-2), decreased renal tubule cell secretion of H^+ (Fig. 17-3), and alveolar hypoventilation. The efficiency of the renal compensatory mechanism is dependent on the presence of cations (sodium, potassium) and chloride (Fig. 17-2 and 17-3). Depletion of these ions as occurs with vomiting impairs the ability of the kidneys to excrete excess HCO_3^-, resulting in incomplete renal compensation for metabolic alkalosis. Hypoventilation in an attempt to compensate for metabolic alkalosis will initially stimulate the medullary chemoreceptors and thus offset the compensatory effect of decreased alveolar ventilation. With time, the CSF pH is normalized by active transport of HCO_3^- into the CSF and the volume of ventilation decreases, despite the persistence of a compensatory increase in the $PaCO_2$.[4] If the $PaCO_2$ again increases, however, the CSF pH will decrease and the same sequence will be repeated. Indeed, respiratory compensation for pure metabolic alkalosis, in contrast to metabolic acidosis, is never more than 75 percent complete. As a result, the pHa remains elevated in patients with primary metabolic alkalosis (Table 17-2). Furthermore, a $PaCO_2$ above 55 mmHg is beyond the normal compensatory mechanism for metabolic alkalosis and reflects concomitant respiratory acidosis.

Table 17-10. Causes of Metabolic Alkalosis

Vomiting or nasogastric suction resulting in excessive loss of hydrogen ions relative to bicarbonate ions
Chronic hypercarbia
Chloride and/or potassium depletion due to diuretics
Metabolism of lactate in lactated Ringer's solution, citrate in stored whole blood, or acetate in hyperalimentation solutions to bicarbonate ions
Hyperaldosteronism leading to increased sodium reabsorption at the distal renal tubule that results in increased hydrogen ion secretion

Table 17-11. Effects of Hypokalemia that Contribute to Metabolic Alkalosis

Increased proximal renal tubule cell reabsorption of bicarbonate ions
Increased distal renal tubule cell secretion of hydrogen ions
Increased distal renal tubule cell synthesis of ammonia

Treatment

Treatment of metabolic alkalosis is directed at resolution of the process responsible for the acid-base derangement (Table 17-10), plus intravenous infusion of potassium chloride which allows the kidneys to excrete excess HCO_3^-.

MEASUREMENT OF ARTERIAL BLOOD GASES

Technological advances that permit the analysis of arterial and mixed venous blood gases as well as pH have contributed greatly to the management of patients during anesthesia and in the intensive care unit (see Chapter 32). Ability to obtain blood gas values within a few minutes permits moment-to-moment adjustments in the care of patients in operating rooms and intensive care units. The small volume of blood required for the measurement (as little as 0.1 ml) extends this technique to the care of premature infants as well as children and adults.

Sampling of Blood

Arterial blood is most often obtained percutaneously from the radial, brachial, or femoral artery. Arterialized venous blood may be an alternative when arterial sampling is not possible. Blood is drawn into a plastic or glass syringe that contains heparin sufficient to fill the dead space of the syringe. Heparin is acidic, and excessive amounts of this anticoagulant in the sampling syringe could falsely lower the measured pH. Elimination of air bubbles from the syringe after obtaining the sample is important, since equilibration of oxygen and carbon dioxide in the blood with the corresponding partial pressures in the air bubble could influence the measured results. Prior to analysis, the blood sample should be placed on ice to retard metabolism which could consume oxygen and produce carbon dioxide.

Temperature Correction

In the past, it was recommended that blood gases and pH should be corrected for temperature if the temperature of the measuring electrode (usually 37 Celsius) differed from the patient's body temperature. This recommendation is based on the knowledge that the solubility of oxygen and carbon dioxide in the blood are temperature-dependent. Therefore, placing blood from a patient with a body temperature less than 37 Celsius into an electrode maintained at 37 Celsius means more molecules enter the gas phase to be sensed as partial pressure than would be present in vivo at the lower body temperature of the patient. Nomograms are available to correct blood gases and pH measurements for temperature. Recently, the need to correct PCO_2 and pH measurements for body temperature has been challenged.[7] It is argued that a normal PCO_2 and pH measured at an electrode temperature of 37 Celsius reflects an unperturbed acid-base status of the patient regardless of the body temperature that existed at the time the sample was drawn. This argument is based on the concept that maintenance of electrochemical neutrality (pH = pOH) requires the pH to rise with reductions in body temperature. Conversely, with increases in body temperature, the neutral point falls and maintenance of electrochemical neutrality requires a decrease in pH. If this concept is accepted, it is unnecessary to correct PCO_2 and pH for variations in body temperature from the temperature of the electrodes which are maintained at 37 Celsius. Temperature correction of the PO_2 remains important, however, to assess oxygenation. As a guideline, the measured PO_2 should be decreased 6 percent for every degree Celsius the patient's body temperature is below the temperature of the electrode (37 Celsius). The PO_2 is increased 6 percent for every degree Celsius the body temperature exceeds 37 Celsius. Furthermore, calculation of the alveolar-to-arterial difference for oxygen (A-aDO$_2$) requires temperature correction of the PaO$_2$ and PaCO$_2$ (Table 17-12).

Blood Gas and pH Electrodes

The oxygen electrode (Clark electrode) used to measure PO$_2$ is a polarographic cell consisting of a silver reference anode and a platinum cathode charged to minus 0.5 volts.[8] The platinum surface is covered with an oxygen permeable membrane (polyethylene) on the other side of which is placed the unknown sample. Electrical current passing through the polaragraphic cell is directly proportional to the PO$_2$ outside the membrane.

The carbon dioxide electrode (Severinghaus electrode) used to measure PCO$_2$ utilizes a carbon dioxide permeable membrane (Teflon) that permits carbon dioxide to diffuse from the unknown sample into a buffer solution containing bicarbonate bathing a conventional glass pH electrode.[9] The measured pH in the bathing solution is altered in direct proportion to the PCO$_2$.

Measurement of pH utilizes a glass electrode which senses the concentration of H$^+$ in the unknown sample. This H$^+$ concentration produces a proportional change in voltage between the glass and reference electrode.

Information Provided by Blood Gases and pH

Minimum information for assessment of oxygenation and ventilation requires the measurement of PaO$_2$ and PaCO$_2$. As an alternative to arterial samples, blood from veins on the back of the hand, which reflects primarily cutaneous blood flow, can be used to estimate arterial blood gases and pH. Indeed, the combination of cutaneous vaso-

---

Table 17-12. Calculation of the Alveolar-to-Arterial Difference for Oxygen

$$A\text{-}aDO_2 = P_AO_2 - PaO_2$$

$$P_AO_2 = (P_B - P_{H_2O})F_IO_2 - \frac{PaCO_2}{0.8}$$

A-aDO$_2$ = alveolar-to-arterial difference for oxygen, mmHg
P$_A$O$_2$ = alveolar partial pressure of oxygen, mmHg
PaO$_2$ = arterial partial pressure of oxygen, mmHg
P$_B$ = barometric pressure, mmHg
P$_{H_2O}$ = partial pressure of water vapor, 47 mmHg at 37 Cclsius
F$_I$O$_2$ = inspired concentration of oxygen
PaCO$_2$ = arterial partial pressure of carbon dioxide, mmHg
0.8 = respiratory exchange ratio to compensate for the fact that less carbon dioxide is transferred into the alveolus than is oxygen removed from the alveolus

Example. Arterial blood gases are PaO$_2$ 310 mmHg and PaCO$_2$ 40 mmHg breathing pure oxygen (F$_I$O$_2$ = 1.0). The P$_B$ is 747 mmHg and the P$_{H_2O}$ is 47 mmHg. The A-aDO$_2$ is:

$$P_AO_2 = (747 - 47)1.0 - 40/0.08$$
$$P_AO_2 = 700 - 50$$
$$P_AO_2 = 650 \text{ mmHg}$$

$$A\text{-}aDO_2 = 650 - 310$$
$$A\text{-}aDO_2 = 340 \text{ mmHg}^a \text{ (normal less than 60 mmHg)}$$

---

[a] Assuming each 20 mmHg A-aDO$_2$ represents venous admixture equivalent to 1% of the cardiac output it can be estimated that 17% of the cardiac output is shunted past the lungs without exposure to ventilated alveoli.
(Modified from LoSasso AM, Gibbs PS, Moorthy SS. Recognition and management of respiratory failure. In: Stoelting RK, Dierdorf SF, eds, Anesthesia and co-existing disease. New York, Churchill Livingstone, 1983; 209–25.)

dilation and increased cutaneous blood flow associated with general anesthesia is sufficient to arterialize peripheral venous blood.[10] As a result, the peripheral venous PCO_2 and pH measured during general anesthesia approximate arterial values closely enough to permit estimation of the adequacy of ventilation and acid-base status. The peripheral venous PO_2, however, does not reliably parallel the PaO_2. Nevertheless, when the peripheral venous PO_2 exceeds 60 mmHg, the absence of arterial hypoxemia is confirmed. Additional measurements and calculations that further define the efficiency of oxygenation and ventilation include the A-aDO_2, arterial-to-alveolar PO_2 ratio (a/A), mixed venous PO_2, arterial and mixed venous content of oxygen, position of the oxyhemoglobin dissociation curve, and deadspace to tidal volume ratio (V_D/V_T). The anesthesiologist must be familiar with these measurements and able to rapidly adjust patient care based on information derived from blood gases and pH measurements.

Oxygenation is assessed by measurement of the PaO_2. Arterial hypoxemia, as reflected by a decrease in PaO_2 below 60 mmHg may be caused by a (1) low PO_2 in the inhaled gas (altitude, inadvertent during anesthesia), (2) hypoventilation, and (3) venous admixture.

Hypoventilation. A reduction in PaO_2 due to hypoventilation reflects encroachment of the $PaCO_2$ on the space available in the alveolus for oxygen. The decrease in PaO_2 is roughly equivalent to the increase in alveolar PCO_2.

Venous admixture, as a cause of decreased PaO_2, may reflect right-to-left intrapulmonary shunt (atelectasis, pneumonia), intracardiac shunt (congenital heart disease), or mismatching of ventilation to perfusion (chronic obstructive airway disease). A right-to-left shunt is defined as passage of blood from the pulmonary circulation to the systemic circulation without coming into contact with alveolar gas. Arterial hypoxemia due to a right-to-left shunt represents dilution of oxygenated arterial blood with shunted and desaturated venous blood. In this instance, inhalation of pure oxygen produces minimal, if any, effect on the PaO_2. Mismatching of ventilation to perfusion as a cause of venous admixture and arterial hypoxemia reflects underventilation of alveoli relative to their blood flow. Inhalation of pure oxygen eventually eliminates residual nitrogen from poorly ventilated alveoli such that blood coming from these alveoli is well oxygenated. This is the reason even small increases in the inhaled oxygen concentration (24 to 30 percent) may correct arterial hypoxemia due to mismatching of ventilation to perfusion characteristic of patients with chronic obstructive airway disease. The therapeutic response to supplemental oxygen helps distinguish arterial hypoxemia that is due to a right-to-left shunt from that which is due to mismatching of ventilation to perfusion. Finally, diffusion limitation to the passage of oxygen from the alveoli to blood has not been documented to be a cause of arterial hypoxemia in man.

A-aDO_2. The magnitude of venous admixture may be estimated in the clinical setting by calculation of the A-aDO_2 (Table 17-12). For example, when the PaO_2 is above 150 mmHg, so that hemoglobin is completely saturated with oxygen, the magnitude of venous admixture can be estimated to be equivalent to 1 percent of the cardiac output for every 20 mmHg of A-aDO_2. Below a PaO_2 of 150 mmHg or when cardiac output is increased relative to metabolism, this guideline will underestimate the actual amount of venous admixture. It must be appreciated that the normal A-aDO_2 breathing air is 5 to 10 mmHg reflecting right-to-left intracardiac shunting of 2 to 5 percent of the

Table 17-13. Calculation of the Ratio of Arterial to Alveolar Oxygen Partial Pressure

$$a/A = PaO_2/P_AO_2$$

Example. Arterial blood gases are PaO_2 310 mmHg and $PaCO_2$ 40 mmHg breathing pure oxygen ($F_IO_2 = 1.0$). The P_B is 747 mmHg and the P_{H_2O} 47 mmHg. The a/A is:

$$P_AO_2 = (747 - 47)1.0 - 40/0.08$$
$$P_AO_2 = 700 - 50$$
$$P_AO_2 = 650 \text{ mmHg}$$

$$a/A = 310/650$$
$$a/A = 0.48 \text{ (normal greater than 0.75)}$$

Table 17-14. Calculation of Arterial and/or Venous Content of Oxygen

CaO_2 = (Hb × 1.39)Sat + PaO_2 (0.003)
CaO_2 = oxygen content of arterial blood, ml O_2/dl blood
$C\bar{v}O_2$ = oxygen content of mixed venous blood, ml O_2/dl blood
Hb = hemoglobin, g/dl
1.39 = oxygen bound to hemoglobin, ml/g
Sat = percent saturation of hemoglobin with oxygen
PaO_2 = arterial partial pressure of oxygen, mmHg
$P\bar{v}O_2$ = mixed venous partial pressure of oxygen, mmHg
0.003 = dissolved oxygen, ml/mmHg

Example. Hb = 15 g/dl and PaO_2 100 mmHg resulting in 100% sat, $P\bar{v}O_2$ 40 mmHg resulting in 75% sat

$$CaO_2 = (15 \times 1.39)100 + 100(0.003)$$
$$= 20.85 + 0.3$$
$$= 21.15 \text{ ml/dl}$$

$$C\bar{v}O_2 = (15 \times 1.39)75 + 40(0.003)$$
$$= 15.63 + 0.12$$
$$= 15.75 \text{ ml/dl}$$

$$CaO_2 - C\bar{v}O_2 = 5.4 \text{ ml/dl}$$

cardiac output via bronchial, pleural, and Thebesian veins.

a/A Ratio. A disadvantage of A-aDO_2 is the normal range changes with varying concentrations of inhaled oxygen. For this reason, the a/A ratio may be more useful because it remains relatively constant regardless of the concentration of inhaled oxygen (Table 17-13). For example, a patient with an a/A ratio of 0.5 will have a PaO_2 equal to 50 percent of the alveolar PO_2 regardless of the inhaled concentration of oxygen. A ratio less than 0.75 suggests that the lung is not working well as an oxygen exchanger.

Mixed Venous PO_2. The mixed venous PO_2 is determined by the cardiac output and tissue oxygen consumption. In the presence of unchanging tissue oxygen consumption, the mixed venous PO_2 varies directly with changes in cardiac output. For example, when the cardiac output is decreased, there is less blood flow available for tissue oxygen extraction. Therefore, the continued extraction of the same amount of oxygen from a decreased blood flow must result in a reduced mixed venous PO_2. Tissue hypoxemia is likely when the mixed venous PO_2 is less than 30 mmHg. Disease states associated with arterial to venous admixture (sepsis, portal hypertension) may result in a high mixed venous PO_2 despite inadequate tissue oxygenation.

Arterial and Mixed Venous Content of Oxygen. The difference between the arterial and mixed venous content of oxygen is an estimate of the adequacy of cardiac output relative to the tissue oxygen consumption (Table 17-14). The normal difference in oxygen content of arterial and mixed venous blood is 4 to 6 ml/dl of blood. When tissue oxygen consumption is constant, a decreased cardiac output is accompanied by an increased oxygen content difference between arterial and mixed venous blood.

Oxyhemoglobin Dissociation Curve. The oxyhemoglobin dissociation curve describes the saturation of hemoglobin with oxygen relative to the PO_2 (Fig. 17-6). Alternatively, this curve may be viewed as depicting the loading and unloading of oxygen from hemoglobin at a varying PO_2. The benefit of the sigmoid shape of the curve is ease

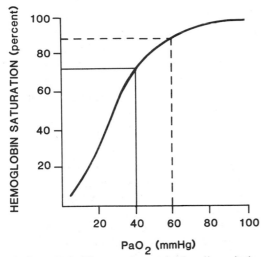

Figure 17-6. The oxyhemoglobin dissociation curve describes the relation of hemoglobin saturation with oxygen (percent) to the PaO_2. The P_{50} is the PaO_2 which results in 50 percent saturation of hemoglobin with oxygen. In the presence of a normal pHa (7.4) and body temperature (37 Celsius) hemoglobin is 50 percent saturated with oxygen at a PaO_2 of 26 mmHg (P_{50}). Events that shift the oxyhemoglobin dissociation curve to the left (P_{50} less than 26 mmHg) may jeopardize tissue oxygenation, since the PaO_2 must decrease further to permit release of oxygen from hemoglobin. Conversely, a shift of the oxyhemoglobin dissociation curve to the right (P_{50} greater than 26 mmHg) permits unloading of oxygen from hemoglobin at a higher PaO_2 and thus favors tissue oxygenation. The mixed venous PO_2 is near 40 mmHg and the associated hemoglobin saturation with oxygen is about 75 percent. Saturation of hemoglobin with oxygen is about 90 percent when the PaO_2 is 60 mmHg. The saturation of hemoglobin with oxygen can be considered to be 100 percent when the PaO_2 exceeds 150 mmHg.

of oxygen loading onto hemoglobin over a wide range of minimally changing PO_2 values (flat upper portion of the curve) and ease of release of oxygen from hemoglobin with small changes in PO_2 values (steep lower portion of curve). A normal oxyhemoglobin dissociation curve is characterized by 50 percent saturation of hemoglobin with oxygen at a PO_2 of 26 mmHg. The PO_2 that

Table 17-15. Events that Shift the Oxyhemoglobin Dissociation Curve

Left Shift (P_{50} less than 26 mmHg)	Right Shift (P_{50} greater than 26 mmHg)
Alkalosis	Acidosis
Hypothermia	Hyperthermia
Decreased 2,3-diphosphoglycerate	Increased 2,3-diphosphoglycerate due to chronic arterial hypoxemia or anemia

results in 50 percent saturation is referred to as the P_{50}. Events that shift the oxyhemoglobin dissociation curve to the left (P_{50} less than 26 mmHg) may jeopardize tissue oxygenation as oxygen is more tightly bound to hemoglobin and the PaO_2 must fall to a lower than normal level before oxygen is released from hemoglobin and becomes available to tissues (Table 17-15). Events that shift the oxyhemoglobin dissociation curve to the right (P_{50} greater than 26 mmHg) facilitate tissue oxygen availability by permitting the unloading of oxygen from hemoglobin at an increased PaO_2 (Table 17-15).

Compensation for Arterial Hypoxemia. Increased cardiac output is the most important compensatory mechanism for correction of arterial hypoxemia. For example, if cardiac output increases and tissue oxygen consumption is unchanged, the result is decreased extraction of oxygen from venous blood. The effect of this decreased oxygen extraction is an increased mixed venous PO_2 that produces less dilution when arterial and shunted venous blood mix. A less efficient compensatory mechanism to offset arterial hypoxemia is hyperventilation. For example, the resulting alveolar PCO_2 decrease is paralleled by a similar increase in the PaO_2. Nevertheless, an accompanying increased oxygen consumption of the respiratory muscles is likely to offset any gain in available oxygen produced by hyperventilation.

Table 17-16. Calculation of the Dead Space to Tidal Volume Ratio

$$V_D/V_T = \frac{PaCO_2 - P_ECO_2}{PaCO_2}$$

V_D/V_T = ratio of dead space to tidal volume
$PaCO_2$ = arterial partial pressure of carbon dioxide, mmHg
P_ECO_2 = mixed exhaled partial pressure of carbon dioxide, mmHg

Example. The $PaCO_2$ is 40 mmHg and P_ECO_2 20 mmHg during controlled ventilation of the lungs. The V_D/V_T is:

$$V_D/V_T = \frac{40 - 20}{40}$$
V_D/V_T = 20/40
V_D/V_T = 0.5 (normal less than 0.3)

(Modified from Lo Sasso AM, Gibbs PS, Moorthy SS. Recognition and management of respiratory failure. In: Stoelting RK, Dierdorf SF, eds, Anesthesia and co-existing disease. New York, Churchill Livingstone, 1983; 209–25.)

Ventilation. The $PaCO_2$ reflects the adequacy of the lung for removing carbon dioxide from pulmonary capillary blood. In the steady state, $PaCO_2$ is directly proportional to the metabolic production of carbon dioxide and inversely proportional to alveolar ventilation. The production of carbon dioxide depends on the metabolic state of the individual and parallels tissue oxygen consumption. Under normal conditions, only 80 percent as much carbon dioxide is produced as oxygen is consumed (respiratory quotient = 0.8). Assuming a tissue oxygen consumption of 250 ml/min, the production of carbon dioxide would be 200 ml/min. When the $PaCO_2$ is above 44 mmHg, the patient is hypoventilating relative to carbon dioxide production while a $PaCO_2$ below 36 mmHg is defined as hyperventilation. Wasted ventilation or increased physiologic deadspace may result in an elevated $PaCO_2$ even when minute ventilation is increased. The V_D/V_T ratio, which depicts areas in the lung that receive adequate ventilation but inadequate or no pulmonary blood flow, should not exceed 0.3 (Table 17-16). In contrast to PaO_2, venous admixture has little to no impact on $PaCO_2$, reflecting the extreme diffusibility of carbon dioxide.

REFERENCES

1. Moorthy SS. Acid-base disturbances. In: Stoelting RK, Dierdorf SF, eds, Anesthesia and co-existing disease. New York, Churchill Livingstone, 1983;227–37.
2. Normal J. An assessment of acid-base balance. Br J Anaesth 1978;50:45–60.
3. Siggard-Andersen O. Blood acid base alignment normogram. Scand J Clin Lab Invest 1963;15:211–7.
4. Mitchell RA, Singer MM. Respiration and cerebrospinal fluid pH in metabolic acidosis and alkalosis. J Appl Physiol 1965;20:905–11.
5. Edelist G, Osorio A. Postanesthetic initiation of spontaneous ventilation after passive hyperventilation. Anesthesiology 1969;31:222–7.
6. Barcenas CG, Fuller TJ, Knochel JP. Metabolic alkalosis after massive blood transfusion. JAMA 1976;236:953–4.
7. Ream AK, Reitz BA, Silverberg G. Temperature correction of PCO$_2$ and pH in estimating acid-base status: An example of the emperor's new clothes? Anesthesiology 1982;56:41–4.
8. Clark LC. Monitor and control of blood and tissue oxygen tensions. Trans Am Soc Artif Intern Organs 1956;2:41–8.
9. Severinghaus JW, Bradley AF. Electrodes for blood PO$_2$ and PCO$_2$ determination. J Appl Physiol 1958;13:515–20.
10. Williamson DC, Munson ES. Correlation of peripheral venous and arterial blood gas values during general anesthesia. Anesth Analg 1982;61:950–2.

18

Fluid and Blood Therapy

The perioperative management of a patient's fluid balance includes preoperative evaluation and intraoperative maintenance and replacement of fluid losses. Preoperative treatment of hypovolemia is helpful, since circulatory changes induced by anesthetics and surgery are augmented by a pre-existing reduction of intravascular fluid volume. Intraoperatively, in addition to blood loss, fluids can shift into various body compartments. Knowledge of these shifts can aid in predicting fluid requirements. Maintaining normal intravascular fluid volume is dependent on knowledge of these compartmental fluid changes, quantitation of blood loss, and selection of the appropriate fluid for treatment.

PATHOPHYSIOLOGY OF CHANGES IN BODY FLUID COMPARTMENTS

Normal Body Fluid Compartments

Total body water can be subdivided into extracellular fluid (ECF) and intracellular fluid (ICF). Approximately 20 percent of the body weight (kg) is represented by ECF and 30 percent by ICF. The ECF is further subdivided into plasma volume (PV) and interstitial fluid (ISF). These latter two compartments are separated by the walls of the blood vessels, with the PV being defined as that fluid contained within the vascular system, but external to the blood cells, while ISF is confined to that compartment which

is external to the blood vessels and internal to the cells. PV represents 5 percent of the body weight and ISF constitutes 15 percent of body weight. If the red cells are added to the plasma volume, a total blood volume of approximately 7.5 percent of body weight results.

Total body water content varies with age, sex, and body habitus. Fifty-five percent of the body weight constitutes body water in adult males, whereas 45 percent of body weight is represented by total body water in adult females. Because fat contains little water, obese adults have less total body water per kg than lean adults. Infants have 80 percent of their body weight represented by total body water.

Preoperative Evaluation

The anesthesiologist should evaluate the patient's mental status, history of input and output, blood pressure in both supine and sitting positions, heart rate, skin turgor, and urinary output with respect to alterations in these parameters produced by changes in intravascular fluid volume and/or concentration of electrolytes. Serum electrolytes should be measured along with, in some situations, serum osmolarity. Volume, concentration, and composition of the ECF are the three steps by which the intraoperative fluid and electrolyte status are evaluated (Table 18-1).[1]

243

Table 18-1 An Outline of Steps for Fluid and Electrolyte Evaluation

Volume
    Blood pressure sitting and supine
    Skin turgor
    Heart rate
    Mucous membrane moisture
    Urine output
Concentration
    Serum sodium
    Serum osmolarity
Composition
    Serum electrolytes
    Blood urea nitrogen (BUN)
    Blood glucose
    Analysis of arterial blood gases and pH

(Data from Giesecke AH Jr. Perioperative fluid therapy—crystalloids. In: Miller RD, ed, Anesthesia. New York, Churchill Livingstone, 1981, 865–84.)

Volume. ECF volume is best determined at the bedside. This volume should be accurately assessed because most anesthetic techniques and drugs can lead to marked circulatory depression in patients who have a deficit of ECF volume. Tachycardia and dry mucous membranes may indicate a mild volume deficit, even though the blood pressure is normal. This type of deficit can be seen in patients who have had extensive preoperative evaluation that required restricted oral intake, enemas for diagnostic radiologic procedures, and blood withdrawal for various laboratory tests.

Determining whether orthostatic (postural) hypotension is present is extremely useful in detecting more severe forms of intravascular fluid volume deficits. If the systolic blood pressure decreases more than 20 mmHg when the patient changes from the supine to standing or sitting position, there is a deficit of 6 to 8 percent of body weight as fluid. Observation of the heart rate is important in differentiating orthostatic hypotension due to autonomic drugs (antihypertensives) from an intravascular fluid volume deficit. If orthostatic hypotension occurs, the heart rate should increase in a compensatory manner. If this does occur, most likely the decrease in blood pressure is due to an intravascular fluid volume deficit. If,

however, the blood pressure decreases and the heart rate does not increase, a defect in autonomic nervous system function should be suspected, which may be a result of antihypertensives the patient is receiving (see Chapter 3).

In severe cases of ECF deficits, the bladder probably should be catheterized to accurately quantitate urinary output. A decrease or absence of urinary output obviously indicates a severe deficit in ECF volume.

Conversely, a volume excess may be present in the surgical patient, either from an iatrogenic cause (excessive fluid administration), or some pathologic cause (cirrhosis of the liver). Soft tissue edema and diuresis (> 100 ml/hr) are usually signs of excessive intravenous fluid administration. The blood pressure will initially increase but will subsequently decrease if the excessive intravascular fluid is sufficiently severe as to induce cardiac failure. In this situation, the patient will exhibit edema, which may manifest initially in the scleral conjunctiva. In severe cases, peripheral edema and even pulmonary edema will result. Treatment of cardiac failure should be undertaken before proceeding with anesthesia and surgery.

Concentration. The concentration of constituents in ECF is determined to a large extent by total body water content. Although some bedside clues may be present, laboratory diagnosis is helpful for diagnosing abnormalities in body fluid concentrations. The two laboratory tests which are most valuable are the serum sodium concentration and, if available, the serum osmolarity. The definition of osmolarity is often confusing to physicians. One *osmole* is defined as one mole of nondissociating substance in one liter of solution. The term *milliosmole* (mOsm) is 1/1000 of an osmole of a substance in solution. *Osmolarity* is the number of osmoles/liter of solution, whereas *osmolality* is the number of osmoles/100 g of solvent. In dilute solutions, as exist in the human body, osmolality is approximately equal to osmolarity. The normal osmolarity of ECF is 285 to 295 mOsml/L. When electrolyte-free water is lost from the body, the serum sodium and serum osmolarity increase. Usually, these increases are due to inadequate water intake or can occur in pathologic situations such as fever and loss of fluid from denuded tissues (e.g., burns).

When water is present in body fluids in excess of the normal ratio, the serum sodium concentration and osmolarity are reduced. Also, the patient can suffer from a hypovolemic/hyponatremic situation in which electrolyte-rich fluids (such as vomitus, diarrhea, or fistula drainage) are lost and are replaced with water. Obviously, proper treatment consists of replacement with crystalloid solutions that are rich in electrolytes, such as lactated Ringer's solution. A normovolemic/hyponatremic condition results from failure of the kidneys to conserve sodium when the intake of sodium is reduced, but volume intake has been adequate. A hypervolemic/hyponatremic condition results from excessive water intake or retention, which, during anesthesia, is most commonly seen following transurethral resection of the prostate (Chapter 22), and when 5 percent dextrose in water is used to correct intravascular fluid volume deficits.

Composition. The composition of the ECF is determined by the presence of various electrolytes. The distribution of electrolytes differs among the fluid compartments of the body (Table 18-2). The major cation in the intravascular fluid is sodium, while the major cation of the intracellular fluid is potassium. The electrophysiology of excitable cells is dependent on the intracellular and extracellular concentrations of sodium, potassium, and calcium.

Hypernatremia (serum sodium concentration exceeds 145 mEq/L) is most often due to a deficit of total body content of water

Table 18-2 Approximate Distribution of Electrolytes

Electrolyte	Extracellular (Plasma) Fluid (mEq/L)	Intracellular Fluid (mEq/L)
Sodium	140	10
Potassium	4.5	150
Calcium	5	1
Magnesium	2	40

and not an excess of total body sodium. Total body sodium can increase, however, when renal function is impaired—as in the patient with kidney disease, cirrhosis of the liver, or congestive heart failure. Peripheral edema is the hallmark of hypernatremia. An expanded intravascular fluid volume may manifest as hypertension. Treatment of hypernatremia due to excess total body sodium content is with renal tubular diuretics.

Hyponatremia (serum sodium concentration below 135 mEq/L) is most often due to an excess of total body water and not to a deficiency of total body sodium. Total body sodium can decrease, however, with vomiting, diarrhea, and third degree burns. Hyponatremia due to sodium loss is characterized by a decreased intravascular fluid volume which manifests as hypotension, tachycardia, oliguria, and hemoconcentration. Central nervous system signs of hyponatremia do not usually occur until the serum sodium concentration decreases below 110 mEq/L. Treatment of hyponatremia rarely requires the intravenous administration of hypertonic saline.

Hyperkalemia (serum potassium concentration above 5.5 mEq/L) can be due to an increased total body potassium content (renal failure) or altered distribution of potassium between intracellular and extracellular sites (respiratory or metabolic acidosis, succinylcholine). Adverse effects of hyperkalemia are likely to accompany acute increases in the serum potassium concentration. In contrast, chronic hyperkalemia is more likely to be associated with a normal gradient between extracellular and intracellular concentrations of potassium. The fact that patients with chronic elevations of potassium are often asymptomatic suggests that the potassium gradient across the cell membrane is more important than the absolute serum concentration of potassium.

The most detrimental effect of hyperkalemia is on the cardiac conduction system, manifesting on the electrocardiogram (ECG) as prolongation of the P–R interval, widening of the QRS complex, and peaking of the T waves. Treatment of acute hyperkalemia is designed to shift potassium from the serum into the cells so as to antagonize the effects of potassium on the heart. This goal can be accomplished by the production of systemic alkalosis (iatrogenic hyperventilation, intravenous administration of sodium bicarbonate) or intravenous injection of glucose (25 grams) combined with regular insulin (10 to 15 units). Insulin is given to ensure that glucose enters the cell and carries potassium with it. Calcium (500 mg) can also be administered slowly intravenously to antagonize the adverse effects of potassium. All these treatments represent temporizing measures until elimination of excess potassium from the body can be accomplished.

Ideally, serum potassium concentrations should be below 5.5 mEq/L before proceeding with elective surgery. Emergency surgery in the presence of hyperkalemia requires careful monitoring of the ECG to detect adverse effects of potassium on the heart. Avoidance of systemic acidosis due to hypoventilation or arterial hypoxemia is important, as this change would accentuate hyperkalemia.

Hypokalemia (serum potassium concentration below 3.5 mEq/L) can be due to a decreased total body potassium content (vomiting, diarrhea, nasogastric suction) or an alteration in the distribution of potassium between intracellular and extracellular sites (respiratory or metabolic alkalosis). Adverse effects of chronic hypokalemia include decreased myocardial contractility and skeletal muscle weakness. There is increased automaticity of the atria and ventricles, manifesting as cardiac dysrhythmias. Alterations in cardiac conduction manifest on the ECG as prolongation of the P–R and Q–T interval and flattening of the T wave. Treatment of chronic hypokalemia is with potassium chloride supplementation given orally, remembering that several days will be necessary to replete potassium stores. Intravenous administration of potassium chloride (0.2 to 0.4 mEq/kg/hr) is recommended when hypokalemia is associated with adverse cardiac changes.

The advisability of proceeding with elective surgery in the presence of serum potassium concentrations below 3.5 mEq/L is controversial. Nevertheless, in the absence of skeletal muscle weakness or abnormal findings on the ECG, elective operations can most likely be safely performed in the presence of moderate hypokalemia. Certainly, events known to acutely lower serum potassium concentration, such as iatrogenic hyperventilation, must be avoided.

Hypercalcemia (serum calcium concentration above 5.5 mEq/L) is typically due to hyperparathyroidism and neoplastic disorders with bone metastases (see Chapter 23). When serum calcium exceeds 8 mEq/L, cardiac conduction disturbances manifest on the ECG as a prolonged P–R interval, wide QRS complex, and shortened Q–T interval. During anesthesia, it is important to maintain hydration and urine output to minimize further increases in the serum calcium concentration.

Hypocalcemia (serum concentration below 4.5 mEq/L) can be due to reduced serum albumin concentrations, hypoparathyroidism, pancreatitis, and renal failure (see Chapter 23). Impaired neuromuscular function in the presence of hypocalcemia reflects decreased presynaptic release of acetylcholine. Decreased myocardial contractility with elevated central venous pressure and hypotension are typical. Skeletal muscle spasm, including laryngospasm, may accompany hypocalcemia. During anesthesia, it is important to remember that respiratory alkalosis due to iatrogenic hyperventilation can rapidly decrease the serum ionized calcium concentration.

ROUTINE INTRAOPERATIVE INTRAVENOUS THERAPY WITHOUT BLOOD LOSS

Solutions administered intravenously are required for maintenance of normal body fluid composition. Available solutions are classified either as crystalloids or colloids (see the section *Other Intravenous Solutions*). Colloids are frequently recommended for specific situations, such as fluid loss from fistulae, weeping or oozing from raw surfaces, and ascitic fluid. Crystalloid solutions are sufficient to maintain normal body fluid composition in the majority of patients (Table 18-3).

Independent of the type of surgery, all patients have insensible losses, which include evaporation of water from the respiratory tract, sweat, stool, and urinary excretion, which need to be replaced. This requires administration of about 1.5 to 2 ml/kg/hr intravenously of crystalloid solution. Febrile patients or children may have a larger insensible loss. Although Giesecke[1] recommends that these insensible losses be replaced with a solution such as 5 percent dextrose in water, probably any crystalloid solution which is reasonably isotonic with plasma is satisfactory (Table 18-3).

In addition to replacing insensible losses, the extent to which surgery is traumatic will dictate how much additional crystalloid solution should be given intravenously. With extreme surgical trauma, which would include bowel resections for intestinal obstruction, an isotonic reduction in ECF volume can occur. In addition isotonic transfer of fluids can occur from functional body fluid compartments to nonfunctional ones. Giesecke[1] and Shires and Canizaro[2] have demonstrated that traumatic surgery causes a transfer of functional ECF into a newly formed acute sequestered edema space, which they have termed "third space." Such a shift in fluid occurs with surgical trauma, blunt trauma, burns, and infections. Thus, this acute sequestered edema is a nonfunctional appendage of the ISF. This loss of fluid from the functional ECF

Table 18-3 Comparison of Various Crystalloid Solutions

Solution	Dextrose (mg/dl)	Na (mEq/L)	Cl (mEq/L)	K (mEq/L)	Mg (mEq/L)	Ca (mEq/L)	Lactate (mEq/L)	Approximate pH	mOsm/L (calculated)
ECF	90–110	140	108	4.5	2.0	5.0	5.0	7.4	290
5% dextrose/water	50	—	—	—	—	—	—	5.0	253
5% dextrose/ 0.45% NaCl	50	77	77	—	—	—	—	4.2	407
5% dextrose/0.9% NaCl	50	154	154	—	—	—	—	4.2	561
0.9% NaCl	—	154	154	—	—	—	—	5.7	308
Lactated Ringer's solution	—	130	109	4.0	—	3.0	28	6.7	273
5% dextrose/ lactated Ringer's solution	50	130	109	4.0	—	3.0	28	5.3	527
Normosol-R	—	140	98	5.0	3.0	—	[a]	7.4	295
5% NaCl	—	855	855	—	—	—	—	5.6	1171

[a] Contains acetate 27 mEq/L and gluconate 23 mEq/L.

Table 18-4. Guidelines for Intraoperative Crystalloid Therapy

Step 1
    Give an isotonic electrolyte containing solution at a rate of 2 ml/kg/hr to replace insensible losses.

Step 2
    In addition to Step 1, the magnitude of surgical trauma should be estimated and an appropriate electrolyte containing solution be given:

Minimal trauma	add	3–4 ml/kg/hr
Moderate trauma	add	5–6 ml/kg/hr
Severe trauma	add	7–8 ml/kg/hr

Step 3
    Replace the volume of blood loss with three times the volume of crystalloid solution or blood.

Step 4
    Monitor vital signs and urine output (about 1 ml/ kg/hr should suffice).

(Adapted from Giesecke AH Jr. Perioperative fluid therapy-crystalloids. In: Miller RD, ed, Anesthesia. New York, Churchill Livingstone, 1981, 865–84.)

needs to be replaced intraoperatively. A guide to routine fluids for intraoperative maintenance and replacement is outlined in Table 18-4.[1] Minimal surgical trauma would include plastic procedures or a craniotomy. Moderate surgical trauma would be exemplified by a hernia repair or thoracotomy. Extreme surgical trauma would be exemplified by a bowel resection for intestinal obstruction.

INTRAOPERATIVE INTRAVENOUS THERAPY WITH BLOOD LOSS

If blood loss is sufficiently large, red blood cells in the form of whole blood or packed red cells will have to be administered. This is true despite compensatory physiologic changes, which occur in response to a loss of intravascular fluid volume, as well as the ability to replace some blood loss with crystalloid solutions. Compensatory changes in response to blood loss include vasoconstriction of the splanchnic system and the venous capacitance vessels. This vasoconstriction can conceal the signs of acute blood loss until at least 10 percent of the blood volume is lost. Healthy patients may lose up to 20 percent of their blood volume before signs occur, such as a reduction in central venous pressure, hypotension, or tachycardia. Anesthetics reduce the ability of the body to compensate for changes in blood loss and attenuate the classic signs of hypovolemia, such as tachycardia.

With acute blood loss, ISF and extravascular protein are transferred to the intravascular space, which tends to maintain PV. For this reason, when crystalloid solutions are utilized to replace blood loss, they must be given in amounts equal to three times the amount of blood loss not only to replenish intravascular fluid volume, but also to replenish that fluid lost from the interstitial spaces.

Arterial blood pressure, heart rate, and central venous pressure should be checked to determine whether intravascular fluid volume is being adequately maintained. Although intravascular fluid volume can be maintained with crystalloid solutions, the underlying question is when should whole blood be administered. In this regard, serial determination of the hematocrit is extremely valuable. Even though the hematocrit is not a reliable guide for assessing adequacy of intravascular fluid volume, it is extremely useful for determining whether the ratio between crystalloid and blood therapy has been appropriate. To maximize oxygen carrying capacity and, conversely, ensure that the viscosity of blood is such that capillary flow will be adequate, a hematocrit of 30 percent is often adequate. Therefore, when intravascular fluid volume is replaced, the hematocrit should be determined to assess whether the appropriate amount of blood has been given. For example, if the hematocrit is 35 to 40 percent, it would be appropriate to continue replacing blood loss with crystalloid solutions alone. If the hematocrit is 25 to 30 percent, it would be appropriate to administer blood as part of the replacement solution. Al-

Table 18-5 ABO Compatibility Testing

Blood Group	Red Blood Cells[a] Tested with		Serum[b] Tested with	
	Anti-A	Anti-B	A cells	B cells
A	+	0	0	+
B	0	+	+	0
AB	+	+	0	0
O	0	0	+	+

Symbols: + = agglutination; 0 = no agglutination.
[a] Using patient's cells.
[b] Using patient's serum.
(Modified from Miller RD, Brzica SM. Blood, blood component, colloid, and autotransfusion therapy. In: Miller RD, ed, Anesthesia. New York, Churchill Livingstone, 1981, 885–922.)

though this approach is a rather simplified description of replacing blood loss, it has served as a useful guide in hectic situations when patients are rapidly losing blood.

ESSENTIALS OF BLOOD THERAPY

Compatability Testing

The ABO-Rh type crossmatch and antibody screen are referred to as a compatability test. These tests were designed to identify antigen-antibody interactions so that in vivo hemolysis could be prevented. Also, in an emergency situation, the clinician must know the potential dangers of giving blood which has not undergone a complete crossmatch. Therefore, knowledge of the terms *type specific* and *type and screen* are essential during blood therapy.

Type specific blood means that only the ABO-Rh has been determined according to the classification listed in Table 18-5. Determination of the patient's correct blood type is exceedingly important in order to avoid the most serious and tragic reactions associated with blood transfusions. These reactions are due to naturally occurring antibodies, which activate complement and lead to rapid intravenous hemolysis. Anti-A and/or anti-B antibodies are formed whenever an individual lacks either or both the A and B antigens. ABO typing is done

by testing red blood cells for the A and B antigens, and the serum for the A and B antibodies, prior to transfusion. If type specific blood is given, the chances for a clinically significant reaction are about 1 in 1,000.

Type and screen refers to blood which has not been crossmatched, but in which the ABO-Rh type has been determined. The presence of most of the commonly found unexpected antibodies is detected by the screen. The serum is tested for the presence of antibodies by adding reagent red blood cells (type O) that possess most of the common antigen determinants. The reagent red cells are made available by companies which obtain the red cells from donors with known antigens. With a negative antibody screen, the chances of a clinically significant reaction occurring are about 1 in 10,000. For this reason, the Bureau of Biologics of the Food and Drug Administration is considering eliminating the federal regulation that all blood given electively undergo a complete crossmatch. Therefore, in the future, blood may be electively given when only the type and screen has been performed, rather than the complete crossmatch. Obviously, when the screen is positive, the crossmatch must be performed.

Crossmatch involves testing the donor red cells with the recipient's serum by methods providing for detection of agglutinating and non-agglutinating antibodies, including the antiglobulin test.[3] This is designated as the major crossmatch.

Blood Storage

Currently, blood is stored either in citrate phosphate dextrose (CPD) preservative or citrate phosphate dextrose-adenine (CPD-A_1) preservative, at a temperature of 1 to 6 Celsius. Blood stored in CPD solution is outdated when it has been stored for 21 days or longer. Blood stored in CPD-A_1 solution is deemed outdated when it has been stored for 35 days or longer. The criteria utilized to determine storage times for blood is the requirement that at least 70 percent of the transfused red blood cells remain viable in the circulation for 24 hours after infusion. For a more detailed description of the influence of storage on various components of blood, see Table 18-6.[3]

Component Therapy

A major advance in the field of blood banking has been the ability to fractionate blood into specific components. Although many components are available, packed red blood cells, platelet concentrates, fresh frozen plasma, and cryoprecipitates are the most commonly administered components.

Packed Red Blood Cells. Essentially, packed red blood cells contain the same amount of hemoglobin as whole blood, but much of the plasma has been removed. The hematocrit of whole blood is approximately 40 percent, and the hematocrit of packed red blood cells is 70 percent. The position of the American Association of Blood Banks has been that transfusion of whole blood is required for blood loss sufficient to cause hypovolemic shock. Less severe degrees of hemorrhage may be effectively treated with packed red blood cells, thus retaining plasma and the components for other patients who need these specific components. Most blood banks have followed the principle that whole blood cannot be obtained in operating rooms except by special request. In essence, blook bankers are saying that, except for rare situations (e.g., hypovolemic shock), whole blood is not necessary.

Complications associated with packed red blood cells are essentially the same as that with whole blood. One exception would be that the chance of developing citrate intoxication would be less with packed red cells than with whole blood, because less citrate is present in packed red blood cells. Conversely, hemorrhage due to dilution of factors V and VIII is more likely than with whole blood because these factors are removed with the plasma when the red blood cells are packed. It should be remembered that the incidence of hepatitis is the same for packed red blood cells and whole blood.

The administration of packed red blood cells is facilitated by reconstituting them in a crystalloid solution. The selection of a particular crystalloid solution should be based on two factors, one being the os-

Table 18-6. Chemical and Hemotologic Changes in CPD Blood with Storage Time

Test	Day			
	1	7	14	21
Blood pH	7.1	7.0	7.0	6.9
Blood PCO_2 (mmHg)	48	80	110	140
Blood lactate (mEq/L)	41	101	145	179
Plasma bicarbonate (mEq/L)	18	15	12	11
Plasma potassium (mEq/L)	3.9	12	17	21
Plasma dextrose (mg/dl)	345	312	282	231
Plasma hemoglobin (mg/dl)	1.7	7.8	13	19
2,3-DPG[a] (μM/ml)	4.8	1.2	1.0	<1.0
Platelets (%)	10	0	0	0
Factors V & VIII (%)	70	50	40	20

[a] 2,3-DPG = 2,3-diphosphoglycerate.

(Modified from Miller RD, Brzica SM. Blood, blood component, colloid, and autotransfusion therapy. In: Miller RD, ed, Anesthesia. New York, Churchill Livingstone, 1981, 885–922.)

molarity, and the other being whether the solution contains calcium. If the solution is hypotonic, hemolysis will occur (Table 18-3, Table 18-7). If the solution contains calcium, small clots will result (Table 18-3, Table 18-7). The most commonly utilized solution to reconstitute packed red blood cells is 0.9 percent saline.

Platelet concentrates are prepared by differential centrifugation, either from freshly drawn units of blood or from donors who specifically donate platelets by plasmapheresis. Platelet function is better maintained in solutions stored at 4 Celsius than at room temperature. Therefore, on a theoretical basis, platelets stored at 4 Celsius are preferred when immediate hemostasis is desired. Platelets stored at room temperature take about 24 hours to establish their hemostatic effect, and probably should be used for patients such as those with chronic thrombocytopenia. Unfortunately, clinicians rarely have the luxury of being able to select platelets according to storage temperature.

Usually, one platelet concentrate will increase the platelet count about 10,000 cells/mm^3 in a 70 kg patient. Therefore, 10 platelet concentrates will have to be given if one wishes to increase a platelet count by 100,000 cells/mm^3.

Fresh Frozen Plasma. When plasma is removed from a donor unit within a short period of time after donation and rapidly frozen, such plasma, when thawed and reused will be as efficacious in the recipient as fresh plasma. Of particular importance is that fresh frozen plasma contains normal levels of all coagulation factors, except platelets. Usually 2 to 4 units of fresh frozen plasma will satisfactorily restore markedly depressed coagulation factors, such as factors V and VIII.

Cryoprecipitate is prepared in such a way that it contains significant levels of factor VIII, which is used in the treatment of factor VIII deficiency or hemophilia A.

COMPLICATIONS OF BLOOD THERAPY

Acid-Base

When blood is introduced into CPD solution, its pH immediately decreases to about 7.1 (Table 18-6). Due to the accumulation of lactic and pyruvic acids from red blood cell metabolism and glycolysis, the pH of stored blood continues to de-

Table 18-7. Compatibility of Blood with Intravenous Solutions

Blood to Intravenous Solution—1:1 Ratio	Hemolysis at 30 min	
	Room Temperature	37°C
5% dextrose in water	1+	4+
Plasmanate*	1+	3+
5% dextrose in 0.2% saline	0	3+
5% dextrose in 0.4% saline	0	0
5% dextrose in 0.9% saline	0	0
0.9% saline	0	0
Normosol-R pH 7.4†	0	0
Lactated Ringer's solution	0 (clotted)	0 (clotted)

* Cutter Laboratories, Inc., Berkeley, CA.
† Abbott Laboratories, Chicago, IL.
(Miller RD, Brzica SM. Blood, blood component, colloid, and autotranfusion therapy. In: Miller RD, ed, Anesthesia. New York, Churchill Livingstone, 1981, 885–922.)

crease to about 6.9 after 21 days of storage. As a result, some clinicians recommend giving one ampule (44.6 mEq) of sodium bicarbonate for every 5 units of blood administered. This has, however, been shown to be an unnecessary procedure. Therefore, bicarbonate should only be given in documented cases of metabolic acidosis as determined by analysis of arterial pH.

Coagulation Abnormalities

A bleeding problem can occur after infusion of multiple units (usually 10 or more) of stored blood. This problem may manifest by oozing into the surgical field, hematuria, gingival bleeding, or bleeding from venous puncture sites. When such bleeding occurs in a patient who did not have a coagulopathy preoperatively, the differential diagnosis is as follows:

1. Dilutional thrombocytopenia
2. Low factors V and VIII
3. Disseminated intravascular coagulation and/or fibrinolysis
4. Hemolytic transfusion reaction

Dilutional thrombocytopenia is probably the most likely cause of a hemorrhagic problem in a patient who has received multiple units of blood. Considering survival time and viability, total platelet activity is only 50 to 70 percent of the original value following 6 hours of storage in CPD solution at 4 Celsius. After 24 hours of storage platelet activity is only 10 percent of normal, and after 48 hours only 5 percent of normal. Therefore, infusion of blood stored for 24 hours or longer will markedly dilute the available platelet pool.

Low Factors V and VIII. Although factors V and VIII are very labile, they rarely decrease to below 20 percent of normal after 21 days of storage (Table 18–6).[3] Because a level of only 20 percent is required for adequate hemostasis, it is highly unlikely that administration of whole blood would cause these factors to decrease sufficiently to cause a bleeding problem. If packed red blood cells are given instead of whole blood, however, much of the plasma and, therefore, factors V and VIII are removed, and a hemorrhagic problem from this cause is more likely.

Disseminated Intravascular Coagulation. With disseminated intravascular coagulation (DIC), the clotting system is stimulated by a toxin or other cause, which results in a hypercoagulable state. This hypercoagulable state causes fibrin to be deposited in the microcirculation of vital organs, such as the kidneys. In an attempt to counteract the hypercoagulable state, the fibrinolytic system is activated to lyse the excessive fibrin. This is termed secondary fibrinolysis. Primary fibrinolysis is very rare and refers to the activation of the fibrinolytic system without concomitant DIC.

Although heparin is the drug treatment for DIC, its efficacy has been challenged by several clinical investigators, including Mant and King.[4] They concluded that although bleeding is common, DIC rarely causes significant organ damage and infarction. Furthermore, heparin is seldom useful and often causes hemorrhage. DIC is associated with high mortality, primarily due to the severity of the patient's underlying disorder. Perhaps DIC is best regarded as an incidental preterminal event in most patients. Without removing the underlying cause or disease, treatment of DIC with heparin is seldom useful.

Differential Diagnosis. With these possible causes of bleeding in mind, the recommended diagnostic tests for determining the cause of the bleeding are as follows:

1. A platelet count
2. Partial thromboplastin time
3. Plasma fibrinogen level
4. Clot on the wall

In a patient who does not have a chronic reason for thrombocytopenia, generally if the platelet count is above 100,000/mm³, bleeding will not occur. Conversely, if the platelet count is below 50,000 cells/mm³, bleeding will occur. Therefore, in the perioperative period when the platelet count begins to approach 100,000 cells/mm³ and more blood transfusions are going to be given, platelets probably should be ordered (e.g., in the form of platelet concentrates, platelet-rich plasma, or fresh blood). A markedly elevated partial thromboplastin time (greater than 55 sec) probably indicates low levels of factors V and VIII, which can be treated by administration of fresh frozen plasma. If the plasma fibrinogen level is markedly reduced (i.e., 100–150 mg/dl), then DIC and/or fibrinolysis is present. Because the incidence of primary fibrinolysis is so rare, fibrinolysis most likely is due to DIC. Presently, we recommend that heparin, in most cases, not be given, but that emphasis be placed on removing the precipitating cause of the DIC. Putting a test tube full of blood on the wall will help determine whether hemolysis has occurred. Obviously from a quantitative view, a coagulopathy is unlikely to be caused by a hemolytic transfusion reaction. If hemolysis is present, however, such a reaction can be catastrophic if not immediately recognized (see the section *Transfusion Reactions*).

Citrate Intoxication

Citrate intoxication is not caused by the citrate ion per se, but because citrate binds calcium and produces hypocalcemia. Thus, the signs of citrate intoxication are those of hypocalcemia (see the section *Hypocalcemia*). Symptomatic hypocalcemia is unlikely to occur unless CPD blood is given at a rate greater than 150 ml/70 kg/min or about 1 unit every 5 minutes to a 70 kg adult. Therefore, the routine administration of calcium is unwarranted. Furthermore, if packed red blood cells are utilized, the chance of citrate intoxication is lessened even more, because much of the citrate has been removed when the plasma was fractionated.

Temperature Reductions

Administration of unwarmed blood which has been stored at 4 Celsius can decrease the patient's body temperature. If the patient's body temperature decreases to less than 30 Celsius, ventricular irritability and even cardiac arrest may occur. Although there are many reasons for a patient to develop hypothermia, we believe that all blood should be warmed prior to its administration so as to minimize reductions in body temperature. Even a decrease of body temperature as little as 0.5 to 1.0 Celsius may induce shivering postoperatively, which in turn may increase oxygen consumption by as much as 400 percent. To meet the demands of an elevated oxygen consumption, cardiac output must be increased. This may be too much stress for a patient with marginal cardiac reserve.

Suggestions that warming stored blood favors the entry of potassium from the plasma back into the red blood cells before the blood is infused have not been confirmed. Indeed, it is likely that warming stored whole blood does not alter the serum concentration of potassium.

Although blood warmed excessively can be hemolyzed, most of the warmers are sufficiently regulated to prevent this possibility from happening.

Infusion of Microaggregates

It has been known for some time that microaggregates accumulate in stored blood. Many clinicians have postulated that these microaggregates are not filtered by the standard 170 micron filter during routine transfusion, and, therefore, enter the recipient's blood stream and end up in the lungs, causing adult respiratory distress syndrome. Although there is no doubt that microaggregates begin to accumulate when blood has been stored for more than 3 days, the documentation that patients are harmed by this debris is lacking. For example, the fundamental question as to whether patients are more likely to develop adult respiratory distress syndrome if they receive stored blood through a 170 micron filter versus a micropore filter (less than 40 microns) has not been established.

Although many investigators have attempted to determine whether microaggregate blood filtration is necessary, recent studies by Snyder et al.[5] seriously question the need to use micropore filters. They studied 50 patients undergoing elective coronary artery bypass surgery. One group received blood via a 170 micron filter and the other received blood via a 20 micron filter. Postoperatively, various pulmonary function tests were performed. They concluded that, even for patients with some degree of pretransfusion pulmonary dysfunction, use of microaggregate filters for 6 to 7 unit transfusions did not provide significant clinical benefit.[5]

Some have argued that because the micropore blood filters cause no harm (platelets not removed) and that the microaggregates can cause no good, perhaps we should still routinely use the micropore filters for blood stored for 3 days or longer. A recent report, however, indicates that hemolysis can occur when micropore filters are utilized on blood stored for more than 14 days.[6] Certainly, these filters increase resistance to flow.

In summary, we are not recommending that the micropore filters not be used, but are saying that there is no evidence that they are necessary. Obviously, further studies are needed to establish the role of infusion of microaggregates on the well-being of patients.

Transfusion Reactions

Hemolytic Reaction. One of the most catastrophic reactions is that arising from hemolysis, which usually occurs because of "clerical errors," in which the wrong blood group has been infused into a patient. Mortality may occur in 20 to 60 percent of patients experiencing severe hemolytic transfusion reactions.

The classic signs and symptoms of a hemolytic transfusion reaction, which include headache, chills, fever, and nausea, are masked by anesthesia. Therefore, under general anesthesia, the three cardinal signs of a hemolytic transfusion reaction are hemoglobinuria, excessive bleeding or oozing, and hypotension.

Haptoglobin is a protein that can bind about 100 mg of hemoglobin/dl of plasma. When the ability of haptoglobin to bind free hemoglobin has been exceeded, free hemoglobin will exist in the circulation to be excreted by the kidney. The most common resultant problems are renal failure and DIC.

Although the exact cause of renal failure is not known, a common hypothesis is that hemoglobin, in the form of acid hematin, precipitates in the distal tubule, causing a mechanical tubular blockage. Nevertheless, renal dysfunction does not occur when stroma free hemoglobin solutions are administered as plasma volume expanders. This observation suggests that renal dysfunction associated with a hemolytic reaction is due to deposition of stromal contents of red blood cells in the renal tubules, rather than precipitation of hemoglobin. Regardless of the mechanism, the treatment is immediate discontinuation of the transfusion, return of the remaining blood to the laboratory for recrossmatching, and maintenance of urine output above 1 ml/kg/hr by generous administration of intravenous fluids and diuretics. Indeed, the magnitude of precipitation in the renal tubules probably is inversely related to the volume of urine flow. Furthermore, intravenous sodium bicarbonate 0.5 to 1 mEq/kg to alkalinize the urine has been recommended to improve the solubility of hemoglobin degradation products.

In summary, any time a patient has hemoglobinuria or hemolysis, a hemolytic transfusion reaction should be assumed until proven otherwise.

Minor Reactions. These reactions to blood transfusion usually are not serious and take the form of either a febrile or allergic reaction. A febrile reaction is characterized by chills, fever, and urticaria, due to antigens to which the recipient has leukocyte antibodies. Allergic reactions are very similar and are characterized by urticaria, or in more severe cases, chills and fever. Supportive therapy may include antihistamines. If a patient desperately needs a transfusion, the appearance of a rash should not stop the clinician from continuing to administer the blood. If the reaction begins with chills, fever, and urticaria, the plasma and urine should be examined for free hemoglobin to rule out the diagnosis of a hemolytic transfusion reaction.

Infectivity of Blood

Hepatitis. Unfortunately, the reduction of posttransfusion hepatitis B through universal screening of blood donors for hepatitis B surface antigen has not brought about an obvious reduction in the overall prevalence of the disease. The reason is that the vast majority of all posttransfusion hepatitis in the United States is due to another virus, currently designated as non-A, non-B, or type C. Currently, by combining icteric and nonicteric hepatitis, the incidence of posttransfusion hepatitis ranges from 5 to 15 percent. Approximately one-half of these cases go on to develop chronic active hepatitis. This statistic has been derived from those patients who have received blood that is from volunteer blood donors, rather than those from commercial sources. Administration of blood from commercial donors would likely be associated with an even higher incidence of hepatitis. Recently, consideration has been given as to whether routine testing of donor blood for alanine aminotransferase activity should be done in order to reduce the transmission of hepatitis. Current results indicate, however, that the benefits from such testing would not be feasible or reasonable.[7] The clinician must recognize that transfusion of stored blood is associated with a significant incidence of hepatitis. Therefore, measures to minimize the need for blood transfusions should be taken, including autotransfusion, and the increased use of other solutions to replace blood loss (see the section, *Other Intravenous Fluids*).

Acquired immunodeficiency syndrome (AIDS) is a secondary immune deficiency often associated with opportunistic infections or a rare form of malignancy, Karposi's sarcoma, or both. Th fatality rate of AIDS is approximately 70 percent, usually within 2 years of diagnosis. AIDS is found in predominantly four groups of individuals, which include promiscuous homosexual males, persons who have resided in Haiti, intravenous drug abusers, and hemophiliacs. The major concern is whether AIDS is transmitted by blood and blood products. Certainly, blood and blood products may be one possible method of transmission, although this possibility remains unproven. It is highly unlikely that AIDS is transmitted by blood routinely given intraoperatively. Isolation of a virus responsible for AIDS offers hope for screening blood for this organism. Until then, increased caution in the use of blood and blood products is warranted.[8]

OTHER INTRAVENOUS FLUIDS

Intravenous solutions other than crystalloids include colloids (5 percent albumin, plasma protein fraction, dextran, starch solutions) and hemoglobin substitutes (stroma-free hemoglobin, Fluosol-DA).[9-13] Hemoglobin substitutes are not yet clinically available.

REFERENCES

1. Giesecke AH Jr. Perioperative fluid therapy-crystalloids. In: Miller RD, ed, Anesthesia. New York, Churchill Livingstone, 1981;865–84.
2. Shires GT, Ganizaro PC. Fluid and electrolyte nutritional management of the surgical patient. In: Schwartz SI, ed, Principles of surgery. Third edition. New York, McGraw Hill, 1979;65–97.
3. Miller RD, Brzica SM. Blood, blood component, colloid and autotransfusion therapy. in: Miller RD, ed, Anesthesia. New York, Churchill Livingstone, 1981;885–922.
4. Mant MJ, King EG. Severe, acute disseminated intravascular coagulation. Am J Med 1979;67:557–63.
5. Snyder EL, Hazzey A, Barash PG, Palermo G. Microaggregate blood filtration in patients with compromised pulmonary function. Transfusion 1982;22:21–5.
6. Schmidt WF III, Kim HC, Tomassini N, Schwartz E. RBC destruction caused by a micropore blood filter. JAMA 1982; 248:1629–32.
7. Hornbrook MC, Dodd RY, Jacobs P, Friedman LI, Sherman KE. Reducing the incidence of non-A, non-B post-transfusion hepatitis by testing donor blood for alanine aminotransferase. N Engl J Med 1982; 307:1315–21.
8. Miller RD, Bove JR. Acquired immunodeficiency syndrome (AIDS) and blood products. Anesthesiology 1983;59:493–4.
9. Tremper KK, Friedman AE, Levine EM, Lapin R, Camarillo D. The preoperative treatment of severely anemic patients with a perflurochemical oxygen-transport fluid, Fluosol-DA. N Engl J Med 1982;307:277–83.
10. Abel WG. Blood substitute oxygen carriers. NY State J Med 1982;82:1429–33.
11. Hauser CJ, Kaufman C, Frantz R, Shippy C, Schwartz S, Shoemaker WC. Use of crystalline hemoglobin as replacement of RBC mass. Arch Surg 1982;117:782–6.
12. Daniels MJ, Strauss RG, Smith-Floss AM. Effects of hydroxyethyl starch on erythrocyte typing and blood crossmatching. Transfusion 1982;22:226–8.
13. Puri VK, Paidipaty B, White L. Hydroxyethyl starch for resuscitation of patients with hypovolemia and shock. Crit Care Med 1981;9:833–7.

Section IV
Special Anesthetic Considerations

19

Cardiac Disease

Management of anesthesia for the patient with cardiac disease requires an understanding of the pathophysiology of the disease process and a careful selection of anesthetics, muscle relaxants, and monitors to match the unique needs introduced by each individual patient.

CORONARY ARTERY DISEASE

Coronary artery disease is present in about 20 percent of the male population of less than 60 years of age.[1] The presence of coronary artery disease in patients who undergo anesthesia for noncardiac surgery is associated with increased morbidity and mortality. The patient history, evaluation of the electrocardiogram (ECG), and interpretation of cardiac catheterization and angiography data are the essential components of the preoperative cardiac evaluation. Ultimately, these data should determine whether the patient is in the best medical condition possible prior to elective cardiac or noncardiac surgery.

Patient History

Important aspects of the history taken from the patient with coronary artery disease prior to noncardiac surgery include cardiac reserve, characteristics of angina pectoris, and the presence of a prior myocardial infarction. Potential interactions of medications used in the treatment of coronary artery disease with drugs used to produce anesthesia must also be considered. A thorough evaluation is especially important, since a patient can remain asymptomatic despite 50 to 70 percent stenosis of a major coronary artery.

Cardiac Reserve. Limited exercise tolerance in the absence of significant pulmonary disease is the most striking evidence of reduced cardiac reserve. If a patient can climb two to three flights of stairs without symptoms, cardiac reserve is probably adequate.

Angina Pectoris is considered to be stable when no change has occurred for at least 60 days in precipitating factors, frequency, and duration. Chest pain produced with less than normal activity or lasting for increasingly longer peiods of time is considered to be characteristic of unstable angina pectoris and may signal an impending myocardial infarction. Dyspnea following the onset of angina pectoris is indicative of acute left ventricular dysfunction due to myocardial ischemia. Angina pectoris due to spasm of the coronary arteries (variant or Prinzmetal's angina) differs from classical angina pectoris in that it may occur at rest but not during vigorous exertion.

Knowledge of the heart rate and/or systolic blood pressure at which angina pectoris or evidence of myocardial ischemia oc-

Table 19-1. Incidence of Perioperative Myocardial Reinfarction

Time Elapsed since Prior Myocardial Infarction	Tarhan et al[2]	Steen et al[3]
<3 months	37%	27%
3–6 months	16%	11%
>6 months	5%	6%

Incidence was not different ($P > 0.05$) between the two studies at any time interval.

(McCammon RL. Coronary artery disease. In: Stoelting RK, Dierdorf SF, eds. Anesthesia and coexisting disease. New York, Churchill Livingstone 1983:1–26.)

curs on the ECG is important preoperative information. These values should not be exceeded intraoperatively. An increased heart rate is more likely than hypertension to produce signs of myocardial ischemia. This is predictable, since a rapid heart rate increases myocardial oxygen requirements and reduces the time during diastole for coronary blood flow and thus delivery of oxygen to occur. Conversely, elevated myocardial oxygen requirements produced by the increased systolic blood pressure are offset by improved perfusion through pressure-dependent atherosclerotic coronary arteries.

Prior Myocardial Infarction. The incidence of myocardial reinfarction in the perioperative period is related to the time elapsed since the previous myocardial infarction (Table 19-1).[2,3] The incidence of a perioperative myocardial reinfarction did not stabilize at 5 to 6 percent until 6 months after the prior myocardial infarction. Thus, elective surgery, especially thoracic and upper abdominal procedures, should be delayed for about 6 months after a myocardial infarction. Even after 6 months, the 5 to 6 percent incidence of myocardial reinfarction is about 50 times greater than the 0.13 percent incidence of perioperative myocardial infarction in patients undergoing similar operations but in the absence of a prior myocardial infarction. None of the myocardial

reinfarctions observed in these studies occurred intraoperatively. Indeed, the greatest incidence of myocardial reinfarction was observed on the third postoperative day.

Several factors influence the incidence of myocardial reinfarction in the perioperative period. For example, the incidence of myocardial reinfarction is increased in patients undergoing intrathoracic or intra-abdominal operations lasting longer than 3 hours. Factors that have not been shown to predispose to a myocardial reinfarction include (1) the site of the previous myocardial infarction, (2) a history of prior aortocoronary bypass graft surgery, (3) the site of the operative procedure if the duration of the surgery is less than 3 hours, and (4) the drugs and/or techniques used to produce anesthesia. Finally, close hemodynamic monitoring using intra-arterial and pulmonary artery catheters and prompt pharmacologic treatment or fluid infusion to treat hemodynamic alterations from a normal range may reduce the risk of perioperative myocardial reinfarction in high-risk patients.[1]

Current Medications. The drugs most likely to be encountered in patients with coronary artery disease are beta antagonists and calcium channel blockers. In addition, patients with coronary artery disease may be receiving drugs classified as antihypertensives and diuretics. A knowledge of the pharmacology of these drugs and potential adverse interactions with anesthetics is an important preoperative consideration (see Chapters 3 and 22). Despite the potential for adverse drug interactions, cardiac medications being taken preoperatively probably should be continued without interruption through the perioperative period.

Electrocardiogram (ECG)

The preoperative ECG should be examined for evidence of (1) myocardial ischemia, (2) prior myocardial infarction, (3) cardiac hypertrophy, (4) abnormal cardiac rhythm and/or conduction disturbances, and (5) electrolyte abnormalities. The resting ECG in the absence of angina pectoris may be normal despite extensive coronary artery disease. Nevertheless, an ECG demonstrating ST segment depression greater than 1 mm, particularly during angina pectoris, confirms the presence of myocardial ischemia. Furthermore, the ECG lead demonstrating changes of myocardial ischemia can help determine the specific diseased coronary artery (Table 19-2).[1] It should be remembered that a prior myocardial infarction, especially if subendocardial, may not be accompanied by persistent changes on the ECG. The presence of premature ventricular beats may signal their likely occurrence intraoperatively. A P-R interval greater than 0.2 seconds is most often related to digitalis therapy. Conversely, blocks of conduction of the cardiac impulse that occur below the atrioventricular node most likely reflect pathological changes rather than drug effect.

Cardiac Catheterization and Angiography

Cardiac catheterization and angiography are highly specialized tests which are not routinely performed in most patients before noncardiac surgery. When available, however, these data provide objective evidence of left ventricular function and facilitate prediction of the patient's response to the stresses of anesthesia and surgery. For example, left ventricular function can be classified as good or impaired, based on the history, physical examination, and measurements obtained during cardiac catheterization (Table 19-3).[1]

Management of Anesthesia

Management of anesthesia in the patient with coronary artery disease is based on maintaining a favorable balance between myocardial oxygen requirements and myocardial oxygen delivery so as to prevent myocardial ischemia (Table 19-4).[1] Any perioperative event associated with persistent tachycardia, systolic hypertension, arterial hypoxemia, or diastolic hypotension can adversely influence this delicate balance. The maintenance of this balance is more important than the specific technique and/or drugs selected to produce anesthesia and skeletal muscle paralysis. It is critical that persistent and excessive changes in heart rate and blood pressure be avoided. Heart rate and blood pressure probably should be maintained within 20 percent of the awake values.

Induction of Anesthesia. Preoperative medication should produce reliable sedation so as to allay anxiety, which if unopposed could lead to secretion of catecholamines and an increase in myocardial

Table 19-2. Area of Myocardial Ischemia as Reflected by the Electrocardiogram

Electrocardiogram Lead	Coronary Artery Responsible for Myocardial Ischemia	Area of Myocardium that May Be Involved
II, III, aVF	Right coronary artery	Right atrium Sinus node Atrioventricular node Right ventricle
V_3–V_5	Left anterior descending coronary artery	Anterolateral aspects of the left ventricle
I, aVL	Circumflex coronary artery	Lateral aspects of the left ventricle

(Adapted from McCammon RL. Coronary artery disease. In: Stoelting RK, Dierdorf SF, eds. Anesthesia and co-existing disease. New York, Churchill Livingstone 1983:1–26.)

Table 19-3. Evaluation of Left Ventricular Function

	Good Function	Impaired Function
Prior myocardial infarction	No	Yes
Evidence of congestive heart failure	No	Yes
Ejection fraction	Above 0.55	Below 0.4
Left ventricular end-diastolic pressure	Below 12 mmHg	Above 18 mmHg
Cardiac index	Above 2.5 L/min/m^2	Below 2 L/min/m^2
Areas of ventricular dyskinesia	No	Yes

(Adapted from McCammon RL. Coronary artery disease. In: Stoelting RK, Dierdorf SF, eds. Anesthesia and co-existing disease. New York, Churchill Livingstone 1983:1–26.)

oxygen requirements due to an elevation of blood pressure and heart rate. A frequent approach is intramuscular morphine plus scopolamine with or without an orally administered benzodiazepine. Scopolamine is valuable because of its profound sedative and amnesic effect without producing undesirable changes in heart rate. It may also be appropriate to apply a transdermal preparation of nitroglycerin at the time the preoperative medication is administered. Furthermore, a continuous intravenous infusion of nitroglycerin (0.25 to 0.5 µg/kg/min) during the perioperative period should also be considered in the patient with known coronary artery disease.

Induction of anesthesia is acceptably accomplished with the intravenous administration of an ultrashort-acting barbiturate or benzodiazepine or by inhalation via a mask. Ketamine increases heart rate and blood pressure and would likely increase myocardial oxygen requirements. Intubation of the trachea is facilitated by the administration of succinylcholine or a nondepolarizing muscle relaxant.

Myocardial ischemia may accompany the hypertension and tachycardia that result from the stimulation of direct laryngoscopy necessary for intubation of the trachea. A short duration of direct laryngoscopy (ideally less than 15 seconds) is important in minimizing the magnitude of these circulatory changes. When the duration of direct laryngoscopy is not likely to be short or when hypertension pre-exists, the addition of other drugs to minimize the pressor response produced by the intubation sequence should be considered. For example, laryngotracheal lidocaine (2 mg/kg) administered just before inserting the tube into the trachea minimizes the magnitude and duration of the blood pressure increase. Likewise, intravenous lidocaine 1.5 mg/kg, administered about 90 seconds before beginning direct laryngoscopy, is efficacious. An alternative to lidocaine is nitroprusside 1 to 2 µg/kg administered intravenously about 15 seconds before beginning direct laryngoscopy or fentanyl 8 µg/kg 2 to 4 minutes before beginning laryngoscopy.[1] None of these pharmacologic interventions, however, reliably prevent the heart rate increase produced by direct laryngoscopy.

Maintenance of Anesthesia. The choice of anesthesia is often based on the patient's left ventricular function (Table 19-3).[1] For example, the patient with coronary artery disease but normal left ventricular function is likely to develop tachycardia and hyper-

Table 19-4. Determinants of Myocardial Oxygen Requirements and Delivery

Myocardial Oxygen Requirements	Myocardial Oxygen Delivery
Heart rate	Coronary blood flow
Systemic blood pressure	Oxygen content of
Myocardial contractility	arterial blood
Ventricular volume	

(Adapted from McCammon RL. Coronary artery disease. In: Stoelting RK, Dierdorf SF, eds. Anesthesia and co-existing disease. New York, Churchill Livingstone 1983:1–26.)

tension in response to intense stimulation. Controlled myocardial depression produced by a volatile anesthetic with or without nitrous oxide may be appropriate if the primary goal is to prevent increased myocardial oxygen requirements. Equally acceptable for the maintenance of anesthesia is the use of a nitrous oxide-narcotic technique, with the addition of a volatile anesthetic as necessary to treat hypertension. When hypertension is treated with a volatile anesthetic, isoflurane lowers blood pressure by decreasing systemic vascular resistance; halothane tends to lower blood pressure by reducing cardiac output (see Chapter 4). Isoflurane may also function as a coronary vasodilator in patients with coronary artery disease.[4] The role of enflurane or halothane as a coronary vasodilator has not been determined.

Patients with impaired left ventricular function, as associated with a prior myocardial infarction, may not tolerate direct myocardial depression produced by a volatile anesthetic. In these patients, the use of a short-acting narcotic such as fentanyl with nitrous oxide may be more appropriate. It must be remembered that nitrous oxide, when administered to patients who have received prior narcotics for anesthesia, may produce undesirable reductions in blood pressure and cardiac output.[1] High dose fentanyl (50 to 100 μg/kg) as the sole anesthetic has been advocated for patients who cannot tolerate even minimal anesthetic induced myocardial depression.[5]

A regional anesthetic is an acceptable technique in patients with coronary artery disease. It is important to realize, however, that flow through coronary arteries narrowed by atherosclerosis is pressure dependent. Therefore, reductions in blood pressure associated with a regional anesthetic that exceed about 20 percent of the preblock value probably should be treated with an intravenous infusion of crystalloid solution and/or sympathomimetic such as ephedrine.

Muscle Relaxant. The choice of nondepolarizing muscle relaxant during maintenance of anesthesia for a patient with coronary artery disease is dictated by the circulatory effects of these drugs and the likely impact of these changes on myocardial oxygen requirements and myocardial oxygen delivery (see Chapter 8). Metocurine, atracurium, and vecuronium are good choices in patients with coronary artery disease, as these drugs do not produce significant changes in heart rate or blood pressure and are, therefore, unlikely to alter myocardial oxygen requirements. Pancuronium increases heart rate and blood pressure, but these changes are usually less than 10 to 15 percent above predrug values, making this drug a possible choice for administration to patients with coronary artery disease. Furthermore, circulatory changes produced by pancuronium can be used to offset negative inotropic and/or chronotropic effects of drugs being used for anesthesia. Beta-adrenergic blockers, often taken by hospitalized patients with coronary artery disease, may attenuate the increase in heart rate normally produced by pancuronium. Reductions in blood pressure produced by d-tubocurarine could jeopardize myocardial oxygen delivery by decreasing coronary blood flow, making this drug an unlikely choice.

Reversal of a nondepolarizing neuromuscular blockade with an anticholinesterase-anticholinergic combination can be safely accomplished in patients with coronary artery disease. Glycopyrrolate apparently has less chronotropic effect than atropine and may be the anticholinergic of choice. Nevertheless, marked increases in heart rate rarely occur with reversal of nondepolarizing muscle relaxants, and, therefore, atropine seems as acceptable as glycopyrrolate for combination with the anticholinesterase.

Monitoring. The intensity of monitoring in the perioperative period is dictated by the complexity of the operative procedure and severity of the coronary artery disease. The ECG is the only way to monitor the balance between myocardial oxygen requirements and myocardial oxygen delivery in unconscious patients (see Chapter 16). When this balance is unfavorably altered, myocardial ischemia occurs, as evidenced on the ECG by at least 1 mm downsloping of the ST segment from the base line. A precordial V_5 lead is the best selection for detecting ST segment changes characteristic of myocardial ischemia of the left ventricle during anesthesia. A pulmonary artery catheter is helpful for monitoring responses to intravenous fluid replacement and the therapeutic effects of drugs on left ventricular function. Right atrial pressure may not reliably reflect left heart filling pressure in the presence of left ventricular dysfunction due to coronary artery disease. Conversely, right atrial pressure correlates with pulmonary artery occlusion pressure in patients with coronary artery disease when the ejection fraction is above 0.5 and there is no evidence of left ventricular dysfunction.[16]

The appearance of signs of myocardial ischemia on the ECG supports the aggressive treatment of adverse changes in heart rate and/or blood pressure. Tachycardia is treated with the intravenous administration of propranolol while excessive increases in blood pressure respond to nitroprusside. Nitroglycerin is a more appropriate choice than nitroprusside when myocardial ischemia is associated with a normal blood pressure. Hypotension should be treated with a sympathomimetic so as to rapidly restore pressure-dependent perfusion through atherosclerotic coronary arteries. In addition to drugs, the intravenous infusion of fluids to restore blood pressure is ideal, since myocardial oxygen requirements for volume work of the heart are less than those for pressure work. The disadvantage of this approach is the time necessary for fluid treatment to be effective.

Recovery from general anesthesia may be associated with evidence of left ventricular dysfunction in patients with coronary artery disease. Preoperative administration of digoxin may prevent this impairment of cardiac function.[7]

VALVULAR HEART DISEASE

The most frequently encountered forms of valvular heart disease produce pressure overload (mitral stenosis, aortic stenosis) or volume overload (mitral regurgitation, aortic regurgitation) of the left ventricle. The net effect of valvular heart disease is interference with forward flow of blood from the heart into the systemic circulation. Selection of anesthetic drugs and muscle relaxants for patients with valvular heart disease are based on the likely effects that drug-induced changes in cardiac rhythm, heart rate, blood pressure, systemic vascular resistance, and pulmonary vascular resistance will have relative to maintenance of cardiac output in these patients. When cardiac reserve is minimal, high doses of fentanyl, 50 to 100 μg/kg, may be used as the sole anesthetic.[5] Patients with valvular heart disease should receive antibiotics in the perioperative period for protection against infective endocarditis.

Mitral Stenosis

Mitral stenosis is characterized by mechanical obstruction to left ventricular diastolic filling secondary to a progressive decrease in the orifice of the mitral valve. The obstruction produces an increase in left atrial and pulmonary venous pressure. Increased pulmonary vascular resistance is likely when the left atrial pressure is chronically elevated above 25 mmHg. Distension of the left atrium predisposes to atrial fibrillation, while stasis of blood in this chamber favors the formation of thrombi which can be displaced as systemic emboli. Mitral stenosis is almost always due to the fusion of the mitral valve leaflets during the healing process of acute rheumatic carditis. Symptoms of mitral stenosis do not usually develop until about 20 years following the initial episode of rheumatic fever. A sudden increase in the demand for cardiac output such as pregnancy or sepsis, however, may unmask previously asymptomatic mitral stenosis.

Patients taking digitalis preoperatively for the control of heart rate should have this drug continued until the time of surgery. Since diuretic therapy is frequent, the serum potassium concentration should be measured preoperatively. Also, patients with mitral stenosis can be more susceptible than normal individuals to the ventilatory depressant effects of sedative drugs used for preoperative medication. When an anticholinergic is included in the preoperative medication, scopolamine or glycopyrrolate has fewer chronotropic effects than atropine.

Management of Anesthesia. Induction of anesthesia in the presence of mitral stenosis can be safely achieved with administration of an ultrashort-acting barbiturate or benzodiazepine followed by succinylcholine to facilitate intubation of the trachea. Ketamine is probably not a good choice for induction of anesthesia because of its propensity to increase heart rate. Drugs used for maintenance of anesthesia should cause minimal changes in heart rate and in systemic and pulmonary vascular resistance. Furthermore, these drugs should not greatly reduce myocardial contractility. These goals can be achieved with combinations of nitrous oxide and short-acting narcotics or low concentrations of volatile anesthetics. Although nitrous oxide can increase pulmonary vascular resistance, it is not enough to justify avoiding this drug in all patients with mitral stenosis (Fig. 19-1).[8] The effect of nitrous oxide on pulmonary vascular resistance, however, seems to be accentuated when pre-existing pulmonary hypertension is severe.

Nondepolarizing muscle relaxants with minimal circulatory effects (metocurine,

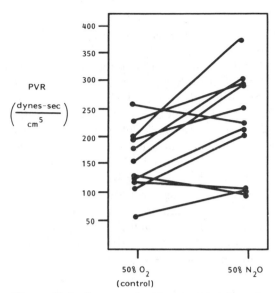

Figure 19-1. Compared with control values for calculated pulmonary vascular resistance (PVR), the inhalation of 50 percent nitrous oxide increased PVR in 8 of 11 patients. Nevertheless, the magnitude of increase in PVR was not sufficient to recommend the routine avoidance of nitrous oxide in patients with co-existing pulmonary hypertension. (Hilgenberg JC, McCammon RL, Stoelting RK. Pulmonary and systemic vascular responses to nitrous oxide in patients with mitral stenosis and pulmonary hypertension. Anesth Analg 1980;59:323–6.)

atracurium, vecuronium) are ideal for use in patients with mitral stenosis. Pancuronium is less appropriate because of its ability to increase the speed of transmission of the cardiac impulse through the atrioventricular node, which could lead to excessive increases in heart rate. Such increases would seem particularly likely in the presence of atrial fibrillation, since the ventricular response to atrial impulses is determined by the degree of atrioventricular conduction. There is no reason to avoid pharmacologic reversal of nondepolarizing muscle relaxants, but the adverse effects of drug-induced tachycardia should be anticipated. Intraoperative fluid therapy must be carefully titrated, as these patients are susceptible to intravascular volume overload and to the development of left ventricular failure and pulmonary edema. Likewise, the head-down position is not well tolerated, since the pulmonary blood volume is already increased. Monitoring right atrial pressure is a helpful guide to the adequacy of intravascular fluid replacement. An increase in right atrial pressure could also reflect nitrous oxide-induced pulmonary vasoconstriction, suggesting the need to discontinue this drug. Postoperatively, patients with mitral stenosis are at high risk for developing pulmonary edema and right heart failure. Mechanical support of ventilation of the lungs is often necessary, particularly following major thoracic or abdominal surgery.

Mitral Regurgitation

Mitral regurgitation is characterized by left atrial volume overload and decreased left ventricular forward stroke volume due to passage of part of each stroke volume through the incompetent mitral valve back into the left atrium. This regurgitant flow is responsible for the characteristic V wave seen on the recording of the pulmonary artery occlusion pressure (Fig. 19-2).[9] Mitral regurgitation is usually due to rheumatic fever and is almost always associated with mitral stenosis. Isolated mitral regurgitation is often acute, reflecting papillary muscle dysfunction following a myocardial infarction or rupture of a chordae tendinae secondary to infective endocarditis.

Management of Anesthesia in patients with mitral regurgitation should be designed to reduce the likelihood of reductions in heart rate or increases in systemic vascular resistance that would lead to a decrease in the forward left ventricular stroke volume. Conversely, cardiac output can be improved by mild increases in heart rate and mild reductions in systemic vascular resistance.

A general anesthetic is the usual choice for patients with mitral regurgitation. Although reductions in systemic vascular resistance are theoretically beneficial, the uncontrolled nature of this response with a regional anesthetic detracts from the use of this technique for other than surgery on periphral sites. Maintenance of anesthesia can be provided with nitrous oxide plus a volatile drug, the concentration of which can be adjusted to attenuate undesirable increases in blood pressure and systemic vascular resistance that can accompany surgical stimulation. Nondepolarizing muscle relaxants—such as metocurine, atracurium, and vecuronium—that lack circula-

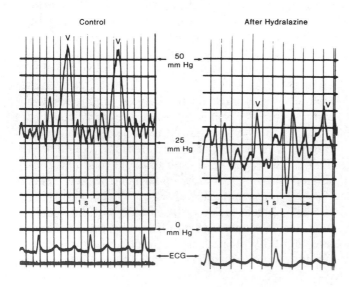

Control   After Hydralazine

50 mm Hg

25 mm Hg

1 s

0 mm Hg

ECG

Figure 19-2. Regurgitant blood flow into the left atrium via an incompetent mitral valve produces a V wave on the trace of the pulmonary artery occlusion pressure. Vasodilation produced by hydralazine reduces impedence to forward ejection of blood from the left ventricle such that regurgitant flow into the left atrium is less and the size of the V wave is decreased. (Greenberg BH, Rahimtoola SH. Vasodilator therapy for valvular heart disease. JAMA 1981;246:269–72. Copyright 1981, American Medical Association.)

tory effects are ideal. Pancuronium is also acceptable, as the mild increase in heart rate produced by this drug could increase forward left ventricular stroke volume. Although d-tobucurarine reduces systemic vascular resistance, the magnitude of this response is not predictable, making this an unlikely drug choice for the patient with mitral regurgitation. Intravascular fluid volume must be maintained by the prompt replacement of blood loss so as to assure adequate cardiac filling and ejection of an optimal forward left ventricular stroke volume.

Aortic Stenosis

Aortic stenosis is characterized by increased left ventricular systolic pressure so as to maintain the forward stroke volume through a narrowed aortic valve. The magnitude of the pressure gradient serves as an estimate of the severity of valvular stenosis. Hemodynamically significant aortic stenosis is associated with a pressure gradient greater than 50 mmHg. The increased intraventricular pressure is associated with a compensatory increase in the thickness of the left ventricular wall. Angina pectoris occurs often in these patients in the absence of coronary artery disease, reflecting increased myocardial oxygen needs due to the increased amounts of ventricular muscle associated with myocardial hypertrophy. Furthermore, myocardial oxygen delivery is decreased due to compression of subendocardial coronary blood vessels by the increased left ventricular systolic pressure.

Isolated nonrheumatic aortic stenosis usually results from progressive calcification and stenosis of a congenitally abnormal (usually bicuspid) valve. Aortic stenosis due to rheumatic fever almost always occurs in association with mitral valve disease. Likewise, aortic stenosis is usually associated with some degree of aortic regurgitation. Regardless of the etiology of aortic stenosis, the natural history of the disease includes a long latent period, often 30 years or more, before symptoms occur. Since many patients with aortic stenosis are asymptomatic, it is important to listen for this cardiac murmur (systolic murmur in the second right intercostal space) in all patients scheduled for surgery. Indeed, the incidence of sudden death is increased in patients with aortic stenosis.

Management of Anesthesia. Goals during management of anesthesia in patients with aortic stenosis are maintenance of normal sinus rhythm and avoidance of extreme and prolonged alterations in heart rate, systemic vascular resistance, and intravascular fluid volume. Preservation of normal sinus rhythm is critical, since the left ventricle is dependent on a properly timed atrial contraction to assure an optimal left ventricular filling and stroke volume. Marked increases in heart rate (above 100 beats/min) can reduce the time for left ventricular filling and ejection, while bradycardia (below 60 beats/min) can lead to acute overdistension of the left ventricle. In view of the obstruction to left ventricular ejection, it must be appreciated that a decrease in systemic vascular resistance may be associated with large reductions in blood pressure and coronary blood flow.

A general anesthetic is usually preferred to a regional anesthetic, since sympathetic nervous system blockade can lead to undesirable decreases in systemic vascular resistance. Maintenance of anesthesia can be with nitrous oxide plus a short-acting narcotic or low concentration of a volatile drug. A potential disadvantage of volatile drugs (especially halothane) is depression of sinus node automaticity, which may lead to junctional rhythm and decreased left ventricular filling due to loss of a properly timed atrial contraction.

Intravascular fluid volume must be maintained by prompt replacement of blood loss and liberal administration of intravenous fluids. If a pulmonary artery catheter is utilized, it should be remembered that the occlusion pressure may underestimate the left ventricular end-diastolic pressure by as much as 7 mmHg, because of the decreased compliance of the left ventricle that accompanies chronic aortic stenosis. A direct current defibrillator should be immediately available when anesthesia is administered to a patient with aortic stenosis, since external cardiac massage is unlikely to be effective in creating an adequate stroke volume across a stenosed valve.

Aortic Regurgitation

Aortic regurgitation is characterized by decreased forward left ventricular stroke volume due to regurgitation of part of the ejected stroke volume from the aorta back into the left ventricle through an incompetent aortic valve. A gradual onset of aortic regurgitation results in marked left ventricular hypertrophy. Increased myocardial oxygen requirements secondary to left ventricular hypertrophy, plus a characteristic decrease in aortic diastolic pressure which reduces coronary blood flow, can manifest as angina pectoris in the absence of coronary artery disease. Acute aortic regurgitation is most often due to infective endocarditis, trauma, or dissection of a thoracic aneurysm. Chronic aortic regurgitation is usually due to prior rheumatic fever. In contrast to aortic stenosis, the occurrence of sudden death with aortic regurgitation is rare. Management of anesthesia for noncardiac surgery in patients with aortic regurgitation is as described for patients with mitral regurgitation.

MITRAL VALVE PROLAPSE

Mitral valve prolapse (click-murmur syndrome, Barlow's syndrome) is characterized by an abnormality of the mitral valve support structure that permits prolapse of the valve into the left atrium during contraction of the left ventricle. Based on the presence of a characteristic systolic mur-

mur best heard at the apex, it is estimated that 5 to 10 percent of the adult population manifests this valve abnormality. Echocardiography is helpful in confirming the diagnosis of mitral valve prolapse. There seems to be an increased incidence of mitral valve prolapse in patients with musculoskeletal abnormalities including Marfan's syndrome, pectus excavatum, and kyphoscoliosis. In addition to mitral regurgitation, complications associated with mitral valve prolapse include supraventricular cardiac dysrhythmias, altered conduction of the cardiac impulse through the atrioventricular node (pre-excitation syndrome), and sudden death.

Management of Anesthesia. The important principle in the management of anesthesia in patients with mitral valve prolapse is the avoidance of events that can increase cardiac emptying and accentuate prolapse of the mitral valve into the left atrium. Perioperative events that can increase cardiac emptying include (1) sympathetic nervous system stimulation, (2) decreased systemic vascular resistance, and (3) performance of surgery with patients in the head-up or sitting position. With this in mind, it is important to optimize the intravascular fluid volume in the preoperative period. Ketamine or pancuronium are not recommended because of their ability to increase cardiac contractility and heart rate. Maintenance of anesthesia is most often with nitrous oxide plus a volatile anesthetic so as to minimize sympathetic nervous system activation due to noxious intraoperative stimulation. The dose of volatile anesthetic must be titrated to avoid excessive reductions in systemic vascular resistance. A regional anesthetic could also produce undesirable reductions in systemic vascular resistance.

CONGENITAL HEART DISEASE

Approximately 8 of every 1000 live births are associated with some form of congenital heart disease. Although more than 100 dif-

Table 19-5. Common Congenital Heart Defects

	Percent of Total Defects
Ventricular septal defect	28
Secundum atrial septal defect	10
Patent ductus arteriosus	10
Tetralogy of Fallot	10
Pulmonary stenosis	10
Aortic stenosis	7
Coarctation of the aorta	5
Transportation of the great vessels	5

(Adapted from Haselby KA. Congenital heart disease. In: Stoelting RK, Dierdorf SF, eds. Anesthesia and co-existing disease. New York, Churchill Livingstone 1983:47–70.)

ferent congenital heart lesions are known, nearly 90 percent of all cardiac defects can be placed in 1 of 10 categories (Table 19-5).[10] From the standpoint of management of anesthesia, it is helpful to categorize congenital heart defects as those lesions that result in a left-to-right intracardiac shunt and those that result in a right-to-left intracardiac shunt. Patients with congenital heart disease should receive antibiotics in the perioperative period for protection against infective endocarditis.

Left-to-Right Intracardiac Shunt

A left-to-right intracardiac shunt may be due to an atrial septal defect or ventricular septal defect. Patent ductus arteriosus is an example of a left-to-right shunt at the level of the aorta. The result of these shunts is increased pulmonary blood flow with pulmonary hypertension, right ventricular hypertrophy, and eventually congestive heart failure.

Atrial Septal Defect. An atrial septal defect is often first suspected when there is a history of frequent pulmonary infections or when a systolic murmur is noted over the area of the pulmonary valve during a routine physical examination. Surgical closure of an atrial septal defect is indicated when the pulmonary blood flow is at least twice the systemic blood flow.

Management of Anesthesia. The presence of an atrial septal defect has only minor implications for the management of anesthesia. For example, as long as systemic blood flow remains normal, the pharmacokinetics of inhaled drugs will not be significantly altered despite increased pulmonary blood flow. Increased pulmonary blood flow means that hemodynamic effects of positive intrathoracic pressure during controlled ventilation of the lungs are well tolerated. Drugs or events that increase systemic blood pressure and/or systemic vascular resistance should be avoided, as this change favors an increase in the magnitude of the left-to-right shunt at the atrial level. Conversely, decreases in these parameters as produced by volatile anesthetics or increases in pulmonary vascular resistance due to positive pressure ventilation of the lungs tend to decrease the magnitude of the shunt. Finally, it is imperative to avoid the entrance of air into the right atrium as can occur via the tubing used to deliver intravenous solutions. This air could bypass the lungs and cross directly into the systemic circulation to enter the coronary and/or cerebral arteries.

Ventricular Septal Defect. A patient with a small ventricular septal defect (ratio of pulmonary to systemic blood flow less than 1.5 to 1) is usually asymptomatic, with the only evidence of the cardiac abnormality being a pansystolic murmur that is of maximum intensity along the left sternal border. A large ventricular septal defect is characterized by a left-to-right intracardiac shunt that results in a pulmonary blood flow that exceeds systemic blood flow by three to five times. Recurrent pulmonary infections and eventually congestive heart failure are typical complications in patients with large ventricular septal defects. Management of anesthesia is as described for atrial septal defect.

Patent Ductus Arteriosus. Failure of the ductus arteriosus to close after birth results in passage of oxygenated blood from the aorta into the pulmonary artery. Most patients are asymptomatic, with the only manifestation being a continuous systolic and diastolic murmur. Management of anesthesia is as described for atrial septal defect.

Right-to-Left Intracardiac Shunt

A right-to-left intracardiac shunt is characterized by decreased pulmonary blood flow and arterial hypoxemia. Tetralogy of Fallot is the most common of the congenital cardiac defects that result in a right-to-left intracardiac shunt.

Tetralogy of Fallot is characterized by the presence of a ventricular septal defect, an aorta that overrides the pulmonary artery outflow tract, obstruction to blood flow through the pulmonary artery outflow tract, and right ventricular hypertrophy. Arterial blood gases and pH are likely to reveal a normal $PaCO_2$ and pH and a markedly reduced PaO_2 (usually below 50 mmHg) even when breathing oxygen. Squatting is a common feature of children with tetralogy of Fallot. Presumably, squatting increases the systemic blood pressure and systemic vascular resistance by kinking the large arteries in the inguinal area. These circulatory changes reduce the magnitude of the right-to-left intracardiac shunt leading to increased pulmonary blood flow and improved arterial oxygenation.

Hypercyanotic attacks ("tet spells") can occur without provocation but are often associated with crying or exercise. The most likely explanation for these attacks is a sudden reduction in pulmonary blood flow due to either a decrease in systemic vascular resistance or spasm of cardiac muscle in the region of the pulmonary artery outflow (infundibular) tract. Phenylephrine is the most effective treatment, presumably because this drug increases systemic vascular resistance and forces more blood through the lungs. A sympathomimetic, such as ephedrine with beta agonist properties, is not se-

lected because sympathetic nervous system stimulation could accentuate spasm of the infundibular cardiac muscle. Propranolol is effective when the hypercyanotic attack is due to cardiac muscle spasm in the region of the pulmonary artery outflow tract.

Management of Anesthesia. The management of anesthesia for a patient with tetralogy of Fallot requires a thorough understanding of those events or drugs which can alter the magnitude of the right-to-left intracardiac shunt. For example, drug-induced responses that decrease systemic vascular resistance and blood pressure (volatile anesthetics, histamine release due to d-tubocurarine) will increase the magnitude of the right-to-left shunt and decrease the PaO_2. Pulmonary blood flow can also be reduced by increases in pulmonary vascular resistance that accompany positive pressure ventilation of the lungs or application of positive end-expiratory pressure. Nevertheless, the advantages of controlled ventilation of the lungs offset the potential hazards, as evidenced by the fact the PaO_2 usually improves.

Preoperatively, it is important to avoid dehydration by maintaining oral feedings in the very young or by providing intravenous fluids before arriving in the operating room. Crying associated with intramuscular administration of drugs used for preoperative medication can lead to a hypercyanotic attack. For this reason, it may be prudent to avoid intramuscular administration of drugs until the patient is in a highly supervised environment and an alpha agonist such as phenylephrine is immediately available for treatment of a hypercyanotic attack.

Induction of anesthesia in a patient with tetralogy of Fallot is best accomplished with intramuscular (4 to 6 mg/kg) or intravenous (1 to 2 mg/kg) ketamine. Indeed, the onset of anesthesia following the injection of ketamine is often associated with an improvement in the PaO_2 which presumably reflects increased pulmonary blood flow due to ketamine-induced elevation in systemic vascular resistance that leads to a decrease in the magnitude of the right-to-left intracardiac shunt.

Maintenance of anesthesia is best achieved with ketamine plus nitrous oxide. Disadvantages of nitrous oxide include the possible increase in pulmonary vascular resistance evoked by this drug and the reduction in inspired concentration of oxygen that is necessitated by use of this anesthetic. Therefore, it would seem prudent to limit the inspired concentration of nitrous oxide to no more than 50 percent. Volatile anesthetics are not recommended for induction or maintenance of anesthesia because of the propensity of these drugs to increase the magnitude of right-to-left intracardiac shunt by decreasing systemic vascular resistance and blood pressure.

Pancuronium is an ideal muscle relaxant selection, as this drug maintains systemic blood pressure. d-Tubocurarine would not be a logical choice, as this muscle relaxant could increase the magnitude of the right-to-left intracardiac shunt by virtue of its ability to decrease systemic vascular resistance secondary to histamine release and the blocking of impulse transmission through autonomic ganglia.

Ventilation of the lungs should be controlled, but it must be appreciated that excessive positive airway pressure may adversely increase resistance to blood flow through the lungs. Intravascular fluid volume must be maintained with intravenous fluid administration, since acute hypovolemia tends to increase the magnitude of the right-to-left intracardiac shunt. In view of co-existing polycythemia, it is not necessary to replace blood loss that is less than 20 percent of the estimated blood volume. It is crucial that care be taken to avoid infusion of air via the tubing used to deliver intravenous solutions, since this could lead to direct air embolization to the coronary and/or cerebral arteries. Finally, phenylephrine should be immediately available to

Table 19-6. Classification of Heart Block

First-degree atrioventricular heart block
Second degree atrioventricular heart block
Mobitz type I (Wenckebach)
Mobitz type II
Unifasicular heart block
Left anterior hemiblock
Left posterior hemiblock
Right bundle branch block
Left bundle branch block
Bifasicular heart block
Right bundle branch block plus left anterior hemiblock
Right bundle branch block plus left posterior hemiblock
Third degree (trifasicular, complete) atrioventricular heart block

(Adapted from Goodloe SL. Abnormalities of cardiac conduction and cardiac rhythm. In Stoelting RK, Dierdorf SF, eds. Anesthesia and co-existing disease. New York, Churchill Livingstone 1983:71–92.)

treat undesirable reductions in systemic vascular resistance and blood pressure.

DISTURBANCES OF CARDIAC CONDUCTION AND RHYTHM

The ECG is the most valuable tool for diagnosing and treating disturbances of cardiac conduction and rhythm. The following questions should be asked when interpreting the ECG:[11]

1. What is the heart rate?
2. Are P waves present and what is their relationship to the ORS complexes?
3. What is the duration of the P–R interval (normal 0.12 to 0.2 seconds)?
4. What is the duration of the QRS complex (normal 0.05 to 0.1 seconds)?
5. Is the ventricular rhythm regular?
6. Are there early cardiac beats or abnormal pauses following a preceding QRS complex?

Heart Block

Disturbances of conduction of the cardiac impulse can be classified according to the site of the conduction block relative to the atrioventricular node (Table 19-6).[11] Heart block occurring above the atrioventricular node is usually benign and transient. Heart block below the atrioventricular node tends to be progressive and permanent.

A theoretical concern in patients with bifasicular heart block is that perioperative events such as alterations in blood pressure, arterial oxygenation, or electrolyte concentrations might compromise conduction in the one remaining intact fasicle, leading to the acute onset intraoperatively of third-degree atrioventricular heart block. There is no evidence, however, that surgery performed during a general or regional anesthetic predisposes to the development of third-degree atrioventricular heart block in patients with co-existing bifasicular block. Therefore, placement of a prophylactic artificial cardiac pacemaker is not recommended prior to anesthesia and surgery.

Treatment of third-degree atrioventricular heart block is with a permanently implanted artificial cardiac pacemaker. A temporary transvenous artificial cardiac pacemaker should be placed before induction of anesthesia for placement of a permanent artificial pacemaker. This recommendation is based on the clinical impression that the incidence of cardiac arrest is increased during induction of anesthesia in patients with third-degree atrioventricular heart block. It must be remembered that the presence of a transvenous artificial cardiac pacemaker creates a situation in which there is a direct connection between external electrical sources and the endocardium. This predisposes the patient to the hazard of ventricular fibrillation from microshock levels of electrical current. A continuous infusion of isoproterenol may be necessary to maintain an adequate heart rate until the artificial cardiac pacemaker can be placed.

Sick Sinus Syndrome

Sick sinus syndrome is characterized by sinus bradycardia complicated by episodes of supraventricular tachycardia. Placement of an artificial cardiac pacemaker is the treatment for patients with symptomatic bradycardia. Artificial cardiac pacing may not suppress a rapid heart rate but does permit the safe use of propranolol and/or digoxin whose depressive effects on the sinus node mandate the presence of an artificial cardiac pacemaker prior to using these drugs to control tachydysrhythmias in patients with sick sinus syndrome.

Ventricular Premature Beats

Ventricular premature beats are recognized on the ECG by virtue of (1) their premature occurrence, (2) the absence of a P wave preceding the QRS complex, (3) a wide and often bizarre QRS complex, (4) an inverted T wave, and (5) a compensatory pause that follows the premature beat. Frequent (more than six per minute) and/or multifocal ventricular premature beats should be treated with the intravenous administration of lidocaine, 1 to 2 mg/kg. At the same time the underlying cause (arterial hypoxemia, hypercarbia, hypertension, hypokalemia, mechanical irritation of the ventricles) should be eliminated.

Ventricular Tachycardia

Ventricular tachycardia is defined as the appearance of at least three consecutive wide QRS complexes on the ECG (duration at least 0.12 seconds) occurring at an effective heart rate greater than 100 beats/min. Ventricular tachycardia not associated with hypotension is initially treated with the intravenous administration of lidocaine. Symptomatic ventricular tachycardia is best treated with external electrical cardioversion. The synchronizer circuit is activated by the QRS complex on the electrocardiogram and the current is delivered 10 msec after the peak of the R wave. Delivery of the shock during the RS segment is important so as to avoid the T wave which corresponds to the vulnerable period of the cardiac action potential when an electrical stimulus can induce ventricular fibrillation. The energy setting for external cardioversion is 20 to 200 joules.

Pre-excitation Syndromes

Pre-excitation syndromes are characterized by activation of a portion of the ventricles by cardiac impulses that travel from the atria via anomalous conduction pathways.[11] These pathways bypass the atrioventricular node such that activation of the ventricles occurs earlier than it would if impulses reached the ventricles by normal pathways.

Wolff-Parkinson-White Syndrome. The Wolff-Parkinson-White syndrome is the most frequent of the pre-excitation syndromes, with an incidence that may approach 0.3 percent of the general population.[11] The lack of a physiologic delay in transmission of the cardiac impulse along the Kent fibers results in the characteristic short P–R interval on the ECG. The wide QRS complex and delta wave on the ECG reflect the composite of cardiac impulses conducted by normal and anomalous pathways. Paroxysmal atrial tachycardia is the most frequent cardiac dysrhythmia associated with this syndrome.

Management of Anesthesia. The goal during management of anesthesia in the presence of a pre-excitation syndrome is to avoid events (anxiety) or durgs (anticholinergics, ketamine, pancuronium) that might increase sympathetic nervous system activity and predispose to tachydysrhythmias. All antidysrhythmics should be continued throughout the perioperative period. Droperidol (0.2 to 0.6 mg/kg) may be uniquely protective in preventing tachydysrhythmias in these patients.[12] Induction of anesthesia can be safely accomplished with the intravenous administration of a barbiturate or benzodiazepine. Intubation of the trachea should be performed only after a sufficient

depth of anesthesia has been achieved with nitrous oxide plus a volatile drug or narcotic. Nondepolarizing muscle relaxants with minimal effects on heart rate (metocurine, d-tubocurarine, atracurium, vecuronium) or succinylcholine are ideal to facilitate intubation of the trachea or to provide skeletal muscle paralysis during surgery.

The onset of paroxysmal atrial tachycardial or atrial fibrillation in the perioperative period can be treated with the intravenous administration of lidocaine, which depresses conduction through the anomalous cardiac conduction pathway. Intravenous propranolol is also useful for slowing an increased heart rate. Electrical cardioversion is indicated when the tachydysrhythmia is life-threatening. Digitalis and verapamil should not be used for the treatment of atrial fibrillation in these patients, as these drugs can accelerate conduction of impulses through the anomalous pathway.[13]

Romano-Ward Syndrome

The Ramono-Ward syndrome is characterized by a prolonged Q–T interval on the ECG that is associated with recurrent cardiac ventricular dysrhythmias and syncopal episodes. Treatment of these patients is with a beta antagonist or left stellate ganglion block. The effectiveness of a left stellate ganglion block supports the hypothesis that this syndrome results from a congenital imbalance of autonomic innervation to the heart produced by a decrease in the right cardiac sympathetic nerve activity.

ARTIFICIAL CARDIAC PACEMAKERS

Preoperatively the adequacy of artificial cardiac pacemaker function must be confirmed. The rate of discharge of an artificial atrial or ventricular asynchronous pacemaker is the most important indicator of pulse generator function. A 10 percent decrease in heart rate from the initial fixed discharge rate is a sign of battery failure.

Proper function of artificial ventricular synchronous and sequential cardiac pacemakers can be confirmed by demonstrating the appearance of captured beats on the electrocardiogram when the artificial cardiac pacemaker is converted to the asynchronous mode by an externally applied converter magnet.

Intraoperative monitoring of the patient with an artificial cardiac pacemaker includes the ECG so as to detect immediately the appearance of asystole. Atropine and isoproterenol should be immediately available should artificial cardiac pacemaker function cease. If electrocautery interferes with the ECG, monitoring a palpable peripheral pulse and/or auscultation through an esophageal stethoscope confirms continued cardiac activity. Inhibition of pulse generator activity by electromagnetic interference, which is interpreted as spontaneous cardiac activity by the artificial cardiac pacemaker, is most likely when the ground plate for electrocautery is placed near the pulse generator. For this reason, the ground plate should be placed as far as possible from the pulse generator. Despite these concerns, it is alleged that improved shielding and circuit design of pulse generators results in conversion of artificial ventricular synchronous pacemakers to the asynchronous mode during continuous use of electrocautery, thus eliminating the hazard of electromagnetic inhibition or the need for an external converter magnet. Finally, selection of drugs or techniques for anesthesia is not influenced by the presence of an artificial cardiac pacemaker, as there is no evidence that the threshold and subsequent response of these devices is altered by drugs administered in the perioperative period.

ESSENTIAL HYPERTENSION

Essential hypertension is defined as a sustained elevation of arterial blood pressure (systolic blood pressure above 160 mmHg and/or a diastolic blood pressure

Table 19-7. Management of Anesthesia for the Patient with Essential Hypertension

Preoperative evaluation
  Determine adequacy of blood pressure control
  Review pharmacology of antihypertensives
  Evaluate associated organ dysfunction (cardiac, CNS, renal)
Induction of anesthesia and intubation of the trachea
  Anticipate exaggerated blood pressure changes
  Minimize pressor response during intubation of the trachea by limiting duration of laryngoscopy to less than 15 seconds.
Maintenance of anesthesia
  Use volatile anesthetic to control blood pressure
  Monitor electrocardiogram for evidence of myocardial ischemia
Postopertive management
  Anticipate excessive increases in blood pressure

(Adapted from Goodloe SL. Essential hypertension. In: Stoelting RK, Dierdorf SF, eds. Anesthesia and co-existing disease. New York, Churchill Livingstone 1983:99–117.)

greater than 95 mmHg) independent of any known cause. It is estimated that one in six American adults have essential hypertension. Less than one-half of these individuals have been diagnosed and even fewer are receiving appropriate drug therapy.

Management of Anesthesia

Management of anesthesia for the patient with essential hypertension includes preoperative evaluation of the treatment and extent of the disease plus a consideration of the implications of exaggerated blood pressure elevations intraoperatively in response to noxious stimulation (Table 19-7).[14]

Preoperative Evaluation. The preoperative evaluation of the patient with essential hypertension begins with a determination of the adequacy of blood pressure control and a review of the pharmacology of the antihypertensives being used for therapy (see Chapter 3). It is important to maintain current therapy with antihypertensives throughout the perioperative period. Evidence of major organ dysfunction (congestive heart failure, coronary artery disease, cerebral ischemia, renal dysfunction) must be sought. The patient with essential hypertension is assumed to have coronary artery disease until proven otherwise. Evidence of peripheral vascular disease must be recognized, particularly when placement of an intra-arterial catheter in the perioperative period is anticipated. It can be assumed that nearly one-half of patients with evidence of peripheral vascular disease will have 50 percent or greater stenosis of one or more coronary arteries even in the absence of angina pectoris and the presence of a normal resting ECG. Essential hypertension is associated with a shift to the right of the curve for the autoregulation of cerebral blood flow, emphasizing that these patients are more vulnerable to cerebral ischemia should perfusion pressure decrease. The detection of renal dysfunction due to chronic hypertension may influence the selection of drugs (possibly avoid enflurane and decrease dose of nondepolarizing muscle relaxants) used during anesthesia.

The value of treating essential hypertension before elective operation is suggested by the observation that the incidence of hypotension and evidence of myocardial ischemia on the ECG during the maintenance of anesthesia is increased in patients who remain hypertensive prior to induction of anesthesia.[14] Nevertheless, blood pressure elevations during the intraoperative period are more likely to occur in patients with a history of essential hypertension regardless of the degree of blood pressure control preoperatively. Furthermore, there is no evidence that the incidence of postoperative cardiac complications is increased when hypertensive patients undergo elective operations, as long as the preoperative diastolic blood pressure does not exceed 110 mmHg.

Induction of anesthesia with the intravenous administration of an ultrashort-acting barbiturate or benzodiazepine is acceptable—remembering that an exaggerated reduction in blood pressure may occur, particularly if hypertension is present preoperatively. This response most likely reflects unmasking of a reduced intravascular fluid volume due to chronic hypertension. Ketamine is rarely selected for induction of anesthesia, as its circulatory effects could adversely increase blood pressure, especially in patients with co-existing hypertension.

Exaggerated blood pressure increases during direct laryngoscopy for intubation of the trachea are predictable in patients with the preoperative diagnosis of essential hypertension. Evidence of myocardial ischemia on the ECG may appear at this time. It would seem logical to assure maximal attenuation of the sympathetic nervous system response evoked by direct laryngoscopy by administering a volatile anesthetic or intravenous fentanyl before intubation of the trachea is attempted. Regardless of the drugs administered before intubation of the trachea is attempted, it must be recognized that an excessive depth of anesthesia can produce reductions in blood pressure that are as undesirable as hypertension. The most important concept for limiting the pressor response elicited by intubation of the trachea is to minimize the duration of direct laryngoscopy to 15 seconds or less.[1] In addition, the administration of laryngotracheal lidocaine immediately prior to placement of the tube in the trachea will minimize any additional pressor response.

Maintenance of Anesthesia. The goal during maintenance of anesthesia is to adjust the depth of anesthesia in appropriate directions so as to minimize wide fluctuations in blood pressure. In this regard, a technique utilizing nitrous oxide plus a volatile anesthetic is ideal for permitting rapid adjustments in depth of anesthesia in response to elevations or decreases in blood pressure. Indeed, the management of intraoperative blood pressure lability by adjusting the inhaled concentration of anesthetic is probably more important than preoperative control of hypertension.

The most likely intraoperative changes in blood pressure are hypertensive episodes produced by surgical stimulation. Volatile anesthetics are ideal for attenuating the activity of the sympathetic nervous system which is responsible for this pressor response. Halothane, enflurane, and isoflurane produce dose-dependent reductions in blood pressure by different primary mechanisms (see Chapter 4). A nitrous oxide-narcotic technique is also acceptable for the maintenance of anesthesia, but the addition of a volatile drug is often necessary to control undesirable elevations in blood pressure, particularly during periods of maximal surgical stimulation. The continuous intravenous infusion of nitroprusside is an alternative to the use of a volatile anesthetic for maintaining normotension during the intraoperative period.

Intraoperative monitors for the patient with co-existing essential hypertension are determined by the complexity of the surgery. The ECG is monitored with the goal of recognizing changes suggestive of myocardial ischemia. Invasive monitoring utilizing an intra-arterial and pulmonary artery catheter is indicated if major surgery is planned and there is evidence preoperatively of left ventricular dysfunction.

There is no evidence that a specific muscle relaxant is the best selection in patients with essential hypertension. Although pancuronium can increase the blood pressure, there are no data suggesting that this mild pressor response is exaggerated by co-existing hypertension.

A regional anesthetic is a questionable choice when high levels of sympathetic nervous system block would be associated with the sensory level necessary for the planned surgery. This caution is based upon the possibility of excessive reductions in blood pressure when vasodilation unmasks a decreased intravascular fluid volume associated with chronic hypertension.

Postoperative Management. Hypertension in the early postoperative period is a frequent response in patients with a preoperative diagnosis of essential hypertension. If hypertension persists despite adequate analgesia, it may be necessary to administer a vascular smooth muscle vasodilator such as hydralazine (5 to 10 mg intravenously every 10 to 20 minutes) or a continuous intravenous infusion of nitroprusside. The ECG should also be monitored for signs of myocardial ischemia.

CONGESTIVE HEART FAILURE

Elective surgery should not be performed in a patient who manifests evidence of congestive heart failure. Indeed, the presence of congestive heart failure has been reported to be the single most important factor for predicting postoperative morbidity. When surgery cannot be delayed, however, the drugs and techniques chosen to provide anesthesia must be selected with the goal of optimizing cardiac output. Ketamine is ideal for the induction of anesthesia in the presence of congestive heart failure (see Chapter 6). The use of a volatile anesthetic for maintenance of anesthesia is not recommended because of the potential for cardiac depression. In the presence of severe congestive heart failure, the use of fentanyl (50 to 100 µg/kg) as the sole anesthetic may be justified.[5] Positive pressure ventilation of the lungs may be beneficial by decreasing pulmonary congestive and improving arterial oxygenation. Invasive monitoring of arterial pressure as well as of cardiac filling pressures is justified when major surgery is necessary. Maintenance of myocardial contractility with a continuous infusion of dopamine or dobutamine may be necessary in the perioperative period.

A regional anesthetic is a consideration for the patient with congestive heart failure requiring peripheral surgery. The mild reduction in systemic vascular resistance secondary to peripheral sympathetic nervous system block could facilitate an increased left ventricular stroke volume. Nevertheless, a regional anesthetic should probably not be selected in preference to a general anesthetic if the only reason is the belief that a regional block will reliably improve cardiac output.

HYPERTROPHIC CARDIOMYOPATHY

Hypertrophic cardiomyopathy (idiopathic hypertrophic subaortic stenosis, IHSS) is characterized by obstruction to left ventricular outflow produced by asymmetric hypertrophy of the intraventricular septal muscle. Associated left ventricular hypertrophy in an attempt to overcome the obstruction may be so massive that the volume of the left ventricular chamber is reduced. Despite these adverse changes, the stroke volume remains normal or increased due to the hypercontractile state of the myocardium.

Management of Anesthesia

The goal during management of anesthesia for patients with hypertrophic cardiomyopathy is to decrease the pressure gradient across the left ventricular outflow obstruction. Reductions in myocardial contractility and increases in preload (ventricular volume) and afterload will decrease the magnitude of left ventricular outflow obstruction (Table 19-8).[15] With this in mind, induction of anesthesia is safely accomplished with thiopental. Nitrous oxide plus halothane is ideal for maintenance of anesthesia, providing mild myocardial depression without undesirable decreases in systemic vascular resistance and blood pressure. Theoretically, enflurane and isoflurane would be less ideal choices than halothane, as these drugs decrease systemic vascular resistance more than does halothane (see Chapter 4). Narcotics are not good choices, as they do not produce myocardial depression and at the same time

Table 19-8. Events that Decrease Left Ventricular Outflow Obstruction in the Presence of Hypertrophic Cardiomyopathy

Decreased myocardial contractility
    Beta-adrenergic block (propranolol)
    Volatile anesthetics (halothane)
Increased preload
    Increased intravascular fluid volume
    Bradycardia
Increased afterload
    Alpha-adrenergic stimulation (phenylephrine)
    Increased intravascular fluid volume

(Adapted from Hilgenberg JC. Cardiomyopathies. In: Stoelting RK, Dierdorf SF, eds. Anesthesia and coexisting disease. New York, Churchill Livingstone 1983:129–33.)

can reduce systemic vascular resistance. Succinylcholine is acceptable to facilitate intubation of the trachea, but administration of nitrous oxide plus halothane should precede direct laryngoscopy so as to minimize the degree of undesirable sympathetic nervous system stimulation that is likely to be evoked by this maneuver. A nondepolarizing muscle relaxant (metocurine, atracurium, vecuronium) with minimal to no effect on the circulation is the best choice when prolonged skeletal muscle paralysis is needed. Pancuronium is not a good selection because of its ability to increase heart rate and myocardial contractility. Likewise, sudden reductions of systemic vascular resistance produced by d-tubocurarine are unacceptable.

Intraoperative hypotension is best treated with intravenous fluids and/or an alpha agonist such as phenylephrine. Drugs with beta agonist activity must not be used to treat hypotension, as any increase in cardiac contractility or heart rate could increase left ventricular outflow obstruction. When hypertension occurs, an increased delivered concentration of halothane is the best treatment. Vasodilators such as nitroprusside or nitroglycerin are not good choices for lowering blood pressure, since reductions in systemic vascular resistance can increase left ventricular outflow obstruction.

COR PULMONALE

Cor pulmonale is the designation for right ventricular hypertrophy and eventual cardiac dysfunction that occurs secondary to chronic pulmonary hypertension. Elective operations in patients with cor pulmonale should not be performed until any reversible component of the co-existing pulmonary disease has been treated.

Goals during management of anesthesia in patients with cor pulmonale are to avoid events or drugs that could increase pulmonary vascular resistance. A volatile anesthetic is ideal for relaxing vascular smooth muscle and attenuating airway responsiveness to stimuli produced by a tracheal tube. Nitrous oxide has been shown to increase pulmonary vascular resistance in the presence of large doses of narcotics but not in the presence of diazepam or a volatile anesthetic.[8] Another disadvantage of nitrous oxide is the associated reduction in the inspired concentration of oxygen necessitated by the administration of this drug. Therefore, the delivered concentration of nitrous oxide is usually limited to 50 percent, and right atrial pressure is monitored to detect any adverse drug-induced effect on pulmonary vascular resistance.

CARDIAC TAMPONADE

Cardiac tamponade is characterized by reductions in (1) diastolic filling of the ventricles, (2) stroke volume, and (3) blood pressure due to increased intrapericardial pressure from accumulation of fluid in the pericardial space. The decreased stroke volume results in activation of the sympathetic nervous system (tachycardia, vasoconstriction) in an attempt to maintain the cardiac output. Cardiac output and blood pressure are maintained as long as the pressure in the central veins exceeds the right ventricular end-diastolic pressure.

Institution of general anesthesia and positive pressure ventilation of the lungs in the presence of cardiac tamponade can lead to profound hypotension, reflecting anesthetic-induced peripheral vasodilation, direct myocardial depression, and decreased venous return. When percutaneous pericardiocentesis cannot be performed using local anesthesia, the induction and maintenance of general anesthesia is ideally achieved with ketamine. The potential adverse effects of increased intrathoracic pressure on venous return must be considered. Perhaps positive pressure ventilation of the lungs should be avoided until the chest is opened and drainage of the pericardial space is imminent. With this in mind, it may be prudent to perform intubation of the trachea using topical anesthesia prior to the induction of anesthesia. Continuous intravenous infusion of a catecholamine (isoproterenol, dopamine, dobutamine) may be necessary to maintain myocardial contractility.

ANEURYSMS OF THE AORTA

Aneurysms of the aorta most often involve the abdominal aorta. A majority of patients are hypertensive and many have associated atherosclerosis. A dissecting aneurysm denotes a tear in the intima of the arota that allows blood to enter and penetrate between the walls of the vessel, producing a false lumen. Ultimately, the dissection may reenter the lumen through another tear in the intima or rupture through the adventia.

Elective resection of an abdominal aneurysm is indicated when the estimated diameter of the aneurysm exceeds 5 cm. The incidence of spontaneous rupture increases dramatically when the diameter of the aneurysm exceeds 5 cm. Extension of the abdominal aneurysm to include the renal arteries occurs in about 5 percent of patients.

Management of Anesthesia

Management of anesthesia for resection of an abdominal arotic aneurysm includes monitoring of arterial and left atrial filling pressures. Patients with co-existing coronary artery disease are likely to develop increases in the pulmonary artery occlusion pressure and evidence of myocardial ischemia during cross-clamping of the abdominal aorta (Fig. 19-3).[17] Treatment of intraoperative myocardial ischemia is by reducing blood pressure and filling pressures to acceptable levels by pharmacologic interventions which may include continuous intravenous infusion of nitroprusside or nitroglycerin. Urine output should be maintained with intravenous infusion of crystalloid solutions and diuretics so as to minimize the likelihood of postoperative renal failure.

Hypotension can accompany unclamping of the abdominal aorta, presumably reflecting a sudden increase in venous capacitance. In addition, the release of acid metabolites that have accumulated in the ischemic extremity can produce myocardial depression and peripheral vasodilation. The blood pressure decrease can be minimized by infusing intravenous fluids to maintain the pulmonary artery occlusion pressure between 10 to 20 mmHg prior to removal of the aortic cross-clamp. Intravenous sodium bicarbonate is indicated if the arterial pH is below 7.2 following unclamping of the abdominal aorta.

CARDIOPULMONARY BYPASS

Cardiopulmonary bypass (extracorporeal circulation) is characterized by gravity drainage of blood from the patient's vena cavae into an oxygenator followed by its return to the arterial system, usually the ascending aorta, by means of a roller pump (Fig. 19-4).[18] In the presence of a competent aortic valve, the heart is excluded from the

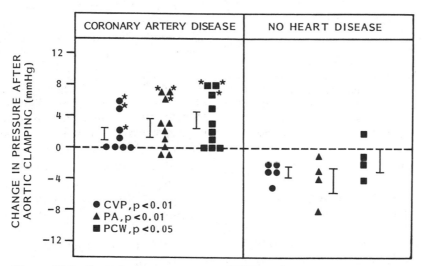

Figure 19-3. Central venous pressure (CVP), pulmonary artery pressure (PA), and pulmonary capillary wedge pressure (PCW) were measured following infrarenal cross-clamping of the abdominal aorta in patients with or without coronary artery disease. Increases in PCW pressure of 7 mmHg or more were always associated with signs of myocardial ischemia on the electrocardiogram (denoted by asterisks). (Attia RR, Murphy JD, Snider M, Lappas DG, Darling RC, Lowenstein E. Myocardial ischemia due to infrarenal aortic cross-clamping during aortic surgery in patients with severe coronary artery disease. Circulation 1976;53:961–5. By Permission of the American Heart Association, Inc.)

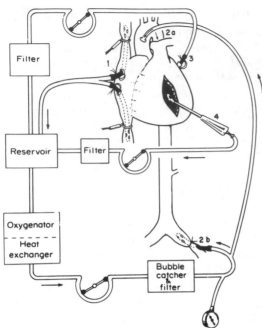

Figure 19-4. Schematic diagram of a cardiopulmonary bypass circuit. Blood from cannulae (1) placed in the superior and inferior vena cava drains by gravity into a reservoir and then to an oxygenator and heat exchanger. A roller pump returns oxygenated blood to the ascending aorta (2a) or rarely the femoral artery (2b). In addition, blood is returned to the reservoir from the left ventricular vent (3) and cardiotomy suction (4). (Nosé Y. Manual on artificial organs. Vol II. The oxygenator. St. Louis, CV Mosby, 1973, as modified in Hug CC. Anesthesia for cardiac surgery. In: Miller RD ed, Anesthesia. New York, Churchill Livingstone 1981:981–1026.)

patient's circulation by tightening occlusive ligatures that have been placed around the superior and inferior vena cava so all returning blood enters the large cannulae in these vessels. If the aortic valve is not competent, it is also necessary to cross clamp the aorta distal to the aortic valve and proximal to the inflow cannula. Otherwise, retrograde blood flow through the incompetent aortic valve would prevent exclusion of the heart from the circulation. When the heart is isolated from the circulation, total cardiopulmonary bypass is present and ventilation of the lungs is no longer necessary

to maintain oxygenation. Elevating the patient above the level of the cardiopulmonary bypass machine facilitates the gravity-dependent venous return.

The roller pump produces nonpulsatile flow into the patient's aorta by compression of the fluid-containing tubing between the roller and curved metal back plate (Fig. 19-4).[18] The required cardiac index delivered by the roller pump depends the patient's body temperature and oxygen consumption. For normothermia or mild hypothermia, a cardiac index of 2 to 2.4 L/min/m² is satisfactory. Mean blood pressure is maintained between 50 and 100 mmHg by increasing or decreasing cardiac index.

Blood is oxygenated in either a bubble or membrane oxygenator. The bubble oxygenator is most popular, consisting of an oxygenating column, a defoaming section to remove air bubbles, and an arterial reservoir. The PaO_2 is maintained between 100 to 150 mmHg by adjusting the flow of oxygen into the oxygenator. It may be necessary to also add carbon dioxide so as to avoid severe hypocarbia. Membrane oxygenators do not utilize a blood-gas interface and produce less trauma to the blood compared with bubble oxygenators. Nevertheless, these more complex and expensive oxygenators have not proven to be more advantageous than the bubble oxygenator.

Heat exchangers are incorporated into oxygenators to control the patient's body temperature by heating or cooling blood as it circulates. Hot or cold water entering the unit at one end with blood entering at the other provides an efficient countercurrent flow system.

Blood from the pericardial cavity and the opened heart as during a valve replacement is returned to a cardiotomy reservoir where it is filtered, defoamed, and returned to the oxygenator for recirculation. The cardiotomy suction is a major cause of hemolysis during cardiopulmonary bypass. When the heart is not opened, as during aortocoronary bypass graft operations, it may be necessary to insert a catheter (vent) into the left ventricle (either through the apex of the left ventricle or via the right superior pulmonary vein) to prevent distension of the left ventricle with blood returning via Thebesian veins or bronchial veins. Filters are incorporated in the oxygen delivery line and arterial delivery system to act as traps for cellular debris.

The tubing used for the cardiopulmonary bypass system is filled with blood and fluid (prime) in a predetermined ratio that is calculated to produce a specific hematocrit with institution of total cardiopulmonary bypass. Because whole body hyopthermia (22 to 28 Celsius) is commonly used, the pump prime usually contains little or no blood such that the hematocrit of blood during bypass is reduced. Hemodilution is important to lessen viscosity during hypothermia. It is mandatory that all air be cleared from the arterial side of the circuit prior to institution of cardiopulmonary bypass. Indeed, pumping of air into the patient by the cardiopulmonary bypass machine is an ever present hazard.

Heparin-induced anticoagulation of the patient is mandatory before placement of the venous and aortic cannulae used for cardiopulmonary bypass. The usual initial dose of heparin administered intravenously is 300 units/kg. The adequacy of anticoagulation is subsequently confirmed by determination of the activated coagulation time (ACT) which should remain above 400 seconds (normal 90 to 120 seconds) during cardiopulmonary bypass.

Monitoring During Cardiopulmonary Bypass

Institution of cardiopulmonary bypass is often associated with a fall in mean arterial pressure, presumably reflecting decreased systemic vascular resistance as the cold priming fluid with low viscosity and oxygen content enters the patient's vascular system. If mean arterial pressure remains below 50 mmHg despite an adequate cardiac index and blood volume, the administration of an alpha agonist such as phenylephrine may be considered. Although supportive evidence is not available, a common goal is to maintain the mean arterial pressure between 50 to 100 mmHg during cardiopulmonary bypass. It is presumed that this perfusion pressure is important for maintenance of cerebral blood flow. A mean arterial pressure above 100 mmHg indicates arterial constriction, which can lead to impairment of tissue perfusion as well as the risk of intracerebral hemorrhage. This hypertension is ideally treated by reducing systemic vascular resistance with the continuous intravenous administration of nitroprusside. Alternatively, the vapor of a volatile anesthetic can be introduced from a vaporizer incorporated into the cardiopulmonary bypass circuit.

A rising central venous pressure with or without facial edema (eyelids and sclera) may reflect improper placement of the vena cava cannulae with obstruction to venous drainage. For example, insertion of a cannula too far into the superior vena cava can obstruct the right innominate vein, leading to an increase of venous pressure in the head with associated cerebral edema. Placement of a cannula to far into the inferior vena cava results in abdominal distension. Confirmatory evidence of misplacement of the vena caval cannulae is inadequate venous return from the patient to the cardiopulmonary bypass machine. Prompt withdrawal of the vena cava cannulae to a more proximal position should immediately improve venous drainage.

A pulmonary artery catheter detects increases in pulmonary artery pressures due to malfunction of the left ventricular vent and the associated inadequate decompression of the left ventricle. Persistent left ventricular distension can result in damage to the contractile elements of the myocardium.

Blood gases and pH are monitored frequently during cardiopulmonary bypass. A mixed venous PO_2 less than 30 mmHg associated with metabolic acidosis suggests inadequate tissue perfusion. Temperature correction of arterial blood gases and pH is probably not necessary (see Chapter 17). Urine output serves as a guide to the adequacy of renal perfusion, with an output of 1 ml/kg/hr being a reasonable expectation.

During total cardiopulmonary bypass the lungs are left quiescent with or without moderate continuous positive airway pressure. The best composition of gases in the lungs during this time is unsettled, although it seems unnecessary to expose unperfused alveoli to high concentrations of oxygen. Continued ventilation of the lungs with oxygen is appropriate when there is some pulmonary blood flow as evidenced by a pulsatile pulmonary artery trace (e.g., partial cardiopulmonary bypass).

Esophageal and rectal temperature are monitored routinely. Drug-induced vasodilation as with nitroprusside may speed the rewarming process, as reflected by more rapid approach of the rectal (peripheral tissues) to esophageal (blood) temperature.

Myocardial Perservation

The goal of myocardial preservation is to reduce myocardial damage introduced by the period of ischemia associated with cardiopulmonary bypass. This goal is achieved by reducing myocardial oxygen consumption by infusing cold (4 Celsius) cardioplegia solution containing potassium (about 20 mEq/L) into the aortic root, which in the presence of a distally cross-clamped aorta and competent aortic valve assures diversion of the solution into the coronary arteries. Potassium blocks the initial phase of myocardial depolarization, resulting in cessation of electrical and mechanical activity. The cold solution produces selective hypothermia of the cardiac muscle. At 37 Celsius, the normally contracting heart muscle consumes oxygen at a rate of 8 to 10 ml/100 g/min. This consumption in the fibrillating

heart at 22 Celsius is 2 ml/100 g/min. The electromechanically quiet heart at 22 Celsius consumes oxygen at a rate of 0.3 ml/100 g/min. The effectiveness of cold cardioplegia is monitored by measuring heart temperature with a temperature probe placed into the left ventricular muscle plus the absence of any visible electrical activity on the electrocardiogram. Cold cardioplegia infusion is supplemented by total body hypothermia and localized epicardial surface cooling using ice or cold irrigation solution placed into the pericardial space. Likewise, avoidance of ventricular distension by use of a vent plus inclusion of mannitol in the cardioplegia solution to prevent myocardial cell edema may be important for preserving subsequent myocardial contractility. Adequate myocardial preservation is suggested by good myocardial contractility without the use of inotropic drugs at the conclusion of cardiopulmonary bypass.

A side effect of cardioplegia solutions is an increased incidence of atrioventricular heart block due to intramyocardial hyperkalemia. This heart block usually resolves in 1 to 2 hours and can be treated temporarily by use of an artificial cardiac pacemaker. Intramyocardial hyperkalemia also produces decreased myocardial contractility. Systemic hyperkalemia is likely to occur when coronary sinus blood containing cardioplegic solution is returned to the oxygenator for subsequent circulation. Decreased renal function during cardiopulmonary bypass will also contribute to hyperkalemia. If hyperkalemia persists at the conclusion of cardiopulmonary bypass, it may be necessary to administer intravenous glucose (25 grams) plus regular insulin (10 to 15 units) in an attempt to shift potassium into the cells.

Maintenance of Anesthesia

Drugs selected for maintenance of anesthesia in patients undergoing cardiopulmonary bypass are determined by the patient's cardiac disease. Institution of cardiopulmonary bypass, however, produces a sudden dilution of circulating drug concentrations that can acutely reduce the depth of anesthesia. For this reason, supplemental intravenous anesthetics such as narcotics may be administered at this time. Likewise, skeletal muscle paralysis may be supplemented with additional nondepolarizing muscle relaxant. Anesthetic depth can also be increased by delivering a volatile anesthetic from a vaporizer incorporated into the cardiopulmonary bypass circuit. It must be appreciated that the impact of hemodilution on drug concentrations is likely to be offset by decreased needs during hypothermia. For reasons that are not clear, anesthetic requirements seem to be minimal following rewarming to a normal body temperature at the conclusion of cardiopulmonary bypass. Therefore, additional anesthesia is not routinely required during rewarming or the early period following the conclusion of cardiopulmonary bypass.

Discontinuation of Cardiopulmonary Bypass

Cardiopulmonary bypass is discontinued when the patient is hemodynamically stable and normothermia has been re-established. When the left side of the heart has been opened as during valve replacement surgery, it is mandatory to remove all air from the cardiac chambers and pulmonary veins before permitting the heart to eject blood into the aorta. Otherwise, systemic air emboli with disastrous cardiac and central nervous system effects can occur. Measurement of cardiac filling pressures, determination of thermodilution cardiac output, and calculation of systemic and pulmonary vascular resistance is necessary to guide intravenous fluid replacement and the appropriate selection of drugs in the early postcardiopulmonary bypass period. On occasion, a continuous intravenous infusion of a vasodilator such as nitroprusside or nitro-

glycerin or an inotrope such as dopamine or dobutamine is necessary to maintain optimal cardiac output. When an adequate blood pressure and cardiac output have been maintained for several minutes, the aortic and vena cava cannulae are removed and protamine is administered intravenously usually over a 3 to 5 minute period to reverse heparin anticoagulation. Occasionally, infusion of protamine is accompanied by hypotension and pulmonary hypertension, possibly reflecting the release of histamine.[19] The administration of nitrous oxide following cardiopulmonary bypass is questionable, since this gas would unmask the presence of air in the heart or coronary arteries. For this reason, anesthesia is most often supplemented when necessary by the intravenous administration of a narcotic or a low inhaled concentration of a volatile anesthetic. The blood and fluid which remains in the cardiopulmonary bypass circuit is washed and collected into plastic bags as packed erythrocytes for possible reinfusion to the patient.

REFERENCES

1. McCammon RL. Coronary artery disease. In: Stoelting RK, Dierdorf SF, eds. Anesthesia and Co-Existing Disease. New York, Churchill Livingstone 1983;1–26.
2. Tarhan S, Moffitt EA, Taylor WF, Guiliani ER. Myocardial infarction after general anesthesia. JAMA 1972;220:1451–4.
3. Steen PA, Tinker JH, Tarhan S. Myocardial reinfarction after anesthesia and surgery. An update: incidence, mortality, and predisposing factors. JAMA 1978;239:2566–70.
4. Reiz S, Balfors E, Sorensen MG, Ariola S, Friedman, A. Truedsson A. Isoflurane—a powerful coronary vasodilator in patients with coronary artery disease. Anesthesiology 1983;59:91–7.
5. Lunn JK, Stanley TH, Eisele J, Webster L, Woodward A. High dose fentanyl anesthesia for coronary artery surgery: plasma fentanyl concentrations and influence of nitrous oxide on cardiovascular responses. Anesth Analg 1979;58:390–5.

6. Mangano DT. Monitoring pulmonary artery pressure in coronary-artery disease. Anesthesiology 1980;53:364–70.
7. Pinaud ML, Blanloeil YAG, Souron RJ. Preoperative prophylactic digitalization of patients with coronary artery disease—a randomized echocardiographic and hemodynamic study. Anesth Analg 1983;62:865–9.
8. Hilgenberg JC, McCammon RL, Stoelting RK. Pulmonary and systemic vascular responses to nitrous oxide in patients with mitral stenosis and pulmonary hypertension. Anesth Analg 1980;59:323–6.
9. Greenberg BH, Rahimtoola SH. Vasodilator therapy for valvular heart disease. JAMA 1981;246:269–72.
10. Haselby KA. Congenital heart disease. In: Stoelting RK, Dierdorf SF, eds. Anesthesia and Co-Existing Disease. New York, Churchill Livingstone 1983;47–70.
11. Goodloe SL. Abnormalities of cardiac conduction and cardiac rhythm. In: Stoelting RK, Dierdorf SF, eds. Anesthesia and Co-Existing Disease. New York, Churchill Livingstone 1983;71–92.
12. Gomez-Arnau J, Marquez-Montes J, Avello F. Fentanyl and droperidol effects on the refractoriness of the accessory pathway in the Wolff-Parkinson-White syndrome. Anesthesiology 1983;58:307–13.
13. Prystowsky EN. Pharmacologic therapy of tachyarrhythmias in patients with Wolff-Parkinson-White syndrome. Herz 1983; 8:133–43.
14. Goodloe SL. Essential hypertension. In: Stoelting RK, Dierdorf SF, eds. Anesthesia and Co-Existing Disease. New York, Churchill Livingstone 1983;99–117.
15. Hilgenberg JC. Cardiomyopathies. In: Stoelting RK, Dierdorf SF, eds. Anesthesia and Co-Existing Disease. New York, Churchill Livingstone 1983;129–40.
16. Lake CL. Anesthesia and pericardial disease. Anesth Analg 1983;62:431–43.
17. Attia RR, Murphy JD, Snider M, Lappas DG, Darling RC, Lowenstein E. Myocardial ischemia due to infrarenal aortic cross-clamping during aortic surgery in patients with severe coronary artery disease. Circulation 1976;53:961–5.
18. Hug CC. Anesthesia for cardiac surgery. In: Miller RD, ed, Anesthesia. New York, Churchill Livingstone 1981;981–1026.
19. Lowenstein E, Johnston WE, Lappas DG, D'Ambra MN, Schneider RC, Daggett WM, Akins CW, Philbin DM. Catastrophic pulmonary vasoconstriction associated with protamine reversal of heparin. Anesthesiology 1983:59–470-3.

20

Pulmonary Disease

The patient with chronic pulmonary disease presents a challenge for management during the intraoperative and postoperative period regardless of the operative site. Nevertheless, thoracic operations are a particular risk for the patient with chronic pulmonary disease.[1] Furthermore, patients with chronic pulmonary disease often manifest co-existing coronary artery disease and/or essential hypertension (see Chapter 19).

OBSTRUCTIVE AIRWAY DISEASE

Obstructive airway disease is the most frequent cause of pulmonary dysfunction. The common pathophysiologic characteristic of all of the obstructive airway disorders is an increased resistance to the flow of gases in the airways. Regional differences in airway resistance lead to areas of mismatching of ventilation to perfusion. As a result, arterial hypoxemia is likely to develop while breathing room air. Retention of carbon dioxide with the development of respiratory acidosis can also occur when regional hypoventilation is severe. All obstructive airway diseases are characterized by dyspnea, reflecting the increased work of breathing introduced by the elevated airway resistance.

Auscultation of the chest will likely reveal wheezing during exhalation, reflecting turbulent gas flow through narrowed airways. The radiograph of the chest shows hyperinflated lungs with increased radiolucency due to decreased pulmonary blood flow. The diaphragm is likely to be depressed. Pulmonary function studies demonstrate reductions in the forced exhaled volume in 1 second (FEV_1) expressed as a percentage of the forced vital capacity (Fig. 20-1).[2] Measurement of the FEV_1 alone can be misleading, as the value may be low if the vital capacity is also reduced.

Bronchial asthma is the classic example of obstructive airway disease that is characterized by acute and reversible elevations of airway resistance. Pulmonary emphysema and chronic bronchitis are examples of obstructive airway diseases characterized by progressive and persistent increases in airway resistance despite treatment.

Bronchial Asthma

Bronchial asthma is estimated to be present in 2.5 percent of the population of the United States. The majority of individuals develop symptoms of asthma before 5 years of age, and male patients outnumber female patients by about two to one. Bronchial asthma is usually, but not always, an inherited disorder in which inhalation of an antigen elicits the elaboration of antibodies of the immunoglobulin E class. The subsequent antigen-antibody interaction causes the release of vasoactive substances

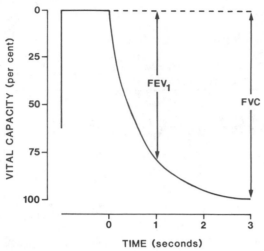

Figure 20-1. Schematic diagram of the forced exhaled volume in 1 second (FEV_1) and forced vital capacity (FVC). The total volume of air exhaled in the first second should be equivalent to at least 80 percent of the FVC. In the presence of obstructive airway disease, the ratio of FEV_1 to FVC is less than 0.8. (LoSasso AM, Gibbs PS, Moorthy SS. Obstructive pulmonary disease. In: Stoelting RK, Dierdorf SF, eds. Anesthesia and co-existing disease. New York, Churchill Livingstone, 1983:171–200.)

including histamine from mast cells in the lungs. These vasoactive substances result in bronchoconstriction, edema of the bronchial mucosa, and secretion of viscous mucus.

Diagnosis. Active bronchial asthma is recognized by the presence of audible wheezing during auscultation of the chest. The ratio of the FEV_1 to the vital capacity is likely to be decreased to less than 80 percent. The administration of a bronchodilator can be expected to improve expiratory flow rates at least 20 percent, emphasizing the reversible aspect of the airway narrowing that is associated with bronchial asthma. The blood eosinophil count is almost invariably elevated above 300 mm^3 in the presence of active immunoglobulin E mediated bronchial asthma. An adequately treated patient with bronchial asthma will usually have a total blood eosinophil count less than 50 mm^3 while a rising count often signals the acceleration of bronchial asthma even before the onset of clinical symptoms. Mild bronchial asthma is usually accompanied by a normal PaO_2 and $PaCO_2$. Further progression of bronchial asthma is associated with a reduction in PaO_2 while the $PaCO_2$ begins to increase. Elevation of the $PaCO_2$ above 50 mmHg in the presence of an acute bronchial asthma attack signals the likely need for intubation of the trachea and mechanical ventilation of the lungs.

Treatment. Drug therapy for bronchial asthma most often includes beta agonists, corticosteroids, and cromolyn. Aerosol adminstration of a beta-2 agonist such as salbutamol or terbutaline is an effective way to deliver high drug concentrations to the airways to produce bronchodilation with minimal likelihood of systemic effects (see Chapter 3). Aminophylline, adminstered as a continuous intravenous infusion, is a frequent treatment for acute bronchial asthma. Corticosteroids are presumably effective in the management of acute exacerbations of bronchial asthma as well as in the maintenance of a stable asymptomatic state by virtue of their anti-inflammatory effects plus their membrane stabilizing actions which reduce the release of histamine from mast cells. Cromolyn is a membrane stabilizer which prevents the degranulation of mast cells and the subsequent release of vasoactive substances responsible for bronchoconstriction. As such, this drug is effective for prophylaxis but is of no value in the management of acute exacerbations of bronchial asthma.

Management of Anesthesia. Preoperatively, the absence of wheezing during quiet breathing and a total blood eosinophil count below 50 cells/mm^3 suggests that the patient is not experiencing an acute exacerbation of bronchial asthma. Bronchodilator drugs should be continued until the time of induction of anesthesia. Supplementation with cortisol may be indicated before major surgery if adrenal cortex suppression from corticosteroids used to treat asthma is a possibility (see Chapter 23). The use of anticholinergics should be individualized, remembering that these drugs can increase the viscosity of secretions, thus making it difficult to remove them from the airway. Adminstration of cimetidine is questionable because antagonism of H-2 mediated bronchodilation could unmask H-1 mediated bronchoconstriction.

A regional anesthetic is an excellent choice when the surgery is superficial or on the extremities. Otherwise, the goal during induction and maintenance of general anesthesia in the patient with bronchial asthma is to depress airway reflexes so as to avoid bronchoconstriction of the hyperreactive airways in response to mechanical stimulation. Induction of anesthesia is with the intravenous adminstration of an ultrashort-acting barbiturate or benzodiazepine. These drugs, however, are unlikely to depress adequately airway reflexes, allowing the precipitation of bronchospasm should intubation of the trachea be attempted. Ketamine, because of its sympathomimetic effects on bronchial smooth muscle, is an alternative selection for induction of anesthesia. Prior to intubation of the trachea, a sufficient depth of anesthesia should be established so as to depress hyperreactive airway reflexes and minimize the likelihood of bronchoconstriction with stimulation of the upper airway. Halothane is a popular drug for administration to patients with bronchial asthma, although enflurane and isoflurane are as effective as halothane in reversing allergic bronchconstriction in a dog model.[3] Furthermore, enflurane and isoflurane, unlike halothane, do not sensitize the heart to the dysrhythmic effects of beta stimulation as produced by beta agonists including aminophylline. Intubation of the trachea is often facilitated by the administration of succinylcholine. Although his-

tamine release has been attributed to succinylcholine, there is no evidence that this drug is associated with the onset of increased airway resistance in patients with bronchial asthma. Skeletal muscle relaxation during maintenance of anesthesia is ideally provided with a nondepolarizing muscle relaxant such as pancuronium, metocurine, atracurium or vecuronium that has minimal ability to elicit the release of histamine. Indeed, d-tubocurarine, which can stimulate the release of histamine, has been shown to increase airway resistance.[4]

Intraoperatively, the PaO_2 and $PaCO_2$ can be maintained at a normal level by mechanical ventilation of the lungs using a slow inspiratory flow rate to optimize distribution of inhaled gases. A slow respiratory rate allows sufficient time for passive exhalation to occur in the presence of increased airway resistance. Positive end-expiratory pressure (PEEP) may not be ideal because adequate exhalation may be impaired in the presence of narrowed airways. Liberal intravenous administration of crystalloid solutions during the perioperative period is important for maintaining adequate hydration and assuring the presence of less viscous secretions that can be more easily expelled from the airway. At the conclusion of elective surgery, it is prudent to extubate the trachea while the depth of anesthesia is still sufficient to suppress hyperreactive airway reflexes. When it is considered unsafe to extubate the trachea until the patient is awake because of the presumed presence of gastric contents, intravenous lidocaine may minimize the likelihood of airway stimulation due to the continued presence of the tracheal tube.

Intraoperative Bronchospasm. Bronchospasm that occurs intraoperatively is rarely due to bronchial asthma but rather reflects other causes such as obstruction of the tracheal tube with secretions or by kinking, endobronchial intubation, pulmonary edema, inhalation of gastric fluid, or pneu-

Table 20-1. Comparative Features of Chronic Obstructive Airway Disease

	Pulmonary Emphysema	Chronic Bronchitis
FEV_1	Decreased	Decreased
Total lung capacity	Marked increase	Moderate increase
Dyspnea	Severe	Moderate
Arterial hypoxemia	Late	Early
Hypercapnia	Late	Early
Cor pulmonale	Late	Early
Prognosis	Good	Poor

(Adapted from LoSasso AM, Gibbs PS, Moorthy SS. Obstructive pulmonary disease. In: Stoelting RK, Dierdorf SF, eds. Anesthesia and co-existing disease. New York, Churchill Livingstone, 1983:171–200.)

mothorax. In the rare instance that bronchospasm is due to bronchial asthma, the cornerstone of treatment is the intravenous administration of aminophylline (5 to 7 mg/kg) administered over 15 minutes followed by a continuous infusion (0.5 to 1 mg/kg/hr). Aerosol administration of a beta-2 agonist such as salbutamol can be achieved by placement of a device in the inspiratory limb of the anesthetic breathing system. When bronchospasm is severe and persists despite intravenous administration of aminophylline and inhalation of salbutamol, the use of intravenous salbutamol (100 μg during 5 minutes) and/or cortisol (4 mg/kg) should be considered.[5]

Pulmonary Emphysema

Pulmonary emphysema (chronic obstructive pulmonary disease, COPD) is characterized by the loss of elastic recoil of the lungs which results in collapse of airways during exhalation leading to increased airway resistance (Table 20-1).[2] Severe dyspnea is typical of emphysema, reflecting the increased work of breathing due to loss of elastic recoil of the lungs. The preoperative evaluation of the patient with emphysema should determine the severity of the disease and elucidate any reversible components such as infection or bronchospasm.

The presence of dyspnea, cough, sputum production, and decreased exercise tolerance suggests the need for preoperative pulmonary function studies. The risk of postoperative respiratory failure is increased if the preoperative ratio of FEV_1 to vital capacity is less than 50 percent. Arterial blood gases are usually normal ("pink puffers"), reflecting a high minute ventilation in an attempt to overcome increased airway resistance. The presence of a $PaCO_2$ above 50 mmHg cautions against performance of elective surgery, as the risk of postoperative respiratory failure is increased. Finally, preoperative detection and treatment of cor pulmonale with supplemental oxygen is essential.

Management of Anesthesia. The presence of pulmonary emphysema does not dictate the use of specific drugs (inhaled or injected) or techniques (regional or general) for the management of anesthesia. More important than the drugs or techniques selected is the realization that these patients are susceptible to the development of acute respiratory failure in the postoperative period.

If a general anesthetic is selected, a volatile anesthetic utilizing humidifcation of the inhaled gases and mechanical ventilation of the lungs is ideal. The need to support ventilation of the lungs is emphasized by the observation that patients with chronic obstructive pulmonary disease, who did not retain carbon dioxide awake, hypoventilated to a greater degree than normal patients during halothane anesthesia.[6] Nitrous oxide is frequently administered in combination with a volatile anesthetic. Potential disadvantages of nitrous oxide include limitation of the inhaled concentration of oxygen and passage of this gas into bullae that result from emphysema. Conceivably, nitrous oxide could lead to enlargement and rupture of a bullae, resulting in the development of a tension pneumothorax. Narcotics, although acceptable, are less ideal for maintenance of anesthesia due to the frequent need for high inhaled concentrations of nitrous oxide (e.g., reduced inhaled concentrations of oxygen) to assure amnesia. Furthermore, narcotics can be associated with prolonged depression of ventilation postoperatively.

Humidification of inhaled gases during anesthesia is important to prevent drying of secretions in the airways. It must be appreciated that systemic dehydration due to inadequate fluid administration during the perioperative period can result in excessive drying of secretions in the airways despite humidification of inhaled gases.

Controlled ventilation of the lungs utilizing large tidal volumes (10 to 15 ml/kg) combined with a slow inspiratory flow rate is ideal for optimizing arterial oxygenation. A slow respiratory rate (6 to 10 breaths/min) allows sufficient time for venous return to the heart and is less likely to be associated with undesirable degrees of hyperventilation. Continued intubation of the trachea and mechanical ventilation of the lungs in the postoperative period is likely to be necessary following major surgery in patients with severe emphysema (see Chapter 32).

Chronic Bronchitis

Chronic bronchitis is characterized by chronic or recurrent secretion of excess mucus into the bronchi, resulting in increased resistance to gas flow through these airways. Patients with chronic bronchitis tend to develop arterial hypoxemia ("blue bloaters"), hypercarbia, and cor pulmonale early in contrast to the delayed onset of these changes with emphysema (Table 20-1).[2] Because the small airways account for only a minor proportion of total airway resistance, chronic bronchitis must be advanced before dyspnea becomes apparent. Cigarette smoking is the major predisposing factor to the development of chronic bronchitis. The preoperative evaluation and management of anesthesia are as described for the patient with pulmonary emphysema.

RESTRICTIVE PULMONARY DISEASE

Restrictive pulmonary disease is characterized by reductions in lung compliance that result in decreased lung volumes (Fig. 20-2).[8] A reduction in vital capacity (normal 50 to 70 ml/kg) in the presence of a normal FEV_1 is the classic evidence of restrictive pulmonary disease.

The patient with restrictive pulmonary disease complains of dyspnea, reflecting the increased work of breathing necessary to expand the poorly compliant lungs. A rapid and shallow pattern of breathing is characteristic, since this minimizes the work of breathing in the presence of decreased lung compliance. A reduction in the $PaCO_2$ reflects hyperventilation produced by the rapid and shallow pattern of breathing. Indeed, the $PaCO_2$ is usually maintained at a decreased to normal value until restrictive pulmonary disease is far advanced.

Acute restrictive pulmonary disease is most often due to leakage of intravascular fluid into the interstitium of the lungs and into the alveoli, manifesting as pulmonary edema. Examples of acute restrictive pulmonary disease include adult respiratory distress syndrome, aspiration pneumonitis, neurogenic pulmonary edema, narcotic-induced pulmonary edema, and high-altitude pulmonary edema. Chronic restrictive pulmonary disease is characterized by the presence of pulmonary fibrosis (sarcoidosis) or processes that interfere with expansion of the lungs (effusion, kyphoscoliosis, obesity, ascites, pregnancy).

Management of Anesthesia

A regional anesthetic is appropriate for peripheral surgery, but it must be appreciated that sensory levels above T10 can be associated with impairment of respiratory muscle activity necessary for the patient with restrictive pulmonary disease to maintain acceptable ventilation. Restrictive pulmonary disease does not influence the choice of drugs used for the induction or

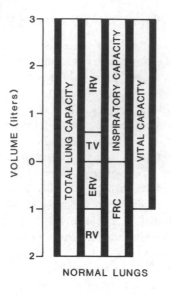

NORMAL LUNGS

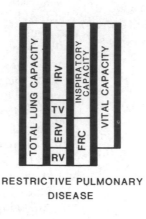

RESTRICTIVE PULMONARY DISEASE

Figure 20-2. Compared with normal lungs, restrictive pulmonary disease is characterized by a decrease in total lung capacity and all the components that comprise this capacity; especially vital capacity. IRV = inspiratory reserve volume, TV = tidal volume, ERV = expiratory reserve volume, RV = residual volume, FRC = functional residual capacity. (LoSasso AM, Gibbs PS, Moorthy SS, Restrictive pulmonary disease. In: Stoelting RK, Dierdorf SF, eds. Anesthesia and co-existing disease. New York, Churchill Livingstone, 1983;201–7.)

maintenance of general anesthesia. The need to minimize depression of ventilation that may persist into the postoperative period should be considered when selecting these drugs. Mechanical ventilation of the lungs is ideal, but high inflation pressures may be necessary to inflate the poorly compliant lungs and/or thorax. Continued ventilation of the lungs in the postoperative period is likely to be necessary when the vital capacity is less than 15 ml/kg or the $PaCO_2$ is above 50 mmHg preoperatively. It should be appreciated that restrictive pulmonary disease contributes to decreased lung volumes, making it difficult to generate an effective cough for removal of secretions from the airway in the postoperative period.

ANESTHESIA FOR THORACIC SURGERY

Anesthesia for thoracic surgery begins with the preoperative performance of pulmonary function tests and evaluation of the adequacy of medical management of chronic pulmonary disease. Choice of drugs to produce anesthesia, selection of monitors, the impact of the lateral decubitus position on respiratory physiology, and indications and techniques for one-lung anesthesia are considerations in planning the management of anesthesia for thoracic surgery. Postoperatively, a high index of suspicion must be maintained for life-threatening complications (hemorrhage, bronchopleural fistula) associated with thoracic surgery. It may be necessary to continue mechanical ventilation of the lungs following thoracic surgery. Finally, methods to provide postoperative analgesia should receive high priority, as pain following thoracic surgery is intense.

Preoperative Preparation

Patients undergoing thoracic surgery are at high risk for developing postoperative pulmonary complications, particularly if there is co-existing chronic pulmonary disease. Specific preoperative findings that make postoperative pulmonary complications likely include dyspnea, cough and sputum production, wheezing, history of cigarette smoking, obesity, and old age. In addition, a recent upper respiratory infection may be associated with increased airway resistance that persists for as long as 5 weeks.[9] Respiratory defense mechanisms against bacteria may also be impaired following a viral respiratory infection.

Table 20-2. Preoperative Prophylactic Measures

Discontinue smoking	— Carboxyhemoglobin levels decrease within 48 hours so as to increase available hemoglobin
Treat pulmonary infection	— Select antibiotics on basis of culture and sensitivity
Treat reversible component of increased airway resistance	— Beta-2 agonists by aerosol with or without aminophylline
Thin and mobilize secretions	— Hydration and chest percussion
Teach deep breathing and coughing exercises	

The main purpose of preoperative testing is to identify patients at risk for complications and to institute appropriate perioperative therapy. Indeed, the incidence of postoperative pulmonary complications can be reduced by preoperative prophylactic measures (Table 20-2).

Pulmonary function tests are helpful for identifying the patient at increased risk for developing pulmonary complications and for evaluating the response to preoperative pulmonary therapy. Patients with findings suggestive of the presence of chronic pulmonary disease on the history, physical examination, or radiograph of the chest and scheduled for upper abdominal or thoracic surgery should have preoperative pulmonary function tests performed. In addition, elderly patients (over 70 years of age) and morbidly obese patients are candidates for preoperative pulmonary function tests.

There are numerous pulmonary function tests that can be used to quantitate pulmonary disease preoperatively. The simplest and often most informative tests are measurements of flow rates during exhalation (see the section *Obstructive Airway Disease*), vital capacity (see the section *Restrictive Pulmonary Disease*), and maximum breathing capacity. The risk of postoperative pulmonary morbidity is predictably increased when preoperatively the (1) FEV_1 is less than 2 liters; (2) ratio of the FEV_1 to forced vital capacity is less than 0.5; (3) vital capacity is less than 15 ml/kg; or (4) maximum breathing capacity is less than 50 percent of the predicted value.

Prophylactic Digitalis. Resection of pulmonary tissue reduces the available pulmonary vascular bed and can cause postoperative right atrial and ventricular enlargement with associated cardiac dysrhythmias, especially atrial fibrillation. For this reason, prophylactic use of digitalis has been recommended, particularly in elderly patients undergoing resection of large amounts of lung tissue. A disadvantage of prophylactic digitalis is confusion with digitalis toxicity should cardiac dysrhythmias develop postoperatively.

Management of Anesthesia

A general anesthetic with controlled ventilation of the lungs is appropriate for thoracic surgery. Use of a volatile anesthetic with or without nitrous oxide is ideal, as these potent drugs reduce irritability of the airways and can be rapidly eliminated at the conclusion of surgery. If nitrous oxide is administered, the inhaled concentration should be limited to 50 percent until the adequacy of oxygenation can be confirmed by measurement of the PaO_2. A nondepolarizing muscle relaxant is usually administered to facilitate controlled ventilation of the lungs, improve surgical exposure by maximizing mechanical separation of the ribs, and to decrease requirements for the volatile anesthetic. Ketamine is ideal for induction of anesthesia for emergency thoracotomy associated with hypovolemia (blunt trauma, gun shot, stab wound). Most patients undergoing thoracotomy should have an intra-arterial catheter in place to permit continuous monitoring of blood pressure and frequent measurement of blood gases and pH. A central venous pressure catheter is helpful for guiding intravenous fluid replacement. Alternatively, a pulmonary artery catheter should be considered if co-existing coronary artery disease or cardiac valvular dysfunction is present. A catheter should be inserted into the bladder of patients who are expected to undergo long operations associated with alterations in blood volume necessitating infusions of large amounts of intravenous fluids.

Lateral Decubitus Position. The lateral decubitus position necessary for thoracic surgery plus the need for mechanical ventilation of the lungs results in an altered distribution of ventilation relative to perfusion (see Chapter 15).

One-lung anesthesia utilizing a double lumen tracheal tube is indicated when one lung can contaminate the other lung with either infected material or blood or when the distribution of ventilation between the two lungs must be separated, as in the presence of a bronchopleural fistula. A relative indication for one-lung anesthesia is to provide a quiet lung and improved operating conditions as during lobectomy, pneumonectomy, resection of a thoracic aneurysm, or operations on the esophagus.

The Robertshaw tube is a frequently used double-lumen tracheal tube (Fig. 20-3).[9] Inflation of the proximal cuff on this tube provides a seal with the tracheal mucosa. Inflation of the cuff on the distal portion of the tube that is present in the left or right mainstem bronchus provides a seal to isolate that lung from the contralateral lung. A left Robertshaw tube is used for operations requiring isolation of the right lung and ventilation of the left lung. When isolation of the left lung is required, either a left or right Robertshaw tube may be used. The nearness of the right upper lobe bronchus to the carina introduces the risk of inadequate ventilation of the right upper lobe when a

right tube is used. To avoid this complication, it is acceptable to use a left Robertshaw tube for all one-lung anesthesias. Should clamping of the left mainstem bronchus be necesary, the left Robertshaw tube is withdrawn into the trachea at the appropriate time. Proper placement of the Robertshaw tube is confirmed by auscultation of the chest during positive pressure ventilation of the lungs and/or direct visualization by passing a fiberoptic bronchoscope through the tube.

The major disadvantage of one-lung anesthesia is the introduction of an iatrogenic right-to-left intrapulmonary shunt by virtue of continued perfusion to both lungs while only one lung is ventilated. For this reason, use of high inhaled concentrations of oxygen and frequent monitoring of the PaO_2 are indicated during one-lung anesthesia. If arterial hypoxemia persists despite inhalation of high concentrations of oxygen, the selective application of a low level of positive end-expiratory pressure (5 to 10 cm H_2O) to the dependent lung can be instituted in an attempt to divert more ventilation to this lung. Ligation of the pulmonary artery during one-lung anesthesia for a pneumonectomy improves oxygenation by removing perfusion to the unventilated lung. Elimination of carbon dioxide is not usually a problem during one-lung anesthesia.

An alternative to one-lung anesthesia utilizing a double-lumen tracheal tube is the use of high frequency positive pressure ventilation.

Conclusion of Surgery. Hyperinflation of the lung is important to exclude air from the pleural space at the conclusion of thoracic surgery. Furthermore, alveoli incised during segmental resection of the lung continue to leak air into the pleural space, necessitating the placement of drainage tubes (chest tubes) to assure removal of this air and continued expansion of the lung. These

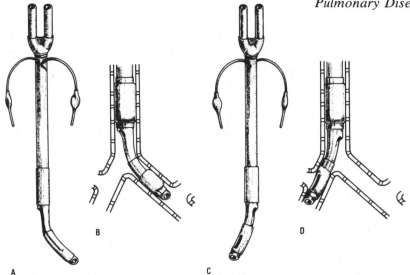

A   C
B   D

Figure 20-3. The Robertshaw double-lumen tracheal tube is available as a left (A) or right (C) design. Placed in the trachea, the distal end of the tube is directed into the left (B) or right (D) mainstem bronchus. The distal end of the right Robertshaw tube incorporates a slotted cuff to permit ventilation of the right upper lobe. (Alfery DD, Benumof JL. Anesthesia for thoracic surgery. In: Miller RD, ed. Anesthesia. New York, Churchill Livingstone. 1981:925–80.)

drainage tubes are connected to a sterile disposable plastic unit which incorporates a one-way valve that permits continuous suction. Chest tubes must not be allowed to kink, since a sudden rise in intrathoracic pressure, as with coughing, may increase the leak and cause a tension pneumothorax if air cannot escape.

Drainage tubes are not necessary following a pneumonectomy. Instead, intrapleural pressure on the operated side is adjusted by aspirating air to slightly below atmospheric pressure. Excessive negative pressure can cause hypotension by shifting the mediastinum and compromising cardiac output.

The trachea may be extubated when the adequacy of spontaneous ventilation is confirmed and protective upper airway reflexes have returned. In otherwise healthy patients, extubation of the trachea may be performed at the conclusion of surgery. Often, however, continued mechanical ventilation of the lungs via a tracheal tube is indicated in the postoperative period (see Chapter 32).

Treatment of Postoperative Pain

Adequate analgesia following thoracic surgery permits patients to breath deeply and cough effectively so as to minimize the likelihood of postoperative atelectasis and/or pneumonia. The intermittent administration of parenteral narcotics is the most frequent approach, adjusting the dose to achieve maximal analgesia without excessive sedation or depression of ventilation. In the early postoperative period the intravenous administration of morphine (1 to 2 mg increments) until adequate analgesia is achieved can be given. Intercostal nerve blocks with a long-acting local anesthetic such as bupivacaine are an alternative to parenteral narcotics for providing analgesia. Intercostal nerve blocks can be performed under direct vision (intrathoracic) by the surgeon prior to closing the chest or postoperatively by the anesthesiologist. Transient hypotension has been associated with intrathoracic performance of the block, presumably reflecting thoracic sympathectomy.[10] Total spinal block has also followed intrathoracic performance of intercostal nerve blocks.[11] Assuming this latter complication represents unrecognized dural puncture or perineural spread of the local anesthetic, it is recommended that the intercostal nerve block be performed at least 8 cm lateral to the intervertebral foramen. Thoracic epidural placement of a local anesthetic is an effective but often impractical method for providing analgesia after a thoracotomy. Alternatively, placement of morphine in the lumbar epidural space has been shown to provide long-lasting analgesia following a thoracotomy.[12] Finally, transcutaneous electrical stimulation provides weak analgesic effects but is devoid of undesirable depressant effects. In the future, continuous intravenous infusion of low doses of narcotic may prove to be an ideal approach for providing optimal analgesia without undesirable side effects.

Mediastinoscopy

Mediastinoscopy is often performed prior to thoracotomy in order to establish the diagnosis and/or resectability of carcinoma of the lung. Hemorrhage and pneumothorax are the most frequently encountered complications of this procedure. If a thoracotomy is not subsequently performed, it is important to maintain a high index of suspicion for penumothorax in the immediate postoperative period. A radiograph of the chest in the recovery room is helpful in detecting the presence of a pneumothorax.

Positive pressure ventilation of the lungs during mediastinoscopy is recommended so as to minimize the risk of venous air embolism. The mediastinoscope can also exert pressure against the right subclavian artery, causing the loss of a pulse distal to the site of compression and an erroneous diagnosis of cardiac arrest. Likewise, unrecognized compression of the right carotid artery has been proposed as an explanation for postoperative neurological deficits following this procedure. Bradycardia during mediastinoscopy may be due to stretching of the vagus nerve or trachea by the mediastinoscope. Treatment is repositioning of the mediastinoscope followed by intravenous atropine if bradycardia persists.

REFERENCES

1. Tarhan S, Moffitt EA, Sessler AD, Douglas WM, Taylor WF. Risk of anesthesia and surgery in patients with chronic bronchitis and chronic obstructive disease. Surgery 1973;74:720–6.
2. LoSasso AM, Gibbs PS, Moorthy SS. Obstructive pulmonary disease. In: Stoelting RK, Dierdorf SF, eds. Anesthesia and coexisting disease. New York, Churchill Livingstone, 1983:171–200.
3. Hirshman CA, Bergman NA. Halothane and enflurane protect against bronchospasm in an asthma dog model. Anesth Analg 1978;57:629–33.
4. Crago RR, Bryan AC, Laws AIC, Winestock AE. Respiratory flow resistance after curare and pancuronium measured by forced oscillations. Can Anaesth Soc J 1972;19:607–14.
5. Petrie GR, Palmer KNV. Comparison of aerosol ipratropium bromide and salbutamol in chronic bronchitis and asthma. Br Med J 1975;1:430–2.
6. Pietak S, Weenig CS, Hickey RF, Fairley HB. Anesthetic effects on ventilation in patients with chronic obstructive pulmonary disease. Anesthesiology 1975;42:160–6.
7. Gold MI, Joseph SI. Bilateral tension pneumothorax following induction of anesthesia in two patients with chronic obstructive airway disease. Anesthesiology 1973;38:93–6.
8. LoSasso AM, Gibbs PS, Moorthy SS. Restrictive pulmonary disease. In: Stoelting RK, Dierdorf SF, eds. Anesthesia and coexisting disease. New York, Churchill Livingstone, 1983:201–7.
9. Alfery DD, Benumof JL. Anesthesia for thoracic surgery. In: Miller RD, ed. Anes-

thesia. New York, Churchill Livingstone, 1981:925–80.

10. Cottrell WM, Schick LM, Perkins HM, Modell JH. Hemodynamic changes after intercostal nerve block with bupivacaine-epinephrine solution. Anesth Analg 1978; 57:492–5.

11. Benumof JL, Semenza J: Total spinal anesthesia following intrathoracic intercostal nerve blocks. Anesthesiology 1975;43:124–5.

12. Nordbert G, Hedner T, Mellstrand T, Dahlstrom B. Pharmacokinetic aspects of epidural morphine analgesia. Anesthesiology 1983; 58:545–51.

21

Hepatic Disease

Management of anesthesia in the presence of liver disease requires an understanding of the physiologic functions of the liver.[1] In addition, the impact of anesthesia and surgery on hepatic blood flow has important implications for the management of anesthesia. Liver function tests are useful for detecting unsuspected liver disease preoperatively and for establishing the diagnosis when postoperative liver dysfunction occurs.

PHYSIOLOGIC FUNCTIONS OF THE LIVER

Physiologic functions of the liver that may be altered by co-existing liver disease include glucose homeostasis, protein synthesis, drug metabolism, and bilirubin formation and excretion. The response of the patient during the perioperative period may be influenced by disease-induced alterations in these important functions of the liver.

Glucose Homeostasis

The liver is responsible for the storage and release of glucose. Glucose enters the hepatocyte, where it is stored as glycogen. Breakdown of glycogen (glycogenolysis) releases glucose back into the systemic circulation to maintain a normal blood glucose concentration. In addition, lactate, glycerol, and amino acids are converted in the liver to glucose by the process known as gluconeogenesis. Exogenous sources of glucose during the fasting period associated with surgery become important when glycogen stores are depleted due to poor preoperative nutrition. Indeed, the patient with cirrhosis of the liver may be vulnerable to the development of hypoglycemia in the perioperative period.

Protein Synthesis

All proteins except gamma globulins and antihemophiliac factor (factor VIII) are synthesized in the liver. Approximately 10 to 15 g of albumin are produced daily to maintain the normal plasma concentration of this protein, between 3.5 to 5.5 g/dl. A plasma albumin concentration less than 3.5 g/dl signifies significant liver disease. The half-time for albumin, however, is about 23 days, emphasizing that acute liver dysfunction will not be reflected by decreased plasma concentrations of this protein.

Protein synthesis in the liver is important for drug binding, coagulation, and production of enzymes necessary for the hydrolysis of ester linkages.

Drug Binding. When liver disease results in decreased albumin production, there will be fewer sites available for drug binding. As a result, the unbound, pharmacologically active fraction of a drug such as thiopental

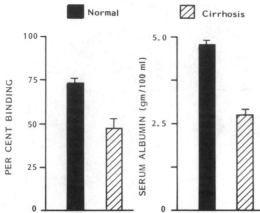

Figure 21-1. The percent binding (mean ± SE) of thiopental to protein is reduced in the presence of cirrhosis of the liver as compared with normal patients. This decreased binding parallels the decrease in the plasma (serum) albumin concentration. (McCammon RL. Diseases of the liver and biliary tract. In Stoelting RK, Dierdorf SF, eds. Anesthesia and co-existing disease. New York. Churchill Livingstone 1983;327–61, with data from ref. 2.).

increases (Fig. 21-1).[2] Increased drug sensitivities due to decreased protein binding are most likely to manifest when plasma albumin concentrations are less than 2.5 g/dl.

Coagulation. Clotting abnormalities must be suspected in any patient with liver disease, since hepatocytes are responsible for the synthesis of most procoagulants. The adequacy of clotting factor levels is evaluated by measuring the prothrombin time, partial thromboplastin time, and bleeding time. Liver function must be dramatically depressed before impaired coagulation is manifest, since many of the coagulation factors require only 20 to 30 percent of their normal levels to prevent bleeding. Nevertheless, the plasma half-time of hepatic-produced clotting factors such as prothrombin and fibrinogen is short and acute liver dysfunction is likely to be associated with clotting abnormalites.

Liver disease associated with splenomegaly can alter the normal coagulation mech-

anism independent of procoagulant synthesis by trapping platelets in the spleen. Another factor predisposing to a bleeding diathesis is the failure of a diseased liver to clear plasma activators of the fibrinolytic system.

Hydrolysis of Ester Linkages. Severe liver disease may decrease the production of cholinesterase enzyme (pseudocholinesterase) enzyme that is necessary for the hydrolysis of ester linkages in drugs such as succinylcholine and ester local anesthetics. As a result, the duration of apnea following the administration of succinylcholine may be prolonged in the presence of liver disease (Fig. 21-2).[3] The plasma half-time for cholinesterase is about 14 days, emphasizing that acute liver failure is unlikely to be associated with a slowed rate of succinylcholine hydrolysis.

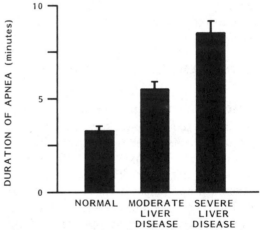

Figure 21-2. The duration of apnea (mean ± SE) following the intravenous administration of succinylcholine (0.6 mg/kg) is prolonged in the presence of moderate and severe liver disease, reflecting decreased hepatic production of cholinesterase enzyme necessary for the hydrolysis of the muscle relaxant. (McCammon RL. Diseases of the liver and biliary tract. In Stoelting RK, Dierdorf SF, eds. Anesthesia and co-existing disease. New York. Churchill Livingstone 1983;327–61, with data from ref. 3.).

Drug Metabolism

Drug metabolism, characterized by the conversion of a lipid soluble drug to a more water soluble and pharmacologically less active substance, is under the control of microsomal enzymes present in the smooth endoplasmic retriculum of the hepatocyte. In chronic liver disease, the number of hepatocytes is reduced such that the amount of drug presented to each cell for metabolism is increased. This may stimulate enzyme activity (enzyme induction), which may accelerate drug metabolism sufficiently to result in resistance to the pharmacologic effects of that drug. Enzyme induction may also be a response to chronic drug therapy or alcohol abuse. In addition, there seems to be cross-tolerance between substances known to produce liver disease (alcohol) and other depressant drugs, including inhaled and injected anesthetics.

A reduced number of hepatocytes could also result in a decreased rate of metabolism of drugs. This could be further exaggerated by reduced delivery of drug to the liver by virtue of decreased hepatic blood flow that predictably accompanies chronic liver disease. Evidence for decreased metabolism of drugs is the demonstration of a prolonged plasma half-time for diazepam, meperidine, and lidocaine in patients with cirrhosis of the liver.[1] Conversely, the plasma half-time of morphine following administration of modest doses of this narcotic is not prolonged, presumably because extrahepatic sites of metabolism (glucuronidation) in the kidneys and gastrointestinal tract offset decreased metabolizing capacity of the liver. Nevertheless, it is important to anticipate cumulative effects of any drug, including morphine, when repeated doses are administered to patients with liver disease.

Bilirubin Formation and Excretion

Bilirubin is produced in the reticuloendothelial system from the breakdown of hemoglobin. This bilirubin is bound to albumin for transport to the liver. Protein-bound bilirubin (unconjugated) is not water soluble and urinary excretion is, therefore, minimal. Conjugation of bilirubin with glucuronic acid in the liver renders bilirubin water soluble. A small amount of conjugated bilirubin enters the circulation and undergoes renal excretion. The remainder is excreted into the biliary canniculi and eventually into the small intestine.

HEPATIC BLOOD FLOW

The liver is unique in that it receives a dual afferent blood supply equivalent to about 25 percent of the cardiac output (Fig. 21-3).[1] The majority of hepatic blood flow (70 percent) is via the portal vein and the remainder is derived from the hepatic artery. Oxygen delivery to the liver may be marginal, since the majority of blood flow is with desaturated hemoglobin delivered via the portal vein. In addition, any reduction in PaO_2 greatly reduces total oxygen delivery to the liver.

Determinants of Hepatic Blood Flow

Hepatic blood flow is determined by perfusion pressure (mean arterial or portal vein pressure minus hepatic vein pressure) and splanchnic vascular resistance. The splanchnic vessels are innervated by sympathetic vasoconstrictor nerve fibers (T3–11). Splanchnic nerve stimulation as produced by arterial hypoxemia or exogenous administration of catecholamines results in increased splanchnic vascular resistance and decreased hepatic blood flow. The hepatic circulation is also supplied with beta receptors, and blockade of these receptors as produced by propranolol is associated with reductions in hepatic blood flow. Positive pressure ventilation of the lungs can decrease hepatic blood flow, presumably by increasing central venous pressure (hepatic vein pressure) and thus decreasing hepatic perfusion pressure. Autoregulation of he-

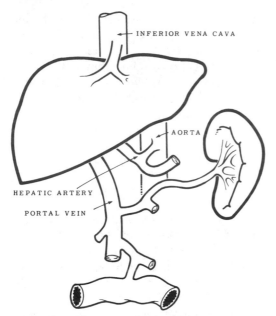

INFERIOR VENA CAVA

AORTA

HEPATIC ARTERY

PORTAL VEIN

Figure 21-3. Schematic diagram of blood flow to the liver. About 70 percent of hepatic blood flow is via the portal vein with the remainder derived from the hepatic artery. Total hepatic blood flow is directly proportional to perfusion pressure across the liver and inversely related to splanchnic vascular resistance. Cirrhosis of the liver increases resistance to flow through the portal vein and decreases hepatic blood flow. (McCammon RL. Diseases of the liver and biliary tract. In: Stoelting RK, Dierdorf SF, eds. Anesthesia and co-existing disease. New York. Churchill Livingstone 1983;327–61.)

patic blood flow is not prominent, emphasizing that drug-induced decreases in blood pressure during anesthesia are likely to be associated with similar reductions in hepatic blood flow. Cirrhosis of the liver that is associated with increased resistance to flow through the liver is predictably accompanied by reductions in hepatic blood flow.

Impact of Anesthetic Drugs on Hepatic Blood Flow. Reductions in perfusion pressure produced by volatile anesthetics as well as spinal or epidural block are associated with similar decreases in hepatic blood flow.[1] Nitrous oxide plus d-tubocurarine and controlled ventilation of the

lungs decreases hepatic blood flow by increasing venous pressure and thus the resistance to flow through the liver. There is no evidence, however, that these drug-induced reductions in hepatic blood flow are associated with inadequate hepatocyte oxygenation. Nevertheless, it is conceivable that underlying liver disease could make the hepatocyte more vulnerable to adverse effects from drug-induced reductions in hepatic blood flow.

Selective hepatic artery constriction has been observed in patients without liver disease during inhalation of halothane or methoxyflurane.[1] The mechanism and clinical significance of this selective hepatic artery constriction are unknown.

Impact of Surgical Stimulation on Hepatic Blood Flow. Surgical stimulation and the nearness of the operative site to the liver are important determinants of the magnitude of decrease in hepatic blood flow during general anesthesia (Fig. 21-4).[4] For example, the greatest reductions in hepatic blood flow occur when the operative site is near the liver, as during a cholecystectomy.

LIVER FUNCTION TESTS

Liver function tests are used to detect the presence of liver disease preoperatively and to establish the diagnosis when postoperative liver dysfunction occurs. It is important to remember that liver function tests are rarely specific. Furthermore, the large reserve of the liver means that considerable hepatic damage can be present before liver function tests are altered. Indeed, cirrhosis may produce little alteration in liver function and only when some additional insult such as surgery produces further deterioration does the underlying liver disease become obvious.

Postoperatively, the magnitude of liver dysfunction as reflected by liver function tests is exaggerated by operations near the liver (Fig. 21-5).[5] The specific anesthetic

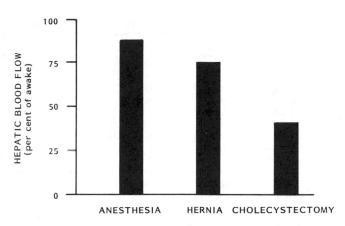

Figure 21-4. The nearness of the operative site to the liver rather than anesthesia (nitrous oxide-halothane) is the most important factor in decreasing hepatic blood flow. (Mc-Cammon RL. Diseases of the liver and biliary tract. In Stoelting RK, Dierdorf SF, eds. Anesthesia and co-existing disease. New York. Churchill Livingstone 1983;327–61, with data from reference 4.)

drug, however, does not influence the magnitude of postoperative liver dysfunction as reflected by liver function tests (Fig. 21-5).[5]

Commonly measured liver function tests include the serum concentrations of albumin, bilirubin, transaminase enzymes, alkaline phosphatase, and prothrombin time (Table 21-1). Based on these tests, postoperative liver dysfunction can be categorized as prehepatic, intrahepatic, and posthepatic (Table 21-2).

Prehepatic Dysfunction

Prehepatic dysfunction as a cause of postoperative jaundice most likely reflects delivery of a bilirubin overload to the patient.

Causes of hyperbilirubinemia include hemolysis, hematoma resorption, or whole blood administration. A 500 ml transfusion of fresh whole blood contains 250 mg of bilirubin. The bilirubin load increases as the age of transfused blood increases. Patients with normal hepatic function can receive large amounts of blood without any appreciable increase in bilirubin. This response can be different in patients with co-existing liver disease.

Overt jaundice is present when the serum bilirubin concentration exceeds 3 mg/dl. The unconjugated fraction of bilirubin is increased more than the conjugated fraction when prehepatic dysfunction is present.

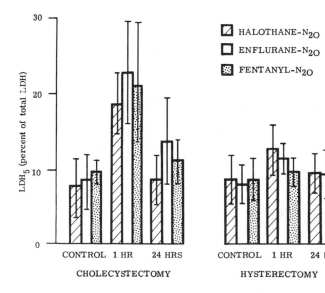

Figure 21-5. The magnitude of elevation of the isoenzyme fraction of lactic dehydrogenase (LDH_5) is determined by the nearness of the operation to the liver and not the drugs used for maintenance of anesthesia. (Viegas OJ, Stoelting RK. LDH_5 changes after cholecystectomy or hysterectomy in patients receiving halothane, enflurane or fentanyl. Anesthesiology 1979;51:556–8.)

Table 21-1. Liver Function Tests

Test	Level[a]
Albumin	3.5–5.5 g/dl
Bilirubin	0.3–1.1 mg/dl
Unconjugated bilirubin (indirect reacting)	0.2–0.7 mg/dl
Conjugated bilirubin (direct reacting)	0.1–0.4 mg/dl
Glutamic oxalacetic transaminase (SGOT) (asparatate aminotransferase)	15–40 units/ml
Glutamic pyruvic transaminase (SGPT) (alanine aminotransferase)	5–35 units/ml
Lactic dyhydrogenase (LDH)	60–100 units/ml
Alkaline phosphatase	10–30 units/ml
Prothrombin time	12–14 seconds

[a] Normal values for each individual hospital laboratory should be consulted when interpreting liver function tests.

(Data from Conn HF, ed. Current Therapy. Philadelphia, WB Saunders, 1980:916–25.)

Intrahepatic Dysfunction

Intrahepatic dysfunction reflects direct hepatocellular damage due to toxic effects of drugs, sepsis, arterial hypoxemia, or viruses. This form of postoperative dysfunction is recognized by hyperbilirubinemia and marked increases in serum transaminase concentrations. Although intraheptic dysfunction can occasionally cause accumulation of unconjugated bilirubin due to impaired hepatic uptake or conjugation, accumulation of conjugated bilirubin is more common, reflecting impaired excretion of bilirubin conjugates into bile. Hepatocytes contain large amounts of transaminase enzymes (glutamic oxalacetic transaminase, glutamic pyruvic transaminase, lactic dehydrogenase) that spill into the circulation when hepatocytes are acutely damaged. Other tissues, however, such as the heart, lung, and skeletal muscle also contain transaminase enzymes. Indeed, postoperative increases in the serum transaminase concentrations may reflect skeletal muscle damage from intramuscular injections given preoperatively or damage to skeletal muscle during surgery. Nevertheless, marked elevations of the serum transaminase enzyme concentrations to three times normal or greater in the postoperative period should suggest acute hepatocellular damage.

Posthepatic Dysfunction

Posthepatic dysfunction reflects bile duct obstruction and is characterized by hyperbilirubinemia (predominately the conjugated fraction) and elevated serum concentrations of alkaline phosphatase. Alkaline phosphatase is present in bile duct cells such that even slight degrees of biliary obstruction are manifested by threefold or greater elevations of the serum concentration of this enzyme. It must be remembered, however, that there are also extrahepatic stores of alkaline phosphatase, particularly in skeletal muscle.

Table 21-2. Classification of Hepatic Dysfunction

	Bilirubin	Transaminases	Alkaline Phosphatase
Prehepatic	Increased (unconjugated fraction)	Normal	Normal
Intrahepatic	Increased (conjugated fraction)	Markedly elevated	Normal to slightly elevated
Posthepatic	Increased (conjugated fraction)	Normal to slightly elevated	Markedly elevated

DRUG-INDUCED HEPATITIS

Many drugs, including isoniazid, phenytoin, sulfonamides, chlorpromazine, and alpha-methyldopa, can cause hepatic cellular changes that are indistinguishable from viral hepatitis. Likewise, administration of halothane, particularly with repeated exposures at short intervals, is occasionally (between 1 in 22,000 to 1 in 35,000 administrations) associated with hepatic dysfunction (see Chapter 5).[6]

There is no evidence that halothane-associated hepatic dysfunction is more likely to occur in patients with co-existing liver disease. However, in view of alternative drugs (enflurane, isoflurane, narcotics), it would seem logical to avoid administering halothane to patients with known liver disease. Furthermore, the magnitude of postoperative hepatic dysfunction is exaggerated in patients with co-existing liver disease regardless of the anesthetic drug administered.[1] Finally, halothane should not be administered to a patient who has experienced postoperative hepatic dysfunction for unknown reasons following a previous operation performed with halothane anesthesia.

CIRRHOSIS OF THE LIVER

Cirrhosis of the liver is a chronic disease process that destroys the hepatic parenchyma and subsequently replaces it with collagen. Excessive use of alcohol is the most frequent cause of cirrhosis. Cirrhosis is associated with a decrease in the number of hepatocytes, leading to an impairment of all the physiologic functions of the liver (see the section *Physiologic Functions of the Liver*). Another important change associated with cirrhosis is a reduction in hepatic blood flow due to increased resistance to blood flow through the portal vein. As a result of this increased resistance, the proportion of hepatic blood flow delivered via the portal vein is decreased and the contri-bution to total hepatic blood flow from the hepatic artery is increased. Therefore, decreases in systemic perfusion pressure or arterial oxygenation during anesthesia and surgery are more likely to jeopardize the adequacy of hepatic blood flow and delivery of oxygen to the liver in patients with cirrhosis as compared with normal patients.

Portal Vein Hypertension

The most striking finding on physical examination related to portal vein hypertension due to cirrhosis is hepatomegaly with or without splenomegaly and ascites. Ascites reflects decreased oncotic pressure secondary to a low plasma albumin concentration, elevated resistance to blood flow through the portal vein, and increased secretion of antidiuretic hormone. Despite the loss of skeletal muscle mass, body weight is often maintained due to accumulation of ascitic fluid.

Gastroesophageal varices are a predictable complication of portal vein hypertension. Chronic bleeding from these varices is reflected by a moderate reduction in the hematocrit.

Extrahepatic Complications of Cirrhosis

A hyperdynamic circulation characterized by an increased cardiac output is often present in patients with cirrhosis.[1] This increased cardiac output may reflect increased intravascular fluid volume, decreased viscosity of the blood secondary to anemia, and generalized peripheral arteriolar vasodilation. In contrast to a hyperdynamic circulation, patients with alcoholic cirrhosis may also develop congestive heart failure due to cardiomyopathy. Megaloblastic anemia is frequent and is probably due to antagonism of folate by alcohol rather than a dietary deficiency.

Arterial hypoxemia is a common finding in the patient with cirrhosis. Indeed, many of these patients have chronic obstructive airway disease associated with cigarette smoking. Furthermore, right-to-left intrapulmonary shunts may develop in the presence of portal vein hypertension, leading to arterial hypoxemia.

Cirrhosis is associated with a reduction in renal blood flow and glomerular filtration rate. Hypoglycemia is a constant threat in the alcoholic patient. The incidence of gallstones is increased, presumably reflecting an elevated bilirubin load due to hemolysis of erythrocytes in the spleen. Peptic ulcer disease is twice as common in patients with cirrhosis. Spontaneous bacterial peritonitis develops in nearly 10 percent of patients with alcoholic liver disease and ascites. Hepatic encephalopathy, presumably due to the systemic accumulation of nitrogenous waste products, is evidenced by asterixis (flapping motion of the hands caused by intermittent loss of extensor muscle tone) and mental obtundation. The development of hepatic encephalopathy is associated with a high mortality.

Management of Anesthesia in the Sober Alcoholic Patient

The best choice of drugs or techniques for anesthesia in the sober patient with alcohol-induced liver disease is not known. Coagulation status should be evaluated preoperatively and parenteral vitamin K administered if the prothrombin time is prolonged. Failure of parenteral vitamin K to improve synthesis of prothrombin suggests the presence of severe hepatocellular disease. Conversely, impaired prothrombin production due to biliary obstruction and absence of bile salts to facilitate gastrointestinal absorption of vitamin K is promptly restored by parenteral vitamin K therapy. All jaundiced patients should receive parenteral vitamin K preoperatively, and if prothrombin time does not return to normal, fresh frozen plasma should be available. It is important to remember that hepatic blood flow is predictably decreased in patients with cirrhosis and any further reduction due to anesthetic-induced depression of cardiac output or blood pressure could jeopardize hepatocyte oxygenation. Furthermore, postoperative liver dysfunction is likely to be exaggerated in any patient with chronic liver disease regardless of the drug or drugs administered for anesthesia.[1]

There is evidence that chronic alcohol abuse increases anesthetic requirements (MAC) for volatile anesthetics (Fig. 21-6).[7] The most likely explanation for this increase is a cross tolerance between depressant drugs. In contrast to resistance to depressant drugs, alcohol-induced cardiomyopathy could make these patients unusually sensitive to the cardiac depressant effects of volatile anesthetics. Likewise, decreased protein binding of drugs in the presence of reduced serum albumin concentrations would increase the pharmacologically active unbound fraction of injected drugs available to act at peripheral receptors.[2] Nevertheless, a study of the pharmacokinetics of thiopental concluded that the risk of prolonged effect following administration of this drug to patients with cirrhosis was unlikely.[8] Finally, jaundiced patients (total serum bilirubin concentration above 8 mg/dl) are more likely to develop acute renal failure and sepsis postoperatively, emphasizing the importance of establishing a diuresis with mannitol preoperatively and initiating antibiotic therapy.[1]

Succinylcholine is an acceptable muscle relaxant, but the dose should be adjusted if liver disease is sufficiently advanced so as to decrease serum cholinesterase activity. Resistance to the effects of d-tubocurarine has been observed in patients with liver disease.[1] Conceivably, this resistance may reflect increased d-tubocurarine binding to gamma globulin and/or increased drug distribution volume due to circulatory changes associated with cirrhosis. Indeed, the dis-

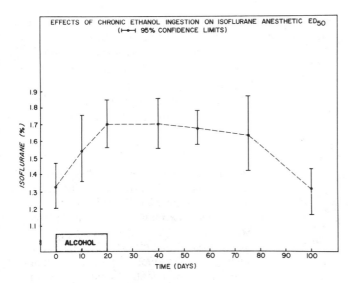

EFFECTS OF CHRONIC ETHANOL INGESTION ON ISOFLURANE ANESTHETIC ED$_{50}$
(I—•—I 95% CONFIDENCE LIMITS)

Figure 21-6. The effect of chronic alcohol ingestion on the anesthetic requirement for isoflurane was determined in mice during and following continuous exposure to ethanol. Isoflurane anesthetic requirements on days 20, 40, 55 and 75 were signifcantly (P < 0.05) elevated above the control value. (Johnstone RE, Kulp RA, Smith TC. Effects of acute and chronic ethanol administration of isoflurane requirement in mice. Anesth Analg 1975;54:277–81.)

tribution volume of pancuronium is increascd and the plasma clearance decreased in patients with alcoholic cirrhosis, as compared with normal patients.[9] Based on these observations, the initial dose of pancuronium necessary to produce adequate skeletal muscle relaxation in the alcoholic patient might be increased, reflecting dilution of the drug in a larger distribution volume. Conversely, the duration of paralysis might be prolonged due to slowed plasma clearance.

Monitoring of intraoperative blood gases, pH, and urine output plus provision of exogenous glucose are important principles. Arterial hypoxemia may be exaggerated intraoperatively if drugs used for anesthesia produce vasodilation of co-existing portasystemic and intrapulmonary shunts.[1] When blood replacement is necessary, it is logical to administer the stored blood as slowly as possible to compensate for decreased clearance of citrate by the diseased liver. A practical point is the avoidance of unnecessary esophageal instrumentation in patients with known esophageal varices.

Manifestations of a severe alcohol withdrawal syndrome (delerium tremens) usually appear 48 to 72 hours after the cessation of drinking. This syndrome represents a medical emergency, as mortality may approach 15 percent. Postoperatively, the patient will manifest tremulousness and hallucinations. There is increased activity of the sympathetic nervous system with catecholamine release leading to diaphoresis, hyperpyrexia, tachycardia, and hypertension. In some patients a grand mal seizure may be the first indication of the alcohol withdrawal syndrome. When seizures occur, hypoglycemia must be ruled out as a possible cause. Initial treatment of delerium tremens consists of sedation with intravenous diazepam (10 mg initially followed by 5 mg every 5 minutes until the patient is calm), propranolol to reduce sympathetic nervous system activity, vitamin replacement including thiamine, and correction of fluid and electrolyte disorders.

Management of Anesthesia in the Intoxicated Alcoholic Patient

In contrast to the chronic but sober alcoholic, the acutely intoxicated patient requires less anesthetic, since there is an additive depressant effect between alcohol and anesthetics. The acutely intoxicated patient also withstands stress and blood loss poorly. Furthermore, the intoxicated patient is more vulnerable to regurgitation of gastric contents, as alcohol slows gastric emptying and reduces the tone of the lower esophageal sphincter.

DISEASES OF THE BILIARY TRACT

Gallstones are reported to be present in 10 percent of males and 20 percent of females between 55 and 65 years of age. Patients who experience repeated attacks of acute cholecystitis eventually develop a fibrotic gallbladder. Liver function tests are usually normal, but an elevated serum bilirubin or alkaline phosphatase concentration suggests the presence of choledocholithiasis (common bile duct stone) or chronic cholangitis.

Management of Anesthesia

Management of anesthesia for cholecystectomy and/or common bile duct exploration is influenced by the effects of drugs used for anesthesia on intraluminal pressures in the biliary tract. Specifically, narcotics (morphine, meperidine, fentanyl, pentazocine) can produce spasm of the choledochoduodenal sphincter, which elevates intrabiliary pressures.[10] This spasm could impair passage of contrast media into the duodenum, erroneously suggesting the need for a sphincteroplasty or the presence of a common bile duct stone. Nevertheless, narcotics have been used in many instances without adverse effects, emphasizing that not all patients respond to narcotics with choledochoduodenal sphincter spasm. Indeed, some feel that the incidence of narcotic-induced sphincter spasm during cholecystectomy is so low that the possibility of this response should not influence the use of narcotics during anesthesia for this operation. The alternative to narcotics for maintenance of anesthesia during a cholecystectomy would be the use of a volatile anesthetic. The possible presence, however, of liver disease is often a concern when selecting a volatile anesthetic for a cholecystectomy. Nevertheless, there is no evidence that hepatic dysfunction after a cholecystectomy is different in patients anesthetized with nitrous oxide plus fentanyl, halothane, or enflurane (Fig. 21-5).[5]

REFERENCES

1. McCammon RL. Diseases of the liver and biliary tract. In: Stoelting RK, Dierdorf SF, eds. Anesthesia and Co-Existing Disease. New York. Churchill Livingstone 1983;327–61.
2. Ghoneim MM, Pandya H. Plasma protein binding of thiopental in patients with impaired renal or hepatic function. Anesthesiology 1975;42:545–9.
3. Foldes FF, Swerdlow M. Lipschitz E, Van Hees GR, Shanor SP. Comparison of the respiratory effects of suxamethonium and suxethonium in man. Anesthesiology 1956;17:559–68.
4. Gelman SI. Disturbances in hepatic blood flow during anesthesia and surgery. Arch Surg 1976;111:881–3.
5. Viegas OJ, Stoelting RK. LDH$_5$ changes after cholecystectomy or hysterectomy in patients receiving halothane, enflurane, or fentanyl. Anesthesiology 1979;51:556–8.
6. Summary of the national halothane study. JAMA 1966;197:775–88.
7. Johnstone RE, Kulp RA, Smith TC. Effects of acute and chronic ethanol administration on isoflurane requirement in mice. Anesth Analg 1975;54:277–81.
8. Pandele G, Chaux F, Salvadori C, Farinotti M, Duvaldestin P. Thiopental pharmacokinetics in patients with cirrhosis. Anesthesiology 1983;59:123–6.
9. Duvaldestin P, Agoston S, Henzel D, Kersten UW, Desmonts JM. Pancuronium pharmacokinetics in patients with liver cirrhosis. Br J Anaesth 1978;50:1131–6.
10. Thompson WL, Johnson AD, Maddrey WL. Diazepam and paraldehyde for treatment of severe delerium tremens: a controlled trial. Ann Intern Med 1975;82:175–80.

22

Renal Disease

The kidneys are essential for maintaining an ideal total body water content and assuring that the solute composition is optimal. Co-existing renal disease can predispose patients to perioperative morbidity and mortality. Furthermore, the possibility of impaired renal function during the perioperative period should be considered in otherwise healthy patients undergoing major operations. Management of patients in the perioperative period with respect to renal function requires an understanding of the (1) anatomy and physiology of the kidney, (2) tests used for evaluation of renal function, (3) effects of anesthetics on renal function, (4) changes characteristic of chronic renal disease, (5) differential diagnosis of postoperative oliguria, and (6) pharmacology of diuretics.

ANATOMY AND PHYSIOLOGY OF THE KIDNEY

The functional unit of the kidney is the nephron (Fig. 22-1).[1] The two components of the nephron are the glomerulus and renal tubule. Physiologic function of the kidney is dependent on renal blood flow, glomerular filtration rate, and responses evoked by nonrenal (parathormone and antidiuretic hormone) and renal (renin and prostaglandins) humoral substances.

Glomerulus

The glomerulus is formed by the invagination of a tuft of capillaries into the dilated and blind end of the nephron, known as Bowman's capsule. Each tuft of capillaries arises from a single afferent arteriole and is drained by an efferent arteriole. The hydrostatic pressure inside these capillaries can be varied by changing the tone of their afferent or efferent arterioles.

Renal Tubule

The renal tubule consists of the proximal convoluted tubule, the loop of Henle, and the distal convoluted tubule. Several distal convoluted tubules join to form the collecting ducts which subsequently drain into the renal pelvis.

Proximal Convoluted Tubule and Loop of Henle.

The proximal convoluted tubule and loop of Henle are a direct continuation of Bowman's capsule. Most of the filtered sodium, chloride, potassium, bicarbonate, protein, and water is reabsorbed from the proximal convoluted tubule and loop of Henle back into the peritubular capillaries. This reabsorption results in an increase in the osmolarity of the filtrate as it travels distally along the renal tubule.

Glucose is actively reabsorbed in the proximal convoluted tubule. When the blood glucose concentration exceeds about 180 mg/dl the reabsorption threshold is exceeded and glucose appears in the urine. Parathormone acts on the proximal convoluted tubule to facilitate reabsorption of calcium and excretion of phosphate.

305

RENAL TUBULE

GLOMERULUS

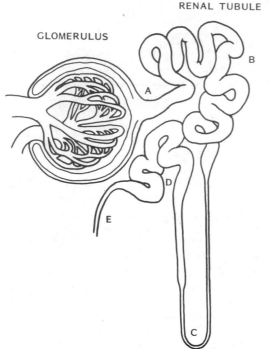

Figure 22-1. Anatomically the nephron consists of the glomerulus and renal tubule. Each glomerulus arises from a single afferent arteriole and the capillaries of this arteriole invaginate the dilated end of the renal tubule known as Bowman's capsule (A). In addition to Bowman's capsule, the renal tubule consists of the proximal convoluted tubule (B), loop of Henle (C), and distal convoluted tubule (D). Several distal convoluted tubules join to form a collecting duct (E) which then drains into the renal pelvis. (Hilgenberg JC. Renal disease. In: Stoelting RK, Dierdorf SF, eds. Anesthesia and co-existing disease. New York, Churchill Livingstone 1983:379–409.)

Distal Convoluted Tubule and Collecting Duct. The distal convoluted tubule and collecting duct are responsible for determining the optimal volume and composition of urine delivered to the renal pelvis. Antidiuretic hormone, released in response to an increase in serum osmolarity, acts on the distal convoluted tubule cells to increase their permeability to water. As a result, water is reabsorbed and the urine becomes more concentrated. Sodium is actively reabsorbed in the distal convoluted tubule, carrying along chloride passively and creating a gradient that favors the secretion of potassium. In general, any event (see the section *Pharmacology of Diuretics*) that increases distal delivery of sodium to the distal tubule will result in increased reabsorption of sodium and secretion of potassium. Hydrogen ion (H^+) secretion and bicarbonate ion (HCO_3^-) reabsorption are also fine-tuned in the distal convoluted tubules. The ability of distal convoluted tubule cells to secrete H^+ is limited because the lowest urine pH that the kidney can achieve by this mechanism is 4.5. However, these same renal tubule cells can also secrete ammonia which combines with H^+ to form ammonium (see Chapter 17). This combination offsets the decrease in urine pH and permits the further secretion of H^+ into the urine.

Renal Blood Flow

Renal blood flow is equivalent to about 20 percent of the cardiac output despite the fact the kidneys represent only 0.5 percent of total body weight. About 25 percent of resting renal oxygen consumption is used for basal metabolism. The majority of oxygen consumption in the kidneys is to support active transport of substances such as sodium and chloride across the renal tubules. It is estimated that two-thirds of the renal blood flow is to the renal cortex. The impact, if any, of anesthetic drugs on distribution of blood flow between the renal cortex and medulla is not known. It is known, however, that positive pressure ventilation of the lungs is associated with a decrease in renal cortical blood flow.[1] Renal blood flow and glomerular filtration rate remain constant at mean arterial pressures ranging from 60 to 160 mmHg. This ability to maintain renal blood flow constant despite changes in perfusion pressure is known as autoregulation. Autoregulation occurs in denervated and isolated-perfused kidneys and, therefore, is under the control of an intrinsic mechanism that has not yet been elucidated. The importance of autoregulation is to protect glomerular capillaries from large increases in pressure during acute hypertensive episodes and to maintain glomerular filtration and renal tubule function during modest decreases in blood pressure. Outside the range of mean arterial pressure associated with autoregulation, renal blood flow becomes pressure-dependent.

Autoregulation does not preclude changes in renal blood flow due to other mechanisms. For example, renal blood flow is influenced by activity of the sympathetic nervous system and the release of renin. Indeed, the kidneys are richly innervated by sympathetic nervous system nerves originating from T4 to L4. Sympathetic nervous system stimulation produces renal vascular vasoconstriction with marked reductions in renal blood flow even if blood pressure is maintained in the range associated with autoregulation. Any reduction in renal blood flow will initiate release of renin which can further reduce renal blood flow (see the section *Humoral Substances*). Release of prostaglandins from the kidney produces vasodilation and can offset the renal artery vasoconstriction that results from release of renin[1] (see the section *Humoral Substances*).

Glomerular Filtration Rate

Hydrostatic pressure in the glomerular capillaries is about 50 mmHg. This pressure acts to force water and other low molecular weight substances such as electrolytes through the glomerular capillaries into Bowman's space. The outward filtration force produced by hydrostatic pressure is opposed by the plasma oncotic pressure. The plasma oncotic pressure is about 25 mmHg at the afferent arteriole and with the filtration of electrolytes increases to about 35 mmHg at the efferent arteriole. Despite the relatively low net filtration pressure, the glomerular capillaries are able to filter plasma at a rate equivalent to about 125 ml/min. Glomerular filtration rate is reduced by decreased mean arterial pressure or reductions in renal blood flow. Ultimately, about 90 percent of the fluid resulting from glomerular filtration is reabsorbed into the circulation during its passage along the renal tubule and thus returned to the circulation.

Humoral Substances

Renin is a proteolytic enzyme secreted by the juxtaglomerular apparatus of the kidney in response to (1) sympathetic nervous system stimulation, (2) decreased renal perfusion pressure, and (3) reductions in the delivery of sodium to the distal convoluted tubule. Renin acts on an alpha-2-globulin in the plasma to form angiotensin I. Angiotensin I is then split by converting enzyme in the lungs to form angiotensin II. Angiotensin II is a potent vasoconstrictor and an important stimulus for the release of aldosterone from the adrenal cortex.

Prostaglandins are produced in the renal medulla and released in response to sympathetic nervous system stimulation and elevated levels of angiotensin II. Prostaglandins designated as PGE_2 and PGI_2 are vasodilators that tend to offset the reductions in renal blood flow produced by vasoconstrictive stimuli.[1]

TESTS USED FOR EVALUATION OF RENAL FUNCTION

Renal function can be evaluated preoperatively by laboratory tests that reflect glomerular filtration rate and renal tubule function (Table 22-1). These tests are not sensitive measurements and significant renal disease can exist despite normal laboratory values. Furthermore, trends are more useful than a single laboratory measurement for evaluating renal function.

Table 22-1. Tests Used for Evaluation of Renal Function

Glomerular Filtration Rate	Renal Tubule Function
Blood urea nitrogen	Urine specific gravity
Serum creatinine	Urine osmolarity
Creatinine clearance	Urine sodium
Proteinuria	

Blood Urea Nitrogen

Blood urea nitrogen concentration (normal 10 to 20 mg/dl) varies with the glomerular filtration rate. Nevertheless, the influence of dietary intake, associated illnesses, and intravascular fluid volume on the blood urea nitrogen concentration make this a potentially misleading test of renal function. For example, the production of urea is increased by a high protein diet or gastrointestinal bleeding, resulting in an elevated blood urea nitrogen concentration despite a normal glomerular filtration rate. Other causes for an increased blood urea nitrogen concentration despite a normal glomerular filtration rate include increased catabolism during a febrile illness and dehydration. An increased blood urea nitrogen concentration in the presence of dehydration most likely reflects increased urea absorption due to slow movement of fluid through the renal tubules. When slow movement of fluid through the renal tubules is responsible for elevation of the blood urea nitrogen concentration, the serum creatinine level remains normal. Blood urea nitrogen concentration can remain normal in the presence of a low protein diet (hemodialysis patients) despite a reduction in glomerular filtration rate. Finally, a low blood urea nitrogen concentration (less than 10 mg/dl) can reflect an excess total body water content. Despite these extraneous influences, a blood urea nitrogen concentration above 50 mg/dl almost always reflects a decreased glomerular filtration rate.

Serum Creatinine

Serum creatinine concentration is a specific indicator of the glomerular filtration rate. In contrast to the blood urea nitrogen concentration, the serum creatinine level is not influenced by protein metabolism or the rate of fluid flow through the renal tubule. As a guide, a 50 percent increase in the serum creatinine concentration reflects a similar decrease in the glomerular filtration rate. Creatinine is a product of skeletal muscle metabolism and its release into the circulation is believed to be relatively constant. The serum creatinine concentration is influenced by skeletal muscle mass such that normal levels (0.7 to 1.5 mg/dl) tend to be higher in muscular males than females. Conversely, the maintenance of normal serum creatinine concentrations in elderly patients with known reductions in glomerular filtration rates reflects decreased creatinine production due to reduced skeletal muscle mass that accompanies aging. Indeed, mild elevations in serum creatinine concentrations in elderly patients should suggest significant renal disease. Likewise, in patients with chronic renal failure, serum creatinine concentrations may not accurately reflect the glomerular filtration rate because of decreased creatinine production in the presence of reduced skeletal muscle mass. Finally, it must be recognized that acute reductions or even cessation of glomerular filtration are not rapidly reflected by measurement of the serum creatinine concentration as it takes 24 to 48 hours for equilibration to occur.[1]

Creatinine Clearance

Creatinine clearance (normal 110 to 150 ml/min) measures the ability of the glomeruli to excrete creatinine into the urine for a given serum creatinine concentration. This measurement does not depend on corrections for age or the presence of a steady state. As such, creatinine clearance is the most reliable measurement of the glomerular filtration rate. The major disadvantage of this test is the need for timed (ideally for 24 hours) urine collections. Preoperatively, the patient with a creatinine clearance between 10 to 25 ml/min must be considered at risk for developing prolonged or adverse responses to drugs, such as the nondepolarizing muscle relaxants, that depend on renal excretion. In these patients, the doses of such drugs should be reduced and fluid and electrolyte replacement carefully monitored.

Proteinuria

Small amounts of protein are normally filtered through glomerular capillaries and then reabsorbed in the proximal convoluted tubules. Proteinuria (excretion of greater than 150 mg/day of protein) is most likely due to abnormally high filtration rather than impaired reabsorption by the renal tubules. At a constant rate of loss, the concentration of protein in the urine will be inversely related to urine volume. Thus, a 2 plus protein in dilute urine signifies a greater excretion rate than 2 plus protein in highly concentrated urine. Intermittent proteinuria occasionally occurs in healthy individuals when standing and disappears when supine. Other nonrenal causes of proteinuria include exercise, fever, and congestive heart failure. Severe proteinuria may result in hypoalbuminemia with associated reductions in plasma oncotic pressure and decreased protein binding of drugs.

Urine Concentrating Ability

The diagnosis of renal tubule dysfunction is established by demonstrating that the kidneys do not produce appropriately concentrated urine in the presence of a physiologic stimulus for the release of antidiuretic hormone. In the absence of diuretic therapy or glycosuria, a urinary specific gravity above 1.018 after an overnight fast, as precedes elective surgery, suggests that the ability of renal tubules to concentrate urine is adequate.[1] High output renal failure following anesthesia with drugs such as methoxyflurane and, rarely, enflurance reflects the inability of renal tubules to concentrate urine in the presence of high serum concentrations of fluoride[1] (see Chapter 5). Other causes of inability of the renal tubules to adequately concentrate urine include (1) hypokalemia, (2) hypercalcemia, (3) chronic pyelonephritis, and (4) treatment with diuretics or lithium.

Sodium Excretion

Urinary excretion of greater than 40 mEq/L of sodium reflects a decreased ability of the renal tubules to reabsorb sodium. Examples of sodium wasting by the renal tubules include (1) drug-induced diuresis (see the section *Pharmacology of Diuretics*), (2) adrenal insufficiency, and (3) hypoaldosteronism.

EFFECTS OF ANESTHETICS ON RENAL FUNCTION

Anesthetics can alter renal function by their effects on the systemic circulation and the sympathetic nervous system. In rare instances, drugs used for anesthesia produce direct nephrotoxicity (see Chapter 5).

Decreased urinary output during anesthesia suggests the release of antidiuretic hormone. However, serum concentrations of antidiuretic hormone have not been shown to change during halothane or morphine anesthesia (Fig. 22-2).[2] Instead, painful stimulation associated with the onset of surgery produces significant increases in circulating levels of antidiuretic hormone. Positive pressure ventilation of the lungs as well as positive end-expiratory pressure can also stimulate the release of antidiuretic hormone presumably by altering left atrial pressure, leading to activation of baroreceptors.[3] Hydration before the induction of anesthesia attenuates the rise in serum antidiuretic hormone concentrations produced by surgical stimulation. Likewise, the increase in circulating renin levels produced by surgical stimulation is attenuated by prior hydration. Like antidiuretic hormone, there is no evidence that anesthetics in the absence of surgical stimulation evoke the release of renin.[4]

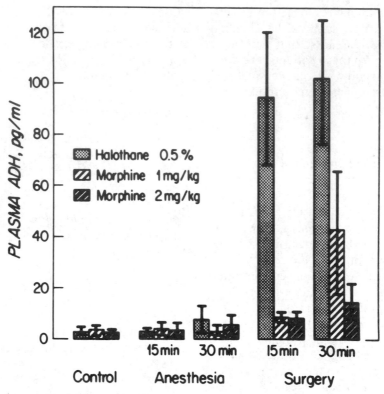

Figure 22-2. Plasma antidiuretic hormone (ADH) levels (mean ± SE) in adult patients were not altered from control measurements during anesthesia. Surgical stimulation increased ADH concentrations particularly in patients receiving halothane. (Philbin DM, Coggins CH. Plasma antidiuretic hormone levels in cardiac surgical patients during morphine and halothane anesthesia Anesthesiology 1978;49:95–8.)

Systemic Circulation

Volatile anesthetics most likely depress renal function by producing dose-dependent decreases in cardiac output and reductions in blood pressure. The net effect is a decrease in renal blood flow, glomerular filtration rate, and urine output during anesthesia. For example, nitrous oxide plus equivalent concentrations of halothane, enflurane or isoflurane produce similar reductions (20 to 40 percent) in renal blood flow and glomerular filtration rate.[1] During administration of halothane, these reductions in renal blood flow and glomerular filtration rate are attenuated by preoperative hydration and administration of low concentra-

tions of the anesthetic (Table 22-2).[5] Although similar data are not available for enflurane or isoflurane, it seems likely that preoperative hydration would produce similar effects.

Alterations in the autoregulation of renal blood flow due to effects produced by volatile anesthetics could exaggerate the changes in renal function that occur in response to blood pressure reductions produced by the anesthetic. Animal studies, however, suggest that halothane, with or without thiopental or nitrous oxide, does not alter autoregulation of renal blood flow (Fig. 22-3).[6] The impact, if any, of enflurane or isoflurane on autoregulation of renal blood flow has not been determined.

Table 22-2. Impact of Inspired Concentration of Halothane and Preoperative Hydration on Renal Function

Inspired Halothane Concentration (%)	Preoperative Hydration	% Decrease from Control	
		Renal Blood Flow	Glomerular Filtration Rate
0.5–1.0	No	61	48
	Yes	12	8
1.2–3.0	No	69	58
	Yes	47	40

(Hilgenberg, JC. Renal Disease. In: Stoelting RK, Dierdorf SF, eds. Anesthesia and Co-Existing Disease. New York, Churchill Livingstone 1983:129–33, with data from ref. 5.)

Changes in renal function during barbiturate-narcotic-nitrous oxide anesthesia are similar to those observed during administration of low concentrations of volatile anesthetics.[1] Droperidol-fentanyl (Innovar) or high dose morphine (2 mg/kg) produced no significant changes in renal blood flow or glomerular rate.[1] The addition of nitrous oxide to droperidol-fentanyl or morphine results in renal function changes similar to those observed during administration of volatile anesthetics. This response most likely reflects a reduction in cardiac output produced by nitrous oxide, leading to a decrease in renal blood flow. Epidural or spinal block results in minimal changes in renal blood flow and glomerular filtration rate. When alterations in renal hemodynamics occur during regional anesthesia, the most likely explanation is a decrease in the systemic blood pressure.

Sympathetic Nervous System

The renal vasculature is richly innervated by the sympathetic nervous system (T4-L4) such that drug-induced changes in systemic vascular resistance can lead to alterations

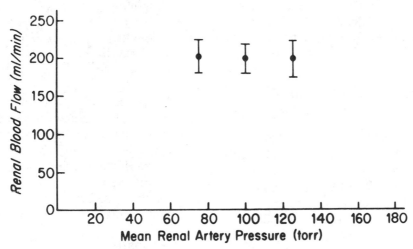

Figure 22-3. Halothane administered to dogs did not alter autoregulation as evidenced by an unchanging renal blood flow despite changes in mean renal artery pressure. (Bastron RD, Perkins FM, Pyne JL. Autoregulation of renal blood flow during halothane anesthesia. Anesthesiology 1977;46:142–4.)

in renal blood flow and glomerular filtration rate. For example, ketamine is associated with decreased renal blood flow and glomerular filtration rate despite increases in cardiac output and mean arterial pressure.[7] Presumably, these changes reflect constriction of renal vasculature by ketamine-induced increases in sympathetic nervous system activity. Conversely, volatile anesthetics that reduce sympathetic nervous system activity might reduce renal vascular resistance. Indeed, low concentrations of halothane partially restore renal blood flow when administered to animals in hemorrhagic shock.[8] It is speculated this change reflects a halothane-induced reduction in sympathetic nervous system activity with a subsequent reduction in renal vascular resistance.

Direct Nephrotoxicity

It could be argued that all anesthetics are direct nephrotoxins since these drugs produce generalized depression of measurable renal function. This depression, however, is transient and usually clinically insignificant. The exception to this generalization is nephrotoxicity produced by fluoride, resulting from metabolic breakdown of some halogenated anesthetics (see Chapter 5).

CHANGES CHARACTERISTIC OF CHRONIC RENAL DISEASE

Chronic renal disease is characterized by a progressive decrease in the number of functioning nephrons, leading to an irreversible reduction in the glomerular filtration rate. Rational management of anesthesia in patients with chronic renal disease requires an understanding of those pathologic changes that accompany renal disease (Table 22-3). Furthermore, the management of anesthesia is influenced by whether the renal disease is sufficient to require hemodialysis (Table 22-4).

Table 22-3. Changes Characteristic of Chronic Renal Disease

Anemia
Increased cardiac output
Decreased platelet adhesiveness
Hyperkalemia
Unpredictable intravascular fluid volume
Metabolic acidosis
Systemic hypertension
Decreased sympathetic nervous system activity
Increased susceptibility to sepsis

Anemia

A hemoglobin concentration in the range of 5 to 8 g/dl (hematocrit 20 to 25 percent) is a hallmark of chronic renal disease. Decreased production of erythropoietin is the most likely explanation for the reduced production of red blood cells. This anemia is well tolerated because of its slow onset which permits time for compensatory increases in cardiac output and to a lesser extent 2,3 diphosphoglycerate concentrations to occur. The greatest hazard of anemia is decreased oxygen carrying capacity, which can result in tissue hypoxia. The importance of increased tissue blood flow in offsetting the effects of anemia emphasizes the need to minimize changes in cardiac output produced by volatile anesthetics (use low concentrations) and positive pressure ventilation of the lungs (use slow ventilatory rate to assure time for venous return between breaths).

Attempts to correct the anemia preoperatively are not recommended unless there is a history of cardiopulmonary dysfunction that limits daily activity. In these patients, the preoperative administration of erythrocytes should be considered. Whole blood is not a logical selection, as the excess volume may contribute to fluid overload.

Coagulopathies

Coagulopathies must be suspected in any patient with chronic renal disease. The most likely coagulation defect is decreased platelet adhesiveness as reflected by a prolonged

Table 22-4. Management of Anesthesia in Patients with Chronic Renal Disease

	Does Not Require Hemodialysis	Requires Hemodialysis
Induction	Thiopental-succinylcholine	Thiopental-succinylcholine
Maintenance	Nitrous oxide plus isoflurane or halothane or fentanyl	Nitrous oxide plus isoflurane or enflurane or fentanyl
Paralysis	d-Tubocurarine or pancuronium or atracurium or vecuronium	d-Tubocurarine or pancuronium or atracurium or vecuronium

bleeding time. Hemodialysis is usually effective in reversing this platelet dysfunction. The possibility of impaired coagulation must be remembered when considering a regional anesthetic technique in patients with chronic renal disease.

Electrolyte and Hydration Status

Hyperkalemia is the most serious electrolyte abnormality associated with chronic renal disease (see Chapter 18). Even when hemodialysis has been performed in the previous 6 to 8 hours, the serum potassium concentration should be measured before induction of anesthesia, since unexpected hyperkalemia can occur rapidly. If surgery cannot be delayed, the serum potassium concentration can be lowered by hyperventilation (a 10 mmHg decrease in $PaCO_2$ or 0.1 unit increase in pH lowers serum potassium about 0.5 mEq/L) and/or intravenous infusion of a glucose-insulin mixture (25 grams of glucose plus 10 to 15 units of regular insulin). Sodium bicarbonate is indicated if metabolic acidosis accompanies hyperkalemia.

Regardless of hydration status, patients with chronic renal disease often respond to induction of anesthesia as if they are hypovolemic. The likelihood of hypotension during induction of anesthesia may be increased if sympathetic nervous system function is attenuated by antihypertensives. Attenuated sympathetic nervous system activity produced by these drugs impairs compensatory peripheral vasoconstriction, such that a small decrease in blood volume, positive pressure ventilation of the lungs, or sudden changes in body position can result in exaggerated reductions in blood pressure.

Metabolic Acidosis

Chronic renal disease interferes with the normal renal excretion of H^+ leading to the appearance of metabolic acidosis. Hemodialysis is effective in restoring the arterial pH (pHa) to nearly normal values. Acidosis in the renal patient is particularly undesirable, since a low pHa favors an extracellular rather than intracellular distribution of potassium.

Systemic Hypertension

Hypertension is a frequent complication of chronic renal disease. Preoperative hypertension is most often due to fluid overload and is best treated by hemodialysis. Refractory hypertension occurs in 10 to 15 percent of patients despite hemodialysis and requires treatment with antihypertensives. Management of hypertension in the perioperative period is with vasodilators such as hydralazine or nitroprusside.

Sepsis

The most common cause of death in patients with chronic renal disease is sepsis often originating from a pulmonary infection. A high incidence of viral hepatitis most likely reflects the frequent use of blood products as well as the effects of immunosuppression. Strict attention to asepsis is important when placing vascular cannulae and tracheal tubes in these patients.

Management of Anesthesia

Patients on hemodialysis undergoing elective surgery should undergo hemodialysis prior to surgery. Regardless of the severity of renal disease, induction of anesthesia and intubation of the trachea can be safely accomplished with the intravenous injection of an ultrashort-acting barbiturate plus succinylcholine. Potassium release following the administration of succinylcholine is not exaggerated in normokalemic patients with chronic renal disease.[9] Caution is necessary, however, when the preoperative serum potassium concentration is in a high normal range, since this combined with a high normal increase of the serum potassium concentration (0.5 to 1 mEq/L) after administration of succinylcholine could result in dangerous hyperkalemia. A theoretical but undocumented concern is the potential for exaggerated potassium release following administration of succinylcholine to patients with neuropathies associated with chronic uremia. Early membranes used for hemodialysis absorbed cholinesterase, leading to the potential for a prolonged response to succinylcholine. Currently used membranes for hemodialysis, however, do not absorb this enzyme.

Maintenance of anesthesia is ideally achieved with nitrous oxide combined with a volatile anesthetic (Table 22-4). Some avoid nitrous oxide so as to permit administration of a higher inspired concentration of oxygen. Potent volatile anesthetics are useful in controlling intraoperative hypertension and reducing the dose of muscle relaxant needed for adequate surgical relaxation. Halothane is often avoided in patients requiring hemodialysis in view of the high incidence of co-existing liver disease due to viral hepatitis in these patients. Likewise, enflurane is an unlikely selection when chronic renal disease is present but not so severe as to require hemodialysis. Anemia reduces blood solubility of the volatile anesthetics, which could speed the rate at which the alveolar concentration can be increased or decreased. Excessive depression of cardiac output is a potential hazard of volatile anesthetics. Narcotics decrease the likelihood of cardiovascular depression, and avoid the concern of hepatotoxicity, but have the disadvantage of being ineffective for controlling intraoperative hypertension.

Meticulous attention must be paid to management of ventilation and intravenous fluid replacement. Normocapnia is ideal, as hyperventilation with associated respiratory alkalosis adversely affects the position of the oxyhemoglobin dissociation curve while respiratory acidosis from hypoventilation could result in acute increases in the serum potassium concentration. Measurement of central venous pressure is useful in guiding fluid replacement. Monitoring of the electrocardiogram is important for recognizing signs of hyperkalemia. Finally, arteriovenous shunts must be carefully protected to assure continued patency during the perioperative period.

Brachial plexus block is useful for the placement of vascular shunts in the arm as are necessary for hemodialysis. The duration of brachial plexus block produced by local anesthetics is shortened by nearly 40 percent in patients with chronic renal disease.[10] It is presumed that increased tissue blood flow due to elevated cardiac output results in a more rapid clearance of the local anesthetic from the active site, leading to a shorter duration of block.

The most perplexing problem regarding altered drug responses in patients with chronic renal disease relates to the use of nondepolarizing muscle relaxants, as many of these drugs undergo extensive renal excretion (see Chapter 8). In favor of the use of d-tubodurarine is its elimination in the bile plus evidence that only about 50 percent of an injected dose is eliminated by the kidneys.[11] The disadvantage of d-tubocurarine is peripheral vasodilation which may produce undesirable hypotension. In contrast, pancuronium is more dependent on renal excretion than is d-tubocurarine but reductions in blood pressure are unlikely. The dependence of atracurium and vecuronium on nonrenal mechanisms for elimination makes these drugs attractive selections for administration to patients with renal dysfunction. Regardless of the muscle relaxant selected, it would seem prudent to reduce the initial dose of drug and to administer subsequent doses based on the response observed using a peripheral nerve stimulator.

A diagnosis of recurarization following reversal of nondepolarizing neuromuscular block with an anticholinesterase should be considered in anephric patients who manifest signs of skeletal muscle weakness in the early postoperative period. In normal patients who are adequately reversed with an anticholnesterase, recurarization does not occur, since continued renal elimination of the muscle relaxant offsets waning effects of the anticholinesterase. Even in anephric patients, there is some protection, since renal elimination of the anticholinesterase is delayed to the same degree as the muscle relaxant. Indeed, other explanations (antibiotics, acidosis, electrolyte imbalance, diuretics) should be considered when recurarization occurs in the patient with renal dysfunction. Finally, caution must be exercised in the use of narcotics for postoperative analgesia in these patients in view of the possibility of exaggerated central nervous system and ventilatory depression after even small doses of narcotics.

DIFFERENTIAL DIAGNOSIS OF PERIOPERATIVE OLIGURIA

Perioperative oliguria (less than 0.5 ml/kg/hr) is classified as prerenal oliguria or acute tubular necrosis.

Prerenal Oliguria

Prerenal oliguria is characterized by excretion of concentrated urine (greater than 400 mOsm/L) containing minimal (less than 40 mEq/L) amounts of sodium. The excretion of a highly concentrated and sodium poor urine confirms that renal tubule function is intact and reflects an attempt by the kidneys to conserve sodium and restore intravascular fluid volume in response to decreased renal blood flow. Decreased renal blood flow most likely reflects an acute reduction in intravascular fluid volume or a decreased cardiac output.

Treatment. A brisk diuresis in response to the rapid infusion of 3 to 6 ml/kg of lactated Ringer's solution (fluid challenge) suggests that an acute reduction in intravascular fluid volume is the cause of prerenal oliguria. Patients with this degree of hypovolemia will need continued intravenous fluid administration, since an extracellular fluid depletion of over 25 percent is required to produce oliguria. When fluid replacement does not result in an improved urine output, the possibility of decreased renal blood flow due to a low cardiac output should be considered. Dopamine (3 to 5 μg/kg/min) is an ideal drug to administer when oliguria is due to a reduced cardiac output. A small dose of furosemide (5 mg) may re-establish urine output in the presence of oliguria due to pain-induced release of antidiuretic hormone. Conversely, this small dose of diuretic is unlikely to reverse oliguria due to decreased renal blood flow. Finally, if a urinary catheter is in place, it is important to confirm its patency.

The use of diuretics to maintain or stimulate urine flow in the perioperative period is controversial. Some feel that prevention of renal tubule urine stasis with a diuretic such as furosemide can prevent prerenal oliguria from progressing to acute tubular necrosis. Nevertheless, supportive evidence for this conclusion is not available.[12] Under any circumstance, it is crucial to restore intravascular fluid volume prior to administration of diuretics, as drug-induced diuresis could exaggerate hypovolemia and further reduce renal blood flow. Measurement of central venous pressure or pulmonary artery occlusion pressure is helpful in evaluating the adequacy of volume replacement prior to administration of a diuretic. Another disadvantage of diuretics is the impairment of sodium reabsorption for at least 6 to 12 hours, making the urine of prerenal oliguria indistinguishable from the urine excreted in the presence of acute tubular necrosis.

Acute Tubular Necrosis

Acute tubular necrosis is another cause of perioperative oliguria. In contrast to oliguria due to hypovolemia, the urine of patients developing acute tubular necrosis contains excessive amounts of sodium (greater than 40 mEq/L) and is poorly concentrated. Hyperkalemia can accompany acute tubular necrosis, reflecting the release of potassium from surgically damaged tissues. In the absence of renal function, the serum potassium concentration increases at a rate of 0.3 to 0.5 mEq/L/day. Following surgery, however, the increase may be 1 to 2 mEq/L/day Furthermore, in patients with extensive tissue injury, the rate of increase in the serum potassium concentration may be as high as 1 to 2 mEq/L/hour. For this reason, the serum concentration of potassium should be monitored frequently when acute tubular necrosis is suspected.

PHARMACOLOGY OF DIURETICS

The frequent administration of diuretics to patients undergoing anesthesia and operation emphasizes the need to appreciate the pharmacology of these drugs. Diuretics are categorized as thiazide diuretics, loop diuretics, potassium-sparing diuretics, carbonic anhydrase inhibitors, and osmotic diuretics.

Thiazide Diuretics

Thiazide diuretics inhibit the reabsorption of sodium and chloride by the renal tubules. This inhibition results in increased urinary loss of sodium, chloride, and water plus augmentation of secretion of potassium. Hypochloremic, hypokalemic metabolic alkalosis is a consequence of prolonged administration of thiazide diuretics. Orthostatic hypotension reflects diuretic-induced reductions in intravascular fluid volume. Thiazide diuretics are most often used in the treatment of ambulatory essential hypertension.

Loop Diuretics

Loop diuretics (ethacrynic acid, furosemide) are the most potent diuretics available. These drugs inhibit sodium and chloride reabsorption and augment secretion of potassium in the loop of Henle and the distal convoluted tubule. These combined effects will result in hypochloremic, hypokalemic metabolic alkalosis. Contraction of the extracellular fluid volume (manifesting as orthostatic hypotension) is rapidly produced by these drugs. Furosemide is primarily used in the treatment of acute pulmonary edema and in the differential diagnosis of acute renal failure. Loop diuretics, however, must not be used to treat oliguria due to decreased intravascular fluid volume, as the drug-induced diuresis may further exaggerate hypovolemia and aggravate renal ischemic changes.

Potassium-Sparing Diuretics

Potassium sparing diuretics (triamterene, spironolactone) are used in combination with thiazide diuretics. Triamterene acts in the distal convoluted tubule to block sodium reabsorption and potassium secretion that is unrelated to aldosterone. Spironolactone acts by antagonizing the effects of aldosterone. Hyperkalemia is a potential adverse effect of potassium-sparing diuretics.

Carbonic Anhydrase Inhibitors

The most commonly used carbonic anhydrase inhibitor is acetazolamide. Acetazolamide inhibits reabsorption of HCO_3^-

and prevents secretion of H^+ by the proximal convoluted tubule. These effects cause urinary loss of HCO_3^- and potassium, resulting in hypokalemic metabolic acidosis.

Osmotic Diuretics

The most frequently administered osmotic diuretic is the six-carbon sugar, mannitol. Mannitol produces diuresis because it is filtered by the glomeruli but not reabsorbed in the renal tubules, leading to the excretion of water. In addition, mannitol increases plasma osmolarity which will then draw fluid from intracellular spaces into extracellular spaces and thus expand, acutely, the intravascular fluid volume. This redistribution of fluid from intracellular to extracellular compartments decreases brain size and may increase renal blood flow. Indeed, mannitol is used most often to reduce intracranial pressure and to protect the kidneys from acute tubular necrosis. In patients who are oliguric secondary to congestive heart failure, however, mannitol-induced increases in extracellular fluid volume may precipitate pulmonary edema.

The preoperative and intraoperative administration of mannitol seems to be particularly beneficial in preventing postoperative renal failure in jaundiced patients (see Chapter 21) or patients undergoing resection of abdominal aortic aneurysms. The value, however, of mannitol after oliguria has developed is not well established.

Urea is an osmotic diuretic that crosses the blood brain barrier more readily than mannitol, resulting in a greater degree of rebound intracranial hypertension. For this reason, urea is not as popular as mannitol for use as an osmotic diuretic.

TRANSURETHRAL SURGERY

Transurethral resection of the prostate (TURP) or bladder tumors entails the excision of tissue and coagulation of bleeding vessels through a modified cystoscope. The use of continuous irrigation with fluid is necessary to improve visibility through the cystoscope, distend the prostatic urethra or bladder, and maintain the operative field free of blood and dissected tissue. Complications of transurethral surgery include (1) intravascular absorption of irrigating fluid, (2) hemorrhage, and (3) perforation of the bladder or urethra.

Intravascular Absorption of Irrigating Fluid

The opening of venous sinuses in association with transurethral surgery leads to intravascular absorption of irrigating fluid. The amount of irrigating fluid absorbed depends on the hydrostatic pressure of the fluid (determined by the height of the fluid container above the patient), the number and size of the venous sinuses opened, and the duration of the resection.

Fluids suitable for irrigation must be non-electrolytic to prevent the dispersion of high frequency electrical current from the operative area. These fluids should also be transparent and nontoxic to tissues. In the past, distilled water was a popular irrigating fluid because of superior visibility. Nevertheless, distilled water cannot be recommended, as intravascular absorption of this hypotonic fluid produces hemolysis. Commonly used irrigating fluids that are nonhemolytic and nearly isotonic include glycine and Cytal. Glycine is an amino acid that normally occurs in the body. A metabolite of glycine is ammonia, but complications from this substance are rarely observed clinically. Nevertheless, prolonged central nervous system depression following use of glycine as the irrigating fluid should suggest the possibility of ammonia toxicity.[13] Cytal is the trade name for the irrigating solution that consists of two sugars, mannitol and sorbitol. The major problem associated with Cytal is the possibility of bacterial contamination, as the sugars provide an excellent culture medium.

Absorption of large volumes of isotonic irrigating fluids produces symptoms of acute increases in intravascular fluid volume and dilution of electrolytes, especially sodium. Early signs of increasing intravascular fluid volume include hypertension and reflex bradycardia. If the transurethral resection continues, pulmonary edema and congestive heart failure eventually occur. Cerebral edema and increased intracranial pressure manifest as headache, restlessness, confusion, and eventually mental obtundation. Seizures are likely when the volume of intravascular fluid absorption is sufficiently large to abruptly reduce the serum sodium concentration below 120 mEq/L.

Management of Anesthesia

Management of anesthesia for transurethral surgery is with a regional or general anesthetic. A T10 sensory level is necessary when a regional anesthetic is selected for transurethral surgery that includes distension of the bladder. Advantages cited for a regional anesthetic include the ability of an awake patient to voice symptoms suggestive of bladder perforation and/or excessive intravascular absorption of irrigating fluid. For example, bladder perforation is often accompanied by complaints of shoulder discomfort that reflects referred pain due to subdiaphragmatic irritation of the diaphragm by extravasated irrigating fluid. Despite the alleged advantages of a regional anesthetic, there is no evidence of differences in morbidity or mortality when a general anesthetic is selected. Regardless of the technique of anesthesia selected, it is important to monitor the patient carefully for signs and symptoms of excessive intravascular absorption of irrigating fluid. In addition to monitoring blood pressure, heart rate, and the electrocardiogram, it may be prudent to measure central venous pressure and obtain periodic blood samples for determination of serum osmolarity and so-dium concentration. Resection time should be limited to as brief a time as possible. Based on an estimated intravascular absorption of irrigating fluid equal to 20 ml/min, the usual recommended resection time is 1 hour. It must be appreciated, however, that times as short as 15 minutes have resulted in symptoms of excessive intravascular absorption of irrigating fluid.[14]

REFERENCES

1. Hilgenberg JC. Renal disease. In: Stoelting RK, Dierdorf SF, eds. Anesthesia and co-existing disease. New York, Churchill Livingstone 1983:379–409.
2. Philbin DM, Coggins CH. Plasma antidiuretic hormone levels in cardiac surgical patients during morphine and halothane anesthesia. Anesthesiology 1974;40:95–8.
3. Fewell J, Bond GC. Role of sinoaortic baroreceptors in initiating the renal response to continuous positive-pressure ventilation in the dog. Anesthesiology 1980;52:408–13.
4. Miller ED, Gianfagra W, Ackerly JA, Peach MJ. Converting enzyme activity and pressure responses to angiotensin I and II in the rat awake and during anesthesia. Anesthesiology 1979;50:88–102.
5. Barry KG, Mazze RI, Schwartz FD. Prevention of surgical oliguria and renal hemodynamic suppression by sustained hydration. N Engl J Med 1964;270:1371–7.
6. Bastron RD, Perkins FM, Pyne JL. Autoregulation of renal blood flow during halothane anesthesia. Anesthesiology 1977;46:142–4.
7. Hirasawa H, Yonezawa T. The effects of ketamine and Innovar on the renal cortical and medullary blood flow of the dog. Anaesthetist 1975;24:349–53.
8. Macdonald AG. The effect of halothane on renal cortical blood flow on normotensive hypotensive dogs. Br J Anaesth 1969;41:644–54.
9. Powell DR, Miller RD. The effect of repeated doses of succinylcholine on serum potassium in patients with renal failure. Anesth Analg 1975;54:746–8.
10. Bromage PR, Gertel M. Brachial plexus anesthesia in chronic renal failure. Anesthesiology 1972;36:488–93.

11. Matteo RS, Nishitateno K, Pua EK, Spector S. Pharmacokinetics of d-tubocurarine in man: effect of an osmotic diuretic on urinary excretion. Anesthesiology 1980;52:335–8.

12. Brown RS. Renal dysfunction in the surgical patient-maintenance of the high output state with furosemide. Crit Care Med 1979;7:63–8.

13. Roesch R, Stoelting RK, Lingeman JE, Kahnoski RJ, Backes DJ, Gephardt SA. Ammonia toxicity due to glycine absorption during a transurethral resection of the prostate. Anesthesiology 1983;58:577–9.

14. Hurlbert BJ, Wingard DW. Water intoxication after 15 minutes of transurethral resection of the prostate. Anesthesiology 1979;50:355–6.

23

Endocrine, Metabolic, and Nutritional Disorders

An understanding of the pathophysiology of endocrine gland function, disorders of metabolism, and abnormalities of nutrition is essential for the management of patients in the perioperative period who manifest disorders related to these symptoms.[1] These disorders may be the primary reason for surgery or may co-exist in patients requiring operations unrelated to these disorders.

THYROID GLAND

Thyroid gland dysfunction reflects over- or underproduction of the two physiologically active thyroid gland hormones, triiodothyronine and thyroxine (tetraiodothyronine). Calcitonin (thyrocalcitonin) is a third hormone released by the thyroid gland in response to elevations of the serum calcium concentration.

Synthesis and Secretion

Synthesis and secretion of triiodothyronine and thyroxine is regulated by thyroid stimulating hormone released from the anterior pituitary. Thyroid stimulating hormone release is controlled by thyrotropin-releasing hormone from the hypothalamus as well as the circulating concentration of thyroid gland hormones. Therefore, thyroid gland dysfunction can reflect disease processes involving the hypothalamus, the anterior pituitary, or the thyroid gland itself.

Laboratory Tests

Total serum thyroxine concentration (normal value 4.4 to 9.9 μg/dl) is the standard screening test for evaluation of thyroid gland function. This value will be elevated in about 90 percent of patients with hyperthyroidism and decreased in 85 percent of patients who are hypothyroid.[1] Serum triiodothyronine concentration (normal 150 to 250 ng/dl) is a sensitive test for detection of hyperthyroidism but not hypothyroidism. Measurement of the serum concentration of thyroid stimulating hormone (normal value up to 7 microunits/ml) is the most sensitive screening test for the detection of hypothyroidism.

Hyperthyroidism

Signs and symptoms of hyperthyroidism (fatigue, weight loss, skeletal muscle weakness, heat intolerance, tachycardia, cardiac dysrhythmias, and congestive heart failure) reflect the impact of excess circulating thyroid gland hormones. Excess sympathetic nervous system activity is suggested by a hyperdynamic circulation manifesting as tachycardia, tachydysrhythmias, and increased cardiac output. Nevertheless, there is no evidence that cardiovascular responsiveness to exogenous catecholamines is altered by increased or decreased activity of the thyroid gland.[2] Adrenal cortex hyperplasia reflects increased production and utilization of cortisol.

Management of Anesthesia. Elective surgery should not be considered until the patient has been rendered euthyroid with antithyroid drugs and the hyperdynamic circulation has been controlled with a beta antagonist as evidenced by a resting heart rate less than 90 beats/min.[1] The combined use of propranolol (60 mg every 8 hours) and potassium iodide is effective in rendering most patients euthyroid in 10 days. Alternatively, treatment for 6 to 8 weeks with a specific antithyroid drug, plus an oral iodide solution for 7 to 10 days before surgery, will produce a euthyroid state and reduce the vascularity of the thyroid gland. When surgery cannot be delayed, the management of anesthesia in the hyperthyroid patient is designed to minimize the effects of excess sympathetic nervous system activity.

Induction of anesthesia can be accomplished with the intravenous administration of thiopental. The chemical structure of thiopental is similar to antithyroid drugs, but it is unlikely that a significant antithyroid effect is produced by an induction dose of thiopental. Ketamine is not a good selection for induction of anesthesia because of the ability of this drug to stimulate the sympathetic nervous system.

The possibility of organ toxicity due to altered or accelerated drug metabolism in the presence of hyperthyroidism must be considered when selecting drugs for the maintenance of anesthesia. In animals pretreated with triiodothyronine and exposed to isoflurane, enflurane, or halothane the incidence of hepatic centrilobular necrosis following exposure to the anesthetic was 28, 24, and 92 percent, respectively.[3] Isoflur-

ane, which provides sufficient potency to offset adverse sympathetic nervous system responses to surgical stimulation and at the same time does not sensitize the myocardium to catecholamines or undergo significant metabolism, would seem an ideal selection to combine with nitrous oxide. In view of the increased oxygen consumption characteristic of these patients, it would seem prudent to limit the inspired concentration of nitrous oxide to 50 percent. Nitrous oxide combined with a narcotic such as fentanyl is an alternative to the use of the volatile drugs but has the disadvantage of not providing inhibition of sympathetic nervous system activity. Prior to intubation of the trachea, it is important to produce a depth of anesthesia sufficient to minimize the sympathetic nervous system response elicited by direct laryngoscopy. Administration of succinylcholine or a nondepolarizing muscle relaxant (metocurine, atracurium, vecuronium) which lacks cardiovascular effects is indicated to facilitate intubation of the trachea.

Controlled studies in animals do not support the clinical impression that anesthetic requirements for inhaled drugs (MAC) are increased in the presence of hyperthyroidism (Fig. 23-1).[4] The discrepancy between clinical impression and objective data is presumed to reflect the increased cardiac output characteristic of hyperthyroidism. For example, the increased cardiac output accelerates uptake of inhaled anesthetics, resulting in the need to raise the inhaled concentration of the drug so as to achieve a brain partial pressure similar to that achieved with a lower inhaled concentration in the euthyroid patient. It should be appreciated that accelerated metabolism of the anesthetic does not alter the partial pressure of the drug necessary in the brain to produce the desired pharmacologic effect. Finally, any elevation in body temperature due to hyperthyroidism would be expected to increase anesthetic requirements about 5 percent for every degree that the body temperature exceeds 37 Celsius.

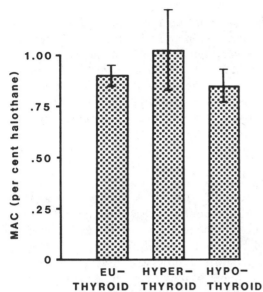

Figure 23-1. The minimum alveolar concentration of halothane (MAC, mean ± SD) measured in dogs was not influenced by the level of activity of the thyroid gland. (Tasch MD. Endocrine diseases. In: Stoelting RK, Dierdorf SF, eds. Anesthesia and co-existing disease. New York, Churchill Livingstone 1983:437–83, with data from reference 4.)

In view of the likely presence of skeletal muscle weakness, it is important to monitor the response produced by muscle relaxants with a peripheral nerve stimulator. When reversal of nondepolarizing neuromuscular blockade is indicated, it may be wise to combine glycopyrrolate rather than atropine with the anticholinesterase so as to minimize the possibility of an excessive increase in heart rate.

Regional anesthesia with its associated block of the sympathetic nervous system is an attractive selection for the hyperthyroid patient requiring surgery on the extremities or lower abdomen. The advantages of a regional anesthetic technique are somewhat offset by the possible need to treat hypotension. Considering the possible sensitivity of these patients to sympathomimetics, it is best to treat hypotension with a reduced dose of phenylephrine if intravenous infusion of fluid is not effective. Epinephrine should not be added to the local anesthetic solution, as systemic absorption of the catecholamine could produce exaggerated circulatory responses.

Constant monitoring of body temperature is mandatory and means to lower body temperature, including cold solutions for intravenous infusion, must be available. The electrocardiogram (ECG) may reveal tachycardia and/or cardiac dysrhythmias, indicating the need for the intravenous administration of propranolol or lidocaine.

Thyroid storm associated with surgery in the hyperthyroid patient can occur intraoperatively but is most likely to manifest in the first 6 to 18 hours after surgery, emphasizing the need to maintain close monitoring of these patients in the early postoperative period. Symptoms of thyroid storm are due to the sudden and excessive release of thyroid gland hormones, leading to hyperthermia, tachycardia, cardiac dysrhythmias, congestive heart failure, dehydration, and shock. Thyroid storm can mimic the onset of malignant hyperthermia.

Treatment of thyroid storm includes intravenous infusion of cold crystalloid solutions, some of which contain glucose, plus administration of drugs to treat specific manifestations of excessive thyroid gland hormone concentrations. Sodium iodide is effective for acutely reducing the release of active hormone from the thyroid gland. Cortisol is indicated to offset the increased endogenous utilization of corticosteroids that could result in acute primary adrenal insufficiency. Propranolol is necessary to alleviate the peripheral effects of thyroid gland hormones on the cardiovascular system. Propylthiouracil is necessary to reduce the synthesis of new thyroid gland hormones, including those that result from the administration of sodium iodide.

Complications Following Total or Partial Thyroidectomy. Damage to the laryngeal nerves, tracheal compression, and inadvertent removal of the parathyroid glands are early complications that can follow thyroid surgery in an euthyroid patient.

Laryngeal Nerves. The entire sensory and motor supply to the larynx is from the two superior and two recurrent laryngeal nerves. The superior laryngeal nerves provide the motor supply to the cricothyroid muscles and sensation above the level of the vocal cords. The recurrent laryngeal nerves supply motor innervation to all the muscles of the larynx except the cricothyroid muscles plus sensation below the level of the vocal cords. Function of the vocal cords following thyroid surgery can be evaluated by asking the patient to say "e." The most common nerve injury following thyroid surgery is damage to the recurrent laryngeal nerve, manifesting as hoarseness and a paralyzed vocal cord which assumes an intermediate position. Bilateral recurrent nerve injury results in aphonia and paralyzed vocal cords that can flap together during inspiration to produce upper airway obstruction. Superior laryngeal nerve paralysis manifests as hoarseness and loss of sensation above the cords, making the patient vulnerable to inhalation of any material present in the pharynx.

Compression of the trachea, leading to airway obstruction, may reflect a hematoma at the operative site or tracheomalacia due to weakening of the tracheal rings by chronic pressure from a goiter. Airway obstruction following extubation of the trachea and in the presence of normal vocal cord function should suggest the diagnosis of tracheomalacia.

Inadvertent Removal of the Parathyroid Glands. Hypoparathyroidism due to inadvertent removal of the parathyroid glands occurs in about 1 percent of patients who undergo a total thyroidectomy. In these patients, signs of hypocalcemia can manifest as early as 1 to 3 hours following surgery but typically do not appear until 24 to 72 hours postoperatively. Laryngeal muscles are very sensitive to hypocalcemia and inspiratory stridor progressing to laryngospasm may be the first suggestion that surgically induced hypoparathyroidism is present (see the section *Hypoparathyroidism*).

Hypothyroidism

Hypothyroidism, as documented by thyroid function tests, is estimated to be present to varying degrees in 0.5 to 0.8 percent of the adult population.[2] Iatrogenic hypothyroidism following surgical or medical treatment of hypothyroidism is responsible for the majority of cases. The development of hypothyroidism in adulthood is insidious and gradual and may go unrecognized, in part because of the associated apathy that minimizes complaints by the patient. Characteristically, there is a generalized reduction in metabolic activity. Lethargy is prominent and intolerance to cold is present. Bradycardia and decreased stroke volume contribute to a significant reduction in cardiac output. Overt congestive heart failure, however, is unlikely and if present may indicate heart disease unrelated to thyroid gland dysfunction. Peripheral vasoconstriction, presumably in an attempt to offset heat loss, leads to the characteristic cool and dry skin in these patients. There is often atrophy of the adrenal cortex and an associated decrease in the production of cortisol. Inappropriate secretion of antidiuretic hormone may result in hyponatremia. Finally, hypothyroidism can be associated with amyloidosis which may include an enlarged tongue, abnormal conduction of the cardiac impulse, and renal disease.

Treatment of hypothyroidism is with exogenous replacement of thyroid gland hormones by oral administration of levo-thyroxine or dessicated thyroid. Intravenous triiodothyronine exerts a physiologic effect within 6 hours, making it the treatment of

Table 23-1. Characteristics of Hypothyroidism Relevant to the Management of Anesthesia

---

Exquisite sensitivity to depressant drugs
Decreased cardiac output
Slowed metabolism of drugs
Decreased intravascular fluid volume
Delayed gastric emptying time
Hyponatremia
Hypothermia
Anemia
Hypoglycemia
Primary adrenal insufficiency
Amyloidosis

---

choice when a rapid response is necessary. Thyroxine requires 10 days to exert a physiologic effect and is, therefore, not effective for emergency treatment of hypothyroidism.

Management of Anesthesia. Elective surgery should not be performed until the patient has been rendered euthyroid.[2] Nevertheless, many cases of hypothyroidism are unrecognized because of the insidious onset of the disease. The possibility of hypothyroidism must be considered in any patient with a history of a previous subtotal thyroidectomy or therapy with radioactive iodine. When surgery cannot be delayed in a known hypothyroid patient, it is important to consider changes characteristic of this disease that have a potential significant impact on management of anesthesia (Table 23-1).

Induction of anesthesia can be accomplished with ketamine. Maintenance of anesthesia is best achieved by inhalation of nitrous oxide plus supplementation if necessary with minimal doses of ketamine, fentanyl, or a benzodiazepine. Volatile anesthetics are not recommended because of the exquisite sensitivity of the hypothyroid patient to drug-induced myocardial depression. The failure of decreases in thyroid activity to reduce anesthetic requirements (MAC) may reflect the maintenance of cerebral metabolic requirements for oxygen that are independent of thyroid activity (Fig. 23-1).[2,4] The reduced skeletal muscle

activity associated with hypothyroidism suggests the possibility of a prolonged response should traditional doses of muscle relaxants be administered to these patients. Pancuronium, because of its mild sympathomimetic effect, would seem an ideal selection for production of skeletal muscle paralysis. Reduced production of carbon dioxide associated with the decreased metabolic rate makes the hypothyroid patient vulnerable to excessive reductions in the $PaCO_2$ during controlled ventilation of the lungs. Since cerebral metabolic requirements for oxygen are not likely to be altered in these patients, it is important to avoid excessive hyperventilation and associated reductions in cerebral blood flow.[2]

Monitoring is directed toward early recognition of congestive heart failure and detection of the onset of hypothermia. Continuous recording of arterial blood pressure and cardiac filling pressures are indicated for invasive operations. In addition to glucose, intravenous solutions should contain sodium so as to prevent the development of hyponatremia. The possibility of acute primary adrenal insufficiency should be remembered when hypotension persists despite intravenous infusion of fluids and/or administration of a sympathomimetic. Maintenance of body temperature is facilitated by increasing the temperature of the operating room and passing intravenous fluid solutions through a warming device.

Recovery from the sedative effects of anesthetics may be delayed in the hypothyroid patient. Support of ventilation of the lungs may be required postoperatively, especially if body temperature is reduced. Postoperative analgesia must be provided with minimal doses of drugs, as these patients are uniquely susceptible to the ventilatory depressant effects of narcotics.

Regional anesthesia is acceptable for management of anesthesia in the hypothyroid patient. Although supporting evidence is not available, it is possible that the dose of local anesthetic necessary for peripheral nerve blocks might be reduced.

PARATHYROID GLANDS

The four parathyroid glands produce the hormone known as parathormone. Parathormone maintains the serum calcium concentration in a normal range (normal value 4.5 to 5.5 mEq/L) by promoting the movement of calcium into the blood from the gastrointestinal tract, kidneys, and bone.

Hyperparathyroidism

Primary hyperparathyroidism results from an excessive secretion of parathormone due to benign parathyroid adenoma (90 percent of patients), carcinoma of a parathyroid gland, or hyperplasia of all four glands. Elevation of the serum calcium concentration above 5.5 mEq/L is the most valuable diagnostic indicator of primary hyperparathyroidism. An elevation of the serum chloride concentration and associated metabolic acidosis reflects the influence of parathormone on renal excretion of bicarbonate ion. The serum phosphorus concentration is usually low due to parathormone-induced renal excretion of phosphorus. Skeletal muscle weakness can be so severe that myasthenia gravis is suspected. Polyuria and polydipsia reflect hypercalcemia. Hypertension is frequently present. Cardiac rhythm is usually normal but the ECG may reveal a prolonged P–R interval and short Q–T interval.

Emergency treatment of hypercalcemia is usually necessary when the serum calcium concentration exceeds 7.5 mEq/L. Initial lowering of the serum calcium concentration is attempted by establishing a diuresis in response to administration of intravenous or oral fluids plus furosemide. When rapid lowering of the serum calcium concentration is necessary, the intravenous administration of mithramycin which inhibits parathormone-induced osteoclastic activity is effective. Rarely, hypercalcemia cannot be managed medically, and emergency parathyroidectomy is required.

Management of Anesthesia. The goal of management of anesthesia for the patient with an elevated serum calcium concentration is the maintenance of hydration and urine output. The possibility of co-existing renal disease and polyuria due to hypercalcemia should be remembered when considering the selection of enflurane. The existence of somnolence and skeletal muscle weakness preoperatively introduces the possibility that intraoperative drug requirements will be reduced. Monitoring the ECG for evidence of adverse effects of hypercalcemia on the heart is important, although the Q–T interval may not be a reliable index of changes in the serum calcium concentration during anesthesia.

Hypoparathyroidism

Hypoparathyroidism due to the absence of parathormone is almost always iatrogenic, reflecting inadvertent removal of the parathyroid glands during thyroidectomy. A decrease in the serum calcium concentration below 4.5 mEq/L is the most valuable diagnostic indicator of hypoparathyroidism. Prolongation of the Q–T interval on the ECG is an indication of hypocalcemia. An acute onset of hypocalcemia as can follow inadvertent removal of the parathyroid glands is likely to manifest as neuromuscular irritability. Facial muscle twitching produced by manual tapping over the area of the facial nerve (positive Chvostek's sign) confirms neuromuscular irritability. Inspiratory stridor reflects neuromuscular irritability of the laryngeal musculature. Treatment of acute hypocalcemia is with the intravenous infusion of calcium until signs of neuromuscular irritability disappear.

ADRENAL CORTEX

The adrenal cortex is responsible for the synthesis of three groups of hormones classified as glucocorticoids (cortisol), miner-

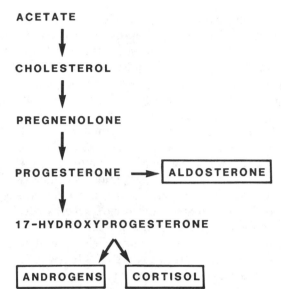

ACETATE

↓

CHOLESTEROL

↓

PREGNENOLONE

↓

PROGESTERONE → ALDOSTERONE

↓

17-HYDROXYPROGESTERONE

ANDROGENS   CORTISOL

Figure 23-2. Steps leading to the synthesis of the three primary hormones secreted by the adrenal cortex. (Tasch MD. Endocrine diseases. In: Stoelting RK, Dierdorf SF, eds. Anesthesia and co-existing disease. New York, Churchill Livingstone 1983:437–83.)

alocorticoids (aldosterone), and androgens (estradiol and testosterone) (Fig. 23-2, Table 23-2).[1] Synthesis and release of glucocorticoids and androgens from the adrenal cortex is regulated by adrenocorticotrophic hormone (ACTH) that is produced in the anterior pituitary. ACTH release is determined by corticotropin-releasing fac-tor from the hypothalamus and a negative feed back mechanism regulated by the serum concentration of cortisol.

Cortisol is the only hormone produced by the adrenal cortex that is essential for life. In addition to its well-known anti-inflammatory effect, cortisol is important for facilitating the (1) conversion of norepinephrine to epinehrine and the subsequent maintenance of blood pressure, (2) retention of sodium and secretion of water and potassium, and (3) breakdown of proteins and subsequent formation of glucose from the amino acids by gluconeogenesis. Hyperglycemia in response to cortisol reflects both gluconeogenesis and inhibition by cortisol of peripheral utilization of glucose by the cells.

Secretion and synthesis of aldosterone by the adrenal cortex are regulated by the renin-angiotension system and the serum concentration of potassium. For example, angiotensin II is a potent stimulus for the release of aldosterone from the adrenal cortex. The mineralocorticoid effects of aldosterone at the renal tubules are reflected by reabsorption of sodium and excretion of potassium. Reabsorption of sodium induced by aldosterone is an important mechanism for regulating the extracellular fluid volume. Indeed, renin release in response to hypovolemia ultimately leads to release of

Table 23-2. Endogenous and Synthetic Corticosteroids

	Glucocorticoid Potency[a] (Anti-Inflammatory Effect)	Mineralocorticoid Potency[a] (Salt-Retaining Effect)	Equivalent Oral or IV Dose (mg)[a]
Cortisol	1	1	20[b]
Cortisone	0.8	0.8	25
Prednisolone	4	0.8	25
Prednisone	4	0.8	5
Methylprednisolone	5	0	4
Dexamethasone	25	0	0.75
Aldosterone		3000	

[a] Potencies and equivalent doses are as compared with cortisol.
[b] Assumed daily endogenous cortisol production.
(Adapted from Tasch MD. Endocrine diseases. In: Stoelting RK, Dierdorf SF, eds. Anesthesia and co-existing disease. New York, Churchill Livingstone 1983:437–83.)

aldosterone and increased reabsorption of sodium in an attempt to restore extracellular fluid volume.

Hyperadrenocorticism (Cushing's Disease)

Hyperadrenocorticism can result from excess production of ACTH, excess production of cortisol, and endogenous administration of corticosteroids. Manifestations of hyperadrenocorticism include fluid retention, hypertension, hypernatremia, hypokalemia, hyperglycemia, skeletal muscle weakness, and osteoporosis. There is a centripetal distribution of fat (truncal obesity and thin extremities) and characteristic moon-facies. The treatment of hyperadrenocorticism is microadenectomy of the pituitary gland when excess ACTH is the cause or adrenalectomy when excess cortisol is responsible.

Management of anesthesia for the patient with hyperadrenocorticism must consider the physiologic effects of excess cortisol secretion. Preoperative evaluation of blood pressure, electrolyte concentrations, and the plasma level of glucose are indicated. The extent of osteoporosis must be considered in terms of subsequent positioning for the operative procedure. The possible impact of co-existing skeletal muscle weakness and/or hypokalemia on the response to muscle relaxants must be remembered when calculating the dose of these drugs. Regional anesthesia is acceptable in these patients, but the likely presence of osteoporosis with possible vertebral body collapse must be appreciated. Continuous intravenous infusion of cortisol at a rate equivalent to 100 mg/day should be started intraoperatively if the surgery is for hypophysectomy or bilateral adrenalectomy.

Hypoadrenocorticism

Hypoadrenocorticism may be due to destruction of the adrenal cortex by disease or hemorrhage, deficiency of ACTH, or prolonged administration of exogenous corticosteroids which suppress the pituitary-adrenal axis. Destruction of the adrenal cortex produces primary adrenal insufficiency or Addison's disease with manifestations reflecting the absence of cortisol and aldosterone. Decreased intravascular fluid volume, hypotension, hyponatremia, hyperkalemia, hypoglycemia, and skeletal muscle weakness can be prominent while cardiovascular collapse may accompany any acute stress such as an upper respiratory tract infection or surgical trauma. Because adrenal insufficiency usually develops slowly, these patients develop a marked pigmentation (from excess ACTH trying to stimulate an unresponsive adrenal cortex) and cardiopenia that is presumed to reflect chronic hypotension. Hypoadrenocorticism due to dysfunction of the anterior pituitary and a deficiency of ACTH is less likely than primary adrenal insufficiency to be associated with severe electrolyte derangements or hypovolemia, since the secretion of aldosterone is maintained.

Treatment of hypoadrenocorticism associated with circulatory collapse is with the intravenous administration of cortisol, 100 mg followed by the continuous infusion of 50 mg every 4 to 6 hours during the first 48 hours following the crisis. Restoration of intravascular fluid volume requires intravenous infusion of glucose in saline. Chronic management of hypoadrenocorticism requires glucocorticoid and mineralocorticoid replacement.

Corticosteroid Therapy before Surgery. Corticosteroid supplementation should be increased whenever the patient being treated for chronic hypoadrenocorticism undergoes a surgical procedure. This recommendation is based on the concern that these patients are susceptible to cardiovascular collapse, since they cannot release additional endogenous cortisol in response to the stress of surgery. More controversial is the management of the patient who may manifest suppression of the pituitary-adrenal axis due to current or previous administration of corticosteroids for treatment of a disease unrelated to pathology in the anterior pituitary or adrenal cortex.[1] The dose of corticosteroid or duration of therapy with a corticosteroid that will produce suppression of the pituitary-adrenal axis is not known. Furthermore, recovery of normal pituitary-adrenal axis function may require as long as 12 months following discontinuation of therapy.[1] Therefore, the tendency empirically is to administer supplemental corticosteroids in the perioperative period when surgery is planned in a patient who is being treated with a corticosteroid or who has been treated for more than 1 month in the past 6 to 12 months. Nevertheless, it should be appreciated that a cause and effect relationship between intraoperative hypotension and acute hypoadrenocorticism in a patient previously treated with corticosteroids has never been documented.

A useful empiric regimen is the administration of intravenous cortisol, 25 mg at the time of induction of anesthesia followed by a continuous intravenous infusion of 100 mg of cortisol during the following 24 hours.[5] This regimen maintains the plasma concentration of cortisol above normal during major surgery in patients receiving chronic treatment with corticosteroids and manifesting a subnormal response to preoperative infusion of ACTH (Fig. 23-3).[5] This regimen should provide adequate plasma concentrations of cortisol in patients considered to be at risk from the presence of a suppressed pituitary-adrenal axis and in whom major surgery is necessary. It is likely that patients undergoing minor operations will need minimal to no additional corticosteroid coverage during the perioperative period.

In addition to low dose intravenous cortisol supplementation, patients receiving daily maintenance doses of a corticosteroid should also receive this dose with the preoperative medication on the day of surgery.

This maintenance dose should be continued following surgery. There is no objective evidence to support increasing the maintenance dose of corticosteroid preoperatively and then gradually decreasing the dose back to maintenance levels during the first few days postoperatively.

Management of anesthesia for the patient with treated hypoadrenocorticism introduces no unique problems other than provision of exogenous corticosteroids and a high index of suspicion for primary adrenal insufficiency should intraoperative hypotension occur. Selection of drugs used for anesthesia is not influenced by the presence of treated hypoadrenocorticism. It should be remembered that an inadequately treated patient may be exquisitely sensitive to drug-induced myocardial depression. Serum concentrations of glucose, sodium, and potassium should be measured frequently during the perioperative period. In view of skeletal muscle weakness, the initial dose of muscle relaxant should be reduced and the response monitored using a peripheral nerve stimulator.

Hyperaldosteronism

Primary aldosteronism (Conn's syndrome) is present when excess secretion of aldosterone from a functional tumor occurs independently of a physiologic stimulus. Increased sodium retention leads to a volume-dependent blood pressure elevation, while increased excretion of potassium results in hypokalemic metabolic alkalosis. Skeletal muscle weakness is presumed to reflect hypokalemia. Hyperaldosteronism should be considered in any patient with hypertension and a serum potassium concentration below 3.5 mEq/L. Confirmation of the diagnosis is by demonstration of an increased plasma concentration of aldosterone and an elevated urinary potassium excretion (greater than 30 mEq/L) despite hypokalemia.

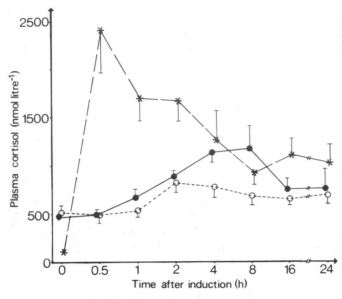

Figure 23-3. Plasma cortisol concentrations (mean ± SE) were measured in patients who had never been treated with cortisol (solid circles), in patients receiving long term corticosteroid treatment but manifesting normal increases in the plasma concentration of cortisol in response to preoperative administration of adrenocorticotrophic hormone (open circles), and in patients receiving long term corticosteroid treatment who manifested subnormal changes in the plasma concentration of cortisol in response to preoperative administration of adrenocorticotrophic hormone (asterisks). Only these latter patients received additional exogenous corticosteroids, consisting of intravenous cortisol 25 mg following the induction of anesthesia plus a continuous intravenous infusion of cortisol 100 mg during the next 24 hours. Plasma concentrations of cortisol were not different between patient groups after the 2 hour measurement. (Symreng T, Karlberg BE, Kagedal B, Schildt B. Physiological cortisol substitution of long-term steroid treated patients undergoing major surgery. Br J Anaesth 1981;53: 949–53.)

Management of anesthesia for excision of an aldosterone-secreting tumor is facilitated by the preoperative correction of hypokalemia. This goal is achieved with the administration of potassium and an aldosterone antagonist such as spironolactone. Hypertension may require management with antihypertensives. Inhaled or injected drugs are acceptable for the maintenance of anesthesia.[1] The use of enflurane, however, may be questionable if hypokalemic nephropathy and polyuria exist preoperatively.

ADRENAL MEDULLA

The adrenal medulla is a specialized part of the sympathetic nervous system capable of synthesizing norepinephrine and epinephrine. The majority of norepinephrine synthesized in the adrenal medulla is methylated to epinephrine by the action of the enzyme phenylethanolamine N-methyl-transferase. The activity of this enzyme is stimulated by cortisol that flows through the adrenal medulla from the adrenal cortex. Thus, cortisol ultimately regulates production of epinephrine.

Pheochromocytoma

Pheochromocytoma is a catecholamine-secreting tumor that originates in the adrenal medulla or aberrant tissue along the paravertebral sympathetic chain. The hallmark of pheochromocytoma is paroxysmal or sustained hypertension. Less than 0.1 percent of all cases of hypertension, however, are due to pheochromocytoma. Other manifestations of pheochromocytoma include weight loss and orthostatic hypotension. Orthostatic hypotension, along with an increased hematocrit, reflects the decrease in intravascular fluid volume associated with sustained hypertension. Myocarditis due to the chronic excess of circulating catecholamines may manifest as ST-T changes on the ECG. Hyperglycemia reflects inhibition of insulin release secondary to catecholamine-produced alpha stimulation.

Definitive diagnosis of pheochromocytoma requires biochemical confirmation of excessive catecholamine production. Measurement of urinary excretion of catecholamines or metabolites of catecholamines, such as metanephrines or vanillylmandelic acid, can be used as an index of catecholamine production. Measurement of total plasma concentrations of catecholamines, however, is the most reliable measurement for the diagnosis of a pheochromocytoma (Fig. 23-4).[6]

Treatment of pheochromocytoma is surgical excision of the catecholamine-secreting tumor or tumors. Before surgical excision, however, it is mandatory to produce alpha blockade with a drug such as phenoxybenzamine which leads to a reduction in blood pressure and a normalization of the blood volume. Alpha blockade also reduces the risk of intraoperative hypertension during the manipulation of the tumor. The persistence of tachycardia and/or cardiac dysrhythmias despite alpha blockade is an indication for the administration of a drug such as propranolol to produce beta blockade. The recommendation that beta blockade not be instituted in the absence of alpha blockade is based on the theoretical concern that a heart depressed by beta antagonists could not maintain an adequate cardiac output should unopposed alpha-mediated vasoconstriction from the release of catecholamines result in abrupt increases in the systemic vascular resistance. Preoperative preparation also includes attempts to localize the anatomical position of the tumor most often with computed tomography and/or arteriography.

Management of anesthesia. Continuation of alpha and beta antagonists is recommended until the induction of anes-

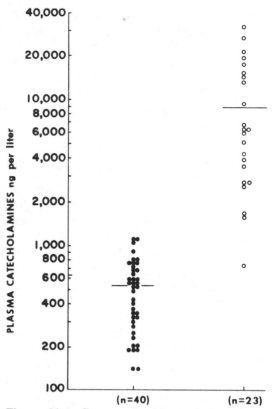

Figure 23-4. Compared with normal patients (open circles), the plasma concentration of catecholamines was above 1000 ng/ml in 22 of 23 patients with pheochromocytoma. (Bravo EL, Tarazi RC, Gifford RW, Stewart BH. Circulating and urinary catecholamines in pheochromocytoma. Diagnostic and pathophysiologic implications. N Engl J Med 1979;301:682–6).

thesia. The goal of preoperative medication is to reduce the likelihood of apprehension-induced activation of the sympathetic nervous system. A catheter should be placed in a peripheral artery to provide continuous monitoring of blood pressure prior to the induction of anesthesia. Induction of anesthesia can be accomplished with the intravenous administration of an ultrashort-acting barbiturate or benzodiazepine. Following the onset of unconsciousness and prior to direct laryngoscopy for intubation of the trachea, the depth of anesthesia should be increased by ventilation of the lungs with nitrous oxide plus enflurane or isoflurane. Selection of enflurane or iso-flurane for maintenance of anesthesia is based on the ability of these drugs to reduce sympathetic nervous system activity. Fur-thermore, these drugs are unlikely to sen-sitize the heart to the dysrhythmic effects of catecholamines. Halothane is not recommended because of the likelihood of cardiac dysrhythmias in the presence of catecholamine release from the pheochromocytoma. Likewise, mainte-nance of anesthesia with nitrous oxide and a narcotic is not ideal, as this drug combi-nation does not suppress activity of the sympathetic nervous system and hyperten-sive responses are likely. The use of In-novar (fentanyl plus droperidol) is ques-tionable, since droperidol has been reported to provoke hypertension in the presence of a pheochromocytoma.[7]

Intubation of the trachea is facilitated by the administration of succinylcholine or a nondepolarizing muscle relaxant with min-imal cardiovascular effects (metocurine, atracurium, vecuronium). The histamine-releasing effects of d-tubocurarine and the vagolytic and possibly mild sympathomi-metic effects of pancuronium would make these drugs unlikely selections. Establish-ment of an adequate depth of anesthesia prior to intubation of the trachea is rec-ommended to minimize the pressor effects cvoked by direct laryngoscopy. It must be remembered that a short duration of direct laryngoscopy (less than 15 seconds) is im-portant for attenuating sympathetic nervous system stimulation associated with intuba-tion of the trachea.

A continuous intravenous infusion of ni-troprusside during surgery will be neces-sary if hypertension persists despite maxi-mum concentrations (about 1.5 to 2 MAC) of enflurane or isoflurane. Subsequent re-ductions in blood pressure may accompany decreases in the plasma concentration of catecholamines that occur as the veins draining the pheochromocytoma are surgi-cally ligated. This hypotension is treated by decreasing the delivered concentration of anesthetic, intravenous infusion of crystal-loid and/or colloid solutions, and, in some patients with persistent reductions in blood pressure, a continuous infusion of norepi-nephrine, dopamine, or dobutamine. A pul-monary artery catheter is helpful in evalu-ating the response of these patients to therapeutic interventions. Monitoring the serum glucose concentration is indicated, as hypoglycemia may occur when plasma catecholamine concentrations decrease fol-lowing removal of the tumor.

Regional anesthesia for excision of a pheochromocytoma has the attractive fea-tures of blocking the sympathetic nervous system and not sensitizing the heart to cat-echolamines. Nevertheless, postsynaptic alpha-adrenergic receptors can still respond to the direct effects of circulating catechol-amines. Furthermore, hypotension that ac-companies ligation of the veins draining a pheochromocytoma cannot be offset by sympathetic nervous system activation in the presence of a regional block. Finally, selection of a regional technique is practical only if the surgical procedure is performed in a supine position.

PITUITARY GLAND

Excessive or deficient function of the pi-tuitary gland can create a number of ana-tomic and physiologic abnormalities. For example, acromegaly occurs when hyperse-cretion of growth hormone occurs in an adult. Airway management and direct lar-yngoscopy for intubation of the trachea may be difficult in these patients due to hyper-trophy of the tongue and facial bones, par-ticularly the mandible. Obviously, a thor-ough preoperative evaluation of the upper airway is mandatory in patients with acro-megaly and often should include neck ra-diographs and possibly indirect laryngos-copy using topical anesthesia.

DIABETES MELLITUS

Diabetes mellitus is a chronic metabolic and systemic disease due to a relative or absolute lack of insulin. Classically, diabetes manifests as hyperglycemia and degeneration of small blood vessels. Diabetes may be considered as juvenile onset (insulin-dependent) or adult onset (noninsulin dependent, nonketoacidosis prone) (Table 23-3).[8] Adult onset diabetes comprises over 90 percent of all diabetics and is almost always associated with obesity.

Complications of Diabetes Mellitus

Complications of diabetes include ketoacidosis, neuropathies, atherosclerosis (coronary artery disease, cerebral vascular disease, peripheral vascular disease) microangiopathy (retinopathy, renal dysfunction), an increased incidence of infection, and decreased postoperative wound tensile strength.

Ketoacidosis is the most serious metabolic complication of diabetes. The finding of metabolic acidosis in the presence of hyperglycemia plus the history of diabetes is sufficient to establish the diagnosis of ketoacidosis. Infection is often responsible for resistance to insulin that leads to the development of ketoacidosis.

Ketoacids have a low renal threshold and about one-half the acid load is excreted in combination with sodium, resulting in hyponatremia. In the presence of acidosis, potassium leaves the cells such that the serum potassium concentration is likely to be elevated despite the presence of a total body potassium deficit. Myocardial contractility and peripheral vascular tone are diminished by ketoacidosis. Hyperglycemia associated with acidosis causes increased serum osmolarity such that water is transferred from cells to extracellular fluid, producing intracellular dehydration. Concomitantly, osmotic diuresis induced by hyperglycemia results in urinary loss of electrolytes, particularly potassium, and depletion of intravascular fluid volume which may be so severe that cardiovascular collapse occurs. Compensatory responses to ketoacidosis are chloride loss via the kidneys and hyperventilation.

The definitive treatment of ketoacidosis is the intravenous administration of insulin. Supplemental potassium infusion may be necessary until acidosis is corrected and potassium re-enters the cells.

Neuropathies. Segmental demyelination associated with diabetes leads to the development of neuropathies. Autonomic nervous system neuropathies that can accompany diabetes are characterized by orthostatic hypotension, resting tachycardia, and delayed gastric emptying time. Compared with nondiabetic patients, the diabetic patient with autonomic nervous system neuropathy manifests minimal heart

Table 23.3. Classification of Diabetes Mellitus

	Juvenile Onset	Maturity Onset
Age of onset (years)	Before 16	After 35
Require exogenous insulin	Yes	Not always
Ketoacidosis prone	Yes	No
Blood glucose concentration	Wide fluctuations	Less marked fluctuations
Nutrition	Thin	Obese
Vascular complications	Rare	Common

(Adapted from Moothy SS. Metabolism and nutrition. In: Stoelting RK, Dierdorf SF, eds. Anesthesia and Co-Existing Disease. New York, Churchill Livingstone 1983:485–521.)

rate responses following the intravenous administration of atropine or propranolol.[9] Painless myocardial infarction and unexplained cardiorespiratory arrest have been reported in diabetic patients with autonomic nervous system neuropathy. Involvement of somatic nerves may manifest as nocturnal sensory discomfort. Further expression of neuropathy is the increased incidence of carpal tunnel syndrome among diabetics.

Management of Anesthesia

The two goals in the management of anesthesia for the patient with diabetes are to prevent hypoglycemia by providing exogenous glucose and to prevent ketoacidosis by assuring an adequate supply of exogenous insulin.[8] The preoperative evaluation should include the adequacy of blood glucose control. The absence of ketoacidosis must be confirmed prior to undertaking any elective surgery. Manifestations of coronary artery disease, cerebral vascular disease, renal dysfunction, and signs of peripheral and autonomic nervous system neuropathies should be noted. Finally, the operation should be scheduled for early in the morning. The choice of drugs for induction and maintenance of general anesthesia is less important than monitoring blood glucose concentrations and treating the potential physiologic derangements associated with diabetes. The effects of anesthetic drugs on the blood glucose concentration and insulin release are varied and probably clinically insignificant with respect to the total management of anesthesia in the diabetic patient. Intubation of the trachea with a cuffed tube seems prudent in view of the decreased gastric emptying time (gastroparesis) associated with autonomic nevous system neuropathy. The high incidence of peripheral neuropathies must be considered and documented in the patient's medical record if a regional anesthetic technique is selected so as to avoid the erroneous assumption postoperatively that the anesthetic caused the pre-existing neurologic deficit.

Management of the Daily Insulin Dose. Traditionally, one-fourth to one-half the usual daily intermediate-acting dose of insulin is administered subcutaneously on the morning of surgery with the preoperative medication. It is usually recommended that an intravenous infusion of glucose be started at the same time insulin is administered. An appropriate fluid selection and infusion rate is 5 percent dextrose in lactated Ringer's solution delivered at 100 ml/hr (5 to 7 g of glucose per hour).

An acceptable alternative to routine administration of preoperative insulin is to withhold insulin and measure the blood glucose concentration every hour during the intraoperative period (Fig. 23-5).[10] Based on this measurement, the blood glucose concentration can be maintained between 100 to 250 mg/dl during the intraoperative period by the intravenous infusion of additional glucose or regular insulin (5 to 10 units).

If oral hypoglycemic drugs are being used, they can be continued until the evening before surgery. It should be remembered, however, that these drugs may produce hypoglycemia as long as 24 to 48 hours following their administration.

Determination of the blood glucose concentration before the induction of anesthesia is recommended. Comparison of the glucose concentration in this blood sample as reported from the laboratory with that glucose value estimated by using a Dextrostix or Chemstrip confirms the accuracy of the latter approach. Estimation of the blood glucose concentration using these commercially available devices can then be repeated with confidence as to their accuracy during surgery. Simultaneous estimates of the blood glucose concentration

Figure 23-5. The mean changes in blood glucose concentration were determined in insulin dependent adult diabetic patients undergoing elective surgery. Group 1 patients received no preoperative insulin or glucose. Group 2 patients received one-fourth to one-half of their usual dose of insulin on the morning of surgery plus the intravenous infusion of 6.25 g of glucose per hour. Group 3 patients did not receive insulin or glucose preoperatively but were treated with intravenous administration of regular insulin if the blood glucose concentration exceeded 200 mg/dl. (Walts LF, Miller J, Davidson MB, Brown J. Perioperative management of diabetes mellitus. Anesthesiology 1981;55:104–9.)

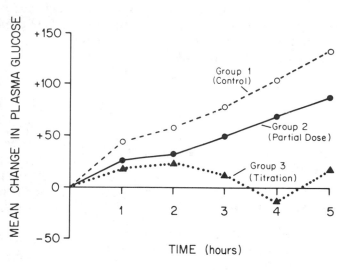

and the presence or absence of ketone bodies in the blood can be determined using a Keto-Diastix.

NONKETOTIC HYPEROSMOLAR HYPERGLYCEMIC COMA

Nonkeotic hyperosmolar hyperglycemic coma occurs most often in elderly patients with an impaired thirst mechanism. Two-thirds of patients who develop this syndrome do not have a history of diabetes mellitus. Typical findings of this syndrome include severe hyperglycemia (usually above 600 mg/dl) that leads to osmotic diuresis with associated loss of sodium, potassium, and intravascular fluid volume. Plasma osmolarity often exceeds 33O mOsm/L. Altered mentation culminating in seizures and coma reflects a decrease in intracellular brain water due to the extreme hyperosmolarity of the plasma. Ketoacidosis does not occur. Treatment is with intravenous regular insulin, potassium supplementation, and restoration of intravascular fluid volume with sodium containing solutions.

HYPOGLYCEMIA

The most important cause of fasting hypoglycemia is an insulinoma (insulin-secreting tumor) of the pancreatic beta cells. The most important aspect of management of anesthesia for surgical resection of an insulinoma is the frequent monitoring of the blood glucose concentration, as profound hypoglycemia can occur intraoperatively particularly during manipulation of the tumor.

PORPHYRIA

Porphyria refers to a group of specific disease entities that result from an abnormality of porphyrin metabolism. Acute intermittent porphyria is the most serious of the porphyrias, affecting both the central and peripheral nervous system.[8] The classic manifestation of acute intermittent porphyria is severe abdominal pain plus variable neurologic deficits occurring in a young to middle-aged patient. Abdominal pain is often mistaken as acute cholecystitis, pancreatitis, appendicitis, or renal colic. The principal neurologic lesion is demyelination leading to skeletal muscle weakness, diminished peripheral reflex responses, and dysfunction of the autonomic nervous system and cranial nerves. Dysfunction of the autonomic nervous system manifests as labile and/or orthostatic hypotension. Death can occur from paralysis of the muscles of respiration. Emotional disturbances may persist between attacks. Patients often have attacks at times of infection, fasting, or menstruation.

Management of Anesthesia

The goal during management of anesthesia in a patient with the diagnosis of acute intermittent porphyria is to avoid provoking an attack with drugs used in the perioperative period. Drugs considered safe for use in patients with this diagnosis include narcotics with the possible exception of pentazocine, inhaled anesthetics, muscle relaxants, anticholinergics, and anticholinesterases. Barbiturates are the drugs most often incriminated in evoking an attack of acute intermittent porphyria, although the safety of benzodiazepines and ketamine has been questioned. Another disadvantage of ketamine is that postoperative psychoses due to the drug might be difficult to differentiate from that which may accompany the disease. Ketamine, however, has been used safely in these patients, while it is equally well-documented that an attack does not always follow administration of barbiturates to patients who are subsequently diagnosed as having acute intermittent porphyria. The use of regional anesthesia is questionable, since a neurologic deficit produced by porphyria might be erroneously attributed to the anesthetic technique. Perioperative monitoring of these patients should consider the frequent presence of autonomic nervous system dysfunction and the possibility of a labile blood pressure. Glucose infusion has been recommended as a method to suppress enzyme activity responsible for the production of porphyrins and thus reduce the likelihood of an acute attack of porphyria.

MORBID OBESITY

Obesity is the most common nutritional disorder in the United States. A body weight of 20 percent above the ideal weight is defined as obesity. Morbid obesity is present when body weight is twice the ideal weight. A metabolic defect to explain obesity has not been found. In adults, the final common pathway leading to obesity is a positive caloric intake.

Adverse Changes Associated with Obesity

Obesity increases the risk for developing medical and surgical disease. Manifestations of adverse changes associated with obesity are metabolic, respiratory, cardiovascular, and hepatic.

Metabolic. Obese individuals are resistant to the effects of insulin, which is consistent with the several-fold increase in the incidence of adult onset diabetes mellitus in obese patients. Oxygen consumption and carbon dioxide production are increased by obesity.

Respiratory. Pulmonary function changes in obese patients suggest restrictive pulmonary disease characterized by reductions in expiratory reserve volume, inspiratory capacity, vital capacity, and functional residual capacity. The diaphragm is elevated and its excursion is markedly limited due to the weight of the abdominal wall. The work of breathing is increased and ventilation becomes diaphragmatic and position dependent.

The PaO_2 is predictably decreased by obesity, presumably reflecting overperfusion of underventilated alveoli. Conversely, the $PaCO_2$ as well as the ventilatory response to carbon dioxide remain normal.

The margin of reserve, however, is small and administration of ventilatory depressant drugs or assumption of the head-down position can lead to the accumulation of carbon dioxide in obese patients.

Obesity-Hypoventilation Syndrome. About 8 percent of morbidly obese patients manifest episodic somnolence and hypoventilation.[8] The elevated $PaCO_2$ is associated with respiratory acidosis, arterial hypoxemia, polycythemia, pulmonary hypertension, and right ventricular failure. The etiology of this syndrome is unknown but may represent a disorder of central nervous system regulation of ventilation.

Cardiovascular. Cardiac output is increased, emphasizing the increased oxygen demand present in an obese individual. There is a positive correlation between increases in blood pressure and weight gain. Increased cardiac output is the presumed cause of increased blood pressure. Pulmonary hypertension is common and most likely reflects the effects of chronic arterial hypoxemia and/or increased pulmonary blood volume. The risk of coronary artery disease is doubled in obese patients. Finally, care should be taken to use a blood pressure cuff of the correct size. As a general rule the width of the blood pressure cuff should be greater than one-third the circumference of the arm. When the cuff is too narrow, a higher amount of pressure will be required to compress the extra tissues and a false high blood pressure will be recorded.

Hepatic. Abnormal liver function tests and fatty infiltration of the liver occur frequently in obese individuals. There is evidence that fluorinated volatile anesthetics are metabolized to a greater extent in obese patients[11] (see Chapter 5).

Management of Anesthesia

The obese patient should be considered at a greater risk of inhalation of gastric contents in view of the increased incidence of gastroesophageal reflux and hiatal hernia in these patients. Furthermore, gastric acidity, gastric fluid volume, and intragastric pressure are increased. The preoperative administration of an H_2-receptor antagonist can be used to increase gastric fluid pH in the obese patient. Finally, drug treatment of obesity with amphetamines can influence anesthetic requirements for volatile anesthetics (see Chapter 2).

The massive amount of soft tissue about the head and upper trunk can impair mandibular and cervical mobility, making maintenance of the upper airway and intubation of the trachea difficult. Following induction of anesthesia, the low functional residual capacity reduces the mixing time for inhaled drugs in the lung. As a result, the rate of increase in the alveolar concentration of an inhaled anesthetic is accelerated. Furthermore, the low functional residual capacity predisposes the obese patient to rapid reductions in the PaO_2 during any period of apnea, as may accompany direct laryngoscopy for intubation of the trachea.

The impact of obesity on the necessary dose of injected drugs is difficult to access. Blood volume is often increased in obese patients, which would tend to reduce the plasma concentration achieved with a single rapid injection of a drug such as thiopental. Conversely, adipose tissue has a low blood flow such that increased doses calculated in an absolute weight basis in obese patients could result in exposing well-perfused tissues to excessive concentrations of drugs. Perhaps the most logical approach is to calculate the initial dose on an ideal rather than actual body weight. Subsequent doses would be based on the patient's response. Repeated injections of drug, however, could result in cumulative effects and prolonged responses reflecting storage of lipid soluble drugs in adipose tissue for subsequent release into the circulation as the plasma concentration of the drug declines.

Present evidence does not make it possible to recommend a specific drug or drug combination for maintenance of anesthesia in obese patients. Nevertheless, the high incidence of co-existing liver disease and altered metabolism of fluorinated anesthetics must be considered when considering selection of a volatile drug. There is no evidence that the high lipid solubility of volatile anesthetics results in delayed postanesthesia awakening in morbidly obese patients.[8] The use of spinal or epidural anesthesia is limited in obese patients because bony landmarks are obscured and predictability of level of anesthesia that will be produced by a given dose of drug is difficult.

Monitoring of arterial blood gases and pH is helpful in evaluating the adequacy of oxygenation and ventilation. Controlled ventilation of the lungs using large tidal volumes to facilitate the maintenance of the functional residual capacity during the intraoperative period is recommended.

Postoperatively, the semisitting position should be employed so as to optimize the mechanics of breathing and to minimize the development of arterial hypoxemia. Supplemental oxygen should be provided, remembering the maximum reduction in PaO_2 typically occurs 2 to 3 days postoperatively.

ANOREXIA NERVOSA

Anorexia nervosa is characterized by weight loss in excess of 25 percent below the ideal body weight associated with orthostatic hypotension, bradycardia, acidosis, hypokalemia, hypomagnesemia, hypocalcemia, dehydration, and hypothermia. Hepatic dysfunction may be due to fatty liver infiltration. Spontaneous pneumodiastinum has been observed. Hemoglobin concentration is usually normal.

ENTERAL AND PARENTERAL NUTRITION

Caloric support in the presence of increased energy requirements is best provided by enteral or total parenteral nutrition (hyperalimentation). It is recommended that patients who have lost more than 20 percent of their body weight should be treated nutritionally before surgery.[12]

Enteral Nutrition

The gastrointestinal tract should be the site used for nutritional supplementation whenever possible. Enteral nutrition is delivered by a nasogastric or orogastric tube. Complications of enteral feedings are not common but can include hyperglycemia leading to osmotic diuresis and hypovolemia. Therefore, blood glucose concentrations should be monitored and exogenous insulin administered when levels exceed 250 mg/dl. The high osmolality of elemental diets is often a cause of diarrhea.

Total Parenteral Nutrition

Total parenteral nutrition (hyperalimentation) is indicated when the gastrointestinal tract is not functioning. Most often a catheter is placed in the subclavian vein so as to permit infusion of a hypertonic solution.

The potential complications of total parenteral nutrition include catheter-related sepsis, hyperglycemia, nonketotic hyperosmolar hyperglycemic coma, hepatic dysfunction, hypomagnesemia, and hyperchloremic metabolic acidosis due to liberation of hydrochloric acid during the metabolism of amino acids present in the parenteral nutrition solution. Concern about catheter-related sepsis is the reason for changing the intravenous delivery tubing for hyperalimentation solutions every 24 hours. Furthermore, this tubing should not be invaded with piggyback injections or stopcocks. Furthermore, blood should not be withdrawn from the catheter and the catheter should not be used to monitor central venous pressure. Hypophosphatemia from the administration of phosphate-depleted solutions can result in a shift of the oxyhemoglobin dissociation curve to the left and decreased release of oxygen from hemoglobin to tissues. The main reason for slowing or discontinuing infusion of parenteral nutrition solutions prior to the induction of anesthesia is to avoid intraoperative hyperosmolarity secondary to rapid infusion of the solution. Abrupt discontinuation, however, should be avoided, as persistence of increased circulating levels of endogenous insulin could contribute to hypoglycemia. Preoperatively, it is important to measure the blood concentration of glucose, phosphate, and potassium. Finally, increased production of carbon dioxide resulting from metabolism of large quantities of glucose may result in the need to initiate artificial ventilation of the lungs or in failure to wean the patient from long term ventilator support. [13]

ENDOCRINE AND METABOLIC CHANGES IN THE PERIOPERATIVE PERIOD

Surgical stimulation produces a profound endocrine and metabolic response that parallels the magnitude of the operative trauma.[8] Conversely, inhaled or injected drugs used to produce anesthesia result in minimal effects on hormone secretion in the absence of surgical stimulation.

The initial endocrine response to surgical stimulation is an increase in the circulating concentrations of cortisol and catecholamines and a decrease in the plasma concentrations of insulin despite hyperglycemia. In view of the latter, excessive infusion of glucose via intravenous solutions could result in intraoperative hyperglycemia.

Surgical trauma evokes protein degradation, reflected by loss of lean body weight and increased urinary excretion of nitrogen postoperatively. Sodium and water retention and excretion of potassium in the postoperative period presumably reflect release of antidiuretic hormone and activation of the renin-angiotensin-aldosterone system.

Attentuation or prevention of the endocrine response to surgery can be produced by afferent neuronal blockade, as with regional anesthesia (T4 sensory level) or by inhibition of hypothalamic function with large doses of narcotics (morphine 4 mg/kg, fentanyl 75 µg/kg).[8] For these reasons, the concept that the administration of the lowest dose of anesthetic is best may not be valid during periods of acute surgical stimulation.[14]

REFERENCES

1. Tasch MD. Endocrine diseases. In: Stoelting RK, Dierdorf SF, eds. Anesthesia and co-existing disease. New York, Churchill Livingstone 1983:437–83.
2. Murkin JM. Anesthesia and hypothyroidism: A review of thyroxine physiology, pharmacology, and anesthetic implications. Anesth Analg 1982;61:371–83.
3. Berman ML, Kuhnert L, Phythyon JM, Holaday DA. Isoflurane and enflurane-induced hepatic necrosis in triiodothyronine-pretreated rats. Anesthesiology 1983;58:1–5.
4. Babad AA, Eger EI. The effects of hyperthyroidism and hypothyroidism on halothane and oxygen requirements in dogs. Anesthesiology 1968;29:1087–93.
5. Symreng T, Karlberg BE, Kagedal B, Schildt B. Physiological cortisol substitution of long-term steroid-treated patients undergoing major surgery. Br J Anaesth 1981;53:949–53.
6. Bravo EL, Tarazi RC, Gifford RW, Stewart BH. Circulating and urinary catecholamines in pheochromocytoma. N Engl J Med 1979;301:682–6.
7. Bitter DA. Innovar-induced hypertensive crises in patients with pheochromocytoma. Anesthesiology 1979;50:366–9.
8. Moorthy SS. Metabolism and nutrition. In: Stoelting RK, Dierdorf SF, eds. Anesthesia and co-existing disease. New York, Churchill Livingstone 1983:485–521.
9. Lloyd-Mostyn RH, Watkins PJ. Defective innervation of heart in diabetic autonomic neuropathy. Br Med J 1975;3:15–7.
10. Walts LF, Miller J, Davidson MB, Brown J. Perioperative management of diabetes mellitus. Anesthesiology 1981;55:104–9.

11. Bentley JB, Vaughan RW, Mille MS, Calkins JM, Gandolfi AJ. Serum inorganic fluoride levels in obese patients during and after enflurane anesthesia. Anesth Analg 1979; 58:409–12.

12. Powell-Tuck J, Goode AW. Principles of enteral and parenteral nutrition. Br J Anaesth 1981;53:169–80.

13. Askanzi J, Nordenstrom J, Rosenbaum SH, Elwyn DH, Hyman AI, Carpentier YA, Kinney JM. Nutrition for the patient with respiratory failure: glucose vs. fat. Anesthesiology 1981;54:373–7.

14. Roizen MF, Horrigan RW, Frazer BM. Anesthetic doses blocking adrenergic (stress) and cardiovascular responses to incision-MAC BAR. Anesthesiology 1981;54:390–8.

24

Neuroanesthesia

Neuroanesthesia requires basic knowledge of the interrelationship between cerebral blood flow (CBF), intracranial pressure (ICP), and the cerebral metabolic rate for oxygen (CMRO$_2$). Various physiologic and pharmacologic influences, many of which are under the control of the anesthesiologist, can alter the fragile relationship between CBF, ICP and CMRO$_2$. Furthermore, neuroanesthesia presents problems which deserve special attention, including deliberate hypotension, venous air embolism, and neuroradiology.

INTRACRANIAL CONTENTS

Approximately 80 to 85 percent of the intracranial contents consist of brain matter and intracerebral water. The remaining contents consist of cerebral blood volume, 3 to 6 percent, and cerebrospinal fluid (CSF), 5 to 15 percent. Because the cranium is a relatively noncompliant space, a volume change in any one of the above compartments requires a reciprocal change to occur in one or more of the remaining compartments. One mechanism for this change is translocation of CSF from intracranial to extracranial storage sites. For example, a patient with a tumor may have an increase in brain matter, and, therefore, a shift of CSF from the cranium into the more compliant spinal subarachnoid space.

CEREBRAL BLOOD FLOW (CBF)

The first measurement of CBF in man was made by Kety and Schmidt in 1945 using a tracer gas. The tracer gas was nitrous oxide with direct jugular bulb puncture or retrograde catheterization of the internal jugular vein providing the venous sample. The metabolic rate could then be calculated by multiplying the arterial to venous difference, for a substrate such as oxygen. In 1961, Lassen and Ingvar measured CBF by monitoring the brain washout of a gamma-emitting isotope, usually xenon following its bolus injection into the internal carotid artery. Columnated external scintillation counters using multiple probes were employed to detect the isotope residue inside the brain, with the CBF then calculated in the same units as the Kety and Schmidt technique. Total CBF is in the range of 50 ml/100 g/min.

Physiologic Determinants of CBF

Physiologic determinants of CBF are the PaCO$_2$, PaO$_2$, systemic blood pressure, and temperature. CBF varies directly with PaCO$_2$ values between 25 and 100 mmHg. For example, CBF decreases about 2 ml/100 g/min for each 1 mmHg decrease in PaCO$_2$. Therefore, hyperventilation will decrease CBF. Conversely, PaO$_2$ has its greatest influence when PaO$_2$ falls below normal physiologic limits. Changes in PaO_2 between 50 to 300 mmHg have little influence in CBF. Below a PaO_2 of 50 mmHg, CBF rapidly increases towards its maximal value.

In man, CBF is autoregulated in that it is maintained constant despite changes in the cerebral perfusion pressure. Autoregulation occurs between a mean arterial pressure of 50 and 100 mmHg. Cerebral perfusion pressure is calculated as mean arterial pressure minus right atrial pressure. When ICP exceeds right atrial pressure, the cerebral perfusion pressure is calculated as the difference between mean arterial pressure and ICP. The ability, however, of autoregulation to maintain CBF constant is modified by cerebral disease states, volatile anesthetics (especially above 0.6 MAC), nonanesthetic cerebral vasodilators (nitroprusside, nitroglycerin), and chronic hypertension.

CBF and $CMRO_2$ vary directly with temperature, decreasing about 7 percent per degree Celsius reduction in body temperature. For this reason, hypothermia is often instituted when CBF is interrupted.

Pharmacologic Determinants of CBF

Inhaled and injected anesthetics can influence CBF and $CMRO_2$ (Fig. 24-1).[1] Volatile anesthetics produce dose-dependent cerebral vasodilation and, therefore, an increase in CBF and depression of $CMRO_2$. Of the volatile anesthetics, halothane is associated with the largest increase in CBF.

Although nitrous oxide increases CBF, it has only been studied at a 70 percent concentration, which could have represented cerebral stress response to the experimental condition, rather than to the anesthetic per se. Still, the addition of 60 percent nitrous oxide to a low concentration of halothane causes a marked increase in CBF and $CMRO_2$ despite electroencelphalographic evidence that CNS depression has occurred.

INTRACRANIAL PRESSURE (ICP)

Control of ICP is a fundamental requirement for successful neuroanesthesia. Perioperatively, methods to monitor ICP and methods to reduce ICP (posture, hyperventilation, osmotic diuretics, tubular diuretics, corticosteroids, barbiturates, CSF drainage) are the same as utilized in the care of a head injury patient in the intensive care unit (see Chapter 32).

Planning the management of neuroanesthesia requires an appreciation of factors that influence ICP. ICP is dependent on the compliance of the CSF space and the resistance to CSF absorption.[1-3] Under pathologic conditions, expansion of an intracranial component results in displacement of some CSF from the head through the foramen magnum into the distensible spinal subarachnoid space. When this mechanism is exhausted, ICP will increase. The intracranial volume/pressure relationship is illustrated in Fig. 24-2.[2] When compensatory

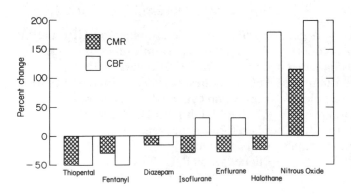

Figure 24-1. The influence of various anesthetic agents on cerebral blood flow (CBF) and cerebral metabolic rate (CMR). (Based on data in Shapiro HM. Anesthesia effects on cerebral blood flow, cerebral metabolism and the electroencephalogram. In: Miller RD, ed., Anesthesia, Churchill Livingstone, New York, 1981;795–824.)

Figure 24-2. Intracranial compliance: An idealized depiction of intracranial volume-pressure relationships. (Shapiro HM. Neurosurgical anesthesia and intracranial hypertension. In: Miller RD, ed., Anesthesia, Churchill Livingstone, New York, 1981;1079–1132.)

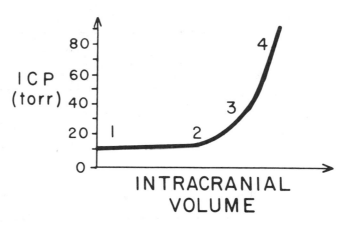

mechanisms are in place (between points 1 and 2), ICP does not change significantly. At point 2, however, compliance is reduced and further increases in volume cause a progressive increase in ICP. When ICP is already elevated (point 3), even small increases in intracranial volume will result in marked intracranial hypertension (between points 3 and 4). In this situation, increases in CBF and/or volume produced by inhaled or injected anesthetics may markedly elevate ICP. When ICP has increased sufficiently, intracranial tissue shifts and localized pressure gradients can develop, leading to vascular compression and regional ischemia.

CLINICAL ANESTHETIC MANAGEMENT

Preoperative Visit

If a craniotomy is planned, the fundamental goal of the preoperative visit is to search for signs of increased ICP. The signs and symptoms most frequently associated with increased ICP are headache, nausea, papilledema, unilateral pupillary dilitation, and oculomotor or abducens nerve palsy. Changes in the level of consciousness and/or irregular ventilatory patterns also indicate advanced stages of increased ICP. A brief neurological examination should be performed the night before surgery. This examination can be used the next morning

as a basis to determine whether the neurological status has changed during the night. When spinal or peripheral neurological surgery is planned, the preoperative neurological examination should focus upon those functions related to the structures involved in the surgical procedure.

Preoperative medication depends on the existing pathology. In general, if a patient has an elevated ICP, sedative drugs should be avoided, especially narcotics and long-acting barbiturates. In patients who do not have increased ICP, such as those with pituitary lesions, occlusive cerebrovascular disease and seizure disorders, preoperative medication is acceptable (see Chapter 10). Furthermore, patients with intracranial aneurysms probably should be heavily sedated to avoid excitation and possible rupture of the aneurysm. Drugs which may cause hypoventilation and hypercarbia should be avoided in patients with brain tumors who have reduced levels of consciousness or the potential to develop an elevated ICP.

Monitors

The recommended monitors for various neurosurgical procedures are summarized in Table 24-1.[2] ICP monitoring is recommended in patients who either have or are likely to have increased ICP. Obviously, anesthesia has been successfully adminis-

Table 24-1. Suggested Monitoring Approach for Neurosurgical and Intracranial Vascular Procedures

Procedure	Blood Pressure (Intra-Arterial)	Cardiac Sounds		CVP	Urine Output	Arterial Gases	End-Tidal CO_2	ICP
		Esophageal Stethoscope	Doppler					
Spinal surgery								
Prone	−	+	−	−	−	±	−	−
Sitting	+	+	+	+[a]	−	±	+	−
Intracranial surgery								
Supratentorial	+	+	−	+	+	+	+ +	+ +
Infratentorial (± sitting)	+	+	+	+[a]	+	+	+ +	+ +
Aneurysm (elective hypotension)	+	+	−	+	+	+	+ +	+ +
Intracranial vascular surgery	+	+	−	−	±	+	+ +	−

Abbreviations: CVP, central venous pressure; ICP, intracranial pressure.
Symbols: + = routine; ± = may or may not be monitored; + + = special risk; − = usually not monitored. Blood pressure, ECG, and temperature monitored in all cases.
[a] CVP tip requires right atrial position.
(Adapted from Shapiro HM: Neurosurgical anesthesia and intracranial hypertension. In: Miller RD, ed, Anesthesia. Churchill Livingstone, New York, 1981;1079–1132.)

tered to these patients without such monitoring, but probably with a lesser margin of safety. The Doppler ultrasound transducer is particularly useful in patients who are vulnerable for venous air embolism (see the section, *Venous Air Embolism*).

Sensory evoked potentials have been advocated by several clinicians.[4] These evoked potentials are the electrophysiologic responses of the nervous system to sensory stimulation. Measurement of sensory evoked potentials requires a controllable stimulus source, a method of amplifying the responses, and data processing that allows storage and averaging of a large number of neuroelectric responses, the latter of which can be accomplished with a storage oscilloscope or by computer. Somatosensory-evoked potentials (for spinal cord surgery), brain stem auditory-evoked potentials (for surgery in the posterior cranial fossa) and visual-evoked potentials (for surgery on the pituitary gland or intracranial aneurysms) have been used for such monitoring. These monitors can detect lack of neurologic function, presumably due to interruption of blood flow or ischemia. When detected, corrective measures such as drug-induced elevations of blood pressure can be immediately taken in an effort to prevent postoperative neurologic deficits.

Anesthetic Choice, Induction, and Maintenance

Several approaches have been used successfully for neuroanesthesia. Preventing an increased ICP is of prime importance. Some measures can be taken prior to induction of anesthesia to reduce ICP. These measures include preoperative administration of corticosteroids, such as dexamethasone or methylprcdnisolone, to patients who have primary or metastatic brain tumors. Also, an osmotic diuretic, such as mannitol, may be given just prior to induction of anesthesia in those patients with a significant shift of intracranial structures and a high ICP.

Ideally, the patient can be persuaded to voluntarily hyperventilate prior to the induction of anesthesia. Induction of anesthesia frequently is accomplished with intravenous thiopental 3 to 5 mg/kg. Thiopental is a cerebral vasoconstrictor and is effective in preventing increases in ICP associated with hypertension that predictably accompanies intubation of the trachea. Lidocaine, which is also a cerebral vasoconstrictor, can be administered intravenously (1.5 mg/kg) at the same time as thiopental to further attenuate potential adverse changes in ICP during intubation of the trachea. Finally, topical anesthesia with lidocaine can be applied to the trachea prior to intubation of the trachea. As soon as the trachea is intubated, hyperventilation and the anesthetic to be used for maintenance should be initiated.

The choice of drug for maintenance of anesthesia is not crucial if measures have been taken to ensure that ICP has not been increased. Cerebral vasodilators, such as halothane, can be used if hyperventilation is induced prior to the anesthetic's administration. Nevertheless, many anesthesiologists prefer to avoid these anesthetics. Instead, they use a combination of nitrous oxide, intravenous ultrashort-acting barbiturates, narcotics, benzodiazepines, and muscle relaxants. Utilization of a volatile anesthetic, however, rather than a combination of intravenous drugs probably allows the postoperative evaluation of the patient to be simpler.

Of prime importance during surgery is the prevention of coughing or gross movement. These events can increase brain engorgement and bleeding. Some anesthesiologists utilize a light level of anesthesia and then induce skeletal muscle paralysis with a muscle relaxant. If this approach is chosen, a peripheral nerve stimulator is valuable for monitoring the effects of muscle relaxants in order to prevent unexpected movement of the patient in response to a painful surgical stimulus. Others hypothesize that since skeletal muscle relaxation per se is not required for the surgery, movement and coughing should be prevented by administering a sufficient dose of anesthetic.

Selection of the specific crystalloid solution and infusion rate is important for patients undergoing neurosurgical procedures. Glucose and water solutions are not recommended, since they are rapidly and equally distributed throughout the total body water. If the concentration of glucose in the blood decreases more rapidly than brain glucose, the brain water becomes hyperosmolar such that water enters and cerebral edema results. For this reason, a hypertonic solution, such as lactated Ringer's solution with or without glucose is preferred (see Chapter 18). Regardless of the crystalloid solution selected, it must be remembered that infusion of large amounts of fluid can increase brain water and possibly elevate ICP. Therefore, the rate of crystalloid infusion should not exceed 1 to 3 ml/kg/hr in the perioperative period.

Recovery from Anesthesia

The patient should be allowed to awaken as smoothly as possible at the conclusion of surgery. Coughing or straining will increase central venous pressure and, therefore, increase ICP. For this reason, it may be advisable to extubate the trachea with the anesthetic level moderately deep. Also, prior administration of thiopental and/or lidocaine may minimize the chances of coughing with extubation of the trachea.

Evaluation of the patient postoperatively for neurological signs (such as impending subdural hematoma) is necessary. If a narcotic has been utilized, it may be necessary to antagonize this drug's effect with naloxone in order to avoid respiratory depression and hypercarbia. Delayed return of consciousness postoperatively or neurologic deterioration in the postoperative period should arouse suspicion of a tension pneumocephalus, especially if nitrous oxide was administered during anesthesia. Subdural accumulation of gases sufficient to cause an adverse elevation in the intracranial pressure can be diagnosed with computed tomography.

SPECIAL PROBLEMS

Air Embolism

An open vein exposed to the atmosphere results in conditions whereby air may be entrained intravascularly.[2,3] Whenever the surgical incision is above the level of the heart, conditions are favorable for a venous air embolism to occur. As a result, the incidence of venous air embolism is as high as 30 to 40 percent in the sitting position, with much lower incidences in the lateral and supine positions. Air that enters a vein travels to the heart where the combination of air and blood in the right ventricle prevents effective cardiac output. The mixing of air and blood produces a characteristic, but unfortunately late occurring, mill-wheel murmur. Pulmonary edema and reflex bronchoconstriction may result from the movement of air into the pulmonary circulation. Air may also pass through a patent foramen ovale (a probe patent foramen ovale is present in up to 25 percent of adults) to reach the coronary and cerebral circulations. It is conceivable, but not documented, that venous air can traverse the pulmonary circulation to reach the left ventricle. Death from venous air embolism is usually secondary to acute cor pulmonale and arterial hypoxemia from obstruction of the pulmonary circulation.

Nonspecific signs of venous air embolism include hypotension, cardiac dysrhythmias, tachypnea, and cyanosis. Central venous pressure is frequently increased, reflecting obstruction of pulmonary vessels with air. Signs of acute pulmonary hypertension may appear on the electrocardiogram (ECG). A sudden deep breath ("gasp reflex") has been noted to occur in animal models during venous air embolism. It is not clear whether the deep breath causes venous air embolism or reflects its occurrence.

Air that reaches the arterial circulation, as via a patent foramen ovale, produces adverse changes by virtue of distribution to the coronary and cerebral arteries. Arterial air embolism to a coronary artery is likely to produce cardiac dysrhythmias and evidence of myocardial ischemia on the ECG. Profound arterial hypotension may reflect decreased myocardial contractility and/or cardiac dysrhythmias. Air embolism to the cerebral circulation may manifest postoperatively as delayed awakening or neurologic deficits.

Specific monitoring devices for venous air embolism include a right atrial catheter, end-expired carbon dioxide determinations, and a Doppler ultrasound transducer. A right atrial catheter is useful both from a diagnostic and therapeutic point of view. Aspiration of air from the right atrium via the catheter will confirm the diagnosis of venous air embolism. Furthermore, air can be removed from the right atrium, minimizing its effect on the pulmonary circulation and cardiac output. The basis upon which monitoring of end-expired carbon dioxide concentrations is useful is the assumption that embolized air will rapidly be ejected into the pulmonary circulation, resulting in capillary obstruction. Thus, the concentration of exhaled carbon dioxide will abruptly decrease. Probably the most sensitive method of detecting venous air embolism is by use of the precordial Doppler ultrasound transducer. With this technique, injected air volumes as little as 0.25 ml can be detected by an abrupt alteration in the quality, intensity, and rhythm of sound as the air enters the heart. Most often the Doppler ultrasound transducer is placed to the right of the sternum at the second or third intercostal spaces. Confirmation that this placement reflects events in the right heart is provided by an audible swishing sound when a bolus of fluid is injected via a right atrial catheter.

When venous air embolism is detected, therapy should be based on prevention of further air entry into the venous system and evacuation of air already embolized. Prevention of further air entry can be accomplished by elevating venous pressure in the surgical wound, which will also aid the surgeon in identifying the site of air entry. Venous pressure can be elevated by jugular vein compression, positive pressure ventilation of the lungs, and lowering of the patient's head. The use of positive end-expiratory pressure for the treatment of venous air embolism is controversial. The increased venous pressure provided by this approach will certainly reduce air entry into the venous circulation but, at the same time, could increase right atrial pressure such that a probe patent foramen ovale opens, allowing passage of air to the systemic circulation. Evacuation of air from the heart can be accomplished in part by aspiration and manipulation of the right atrial catheter. If hypotension occurs, a sympathomimetic with a positive inotropic effect can be administered to encourage movement of air out of the heart. If nitrous oxide is being used, it should be discontinued immediately in order to prevent volume expansion of the embolized air due to the different solubilities of nitrous oxide and nitrogen in blood (see Chapter 2).

Deliberate Hypotension

Controversy regarding the use of deliberate hypotension for surgical procedures has existed for several years. Although blood loss can be decreased and the conditions of the surgical field possibly improved (less blood obscuring the surgeon's view) by its use, the possible increased risk of tissue damage from hypotension-induced hypoperfusion exists. Deliberate hypotension is used for several surgical procedures, but in neuroanesthesia it is often requested to diminish the risk of intraoperative rupture of a cerebral aneurysm. Ultimately, benefits of hypotension must be weighed against the risk of causing cerebral ischemia, or ischemia in other organ systems.

Several studies indicate that the brain can safely tolerate a mean arterial pressure of 55 mmHg.[5] The lower limit of tolerability

and the influence of specific disease states, however, have not been defined. In general, patients who have had a cerebrovascular accident or cerebral ischemic episodes, myocardial infarction within the preceding 3 years, renal disease as indicated by increased serum creatinine level, previous renal transplantation, a systolic blood pressure greater than 170 mmHg, or a diastolic pressure greater than 110 mmHg probably should be excluded from consideration for deliberate hypotension.[5]

Monitoring. In addition to the usual monitors, an intra-arterial catheter is essential during deliberate hypotension to monitor continuously arterial blood pressure. Another monitoring device that is very helpful is an indwelling urethral catheter with a device for measurement of urinary output. A marked decrease in urinary output would imply that the kidney is receiving inadequate perfusion. Although some anesthesiologists may recommend the use of the electroencephalogram, deliberate hypotension has been used in hundreds of cases successfully without such a monitor. Furthermore, this monitor is usually unavailable in the routine operating room setting.

Drugs and Maintenance. Deliberate hypotension can be induced by (1) position (e.g., head up), (2) continuous intravenous infusion of a short-acting vasodilator such as trimethaphan, nitroglycerin or nitroprusside, or (3) by use of a volatile anesthetic. Most often, a combination of these three approaches is used to produce the desired degree of hypotension. Nitroglycerin tends to reduce preload and, thus, cardiac output. As a result, sensitivity to this drug is directly dependent on the patient's blood volume. Trimethaphan is an effective hypotensive drug, by virtue of its direct vasodilator action as well as ganglionic blockade. Ganglionic blockade from trimethaphan can produce persistent mydriasis, which, in the postoperative period can interfere with the neurologic evaluation. Like nitroglycerin, trimethaphan may reduce cardiac output as well as blood pressure. Nitroprusside is a potent vasodilator that decreases blood pressure by peripheral vasodilation while cardiac output is maintained or even increased. The hypotensive effect of nitroprusside is easily reversed by slowing or discontinuing the drug infusion. Although nitroprusside is converted to cyanide and then to thiocyanate, the doses (maximum recommended dose is 8 to 10 µg/kg/min not to exceed 1.5 mg/kg for a 1 to 3 hour administration) required for deliberate hypotension, especially in the presence of a volatile drug for maintenance of anesthesia, are unlikely to result in cyanide intoxication. Nevertheless, arterial pH should be monitored and a high index of suspicion maintained for cyanide toxicity should an unexplained metabolic acidosis accompany infusion of nitroprusside. Compensatory tachycardia may offset the blood pressure lowering effects of all vasodilators that are used to produce controlled hypotension. Propranolol has been recommended to prevent this tachycardia. Oxygenation should be monitored during administration of vasodilators, as these drugs may inhibit hypoxic pulmonary vasoconstriction, resulting in arterial hypoxemia.

Volatile anesthetics used to facilitate deliberate hypotension reduce blood pressure by different mechanisms (see Chapter 4). For example, halothane lowers blood pressure primarily by decreasing cardiac output, while isoflurane acts by decreasing systemic vascular resistance.

In previously normotensive patients, mean arterial blood pressure can be maintained between 55 to 65 mmHg without substantive ischemia to vital organs. Hypotension should be terminated prior to closure of the wound to assure that all bleeding sites have been isolated. For neurosurgery, the duration of deliberate hypotension may be brief, as during isolation and clipping of a cerebral aneurysm.

Hypothermia

Hypothermia will reduce $CMRO_2$ and edema. Therefore, when the cerebral circulation is temporarily interrupted, such as during the clipping of a cerebral aneurysm, hypothermia is sometimes introduced. Hypothermia is protective if induced prior to or during an ischemic insult. The purpose of hypothermia is to reduce metabolism so that tissues may better tolerate a reduction in blood flow. Oxygen consumption is reduced about 7 percent per degree Celsius decrease in body temperature.

Induction of hypothermia is unpleasant for a conscious patient. Therefore, the majority of patients are anesthetized prior to reduction of their body temperature. The techniques of cooling vary from surface application of cold to the direct cooling of blood as it passes from an arterial cannula through coils immersed in ice water back to a vein. Cooling blankets are also helpful, especially if the patient lies between two blankets.

Many physiologic alterations accompany hypothermia. Cardiac output, blood pressure, and heart rate decrease and blood viscosity increases. Cardiac irritability increases and spontaneous ventricular fibrillation may occur at temperatures below 29 Celsius. The affinity between hemoglobin and oxygen is increased, as reflected by a leftward shift in the oxyhemoglobin dissociation curve. Most of these described complications, however, do not occur if temperature is not reduced below 31 Celsius. Lastly, it should be remembered that the anesthetic requirement for the inhaled anesthetics decreases with hypothermia at a rate that parallels the reduction in oxygen consumption.

When inducing hypothermia, it must be realized that temperature continues to drift downward even after the cooling blankets have been turned off. Therefore, if a temperature of 31 Celsius is desired, it probably is advisable to turn the blankets off at about 32.5 Celsius.

Pituitary Surgery

The transphenoidal approach is usually used for pituitary surgery. Special requirements of this approach include oral pharyngeal packing and use of epinephrine-containing solutions, sometimes in large amounts.[6] Therefore, if an anesthetic is used which sensitizes the myocardium to exogenously administered epinephrine, cardiac dysrhythmias may occur.

In about 10 to 20 percent of patients, diabetes insipidus transiently occurs in the first 24 hour period. The diagnosis of diabetes insipidus is based on serum sodium and osmolarity determinations, both of which should be high if diabetes insipidus is present. Also, a dilute polyuria is present. Treatment of diabetes insipidus in the immediate postoperative period includes administration of 5 percent dextrose in water or fluids orally in quantities sufficient to replace urine and insensible losses. Before the volume of intravenous or oral fluids required becomes prohibitive, however, replacement with antidiuretic hormone should be initiated.

Cerebral Aneurysm Surgery

Management of anesthesia for patients with a cerebral aneurysm is based on trying to minimize the chances of a rupture or re-rupture of the aneurysm and to ensure adequate oxygenation to the tissues. A cerebral aneurysm is either reinforced by wrapping it with tissues or adhesives, or obliterated with a clip placed at its origin from the artery. Preoperative medication in a patient who is neurologically normal should be designed to prevent apprehension or excitement or any other factor which may increase ICP and thus increase the chances of the cerebral aneurysm rupturing. If a patient is obtunded or has an increased ICP, however, preoperative medication should be avoided.

The goal for induction of anesthesia is to avoid marked changes in CBF. This can be done by ensuring that deep anesthesia exists prior to intubation of the trachea and cautious replacement of intravascular fluid volume. During maintenance of anesthesia, especially while the cerebral aneurysm is being isolated and clipped, deliberate hypotension will probably be requested.

Vasospasm of the cerebral vessels is a special problem in patients in whom a cerebral aneurysm has ruptured. It apparently occurs in 15 to 20 percent of patients after the bleeding episode and can proceed to cerebral ischemia and infarction. The etiology is questionable, but probably includes mechanical disruption of the vessel, which results in immediate vasospasm and release of vasoactive substances from the blood into the CSF. In any event, vasospasm of the cerebral vessels probably should be treated with intravascular volume expansion, maintenance of adequate cerebral perfusion pressure, and improvement of the rheology by possibly retarding clot fibrinolysis with epsilon aminocaproic acid. Independent of vasospasm in a patient who experiences rebleeding, overly aggressive removal of CSF and reduction of ICP should be avoided because it may negate the tamponade effect.

Carotid Endarterectomy

Carotid endarterectomy is the most commonly performed operation for treatment of patients with a history of transient ischemic attacks or a documented occlusive lesion of greater than 80 percent in the carotid artery. The critical period during surgery is cross clamping of the diseased carotid artery when the patient is dependent on collateral circulation for perfusion of the ipsilateral brain. Rather than rely on collateral circulation, some surgeons routinely place an intraluminal shunt across the surgically clamped carotid artery. Alternatively, a shunt may be placed only when monitors (electroencephalogram, somatosensory evoked potentials, stump pressure) suggest cerebral ischemia. Stump pressure is the pressure in the carotid artery distal to the surgical clamp. Therefore, stump pressure reflects the transmitted pressure via the circle of Willis which implies adequate or inadequate collateral circulation. Available data suggests that a stump pressure above 60 mmHg assures adequate collateral circulation.

Anesthesia for carotid endarterectomy can be performed with local or general anesthesia. Local anesthesia includes a cervical plexus block combined with regional infiltration of local anesthetic. This approach provides the advantage of being able to monitor cerebral function of the patient by voice contact when the carotid artery is occluded. Nevertheless, strokes still can occur postoperatively despite the apparent maintenance of normal cerebral function.

General anesthesia can be acceptably produced with nitrous oxide and combinations of narcotics and/or volatile anesthetics. Regardless of the selection of drugs for anesthesia, the goal must be to maintain blood pressure in a normal range for that patient. For example, hypotension may jeopardize cerebral perfusion pressure and the adequacy of CBF via collaterals. Conversely, hypertension may result in cerebral edema, particularly in diseased areas of brain with altered ability to autoregulate CBF. Ventilation of the lungs should be controlled so as to maintain $PaCO_2$ near 35 mmHg. Attempts to increase CBF by manipulating the $PaCO_2$ are not recommended, as unpredictable and even paradoxical responses can occur in individual patients. Specifically, attempts to increase CBF by allowing the $PaCO_2$ to increase and produce cerebral vasodilation may result in vasodilation only in normal vessels while those already maximally dilated in areas of ischemia cannot respond. The net effect could be a change in the pressure gradient such that blood flow is diverted away from ischemic areas. This phenomenon has been termed the intracerebral steal syndrome.

Conversely, hypocapnia produced by iatrogenic hyperventilation of the lungs would constrict normal cerebral vessels while those manifesting vasomotor paralysis are not altered, leading to a change in the pressure gradient that favors flow to the ischemic area. This response is referred to as the inverse steal or Robin Hood phenomenon. Nevertheless, this response is not predictable and the prudent compromise is to maintain $PaCO_2$ in a low normal range.

Postoperative problems following carotid endarterectomy include lability of blood pressure, loss of carotid body function, myocardial infarction, and stroke. Hypertension may reflect loss of carotid sinus function due to denervation at the time of surgery. Likewise, hypotension could reflect increased activity of a carotid sinus previously shielded by an atheromatous plaque. The significance of loss of carotid body function is the possibility of an impaired ventilatory response to arterial hypoxemia.

Spinal Cord Transection

Spinal cord transection is the damage to the spinal cord that manifests as paralysis of the lower extremities (paraplegia) or all the extremities (quadriplegia). Anatomically, the spinal cord is not divided, but the effect physiologically is the same as if it were transected. The most common cause of spinal cord transection is trauma.

The patient with acute spinal cord transection who requires surgery presents unique problems during the management of anesthesia. For example, further damage to the spinal cord could result from extension of the head in the presence of a cervical fracture. The absence of sympathetic nervous system activity below the level of spinal cord transection makes these patients vulnerable to hypotension, particularly in response to acute changes in body posture, blood loss, or positive airway pressure. Hypothermia is a hazard, as these patients tend to become poikilothermic below the spinal cord transection. Respiration is best managed by mechanical ventilation of the lungs because abdominal and intercostal muscle paralysis, combined with general anesthesia, makes maintenance of adequate spontaneous ventilation unlikely. Succinylcholine must not be administered, since drug-induced hyperkalemia is a hazard (see Chapter 8). Minimal concentrations of anesthetics are required, as the patient is often anesthetic in the operative area.

The most important goal during management of anesthesia for the patient with a chronic transection of the spinal cord is prevention of autonomic hyperreflexia. Autonomic hyperreflexia manifests as abrupt arterial hypertension with an associated compensatory bradycardia due to activation of the carotid sinus. Spinal cord transection above T6 is most likely to be associated with autonomic hyperreflexia with up to 85 percent of patients manifesting this response. Autonomic hyperreflexia is initiated by cutaneous or visceral stimulation below the level of the spinal cord transection. Distension of a hollow viscus, such as the bladder, during cystoscopy is a common initiating event. Stimulation elicits reflex sympathetic activity and vasoconstriction below the level of the spinal cord transection resulting in hypertension. Vasoconstriction and hypertension persist because vasodilatory impulses from the central nervous system cannot traverse the spinal cord to reach the area below the cord transection. Spinal anesthesia is particularly effective in preventing autonomic hyperreflexia. General anesthesia with a volatile drug or epidural block are also effective but less so than a spinal block. Treatment of hypertension with nitroprusside is necessary if autonomic hyperreflexia occurs despite preventive steps.

Neuroradiology

General anesthesia in the neuroradiology area is often fraught with difficulties because the radiology suite has not been designed with anesthesia function in mind. This makes it essential that careful preparation be taken and appropriate anesthetic apparatus and monitoring equipment be available. Other problems may include anesthetizing a patient who is comatose from an unknown etiology. The darkened environment of the radiology suite makes it difficult to assess color, ventilation, and even to read the dials on the anesthetic machine. Maintenance of the airway may be complicated by numerous changes in position and poor access to the head. Lastly, these procedures are often long and performed in a poorly ventilated room, leading the anesthesiologists to have fatigue, boredom, and exposure to trace anesthetics.

Because contrast media are often injected into arteries, veins, or CSF, allergic and toxic reactions can occur. When a history of a previous reaction of iodine compounds is present, corticosteroids, diphenhydramine, and possibly cimetidine should be administered prior to the procedure.

Pneumoencephalography is performed by the slow, incremental injections of air or oxygen into the lumbar subarachnoid space with the patient in the sitting position. When general anesthesia is required, a number of problems result. Due to the high solubility of nitrous oxide in blood, relative to nitrogen, it will rapidly equilibrate into an air-filled ventricle, thereby adding to the intracranial volume with a resulting increase in intracranial pressure (see Chapter 2). Probably, nitrous oxide should not be used for air encephalography. Because the intraventricular air may last as long as 7 days after the procedure, its presence should be ruled out by a skull roentgenogram prior to the subsequent anesthetic administration of nitrous oxide.

REFERENCES

1. Shapiro HM. Neurosurgical anesthesia and intracranial hypertension. In: Miller RD, ed., Anesthesia. New York, Churchill Livingstone, 1981;795–824.

2. Shapiro HM. Anesthesia effects on cerebral blood flow, cerebral metabolism and the electroencephalogram. In: Miller RE, ed., Anesthesia. New York, Churchill Livingstone, 1981;1079–1132.
3. Cottrell JE, Turndorf TH. Anesthesia and neurosurgery. St. Louis, C.V. Mosby Company, 1980.
4. Grundy BL. Intraoperative monitoring of evoked potentials. Anesthesiology 1983; 58:72–87.
5. Thompson GE, Miller RD, Stevens WC, Murray WR. Hypotensive anesthesia for total hip arthroplasty. Anesthesiology 1978;48:91–6.
6. Messick JM Jr, Laws ER Jr, Abbound CF. Anesthesia for transphenoidal surgery of the hypophyseal region. Anesth Analg 1978;57:206–15.

25

Ophthalmic and Otolaryngologic Surgery

Anesthesia for ophthalmic or otolaryngologic surgery requires an appreciation of the anatomy and physiology of structures present in the operative area as well as the unique requirements of specific operative procedures. Most of the operative procedures are elective and often the patients represent extremes of age, being very young or elderly.

OPHTHALMIC SURGERY

Management of anesthesia for the patient undergoing ophthalmic surgery requires an understanding of factors that influence intraocular pressure (IOP), a consideration of adverse drug interactions between ophthalmic drugs and drugs administered perioperatively, and an appreciation of the oculocardiac reflex.

Intraocular Pressure

Normal IOP is 10 to 22 mmHg. The greatest increase in IOP (as much as 35 to 50 mmHg) occurs when venous pressure is acutely elevated as during vomiting or coughing. Direct laryngoscopy for intubation of the trachea can increase IOP even in the absence of coughing or hypertension.[1] Nevertheless, an increase in IOP is most likely when coughing accompanies in-

tubation of the trachea. Succinylcholine increases IOP an average of 6 to 8 mmHg with a return to predrug levels within 5 to 7 minutes.[2] This ocular hypertensive response occurs whether succinylcholine is given as a single intravenous injection, as a continuous infusion, or intramuscularly. In contrast to intravenous succinylcholine, it appears that intramuscular succinylcholine results in a longer duration of increased IOP, necessitating at least a 15 minute wait before the globe is opened. Prolonged tonic contraction of the extraocular muscles produced by succinylcholine is the most likely mechanism for the increase in IOP. Administration of a nonparalyzing dose of a nondepolarizing muscle relaxant (pretreatment) prior to the injection of succinylcholine does not reliably prevent this drug-induced increase in IOP.[1] Conversely, paralyzing doses of nondepolarizing muscle relaxants in the absence of succinylcholine reduce IOP, presumably via their relaxant effects on the extraocular muscles. Inhaled anesthetics are alleged to produce dose-dependent reductions in IOP. Barbiturates, narcotics, neuroleptics, and tranquilizers tend to lower IOP. Ketamine was originally reported to increase IOP but more recent studies have not demonstrated any change.[3] Ketamine may, however, be considered objectionable for ophthalmic anesthesia for other reasons such as blepharospasm and nystagmus. Finally, changes in arterial blood pressure or the $PaCO_2$ within a normal physiologic range have minimal effect on IOP.

Carbonic anhydrase inhibitors (acetazolamide) and osmotic diuretics (mannitol, urea, glycerol) are used in the perioperative period to acutely reduce IOP. Acetazolamide lowers IOP by interfering with the secretion of aqueous humor. Glycerol is effective orally but introduces the hazard of an increased gastric fluid volume in the perioperative period.

Adverse Drug Interactions

Ophthalmic medications applied topically to the cornea may undergo sufficient absorption to produce systemic effects. Unexpected drug interactions during and after surgery may reflect systemic effects of these drugs. For example, topical application of a beta-antagonist, timolol, to treat glaucoma has been associated with bradycardia and bronchospasm.[4] Rarely, a long-acting anticholinesterase, echothiophate, is used to treat glaucoma. Systemic absorption of this drug reduces cholinesterase activity, resulting in marked prolongation of the duration of action of succinylcholine should usual doses of this muscle relaxant be administered. At least 3 weeks is required after cessation of echothiophate therapy for cholinesterase activity to return to 50 percent of predrug levels. Topical application of phenylephrine to produce capillary decongestion and mydriasis can result in severe hypertension if systemic absorption is sufficient. A 2.5 percent phenylephrine solution is recommended to minimize the adverse effects should systemic absorption occur. Chronic treatment with acetazolamide can be associated with renal loss of bicarbonate ion and potassium, leading to metabolic acidosis with hypokalemia.

Oculocardiac Reflex

The oculocardiac reflex consists of a trigeminal-vagal reflex arc that is characterized by a 10 to 50 percent reduction in heart rate. Pressure on the globe and surgical traction (stretch) of extraocular muscles, particularly the medial rectus muscle, are the most likely stimuli to elicit this reflex. Hypercarbia or arterial hypoxemia may also increase the incidence and severity of this reflex. In addition to bradycardia, other manifestations of this reflex include junctional rhythm and premature ventricular contractions. Cardiac arrest has been attributed to the oculocardiac reflex but the evidence to support this is not convincing. Indeed, the importance of this reflex is controversial, with the most important principle being continuous monitoring of the electrocardiogram so as to detect the appearance of bradycardia or cardiac dysrhythmias. Removal of the surgical stimulus is usually sufficient treatment. Furthermore, this reflex tends to fatigue such that the subsequent stimulation is less likely to elicit the same response. Premedication with intramuscular atropine is of no value in preventing this reflex. Prophylactic use of intravenous atropine may, however, be justified in pediatric patients having strabismus correction because of the more active vagal reflexes in children. Should bradycardia persist after removal of the surgical stimulus, the appropriate treatment is the intravenous administration of atropine.

Management of Anesthesia

Management of anesthesia for ophthalmic surgery requires maintenance of an unchanging IOP, early recognition of the oculocardiac reflex. the presence of a motionless eye, and recovery from anesthesia that is not associated with reaction to the tracheal tube, nausea, or vomiting. Intubation of the trachea to assure control of the airway is necessary because of the proximity of the surgical field and draping. Co-existing disease may influence the management of anesthesia independent of the ophthalmic surgery. For example, elderly patients requiring ophthalmic surgery often have associated illnesses such as diabetes mellitus, coronary artery disease, essential hypertension, or chronic obstructive airway disease. Finally, selection of drugs used for anesthesia must consider potential adverse interactions with medications being used to treat ocular disease, particularly glaucoma.

During operations in which the globe is not opened, there can be more flexibility in surgical conditions, but for intraocular procedures, perfection is required. For example, when the globe is open any uncontrolled elevation of IOP can lead to an extrusion of ocular contents and permanent damage. Certainly, the intraoperative use of succinylcholine should be avoided while the eye is open or in patients who have undergone recent eye surgery. Otherwise, increases in IOP produced by succinylcholine are transient, allowing this drug to be safely administered to most patients undergoing ophthalmic surgery.

Nitrous oxide must be used with caution when an intravitreal injection of air and sulfur hexafluoride is performed to compensate for loss of vitreous volume during surgery, as for repair of a retinal detachment. Sulfur hexafluoride is included with air since the low water solubility of this gas ensures persistence of the intraocular bubble for several days postoperatively. Nitrous oxide, which is 34 times more soluble than nitrogen, can diffuse into the intraocular bubble more rapidly than nitrogen can leave, resulting in an enlargement of the bubble and increased IOP.[5] This increased IOP may be sufficient to compromise retinal blood flow, particularly if systemic blood pressure is reduced. When nitrous oxide is discontinued, a fall in IOP occurs to below awake levels, which presumably reflects loss of aqueous humor while the IOP was elevated. This rapid fall in IOP may jeop-

ardize the surgical repair, as for a retinal detachment. For these reasons, it may be prudent to discontinue the inhalation of nitrous oxide about 15 minutes before the creation of an intraocular bubble. Furthermore, nitrous oxide should be avoided for up to 10 days following intravitreal injection of sulfur hexafluoride.[5]

Available data has not demonstrated a significant difference in ocular morbidity between local and general anesthesia. Nevertheless, an impressive record of safety is associated with local anesthesia for ophthalmic surgery in patients with heart disease.[6] When local anesthesia is selected, the ophthalmologist is responsible for the management of the patient, although the anesthesiologist may be consulted regarding selection of sedative drugs. Furthermore, the anesthesiologist may be asked to monitor the patient receiving a local anesthetic. When general anesthesia is selected, it is mandatory to avoid coughing during intubation of the trachea, as any elevation in venous pressure will increase IOP. Short duration laryngoscopy in the presence of adequate anesthesia and skeletal muscle relaxation plus the use of topical tracheal lidocaine (2 mg/kg) or intravenous lidocaine (1.5 mg/kg) are helpful for assuring minimal changes in IOP in response to intubation of the trachea. Likewise, emergence from anesthesia should not be associated with any reaction to the tracheal tube. Maintenance of anesthesia with a volatile drug with or without nitrous oxide is ideal to provide an adequate depth of anesthesia plus rapid awakening and a low incidence of postoperative nausea and vomiting. The eye is a highly innervated pain-sensitive organ and ophthalmic surgery requires surgical levels of anesthesia. Monitoring the electrocardiogram is essential for early recognition of the oculocardiac reflex. Administration of a nondepolarizing muscle relaxant to maintain nearly complete suppression of the twitch response elicited by a peripheral nerve stimulator is useful to prevent unexpected patient movement. Large doses of atropine used in conjunction with an anticholinesterase to reverse neuromuscular block do not alter IOP. The intravenous administration of an antiemetic, such as droperidol (1.25 mg), near the end of general anesthesia in an attempt to minimize the incidence of postoperative nausea and vomiting may be indicated. This may be more important if a narcotic has been included in the preoperative medication. Indeed, a surgical repair may be jeopardized by acute elevations in IOP produced by vomiting. Passage of an orogastric tube to decompress the stomach before awakening from anesthesia may also be helpful in reducing the incidence of postoperative vomiting. A catheter placed in the bladder may be indicated if an osmotic diuretic is administered to lower IOP.

Strabismus Surgery. Special considerations in the management of anesthesia for strabismus surgery include the (1) questionable use of succinylcholine, (2) increased incidence of the oculocardiac reflex, and (3) possible susceptibility to malignant hyperthermia. For example, succinylcholine may produce sustained contraction of the extraocular muscles, making interpretation of the forced duction test unreliable for 15 to 20 minutes.[7] Intravenous atropine (0.007 mg/kg) or local infiltration of the extraocular muscle with lidocaine may be useful in preventing or treating the oculocardiac reflex. Malignant hyperthermia has been reported in patients undergoing strabismus surgery, suggesting a possible generalized skeletal muscle system disturbance in these patients.

Glaucoma. Special considerations in the management of anesthesia for the patient with glaucoma include (1) maintenance of drug-induced miosis throughout the perioperative period, (2) avoidance of venous congestion, and (3) awareness of potential adverse interactions between drugs used to treat glaucoma and those administered during anesthesia (see the section *Adverse Drug Interactions*). Topical application of pilocarpine on the morning of surgery is appropriate. Inclusion of an anticholinergic in the preoperative medication is acceptable, since the amount of drug reaching the eye is too little to dilate the pupil. Likewise, the use of an anticholinergic in combination with an anticholinesterase to reverse a nondepolarizing muscle relaxant is safe since only a small amount of drug reaches the eye. The implications of transient elevations in IOP produced when succinylcholine is adminstered to patients with glaucoma are not known. Presumably, the patient with adequate medical control of glaucoma would not be jeopardized by this transient drug-induced elevation in IOP. Finally, prolonged hypotension may predispose to retinal artery thrombosis in these patients.

Cataract Extraction. Special considerations in the management of anesthesia for cataract extraction include the (1) likely presence of co-existing disease in an elderly patient, (2) need for absolute immobility during the operative procedure, and (3) steps to minimize the occurrence of postoperative nausea and vomiting. Sudden movement or attempts to cough when the globe is open can result in extrusion of ocular contents and permanent damage. For these reasons, when general anesthesia is selected for cataract surgery, it is essential to maintain an adequate depth of anesthesia. In addition, skeletal muscle paralysis is often included to minimize the chance of sudden unexpected movement. Succinylcholine, to facilitate intubation of the trachea, is acceptable since IOP has returned to normal by the time surgery begins.

Open Eye Injury. Special considerations in the management of anesthesia for open eye injury include the (1) possibility of recent ingestion of food, and the (2) need to avoid even minimal increases in IOP if the injured eye is considered salvagable. Therefore, rapid intubation of the trachea facilitated by succinylcholine must be balanced against the possible hazards of drug-induced elevations in IOP. An awake intubation of the trachea, although attractive from the standpoint of airway protection, would be unacceptable since patient reaction to placement of the tube in the trachea would elevate IOP. An alternative to the administration of succinylcholine is the injection of an intubating dose of nondepolarizng muscle relaxant. The disadvantage of this approach is a prolonged duration of skeletal muscle paralysis for what may be a short operation. Regardless of the muscle relaxant selection, it is mandatory to confirm the presence of skeletal muscle paralysis by the use of a peripheral nerve stimulator before initiating direct laryngoscopy for intubation of the trachea. Premature placement of the tube in the trachea will provoke movement of the patient and defeat all the prior attempts to minimize the occurrence of vomiting or elevations in IOP.

Corneal Abrasion

Corneal abrasion is the most common ocular complication associated with general anesthesia. Abrasions typically occur in the inferior one-third of the cornea corresponding to the area exposed when the eyes are not mechanically closed. Reduction in tear production by general anesthetics plus the loss of protective eyelid closure renders patients susceptible to corneal abrasions during anesthesia. For these reasons, ophthalmic ointment is often applied to the cornea following induction of anesthesia. Disadvantages of using ointment are the possible introduction of contaminated material into the eye and the frequent complaint by the patient in the early postoperative period of blurred vision. Alternatively, mechanical closure of the eyelids by gentle application of adhesive strips protects the cornea and avoids the disadvantages of ophthalmic ointment.

The patient who sustains a corneal abrasion will complain of the sensation of a foreign body, tearing, photophobia, and pain that is aggravated by blinking and eye movement. When a corneal abrasion is suspected, it is desirable to obtain an ophthalmology consultation while the patient is still in the recovery room. Following gross examination, a local anesthetic should be instilled and the eye examined with fluorescein to demonstrate the injured area. Corneal abrasions are usually treated by patching the injured eye and applying a prophylactic antibiotic ointment such as erythromycin. Repeated instillation of local anesthetic to control pain is not recommended as these drugs inhibit corneal healing. Healing normally occurs within 48 hours.

OTOLARYNGOLOGIC SURGERY

Optimal management of anesthesia for otolaryngologic surgery is based on reliable control of the upper airway. These patients may present with compromised airways before surgery because of edema, infection, or tumor invasion of the upper airway. Following intubation of the trachea, monitoring with a precordial or esophageal stethoscope is essential because the anesthesiologist is often situated away from direct access to the airway. Monitoring the electrocardiogram is necessary to detect cardiac dysrhythmias that frequently accompany surgical manipulation in the larynx, pharynx, and neck. Blood loss during major otolaryngologic surgery can be substantial and is often underestimated due to hidden losses onto drapes or into the patient's stomach. A posterior pharyngeal pack will keep secretions and blood from pooling in the posterior pharynx and being swallowed into the stomach. Extubation of the trachea may be hazardous following otolaryngologic surgery, especially when the airway is compromised—as due to edema or bleeding following endoscopy or upper airway surgery.

Ear Surgery

Special considerations in the management of anesthesia for ear surgery include (1) facial nerve preservation, (2) the use of epinephrine by the surgeon, and (3) the effect of nitrous oxide on middle ear pressure.

Facial Nerve Preservation. Surgical identification and preservation of the facial nerve is essential during ear surgery and many other otolaryngologic operations. This requirement necessitates maintenance of some skeletal muscle activity if muscle relaxants are administered. Ideally, the twitch response produced by stimulation of the ulnar nerve using a peripheral nerve stimulator should remain 10 to 20 percent of control when muscle relaxants are administered. A volatile anesthetic is ideal because muscle relaxants to prevent unexpected patient movement are not routinely required, thus preserving the ability to easily identify the facial nerve by virtue of skeletal muscle response to electrical stimulation of tissue presumed to be nerve. Futhermore, if nitrous oxide must be discontinued, the patient remains adequately anesthetized by increasing the inhaled concentration of the volatile anesthetic. Another advantage of a volatile anesthetic is the ability to maintain systolic blood pressure between 80 to 85 mmHg so as to minimize intraoperative blood loss if this is deemed important for the success of the surgery.

Use of Epinephrine. Epinephrine is often infiltrated in the operative area by the surgeon to produce vasoconstriction and thus decrease blood loss. Concentrations of epinephrine greater than 1:50,000 (20 μg/ml) do not provide additional vasoconstrictive effect. It must be remembered that halothane is more likely than enflurane or isoflurane to evoke cardiac dysrhythmias in the presence of exogenous epinephrine.

Nitrous Oxide and Middle Ear Pressure. Nitrous oxide, which is 34 times more soluble than nitrogen, enters air-filled cavities such as the middle ear more rapidly than air can leave, resulting in an elevation of middle ear pressure (Fig. 25-1).[8] Under normal conditions, any pressure elevation in the middle ear is passively vented via the eustachian tube into the nasopharynx. Narrowing of the eustachian tube by acute inflammation or the presence of scar tissue, as is likely after an adenoidectomy, impairs the ability of the middle ear to vent passively any pressure increase produced by nitrous oxide. Tympanic membrane rupture, manifesting as bright red blood in the external auditory canal, has been attributed to pressure increases produced by nitrous oxide.[9] Disruption of previous middle ear reconstructive surgery has been reported when nitrous oxide is administered at a later date for operative procedures not involving the ear.[10] During tympanoplasty surgery, the effect of nitrous oxide on middle ear pressure may cause displacement of the tympanic membrane graft. Therefore, the inhaled nitrous oxide concentration should be limited to 50 percent, with discontinuance 15 minutes prior to placement of the graft.[18] Finally, postoperative nausea and vomiting could be due to increased middle ear pressure that persists following the administration of nitrous oxide.

Rapid reabsorption of nitrous oxide when administration of this gas is discontinued can produce negative pressure in the middle ear, manifesting as serous otitis or transient postoperative hearing loss (Fig. 25-2).[8]

Nasal and Sinus Surgery

Special considerations in the management of anesthesia for nasal and sinus surgery include the (1) intraoperative application of topical cocaine to produce maximal vasoconstriction in the operative area, (2) use of a posterior pharyngeal pack, (3) possibility of large intraoperative blood loss,

INTRATYMPANIC PRESSURE CHANGES

L. C. DECEMBER 1974
STARTING PRESSURE 50

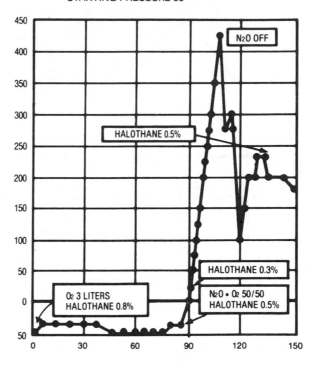

Figure 25-1. Measurements in a single patient demonstrate an abrupt increase in middle ear pressure (mmH_2O) when nitrous oxide is added to the inhaled gases. (Patterson ME, Bartlett PC. Hearing impairment caused by intratympanic pressure changes during general anesthesia. Laryngoscope 1976; 86:402.)

and (4) the need for extubation of the trachea only when protective upper airway reflexes have returned. Systemic absorption of cocaine may manifest as tachycardia and hypertension. The maximum safe dose of topical cocaine is about 3 mg/kg. The use of a combination of topical cocaine and epinephrine has not been shown to increase the vasoconstrictive effectiveness of cocaine. Furthermore, topically applied epinephrine does not retard the systemic absorption nor prolong the anesthetic action of cocaine. Maintenance of anesthesia is acceptably provided by using a volatile anesthetic, which offers the advantage of providing better control of the blood pressure than a narcotic technique. Alternatively, a nitrous oxide-narcotic technique may be selected with intermittent administration of a volatile anesthetic to control blood pres-

sure. Although nasal sinuses represent air-filled cavities, there is no evidence that nitrous oxide produces adverse increases in pressure in these structures (see the section *Nitrous Oxide and Middle Ear Pressure*). Before extubation of the trachea, the pharynx should be suctioned, the posterior pharyngeal pack removed, and the return of protective upper airway reflexes confirmed.

Endoscopy

Special considerations in the management of anesthesia for endoscopy (laryngoscopy, laser surgery, bronchoscopy, esophagoscopy) include the (1) possibility of co-existing airway pathology, (2) management of an upper airway that is shared with the surgeon, (3) need for elimination of

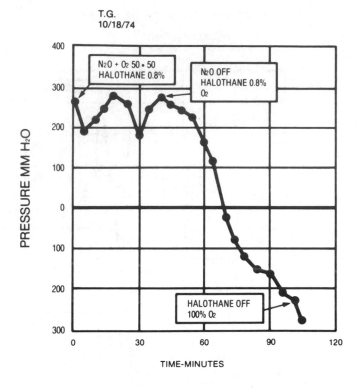

T.G.
10/18/74

N₂O + O₂ 50 · 50
HALOTHANE 0.8%

N₂O OFF
HALOTHANE 0.8%
O₂

HALOTHANE OFF
100% O₂

PRESSURE MM H₂O

TIME-MINUTES

Figure 25-2. Measurements in a single patient demonstrate an abrupt decrease in middle ear pressure (mmH₂O) to below normal when inhalation of nitrous oxide is discontinued. (Patterson ME, Bartlett PC. Hearing impairment caused by intratympanic pressure changes during general anesthesia. Laryngoscope 1976; 86:402.)

cough and laryngeal reflexes, (4) need for a relaxed mandible, (5) protection of teeth with a dental guard, and (6) need for rapid awakening with return of protective upper airway reflexes. Cardiac dysrhythmias are frequently associated with the stimulus of endoscopy. In some patients, endoscopy is best performed with the patient awake utilizing local anesthesia.

Laryngoscopy. General anesthesia for laryngoscopy may be performed with a small (5 mm internal diameter) tracheal tube. This approach permits the use of muscle relaxants to assure optimal surgical working conditions and facilitates ventilation of the lungs. The disadvantage of using a tracheal tube is interference with the surgeon's view of the larynx, especially the posterior commissure. Intermittent injections or a continuous intravenous infusion of succinylcholine is an effective method to produce skeletal muscle relaxation for these short procedures. General anesthetic tech-

niques in the absence of intubation of the trachea utilize spontaneous ventilation during the administration of a volatile anesthetic in oxygen or intermittent high-pressure insufflation of gases through a ventilating (Sanders) bronchoscope. High-pressure insufflation techniques require profound skeletal muscle relaxation to permit adequate ventilation of the lungs. Small children and patients with bullous lung disease do not tolerate the increased airway pressure associated with this technique. High frequency ventilation is an alternative mode for ventilation of the lungs during laryngoscopy (see Chapter 32).

Laser Surgery. Endoscopic laser surgery is used to vaporize papillomas and other tumors. The laser provides a high energy source focused to a fine point that destroys tissue by a thermal effect. A metal tracheal tube or a red rubber (non-portex) tube wrapped with thin metallic tape or moist gauze to prevent its ignition is used.

Nearby, nontarget tissue is also protected by moist gauze. Operating room personnel must wear safety glasses and the patient's eyes are taped shut to prevent damage from any reflected laser beam. The patient must remain absolutely immobile as the laser is critically focused on a specific target tissue and any amount of patient movement may divert the beam to adjacent normal tissue.

Bronschoscopy. Methods of general anesthesia and management of ventilation of the lungs for bronchoscopy do not differ from those for laryngoscopy. A volatile anesthetic is ideal to provide adequate suppression of upper airway reflexes and also permit use of high inhaled concentrations of oxygen. Bronchoscopes in current use include the (1) flexible fiberoptic, (2) rigid-ventilating, and (3) rigid-Venturi (Sanders injector) type. The flexible fiberoptic bronchoscope offers the advantage of being placed via a large (8 mm internal diameter or larger) tracheal tube, permitting reliable ventilation of both lungs during endoscopy. Patient movement or excessive airway pressures during bronchoscopy performed with a rigid bronchoscope may result in a tracheal tear and/or pneumothorax. Trauma associated with bronchoscopy can manifest as airway edema, which may warrant the use of intravenous dexamethasone (0.1 mg/kg).

Head and Neck Surgery

Head and neck surgery such as laryngectomy or radical neck dissection may last 6 to 8 hours and involve substantial blood loss. Patients with carcinoma of the larnyx are often heavy smokers with chronic obstructive airway disease. Patency of the upper airway may be compromised by tumor, necessitating placement of a tracheal tube or performance of a tracheostomy prior to the induction of anesthesia. Surgery near the carotid sinus can elicit a vagal response, manifesting as bradycardia and hypotension. During head and neck surgery open neck veins create the possibility of venous air embolism. Positive pressure ventilation of the lungs decreases the likelihood of venous air embolism by maintaining an elevated pressure in the veins. Maintenance of blood pressure in a low normal range by varying the inhaled concentration of a volatile anesthetic plus a 10 to 15 degree head-up tilt is helpful in minimizing intraoperative blood loss. Blood and intravenous fluids can be warmed to help maintain body temperature during prolonged operations. Finally, a catheter placed in the bladder is indicated if it is anticipated that large volumes of fluid replacement will be necessary.

Tonsillectomy

Special considerations in the management of anesthesia for tonsillectomy include (1) preoperative evaluation of coagulation, (2) determination of the presence of loose teeth, (3) provision of mandibular and pharyngeal muscle relaxation, (4) suppression of laryngeal reflexes, and (5) rapid awakening and return of protective upper airway reflexes. Blood loss during tonsillectomy averages 4 ml/kg, but is usually underestimated due to an undetermined amount of blood draining into the stomach. Maintenance of anesthesia for these short surgical procedures is acceptably achieved with nitrous oxide plus a volatile drug delivered via a tracheal tube. Postoperatively, the patient is often placed in the lateral position with the head lower than the hips (tonsil position) so that blood drains out the mouth. As a result, blood loss is less likely to irritate the vocal cords or to be masked by unrecognized accumulation in the stomach.

Reoperation for continued bleeding from the tonsil bed is a major anesthetic challenge. These patients are often hypovolemic, as reflected by tachycardia and orthostatic hypotension. Rehydration with lactated Ringer's solution (15 to 20 ml/kg) is mandatory prior to the induction of anesthesia. Since large volumes of blood may have been swallowed, it is important to treat these patients as if they have a full stomach. A rapid sequence induction of anesthesia utilizing thiopental and succinycholine plus cricoid pressure is acceptable. The dose of thiopental should be reduced, since the possibility of hypovolemia exists despite attempts at rehydration. Alternatively, awake intubation of the trachea may be performed. The stomach should be emptied via an orogastric tube following placement of the tracheal tube. After the completion of the surgery, the patient is allowed to awaken and protective airway reflexes return before the trachea is extubated.

Tracheostomy

Tracheostomy must be regarded as a procedure that is best performed electively in the operating room. Ideally, a translaryngeal tracheal tube should be in place to facilitate ventilation of lungs and permit an unhurried surgical procedure. Cricothyroidotomy can be performed rapidly as a lifesaving procedure when acute upper airway obstruction occurs and translaryngeal intubation of the trachea is not possible. Early complications of tracheostomy include tube displacement, hemorrhage, and pneumothorax.

REFERENCES

1. Myers EF, Krupin T, Johnson M, Zink H. Failure of nondepolarizing neuromuscular blockers to inhibit succinylcholine-induced intraocular pressure—a controlled study. Anesthesiology 1978;48:149–51.
2. Pandey K. Badola RP, Kumar S. Time course of intraocular hypertension produced by suxamethonium. Br J Anaes 1972; 44:191–5.
3. Ausinisch B, Rayburn LR, Munson ES, Levy NS. Ketamine and intraocular pressure in children. Anesth Analg 1976;55:773–5.
4. Kim JW, Smith PH. Timolol-induced bradycardia. Anesth Analg 1980;59:301–3.
5. Wolf GL, Capuano C, Hartung J. Nitrous oxide increases intraocular pressure after intravitreal sulfur hexafluoride injection. Anesthesiology 1983;59:547–8.
6. Backer CL, Tinker JH, Robertson DM. Myocardial reinfarction following local anesthesia. Anesthesiology 1979;51:S61.
7. Smith RB. Succinylcholine and the forced duction test. Ophthalmol Surg 1974;5:53–5.
8. Patterson ME, Bartlett PC. Hearing impairment caused by intratympanic pressure changes during general anesthesia. Laryngoscope 1976;86:399–404.
9. Owens WD, Gustave F, Sclaroff A. Tympanic membrane rupture with nitrous oxide anesthesia. Anesth Analg 1978;57:283–6.
10. Man A, Segal S, Ezra S. Ear injury caused by elevated intratympanic pressure during general anesthesia. Acta Anaesth Scand 1980;24:224–6.

26

Obstetrics

Optimal analgesia and/or anesthesia for labor, vaginal delivery, or cesarean section requires an understanding of the physiologic changes in the parturient during pregnancy and labor, the effects of anesthetics on the fetus and neonate, the benefits and risks of various techniques of anesthesia, and the significance of obstetric complications on the management of anesthesia.[1] Unlike the patient scheduled for elective surgery, the parturient is rarely in optimal condition at the time anesthetic care becomes necessary. For example, the parturient must always be considered to represent a full stomach and to be at increased risk for inhalation (pulmonary aspiration) of gastric contents. During labor, emergencies such as fetal distress, maternal hemorrhage, and prolapsed cord demand immediate anesthesia.

PHYSIOLOGIC CHANGES IN THE PARTURIENT

Pregnancy and subsequent labor and delivery are accompanied by predictable physiologic changes.

Cardiovascular System

Changes in the cardiovascular system during pregnancy provide for the needs of the developing fetus and prepare the mother for events that will occur during labor and delivery. These changes include alterations in (1) the intravascular fluid volume and its constituents, (2) cardiac output, and (3) peripheral circulation (Table 26-1). The supine hypotension syndrome reflects circulatory changes due to the impact of the enlarging gravid uterus.

Intravascular Fluid Volume. The increase in maternal intravascular fluid volume begins in the first trimester and at term results in an average expansion of about 1000 ml. Plasma volume increases 45 percent and the erythrocyte volume increases 20 percent. This disproportionate increase in plasma volume accounts for the relative anemia of pregnancy. The increased intravascular fluid volume offsets the 400 to 600 ml blood loss that accompanies vaginal delivery and the average 1000 ml blood loss that accompanies cesarean section. Total plasma protein concentration is reduced, reflecting the dilutional effect of the increased intravascular fluid volume. Nevertheless, protein binding of a drug such as thiopental has not been shown to be altered in the parturient.[2]

Cardiac Output is increased about 40 percent above nonpregnant levels by the 10th week of gestation and is maintained at this level throughout the second and third trimesters. This augmentation of cardiac output is primarily due to an elevated stroke volume, as heart rate is not greatly in-

Table 26-1. Changes in the Cardiovascular System during Pregnancy

Variable	Compared with Nonpregnant Value
Intravascular fluid volume	Increased 35 percent
Plasma volume	Increased 45 percent
Erythrocyte volume	Increased 20 percent
Cardiac output	Increased 40 percent
Stroke volume	Increased 30 percent
Heart rate	Increased 15 percent
Peripheral circulation	
Systolic blood pressure	No change
Systemic vascular resistance	Decreased 15 percent
Central venous pressure	No change
Femoral venous pressure	Increased 15 percent

(Adapted from Campbell C, Ravindran RS. The pregnant patient. In Stoelting RK, Dierdorf SF, eds. Anesthesia and co-existing disease. New York, Churchill Livingstone, 1983;683–739.)

creased. Earlier studies suggesting return of cardiac output toward nonpregnant levels during the third trimester were in error. Instead, this decrease reflected reduced venous return due to compression of the inferior vena cava by the gravid uterus when the supine position was assumed.

The onset of labor is associated with further increases in cardiac output which may reach 45 percent above the prelabor value. The greatest increase in cardiac output occurs immediately after delivery when output is elevated as much as 60 percent above prelabor values. A regional anesthetic is capable of attenuating increases in cardiac output during labor and may therefore be an ideal way of protecting a compromised cardiovascular system during the peripartum period. Typically, cardiac output returns to nonpregnant values by 2 weeks postpartum.

Peripheral Circulation. Systolic blood pressure never increases above nonpregnant levels during an uncomplicated pregnancy. Since cardiac output is elevated, the systemic vascular resistance must decrease for the blood pressure to remain normal. There is no change in the central venous pressure during pregnancy, while femoral venous pressure is increased about 15 percent, presumably reflecting compression of the inferior vena cava by the gravid uterus.

Supine Hypotension Syndrome. Reductions in maternal blood pressure associated with the supine position occur in about 10 percent of parturients near term.[1] Diaphoresis, nausea, vomiting, and changes in cerebration may accompany this hypotension. These symptoms are termed the supine hypotension syndrome.

The mechanism for the supine hypotension syndrome is decreased venous return due to compression of the inferior vena cava by the gravid uterus when the parturient assumes the supine position (Fig. 26-1). The resulting decrease in venous return leads to a reduction in cardiac output and a decline in blood pressure. Fortunately, the majority (about 90 percent) of parturients are able to initiate compensatory responses on assuming the supine position. These compensatory responses prevent the appearance of the supine hypotension syndrome. For example, increased venous pressure below the level of compression of the inferior vena cava serves to divert venous blood from the lower half of the body via the paravertebral venous plexuses to the azygos vein. Flow from the azygos vein enters the superior vena cava, and venous return is maintained. This compensatory response means that inadvertent intravascular injection of a local anesthetic during an attempted lumbar epidural block can result in bolus delivery of the drug to the heart with resulting profound myocardial depression. An additional compensatory response that offsets inferior vena cava compression by the gravid uterus is an increase in peripheral sympathetic nervous system activity. This increased activity results in elevation of systemic vascular resistance which permits blood pressure to

Figure 26-1. Schematic diagram showing compression of the inferior vena cava (IVC) and abdominal aorta (Ao) by the gravid uterus when the parturient assumes the supine position.

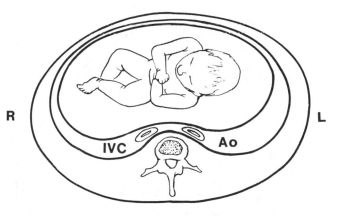

be maintained despite a diminished cardiac output. It is important to recognize that compensatory increases in systemic vascular resistance are impaired by regional anesthetic techniques. Indeed, arterial hypotension is more common and profound during a regional anesthetic administered to a parturient compared with a nonpregnant patient.

In additional to compression of the inferior vena cava, the gravid uterus may also compress the lower abdominal aorta (Fig. 26-1). This compression leads to arterial hypotension in the lower extremities but maternal symptoms or a reduction in blood pressure as measured in the arm do not occur.

The significance of aortocaval compression is the associated reduction in uterine and placental blood flow. Even in the presence of a healthy uteroplacental unit, reductions in maternal blood pressure to less than 100 mmHg that persist for longer than 10 to 15 minutes may be associated with progressive fetal acidosis and bradycardia.

The incidence of the supine hypotension syndrome can be minimized by nursing the parturient in the lateral position. Alternatively, left uterine displacement is effective by moving the gravid uterus off the inferior vena cava or aorta. Displacement of the uterus to the left can be accomplished manually or by elevation of the right hip 10 to 15 cm with a blanket or foam-rubber wedge (Fig. 26-2).

Respiratory System

Changes in the respiratory system during pregnancy are manifest as alterations in (1) the upper airway, (2) minute ventilation, (3) lung volumes, and (4) arterial oxygenation (Table 26-2).

Upper Airway. Capillary engorgement of the mucosal lining of the upper respiratory tract accompanies pregnancy and emphasizes the need for gentleness during intrumentation (suctioning, placement of nasal or oral airways, direct laryngoscopy) of the upper airway. It is prudent to select a smaller size cuffed tracheal tube (6.5 to 7.0 mm internal diameter) since the false vocal cords and arytenoids are often edematous.

Minute ventilation is increased about 50 percent above nonpregnant levels during the first trimester and maintained at this elevated level for the remainder of pregnancy. This increased minute ventilation is achieved by an increased tidal volume as respiratory rate is not greatly altered (Table 26-2). Increased circulating levels of progesterone are presumed to be the stimulus for increased minute ventilation.

The resting maternal $PaCO_2$ decreases from 40 mmHg to about 30 mmHg during the first trimester as a reflection of increased minute ventilation. Arterial pH, however, remains near normal because of increased renal excretion of bicarbonate

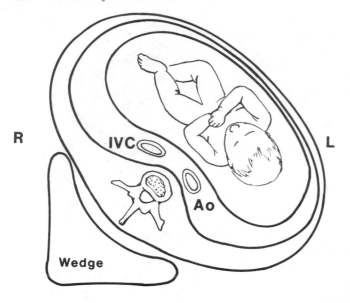

R

IVC

L

Ao

Wedge

Figure 26-2. Schematic diagram depicting left uterine displacement by elevation of the parturient's right hip with a foam-rubber wedge. This position moves the gravid uterus off the inferior vena cava (IVC) and aorta (Ao).

ion. Pain associated with labor and delivery results in further hyperventilation which can be attenuated by lumbar epidural block.

Lung Volumes, in contrast to the early appearance of increased minute ventilation, do not begin to change until about the fifth month of pregnancy (Table 26-2). With in-

Table 26-2. Changes in the Respiratory System during Pregnancy

Variable	Compared with Nonpregnant Value
Minute ventilation	Increased 50 percent
Tidal volume	Increased 40 percent
Respiratory rate	Increased 10 percent
Lung volumes	
Expiratory reserve volume	Decreased 20 percent
Residual volume	Decreased 20 percent
Functional residual capacity	Decreased 20 percent
Vital capacity	No change
Total lung capacity	No change
Arterial blood gases and pH	
PaO_2	Increased 10 mmHg
$PaCO_2$	Decreased 10 mmHg
pH	No change
Oxygen consumption	Increased 20 percent

creasing enlargement of the uterus, the diaphragm is forced cephalad. This change is largely responsible for the 20 percent reduction in functional residual capacity present at term. Vital capacity is not significantly changed.

The combination of increased minute ventilation and decreased functional residual capacity speeds the rate at which changes in the alveolar concentration of an inhaled anesthetic can be achieved. Indeed, induction of anesthesia, emergence from anesthesia, and changes in depth of anesthesia are notably faster in the parturient.

Arterial Oxygenation. Maternal PaO_2 while breathing room air normally exceeds 100 mmHg, reflecting the presence of hyperventilation (Table 26-2). Induction of general anesthesia, however, in the parturient may be associated with marked reductions in the PaO_2 if apnea, as during intubation of the trachea, is prolonged. This tendency for a rapid decrease in PaO_2 reflects a decreased oxygen reserve secondary to the reduction in functional residual capacity. A reduction in cardiac output due to aortocaval compression and increased oxygen consumption may also contribute to a rapid decrease in PaO_2 during apnea. For

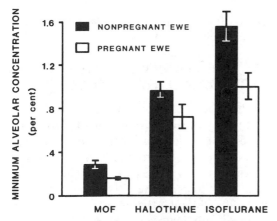

Figure 26-3. The minimum alveolar concentration (MAC) was reduced in the pregnant ewe as compared with the nonpregnant ewe. (Campbell C, Ravindran RS. The pregnant patient. In: Stoelting RK, Dierdorf SF, eds. Anesthesia and co-existing disease. New York, Churchill Livingstone, 1983;683–739, with data from reference 3.)

these reasons, the administration of oxygen (preoxygenation) before any anticipated period of apnea or during a regional anesthetic is important Likewise, it is prudent to provide routinely left uterine displacement.

Nervous System Changes

Central nervous system changes during pregnancy are reflected by decreased MAC for volatile anesthetics, as demonstrated in animals (Fig. 26-3).[3] It is presumed, but not documented, that similar changes occur in humans. Sedative effects produced by progesterone may be partially responsible for this reduction in MAC. The important clinical implication of decreased MAC is that alveolar concentrations of inhaled drugs that would not produce unconsciousness in nonpregnant patients may approximate anesthetizing concentrations in the parturient. This degree of central nervous system depression may also impair protective upper airway reflexes and subject the parturient to the hazards of pulmonary aspiration. Furthermore, the decreased functional residual capacity speeds the rate at

which a potential excessive alveolar concentration of anesthetic can be achieved.

Engorgement of epidural veins as intra-abdominal pressure increases with progressive enlargement of the uterus decreases the size of the epidural space and reduces the volume of cerebrospinal fluid in the subarachnoid space. Decreased volume of these spaces facilitates the spread of the local anesthetic and is consistent with the 30 to 50 percent reduction in dose requirements of local anesthetics necessary for epidural or spinal anesthesia in the parturient at term.[1] Nevertheless, there are also data that do not demonstrate a difference in the level of sensory anesthesia achieved when equal volumes of local anesthetic are injected into the epidural space of pregnant and nonpregnant patients.[4]

Renal Changes

Renal blood flow and glomerular filtration rate are increased about 50 percent by the fourth month of pregnancy. Therefore, the normal upper limits of the blood urea nitrogen and serum creatinine concentration are reduced about 50 percent in the parturient.

Hepatic Changes

Serum bilirubin concentrations and hepatic blood flow are unchanged during pregnancy. Nevertheless, most parturients manifest abnormal bromsulfalein excretion tests. Total protein concentration and pseudocholinesterase activity are decreased. Despite the latter, the response of parturients to moderate doses of succinylcholine is not prolonged.[1] For unknown reasons, serum transaminase concentrations and the circulating levels of alkaline phosphatase are often elevated during pregnancy.

Gastrointestinal Changes

Gastrointestinal changes during pregnancy make the parturient vulnerable to regurgitation of gastric contents and to the development of acid pneumonitis should pulmonary aspiration occur. For example, the enlarged uterus displaces the pylorus upward and backward, which retards gastric emptying. As a result, the gastric fluid volume tends to be elevated, even in the fasting state. In addition, gastrin, which is secreted by the placenta, stimulates gastric hydrogen ion secretion such that the pH of gastric fluid is predictably low in the parturient. Finally, the enlarging uterus changes the angle of the gastroesophageal junction, leading to relative incompetence of the physiologic sphincter mechanism. As a result, gastric fluid reflux into the esophagus and subsequent esophagitis are common in the parturient.

Regardless of the time interval since ingestion of food, the parturient in labor must be treated as having a full stomach. Pain, anxiety, and drugs administered during labor can all significantly retard gastric emptying beyond an already prolonged transit time.

The increased risk for pulmonary aspiration of gastric contents is the reason for recommending the placement of a cuffed tube in the trachea of every parturient who is rendered unconscious by anesthesia. The recognition that the pH of inhaled gastric fluid is important in the production and severity of acid pneumonitis is the basis for the administration of oral antacids (15 to 20 ml every 2 to 4 hours) to the parturient during labor and prior to delivery. The routine use of antacids, however, has not been conclusively proven to reduce morbidity or mortality despite the accepted ability of these drugs to elevate the pH of gastric fluid. It must be appreciated that inhalation of antacids containing particulate matter can produce adverse pulmonary changes. In an attempt to obviate the hazards of inhalation of particulate antacids, the use of the nonparticulate antacid, sodium citrate, has been recommended. Alternatively, the histamine H_2-receptor antagonist, cimetidine, has been shown to reliably elevate

gastric fluid pH in parturients without producing neonatal effects.[5]

PHYSIOLOGY OF UTEROPLACENTAL CIRCULATION

The placenta provides for the union of maternal and fetal circulations for the purpose of physiologic exchange. Maternal blood is delivered to the placenta by the uterine arteries while fetal blood arrives via two umbilical arteries. Nutrient-rich and waste-free blood is delivered to the fetus via a single umbilical vein. The most important determinants of placental function are uterine blood flow and the characteristics of substances available for exchange across the placenta.

Uterine Blood Flow

Maintenance of uterine blood flow at term (500 to 700 ml/min) is critical, as this flow determines the adequacy of placental circulation and fetal well-being. In the presence of a normal placenta, it is estimated that uterine blood flow can decrease about 50 percent before fetal distress, as reflected by acidosis, is detectable.

Uterine blood flow is not autoregulated and is, therefore, directly proportional to mean perfusion pressure across the uterus and inversely proportioned to uterine vascular resistance. Therefore, uterine blood flow is reduced by drugs or events that decrease perfusion pressure (decreased systemic blood pressure or increased venous pressure) or increase uterine vascular resistance.

Hypotension due to aortocaval compression or peripheral sympathetic nervous system blockade decreases uterine blood flow by reductions in perfusion pressure. Drugs administered to the parturient to produce analgesia and anesthesia during labor and delivery could reduce uterine blood flow via drug-induced changes in blood pressure. For example, when the concentration of

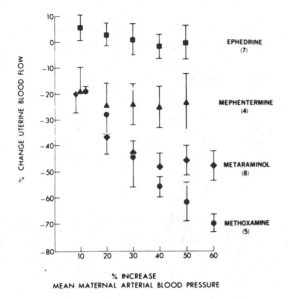

Figure 26-4. Uterine blood flow (mean ± SE) was measured in pregnant ewes (number of animals studied in parentheses) before and after increases in maternal blood pressure produced by the intravenous administration of a sympathomimetic. With the exception of ephedrine, these drugs decreased uterine blood flow despite increasing mean arterial pressure. (Ralson DH, Shnider SM, deLorimer AA. Effects of equipotent ephedrine, metaraminol, mephentermine and methoxamine on uterine blood flow in the pregnant ewe. Anesthesiology 1974;40:354–70.)

volatile anesthetics administered to pregnant ewes exceeds 1 MAC, fetal acidosis develops, suggesting decreased uterine blood flow in association with drug-induced hypotension.[1] Epidural or spinal block does not alter uterine blood flow as long as maternal hypotension is avoided.[1]

Uterine Vascular Resistance. Alpha-adrenergic stimulation produced by methoxamine and metaraminol can increase uterine vascular resistance and decrease uterine blood flow (Fig. 26-4).[6] Conversely, ephedrine is considered the best sympathomimetic to use to raise blood pressure in the parturient because uterine blood flow is maintained in the presence of this vasopressor (Fig. 26-4).[6] Increased uterine vas-

cular resistance with reductions in uterine blood flow can result from maternal stress or pain that stimulates the endogenous release of catecholamines (Fig. 26-5).[7] This response suggests that a regional or general anesthetic may be protective to the fetus. Finally, uterine contractions reduce uterine blood flow secondary to elevated uterine venous pressure.

Placental Exchange

Placenta exchange of substances is principally by diffusion from the maternal circulation to the fetus and vice versa. Diffusion of a substance across the placenta to the fetus depends on the maternal-to-fetal concentration gradient, maternal protein binding, molecular weight, lipid solubility, and degree of ionization of that substance (Table 26-3). Minimizing the maternal blood

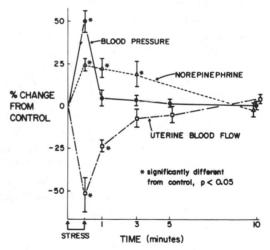

Figure 26-5. Electrically-induced stress in pregnant ewes lasting 30 to 60 seconds resulted in increased maternal blood pressure and serum norepinephrine concentrations (mean ± SE). Uterine blood flow was reduced about 50 percent at the time of maximum blood pressure and catecholamine elevation. (Shnider SM, Wright RG, Levinson G, Roizen MF, Wallis KL, Robbin SH, Craft JB. Uterine blood flow and plasma norepinephrine changes during maternal stress in the pregnant ewe. Anesthesiology 1979;50:524–7.)

Table 26-3. Determinants of Diffusion across the Placenta

	Rapid Diffusion	Slow Diffusion
Maternal protein binding	Low	High
Molecular weight	<500	>1000
Lipid solubility	High	Low
Ionization	Minimal	Maximum

(Campbell C, Ravindran RS. The pregnant patient. In Stoelting RK, Dierdorf SF, eds. Anesthesia and co-existing disease. New York, Churchill Livingstone 1983;683–739.)

concentration of a drug is the most important method for limiting the amount of that drug which ultimately reaches the fetus. Furthermore, transfer to the fetus can be decreased by intravenous injection of a drug during a uterine contraction since maternal blood flow to the placenta is markedly reduced at this time.

Maternal protein binding of local anesthetics is important since only that portion of the drug not bound to protein is available for diffusion across the placenta. At typical clinical concentrations, 50 to 70 percent of lidocaine is bound to protein, compared with 95 percent for bupivacaine. The greater degree of protein binding for bupivacaine could impair placental transfer by reducing the amount of free drug available for diffusion. This is consistent with the observation that the ratio of umbilical vein-to-uterine artery concentration of bupivacaine is lower than the ratio measured for lidocaine.[1]

Molecular Weight and Lipid Solubility. The large molecular weight and poor lipid solubility of nondepolarizing muscle relaxants are consistent with the fact that these drugs cross the placenta only to a limited extent. Succinylcholine has a low molecular weight but is highly ionized and, therefore, does not readily cross the placenta. Conversely, placental transfer of ultrashort-acting barbiturates, local anesthetics, and narcotics is facilitated by the relatively low molecular weight of these substances.

FETAL UPTAKE AND DISTRIBUTION OF DRUGS

Fetal uptake of a substance that crosses the placenta is facilitated by the lower pH (0.1 unit) of fetal compared with maternal blood. The lower fetal pH means that weakly basic drugs (local anesthetics, narcotics) which cross the placenta in the non-ionized form will become ionized in the fetal circulation. Since an ionized drug cannot readily cross the placenta back to the maternal circulation, it follows that this drug will accumulate in the fetal blood against a concentration gradient. This phenomena is known as ion trapping, and may explain the higher concentrations of lidocaine found in the fetus when acidosis due to fetal distress is present (Fig. 26-6).[8] Furthermore, conversion of lidocaine to the ionized fraction maintains the concentration gradient from mother to fetus for the continued passage of non-ionized lidocaine to the fetus. Despite reduced enzyme activity compared with adults, the neonatal enzyme systems are adequately developed to metabolize most drugs with the possible exception of mepivacaine.[1]

The unique characteristics of the fetal circulation influence the distribution of drugs in the fetus and protect the vital organs of the fetus from exposure to high concentrations of drugs initially present in the umbilical venous blood. For example, about 75 percent of umbilical venous blood passes through the liver such that a significant portion of a drug can be metabolized before reaching the fetal arterial circulation for delivery to the heart and brain. Furthermore, a drug in that portion of the umbilical venous blood which enters the inferior vena cava via the ductus venosus will be diluted by drug-free blood returning from the lower extremities and pelvic viscera of the fetus.

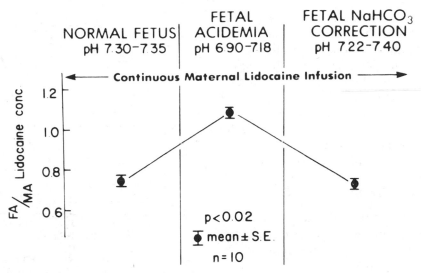

Figure 26-6. Fetal-to-maternal arterial (FA/MA) lidocaine ratios were higher during fetal acidemia than during control (normal fetus), or during pH correction with sodium bicarbonate. This reflects ion trapping of the ionized fraction of lidocaine in the fetus in the presence of acidosis. (Biehl D, Shnider SM, Levinson G, Callender K. Placental transfer of lidocaine: effects of fetal acidosis. Anesthesiology 1978;48:409–12.)

MATERNAL MEDICATION DURING LABOR

Despite the increasing use of epidural block to provide pain relief during labor and vaginal delivery, there is still an occasional role for systemic medications to reduce pain and anxiety. There is no ideal drug, as all systemic medications cross the placenta to some extent and produce depressant effects on the fetus. The amount of fetal depression depends primarily on the dose of drug and route and time of administration before delivery. The drugs likely to be administered as systemic medications are benzodiazepines, narcotics, and dissociative drugs. Barbiturates or scopolamine are no longer popular.

Benzodiazepines

Diazepam readily crosses the placenta barrier. When the maternal dose of diazepam exceeds 30 mg, there is associated fetal hypotonia, decreased feeding, and hypothermia. Beat-to-beat variability of the fetal heart rate is decreased with small intravenous doses (5 to 10 mg) of diazepam but there are no detectable adverse effects on the fetus. Therefore, small doses of intravenous diazepam are acceptable for relieving anxiety, as during cesarean section performed with epidural block.

Narcotics

Narcotics are the most effective systemic medications for the relief of pain during labor and vaginal delivery. All narcotics rapidly cross the placenta and may be responsible for depression of ventilation immediately after birth. Meperidine is the most popular narcotic used in obstetrics, while morphine is rarely administered primarily because of the apparent greater sensitivity of the respiratory center of the newborn to morphine as compared with meperidine. It should be appreciated that the incidence of neonatal depression associated with maternal administration of intramuscular meperidine (50 to 100 mg) is greatest in neonates born 2 to 4 hours after injection.[1] Depression of the neonate is less when delivery occurs within 1 hour or more than 4 hours after injection. The reason for the apparent safe period with intramuscular meperidine is not known.

Dissociative Drugs

Intermittent intravenous doses of ketamine (10 to 15 mg) can be titrated to produce the rapid onset of intense analgesia in the parturient without resulting in loss of consciousness. The dose should not exceed 100 mg in 3 minutes or a total dose of 3 mg/kg. This low-dose approach is particularly useful for parturients in whom vaginal delivery is imminent or when regional anesthesia is incomplete. Ketamine readily crosses the placenta but in low doses does not cause neonatal depression. Nevertheless, adverse maternal psychological changes may accompany even these low doses of ketamine.

PROGRESS OF LABOR

Progress of labor refers to increasing cervical dilation, effacement, and descent of the fetal presenting part through the vagina with time (Fig. 26-7).[9] The onset of regular contractions signals the beginning of the first stage of labor. This stage is subdivided into the latent and active phases, lasting 7 to 13 hours in the primigravida and 4 to 5 hours in the multigravida. The second stage of labor begins with complete dilatation of the cervix. The third stage extends from delivery of the baby until the placenta is expelled.

The progress of labor is unpredictable, being influenced by many variables including maternal pain, parity, size and presentation of the fetus, and drugs and techniques used to provide analgesia or anesthesia. Excessive sedation or the premature initiation

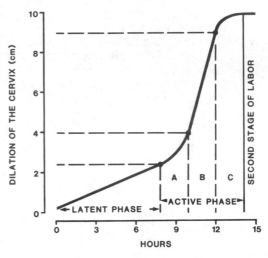

Figure 26-7. The progress of labor is divided into the first and second stages of labor depending on the dilatation of the cervix. The first stage of labor is further subdivided into a latent and an active phase. The active phase consists of the accelerated phase (A), the phase of maximum slope (B), and the deceleration phase (C). (Campbell C, Ravindran RS. The pregnant patient. In: Stoelting RK, Dierdorf SF, eds. Anesthesia and co-existing disease. New York, Churchill Livingstone 1983;683–739, as adapted from Friedman EA. Primigravid labor. A graphicostatistical analysis. Obstet Gynecol 1955;6:567–89. Reprinted with permission from the American College of Obstetricians and Gynecologists.)

of a regional anesthetic is the most common cause for prolongation of the latent phase. During the active phase the most likely causes of delayed progress of labor are cephalopelvic disproportion and fetal malpresentation.

During the active phase a T10 sensory level produced by a spinal or epidural block has no significant effect on progress of labor provided fetal malpresentation is absent and hypotension is avoided. However, a regional anesthetic, by removing the reflex urge to bear down, may prolong the second stage of labor. Nevertheless, even if labor is prolonged by a regional anesthetic there is no evidence this is harmful to the fetus.

Volatile anesthetics produce dose-dependent decreases in uterine activity. Analgesia provided with low inhaled concentrations of halothane (0.5 percent) or enflurane (1 percent) during vaginal delivery does not decrease uterine activity, prolong labor, increase postpartum blood loss, or interfere with the uterine response to oxytocin.[1] Greater inhaled concentrations of volatile anesthetics relax the uterus and are the most reliable way of rapidly producing uterine relaxation when necessary.

REGIONAL ANESTHESIA FOR LABOR AND VAGINAL DELIVERY

Compared with analgesia produced by inhaled or parenteral drugs, the use of regional anesthetic techniques for labor and vaginal delivery reduces the likelihood of fetal drug depression and maternal pulmonary aspiration.

Regional blocks effective during the first stage of labor include paracervical block, lumbar epidural block, and caudal block (Table 26-4). Intraspinal narcotics (epidural or subarachnoid injection) have also been evaluated for relief of pain during the first stage of labor. Pain during the second stage of labor is relieved by lumbar epidural, caudal, spinal, and pudendal nerve blocks (Table 26-4).

Pain During Labor and Delivery

Parturition is associated with two distinct kinds of pain. The first type of pain is visceral in origin caused by uterine contrac-

tions plus dilatation of the cervix. The other type of pain is somatic due to stretching of the vagina and perineum by descent of the fetus. The parturient has an uncontrollable urge to bear down as the presenting fetal part begins its descent through the vagina. It is customary to consider visceral pain as part of the first stage and somatic pain as part of the second stage of labor.

Rational use of regional anesthetic techniques requires an understanding of the pathways responsible for the transmission of visceral and somatic pain during labor and vaginal delivery (Fig. 26-8).[1] During the first stage of labor, afferent visceral pain impulses from the uterus and cervix travel in nerves that accompany sympathetic nervous system fibers and enter the spinal cord at T10 to L1. In the late first stage and the second stage of labor, somatic pain impulses originate primarily from receptors in the vagina and perineum and travel via the pudendal nerves to the spinal cord at S2 to S4.

Paracervical Block

Injection of local anesthetic into the fornix of the vagina lateral to the cervix (3 and 9 positions) eliminates visceral pain by anesthetizing the sensory fibers from the uterus, cervix, and upper vagina. Somatic pain and the urge to bear down are not obtunded. Maternal hypotension does not re-

Table 26-4. Types of Regional Anesthesia for Labor and Vaginal Delivery

Technique	Area of Anesthesia	Type of Pain Blocked
Paracervical block	T10–L1	Visceral
Intraspinal narcotics	No distinct sensory loss	Visceral
Lumbar epidural block		
Segmental	T10–L1	Visceral
Standard	T10–S5	Visceral and somatic
Caudal block	T10–S5	Visceral and somatic
Spinal block		
Saddle	S1–S5	Somatic
Modified	T10–S5	Visceral and somatic
Pudendal nerve blocks	S2–S4	Somatic

(Adapted from Campbell C, Ravindran RS. The pregnant patient. In Stoelting RK, Dierdorf SF, eds. Anesthesia and co-existing disease. New York, Churchill Livingstone 1983;683–739.)

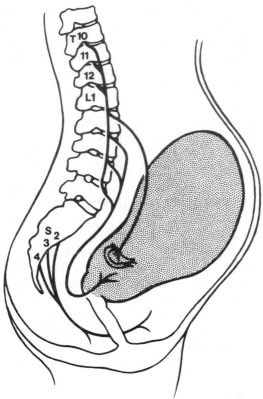

Figure 26-8. Schematic diagram of pain pathways during parturition. Visceral pain during the first stage of labor is due to uterine contraction and dilation of the cervix. Afferent pain impulses from the uterus and cervix are transmitted by nerves which accompany sympathetic nervous system fibers and enter the spinal cord at T10 to L1. Somatic pain during the second stage of labor is vaginal and perineal in origin and impulses travel via the pudendal nerves to S2-4. (Campbell C, Ravindran RS. The pregnant patient. In: Stoelting RK, Dierdorf SF, eds. Anesthesia and co-existing disease, New York, Churchill Livingstone 1983;683–739.)

sult, since sympathetic nervous system block does not occur. Paracervical block is not effective during the second stage of labor, since sensory fibers from the perineum are not blocked. The major disadvantage of a paracervical block is the 8 to 40 percent incidence of fetal bradycardia that develops 2 to 10 minutes after injection of local anesthetic.[1] The cause of brady-

cardia is not known but is probably related to decreased uterine blood flow secondary to uterine vasoconstriction from local anesthetic applied in close proximity to the artery plus direct cardiac toxicity due to high fetal blood levels of the local anesthetic. Bradycardia produced by paracervical block is often associated with fetal acidosis. It would seem prudent to avoid this block in parturients with uteroplacental insufficiency or when there is co-existing fetal distress.

Intraspinal Narcotics

The efficacy of epidural or subarachnoid injection of narcotics for the relief of pain during the first stage of labor is not well-defined. Subarachnoid placement seems to be more effective than epidural injection. Maternal side effects include a high incidence of pruritus, somnolence, and the potential for the delayed onset of depression of ventilation. Neonatal depression does not seem to occur. Narcotics administered by epidural or subarachnoid routes are not reliably effective for pain relief during the second stage of labor.

Lumbar Epidural Block

Advantages of a continuous lumbar epidural block via an appropriately placed plastic catheter include the (1) ability to achieve segmental bands of analgesia (T10–L1) during the first stage of labor when total anesthesia is not required, (2) minimal local anesthetic requirements, and (3) maintenance of pelvic muscle tone so rotation of the fetal head is more easily accomplished. The visceral pain of the first stage of labor can be relieved by injection of 6 to 8 ml of 0.25 percent bupivacaine into the lumbar epidural space. Initially, a 2 ml test dose is injected and 3 minutes allowed to elapse before injecting the remaining drug. This small test dose is utilized to detect an unrecognized subarachnoid injection. Assuming the absence of signs of a spinal block after the test dose, the remaining 4 to 6 ml are injected. The low dose of local anesthetic utilized produces a sensory band of analgesia that is unlikely to produce sufficient peripheral sympathetic block to result in maternal hypotension. Nevertheless, the parturient should be encouraged to remain in the lateral position. Blood pressure should be monitored every 1 to 2 minutes for the first 10 minutes after injection of local anesthetic, then every 5 to 10 minutes until the block dissipates. During the first 20 minutes after the initial dose of local anesthetic and after any additional doses, the parturient should be under continuous surveillance. If hypotension occurs (systolic blood pressure less than 100 mmHg or greater than a 30 percent decrease in a previously hypertensive parturient) left uterine displacement must be confirmed, intravenous fluids infused rapidly, the parturient placed in a 10 to 20 degree head-down position and oxygen administered via a face mask. If blood pressure is not restored in 1 to 2 minutes, intravenous ephedrine (5 to 10 mg) should be administered every 1 to 2 minutes until an appropriate blood pressure response occurs. Ideally, fetal heart rate is continuously monitored electronically before and after the epidural block is instituted.

Supplemental doses of local anesthetic (about two-thirds the initial dose) are administered if the epidural block wanes during the first stage of labor. Additional local anesthetic is injected to provide perineal analgesia as labor progresses. This is accomplished by placing the parturient in the sitting position and injecting slowly 10 to 20 ml of local anesthetic solution. Furthermore, an epidural block can be supplemented to provide adequate anesthesia should a cesarean section become necessary.

Institution of a continuous lumbar epidural block is appropriate when the first stage of labor is well established as evidenced by dilatation of the cervix (6 to 8 cm in a primipara or 4 to 6 cm in a multipara) and uterine contractions are strong and regular.

Caudal Block

Caudal block is produced by injection of a local anesthetic (10 to 12 ml of 0.25 percent bupivacaine) into the sacral epidural space. Compared with a continuous lumbar epidural block, there is a lower incidence of inadvertent dural puncture and perineal analgesia is more profound. Disadvantages of caudal block include difficulty in keeping the sacral area sterile, technical difficulties in identifying the sacral hiatus, and accidental injection of local anesthetic into the fetal head. Finally, it may not be possible to produce a sufficient level of anesthesia with a caudal block should cesarean section become necessary.

Spinal (Saddle) Block

A spinal block is administered immediately before vaginal delivery by injecting a small dose of hyperbaric tetracaine (2 to 4 mg) or lidocaine (20 to 30 mg) into the lumbar subarachnoid space with the parturient in the sitting position. The sitting position is maintained for 2 to 3 minutes to assure that only perineal analgesia (area of the body that would be in contact with a saddle) occurs. A true saddle block does not produce complete pain relief as afferent fibers from the uterus are not blocked.

A modified saddle block is achieved by the subarachnoid injection of 4 to 6 mg of tetracaine or 30 to 50 mg of lidocaine with the sitting position maintained for 30 seconds. With this approach the sensory block typically extends to T10 which prevents pain from contractions of the uterus.

The major disadvantage of a spinal block for vaginal delivery is the subsequent appearance of a headache which is presumably due to loss of fluid through the hole in the dura produced during performance of the block (see Chapter 13).

Pudendal Nerve Block

A pudendal nerve block is typically administered transvaginally by the obstetrician to provide perineal analgesia for normal vaginal delivery. Overlaping innervation of the perineum means the urge to bear down is not completely abolished. Alone, this block provides complete analgesia for episiotomy and repair and is usually sufficient for low forceps delivery. Supplementation with inhalation analgesia is required for mid forceps delivery. A pudendal nerve block is not associated with peripheral sympathetic nervous system blockade and labor is not prolonged.

INHALATION ANALGESIA FOR VAGINAL DELIVERY

The goal of inhalation analgesia is to maintain the parturient in an awake but comfortable state with intact laryngeal reflexes during the first and second stages of labor. The major risk of inhalation analgesia is loss of protective airway reflexes made more likely by the reduced functional residual capacity and decreased MAC associated with pregnancy. Since all inhaled anesthetics readily cross the placenta, the possibility of neonatal effects must also be considered. However, analgesic concentrations of inhaled anesthetics (about 0.3 to 0.4 MAC) are free from excessive depressant effects on the fetus even if admistered for a prolonged period.[1]

An effective form of inhalation analgesia is the continuous administration of 30 to 40 percent nitrous oxide. Less satisfactory analgesia results when nitrous oxide is administered only during the uterine contraction since about 50 seconds are necessary to achieve an effective analgesic concentration of this drug. Intermittent inhalation of methoxyflurane (0.1 to 0.3 percent inhaled) by self-administration or passively from an anesthetic machine is an alternative to the continuous administration of nitrous oxide. It must be appreciated that maternal and neonatal serum fluoride concentrations are increased following the administration of methoxyflurane.[1] Methoxyflurane should not be used in patients with co-existing renal disease as may accompany toxemia of pregnancy. Enflurane (0.5 percent inspired) provides analgesia during the second stage of labor similar to that achieved with nitrous oxide.[10]

ANESTHESIA FOR CESAREAN SECTION

The decision to select a general or regional anesthetic to provide anesthesia for cesarean section depends on the desires of the patient and the presence or absence of fetal distress. When fetal distress is present, a general anesthetic may be preferable since anesthesia can be established quickly and maternal hypotension is less likely. A regional anesthetic is more often chosen for elective cesarean section, particularly when maternal awareness is desirable. Furthermore, a regional anesthetic minimizes the likelihood of maternal pulmonary aspiration and fetal depression.

General Anesthetic

Preoperative medication should include pharmacologic attempts to increase gastric fluid pH. It is common practice to administer antacids for this purpose although cimetidine is also effective for increasing gastric fluid pH (see the section *Gastrointestinal Changes*). If an anticholinergic is judged to be necessary, glycopyrrolate is preferred, since its quaternary ammonium structure prevents significant transfer across lipid barriers such as the placenta. If the cesarean section is elective, diazepam or hydroxyzine may be administered if the parturient is particularly apprehensive.

Following preoxygenation, induction of anesthesia is typically accomplished with thiopental (2 to 4 mg/kg) plus succinylcholine to facilitate intubation of the trachea with a cuffed tube. Cricoid pressure should be applied until the trachea is protected with the cuffed tube. The administration of a small dose of nondepolarizing muscle relaxant (d-tubocurarine 3 mg) prior to succinylcholine is often utilized to prevent skeletal muscle fasiculations. The fetal brain will not be exposed to high concentrations of thiopental if the maternal dose is limited to about 4 mg/kg, reflecting clearance of the drug by the fetal liver and dilution by blood from the viscera and lower extremities. There is no advantage of accelerating or delaying delivery based on a presumed distribution of thiopental in the mother and fetus.

Maintenance of anesthesia until delivery of the fetus is often with nitrous oxide (50 to 60 percent inspired) in oxygen plus succinylcholine for skeletal muscle paralysis. The major disadvantage of using only nitrous oxide is patient awareness during the surgery. Maternal unconsciousness can be assured by the administration of about 0.5 MAC of a volatile anesthetic plus nitrous oxide. This low dose of a volatile anesthetic does not increase maternal blood loss, alter the response of the uterus to oxytocin, or produce neonatal depression. Finally, nitrous oxide supplemented with a volatile anesthetic is associated with a reduced sympathetic nervous system response to surgical stimulation and a better maintenance of uterine blood flow. This response is presumed to reflect inhibition of endogenous norepinephrine secretion by the volatile anesthetic. Excessive hyperventilation must be avoided as the effects of positive pressure can reduce uterine blood flow.

There is controversy regarding the optimal time for delivery when a general anesthetic is used for cesarean section. More important than duration of anesthesia before delivery is the time to delivery following incision into the uterus. Apgar scores are often decreased when the incision to delivery time exceeds 90 seconds, presumably reflecting impaired uteroplacental blood flow.

Following delivery, anesthesia can be supplemented with additional volatile drug or a narcotic. It would seem reasonable to

Table 26-5. Dose of Local Anesthetic for Spinal Block prior to Cesarean Section

Height (cm)	Tetracaine (mg)	Lidocine (mg)
Below 155	7	50
155 to 170	8	60
Above 170	9	70

(Adapted from Campbell C, Ravindran RS. The pregnant patient. In Stoelting RK, Dierdorf SF, eds. Anesthesia and co-existing disease. New York, Churchill Livingstone 1983;683–739.)

pass an oral tube into the stomach to evacuate gastric fluid prior to the conclusion of surgery. The cuffed tube should not be removed from the trachea until it is assured that maternal laryngeal reflexes have returned.

Spinal Block

Spinal block used for cesarean section must provide a sensory level of T4 to T6. A convenient guide for judging the appropriate dose of local anesthetic to be injected into the subarachnoid space is based on the height of the parturient (Table 26-5). Following injection of the local anesthetic in the sitting or lateral position, the parturient is placed supine with leftward displacement of the uterus to minimize aortocaval compression.

The T4 to T6 sensory level necessary for cesarean section is associated with significant peripheral sympathetic nervous system block and the likelihood of maternal hypotension. Hypotension is hazardous, since a decrease in maternal blood presure is associated with a comparable fall in uterine blood flow and placental perfusion, leading to fetal hypoxemia and acidosis. The incidence and magnitude of hypotension may be minimized by continuous left uterine displacement and intravenous hydration with 500 to 1000 ml of lactated Ringer's solution 15 to 30 minutes before performing the spinal block. If hypotension occurs (systolic blood pressure below 100 mmHg or a 30 percent decrease in a previously hypertensive parturient) despite the above measures an intravenous dose of ephedrine (5 to 10 mg) is indicated.

Lumbar Epidural Block

The sensory level necessary for a cesarean section is more controllable and hypotension less precipitous with a continuous lumbar epidural block. Presumably, the slower onset of peripheral sympathetic nervous system block is responsible for the more gradual decrease in blood pressure. Unlike spinal block, anesthesia provided with a lumbar epidural block requires doses of local anesthetic that are associated with significant systemic absorption of the drug. Technically, a lumbar epidural block is more difficult to perform than a spinal block. However, postoperative headache does not occur since the dura is not punctured.

Bupivacaine concentrations must be at least 0.5 percent to assure adequate anesthesia for the surgical stimulus associated with cesarean section. Concentrations of bupivacaine greater than 0.5 percent are not recommended by the manufacturer. This recommendation is based on the concern that inadvertent systemic injection of greater than 0.5 percent bupivacaine could result in cardiovascular collapse due to cardiotoxicity of this local anesthetic.[1] Initially, a test dose of bupivacaine (2 ml) is injected to assure the absence of unrecognized subarachnoid placement of the catheter. Assuming the absence of evidence of a spinal block 3 minutes following the test dose, an additional amount (about 15 to 20 ml) of bupivacaine is injected through the lumbar epidural catheter so as to produce a T4 to T6 sensory level. When a rapid onset of analgesia is necessary, 3 percent 2-chloroprocaine-CE can be used. When chloroprocaine is used, it is imperative that subarachnoid injection be avoided, since permanent neurologic damage has been reported following inadvertent subarachnoid injection of large volumes of this local anesthetic.[12] Lidocaine, 2 percent, is an acceptable alternative to either bupivacaine or chloroprocaine.

ABNORMAL PRESENTATIONS AND MULTIPLE BIRTHS

Description of fetal position is based on the relationship of the fetal occiput, chin, or sacrum to the left or right side of the parturient. Approximately 90 percent of deliveries are cephalic presentation in either the occiput transverse or occiput anterior position. All other presentations and positions are considered abnormal.

Persistent Occiput Posterior

During active labor, the occiput undergoes internal rotation to the occiput anterior position. If this rotation does not occur, the persistent occiput posterior position results in prolonged and painful labor. For example, severe back pain reflects pressure on the posterior sacral nerves by the fetal occiput. Regional anesthetic techniques which relax the maternal perineal muscles are best avoided until spontaneous internal rotation of the fetal head occurs.

Breech Presentation

Breech deliveries are associated with increased maternal (cervical lacerations, retained placenta, hemorrhage) and neonatal (intracranial hemorrhage, prolapse of the umbilical cord) morbidity. There is a growing tendency to deliver breech presentations by elective cesarean section. If cesarean section is planned, either a regional or general anesthetic may be selected. It should be appreciated that during a regional anesthetic there may be difficulty in extracting the infant through the uterine incision. If uterine hypertonus is the cause, it will be necessary to rapidly induce general anesthesia, intubate the trachea, and administer a volatile anesthetic to relax the uterus.

When vaginal delivery is planned for a breech presentation, a frequent approach is infiltration of the perineum with a local anesthetic plus inhalation analgesia. Rapid induction of general anesthesia and intubation of the trachea may be necessary to permit administration of a volatile anesthetic should perineal muscle relaxation be inadequate for delivery of the aftercoming fetal head or if the lower uterine segment contracts and traps the head. An alternative to infiltration and inhalation analgesia is the use of a continuous lumbar epidural block. For example, a lumbar epidural block provides the best analgesia and maximal perineal relaxation for delivery of the fetal head. The ability of the parturient to push during the delivery can be preserved by using low concentrations of local anesthetic (0.25 percent bupivacaine) and providing constant maternal encouragement. However, if uterine relaxation is required for facilitation of a breech extraction during vaginal delivery, it will be necessary to induce general anesthesia.

Multiple Gestations

Choice of anesthesia in the presence of multiple gestations must consider the frequent occurrence of prematurity and breech presentation. Inhalation analgesia plus local infiltration or continuous lumbar epidural block are acceptable methods of anesthesia in these patients. Systemic medications such as narcotics should be minimized, particularly if the fetus is premature.

PREGNANCY AND HEART DISEASE

Detection and evaluation of heart disease in the parturient is crucial for planning management of anesthesia during labor and delivery. Increased cardiac output during pregnancy and following delivery may re-

sult in congestive heart failure in the parturient with co-existing heart disease. For example, each uterine contraction increases cardiac output and central blood volume 10 to 25 percent. Subsequent delivery of the fetus and emptying of the uterus relieves compression of the inferior vena cava and aorta, resulting in a marked increase in blood volume.

For most types of heart disease, no single technique of anesthesia is specifically indicated or contraindicated. Nevertheless, analgesia produced by a continuous lumbar epidural block can minimize the adverse effects of increased cardiac output, particularly when this increase is exaggerated by pain or anxiety. Inhalation analgesia is usually selected when sudden reductions in systemic vascular resistance and blood pressure would be detrimental.

TOXEMIA OF PREGNANCY

Toxemia of pregnancy refers to either preeclampsia or eclampsia. Preeclampsia is a syndrome manifesting after the 20th week of gestation characterized by hypertension (above 140/90 mmHg), proteinuria (greater than 2 g/day), generalized edema, and complaints of headache. Manifestations of preeclampsia usually abate within 48 hours after delivery. Eclampsia is present when convulsions are superimposed on preeclampsia. Eclampsia occurs in about 5 percent of patients with preeclampsia and is associated with a maternal mortality of about 10 percent.

The etiology of toxemia of pregnancy is unknown but may involve an antigen-antibody reaction between fetal and maternal tissues in the first trimester that initiates a placental vasculitis. This vasculitis is presumed to decrease placental perfusion which initiates the release of vasoactive substances (renin, angiotensin, aldosterone) responsible for clinical manifestations of toxemia of pregnancy. Indeed, the path-

Table 26-6. Pathophysiology of Toxemia of Pregnancy

Cardiovascular system
  Generalized vasoconstriction
  Increased vascular responsiveness to sympathetic
    nervous system stimulation
  Decreased colloid oncotic pressure
  Decreased uteroplacental perfusion

Hepatorenal system
  Decreased hepatic blood flow
  Decreased glomerular filtration rate
  Decreased renal blood flow
  Retention of sodium and water

Respiratory system
  Interstitial accumulation of fluid
  Decreased PaO_2
  Exaggerated edema of upper airway and larynx

Central nervous system
  Hyperreflexia
  Cerebral edema
  Seizure activity

Intravascular fluid volume
  Hypovolemia

Coagulation
  Decreased platelet count
  Increased fibrin split products

Uterus
  Hyperactive
  Premature labor

---

ophysiology of toxemia of pregnancy involves nearly every organ system (Table 26-6).

Treatment

Definitive treatment of toxemia of pregnancy is delivery of the fetus and placenta. In the interim, magnesium and antihypertensives may be required. A general or regional anesthetic should not be used in an attempt to lower blood pressure.

Magnesium is effective in the parturient with toxemia of pregnancy by decreasing the irritability of the central nervous system which reduces the likelihood of convulsions. Magnesium also decreases hyperactivity at the neuromuscular junction, presumably by reducing the presynaptic release of acetylcholine as well as by decreasing the sensitivity of the postjunctional membrane to acetylcholine. In addition, magnesium relaxes uterine and vascular smooth muscle which contributes to an increase in uterine blood flow.

Clinically, the therapeutic effects of magnesium therapy are estimated by the responsiveness of deep tendon reflexes. Marked depression of these reflexes is an indication of impending magnesium toxicity. Periodic determination of the serum magnesium concentration is also helpful in adjusting supplement doses of magnesium so as to keep the level in a therapeutic range of 4 to 6 mEq/L. Serum magnesium levels in excess of this range can lead to severe skeletal muscle weakness, hypoventilation, and cardiac arrest. Intravenous calcium is the antidote for toxic effects of magnesium. Finally, magnesium is excreted by the kidneys and must be used with caution when renal function is impaired.

Potentiation of depolarizing and nondepolarizing muscle relaxants is produced by magnesium. This potentiation introduces the need for careful titration of the dose of the muscle relaxant and monitoring the effects produced by these drugs at the neuromuscular junction. Likewise, the doses of sedatives and narcotics should be reduced, as magnesium can also potentiate their effects. Since magnesium readily crosses the placenta, neonatal muscle tone can be decreased at birth.

Antihypertensives are likely to be administered when the diastolic blood pressure exceeds 110 mmHg. Hydralazine is frequently selected because of its rapid onset and ability to maintain or even increase renal blood flow. A continuous intravenous infusion of trimethaphan may be lifesaving in the parturient with a hypertensive crisis. Nitroprusside is not recommended because of the fact that cyanide can cross the placenta and the theoretical concern that this passage could produce adverse effects on the fetus. The goal is to reduce diastolic blood pressure to about 100 mmHg. Fetal heart rate should be continuously monitored during reduction of maternal blood pressure with drugs to insure an early warning if the uteroplacental circulation is being jeopardized by the reduced perfusion pressure.

Management of Anesthesia

Continuous lumbar epidural block is acceptable for vaginal delivery of the preeclamptic patient in good medical control. Epidural block negates the need for maternal narcotics and the possible adverse effects of these drugs on a premature fetus. The absence of the maternal urge to bear down reduces the likelihood of associated blood pressure increases. Before the lumbar epidural block is instituted the patient should be hydrated with intravenous fluids (balanced salt solution or plasmanate) until the central venous pressure is 4 to 6 mmHg or the pulmonary artery occlusion pressure is 6 to 10 mmHg. Furthermore, coagulation studies should be performed prior to the placement of the lumbar epidural catheter. Initially, a segmental band of anesthesia (T10–L1) will provide analgesia for the uterine contractions. As the second stage of labor is entered, the lumbar epidural block can be extended to provide perineal anesthesia. If hypotension occurs, the hypersensitivity of the maternal vasculature to catecholamines must be considered and a reduced intravenous dose of ephedrine (2.5 mg) administered.

Cesarean section is necessary when fetal distress reflecting deterioration of uteroplacental circulation accompanies toxemia of pregnancy. A general anesthetic is usually selected, since a regional anesthetic would be associated with extensive peripheral sympathetic nervous system block. Before induction of anesthesia, an attempt must be made to restore intravascular fluid volume. Continuous monitoring of intra-arterial pressure, cardiac filling pressures, urine output, and fetal heart rate is indicated. Induction of anesthesia is often with thiopental (2 to 4 mg/kg) plus succinylcholine to facilitate rapid intubation of the trachea. The use of a defasiculating dose of a nondepolarizing muscle relaxant prior to the administration of succinylcholine may not be necessary, since magnesium therapy is likely to attenuate skeletal muscle fasiculations produced by the depolarizing drug. Exaggerated edema of the upper airway structures may require the use of a smaller tracheal tube than anticipated. The blood pressure increase elicited by direct laryngoscopy and intubation of the trachea is predictably exaggerated in these patients. A short duration of direct laryngoscopy is helpful for minimizing the magnitude and duration of the blood pressure increase. Hydralazine (5 to 10 mg) administered intravenously 10 to 15 minutes before the induction of anesthesia or intravenous nitroglycerin (1 to 2 µg/kg) just before starting direct laryngoscopy has also been recommended for attenuating this blood pressure response.[1] A volatile anesthetic can be used to control intraoperative hypertension. The potentiation of all muscle relaxants by magnesium must be remembered and a peripheral nerve stimulator used to monitor the effect of a reduced dose of muscle relaxant at the neuromuscular junction.

HEMORRHAGE IN THE PARTURIENT

Hemorrhage in the parturient is the leading cause of maternal mortality. Placenta previa and abruptio placenta are the major causes of bleeding during the third trimester. Uterine rupture can be responsible for uncontrolled hemorrhage that manifests during labor. Postpartum hemorrhage occurs in 3 to 5 percent of all vaginal deliveries and is typically due to retained placenta, uterine atony, or cervical or vaginal lacerations.

Placenta Previa

Placenta previa is the abnormally low implantation of the placenta in the uterus. The cardinal symptom of placenta previa is painless vaginal bleeding that typically manifests around the 32nd week of gestation when the lower uterine segment is beginning to form. When this diagnosis is suspected, the position of the placenta should be confirmed by ultrasonography or radioisotope scan. If these tests are not conclusive and vaginal bleeding persists, the diagnosis is made by direct examination of the cervical os. This examination should be done in the delivery room, only after preparations have been taken to replace acute blood loss and to proceed with an emergency cesarean section. Ketamine is an ideal drug for induction of anesthesia in the presence of acute hemorrhage due to placenta previa. Maintenance of anesthesia prior to delivery is typically with 50 percent nitrous oxide plus succinylcholine to produce skeletal muscle relaxation. The neonate delivered from a parturient in hemorrhagic shock is likely to be acidotic and hypovolemic.

Abruptio Placenta

Abruptio placenta is the separation of a normally implanted placenta after 20 weeks of gestation. When the separation involves only the placental margin, the escaping blood can appear as vaginal bleeding. Alternatively, large volumes of blood loss can remain entirely concealed in the uterus. Severe blood loss from abruptio placenta manifests as maternal hypotension, uterine irritability, and hypertonia plus fetal distress. Clotting abnormalities, resembling disseminated intravascular coagulation, can occur.

The definitive treatment of abruptio placenta is to empty the uterus. If there are no signs of maternal hypovolemia, clotting abnormalities, or fetal distress, the use of a continuous lumbar epidural block is ideal to provide anesthesia for labor and vaginal delivery. However, when the magnitude of hemorrhage is severe, an emergency cesarean section is necessary using a general anesthetic with ketamine for induction and nitrous oxide for maintenance of anesthesia. It is predictable that the neonate born under these circumstances will be acidotic and hypovolemic.

Uterine Rupture

Uterine rupture can be associated with separation of a previous uterine scar, rapid spontaneous delivery, or excessive oxytocin stimulation. Manifestations of uterine rupture include complaints of severe abdominal pain, maternal hypotension, and disappearance of fetal heart tones.

Retained Placenta

Retained placenta occurs in about 1 percent of all vaginal deliveries, and usually necessitates manual exploration of the uterus. If a lumbar epidural or spinal block was not used for vaginal delivery, manual removal of the placenta may be initially attempted under continuous inhalation analgesia. Induction of general anesthesia with intubation of the trachea and administration of a volatile drug to provide uterine relaxation will be necessary if the uterus remains firmly contracted around the placenta.

Uterine Atony

Uterine atony as a cause of postpartum hemorrhage can occur immediately after delivery or manifest several hours later. Retained placenta is a common accompaniment of uterine atony. Treatment is with synthetic oxytocins (Pitocin, Syntocinon) which do not contain vasopressin as present in earlier preparations. Dilute solutions of synthetic oxytocins exert no cardiovascular effects but bolus injections may be associated with tachycardia, vasodilation, and hypotension. These cardiovascular effects are avoided by infusion of 10 to 15 units of snythetic oxytocin in 500 ml of balanced salt solution until uterine contraction is adequate. Finally, synthetic oxytocins, because they lack vasopressin, do not produce exaggerated blood pressure increases in the parturient who has been previously treated with a sympathomimetic.

AMNIOTIC FLUID EMBOLISM

Amniotic fluid embolism is signalled by the sudden onset of respiratory distress, hypotension, and arterial hypoxemia, reflecting the cardiopulmonary effects of entrance of amniotic fluid into the circulation. Multiparous parturients who experience a tumultous labor are most likely to experience an amniotic fluid embolism. Definitive diagnosis is made by demonstrating amniotic fluid material in maternal blood that has been aspirated from a central venous catheter. Treatment is directed toward cardiopulmonary resuscitation and correction of arterial hypoxemia. Conditions that can mimic an amniotic fluid embolism include inhalation of gastric contents and pulmonary embolus.

ANESTHESIA FOR NONOBSTETRIC SURGERY DURING PREGNANCY

The objectives for management of anesthesia in parturients undergoing nonobstetric surgery such as excision of an ovarian cyst or appendectomy are avoidance of teratogenic drugs, avoidance of intrauterine fetal hypoxia and acidosis, and prevention of premature labor.

Avoidance of Teratogenic Drugs

Most drugs, including anesthetics, have been demonstrated to be teratogenic in at least one animal species. In humans, the critical period of organogenesis is between 15 and 56 days of gestation. Nevertheless, there is no evidence that anesthetics administered during pregnancy are teratogenic.[1] Furthermore, there is no evidence in humans that drugs administered to produce analgesia during labor and vaginal delivery adversely affect later mental and neurological development of the offspring.[13]

Avoidance of Intrauterine Fetal Hypoxia and Acidosis

Intrauterine fetal hypoxia and acidosis are prevented by avoiding maternal hypotension, arterial hypoxemia, and excessive changes in the $PaCO_2$. High inspired concentrations of oxygen do not produce in-utero retrolental fibroplasia because high oxygen consumption of the placenta plus uneven distribution of the maternal and fetal blood flow in the placenta prevents fetal PaO_2 from exceeding about 45 mmHg.

Prevention of Premature Labor

It is the underlying pathology necessitating the surgery and not the anesthetic or technique of anesthesia that determines the onset of premature labor. After successful completion of surgery, it is advisable to continue monitoring the fetal heart rate and maternal uterine activity. Premature labor can be treated with a beta-2 agonist such as terbutaline or ritoridine. These drugs relax uterine smooth muscle, resulting in inhibition of uterine contractions.

Management of Anesthesia

Elective surgery should always be deferred until after delivery. When surgery is necessary, it is best to delay the operation until the second or third trimester. Emergency surgery in the first trimester is ideally performed with a lumbar epidural block or spinal block. Spinal block is ideal, as this technique limits fetal drug exposure to a minimum. Continuous intraoperative monitoring of fetal heart rate, after the 16th week of gestation, is helpful in providing early warning of fetal distress due to impaired uteroplacental perfusion (see the section *Diagnosis and Management of Fetal Distress*). When a general anesthetic is chosen, it should be appreciated that low concentrations of volatile drugs are not associated with significant reductions in uterine blood flow. Regardless of the technique of anesthesia selected, it is recommended that the inhaled concentration of oxygen be at least 50 percent.

DIAGNOSIS AND MANAGEMENT OF FETAL DISTRESS

Fetal well-being is often determined by evaluation of beat-to-beat variability in fetal heart rate as computed from R wave intervals on the fetal electrocardiogram. The fetal electrocardiogram is obtained via an electrode placed on the presenting fetal part or indirectly via ultrasound utilizing a sensor placed on the maternal abdomen. Another useful method for monitoring fetal well being is evaluation of fetal heart rate decelerations associated with contractions of the uterus. Fetal heart rate decelerations are classified as early, late, and variable. Fetal scalp sampling is indicated when abnormal fetal heart rate patterns occur. It has been observed[1] that the fetus is usually depressed when one or more fetal scalp pH values are below 7.21.

Beat-to-Beat Variability

Fetal heart rate varies 5 to 20 beats/min with a normal heart rate ranging between 120 to 160 beats/min. This normal variability is thought to reflect the integrity of the neural pathway from the fetal cerebral cortex through the medulla, vagus nerves, and cardiac conduction system. Fetal well-being is assured when beat-to-beat variability is present. Conversely, fetal distress due to arterial hypoxemia, acidosis, or central nervous system damage is associated with minimal to absent variability of the heart rate. Drugs (local anesthetics used for continuous lumbar epidural block, benzodiazepines, narcotics, anticholinergics) administered to the parturient may eliminate

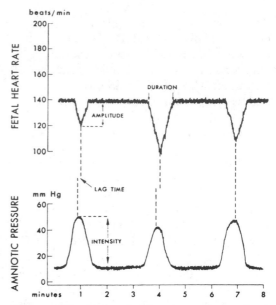

Figure 26-9. Early decelerations of the fetal heart rate are characterized by a short lag time between the onset of the uterine contraction and the beginning of heart rate slowing. The maximum fetal heart rate slowing occurs at the peak intensity of the contraction. Fetal heart rate is back to normal by the time the contraction has ceased. The most likely explanation for this fetal heart rate slowing is vagal stimulation due to compression of the fetal head. (Shnider SM. Diagnosis of fetal distress: fetal heart rate. In: Shnider SM, ed. Obstetrical anesthesia: current concepts and practice. © 1970 The Williams and Wilkins Co, Baltimore; 197–203.)

fetal heart rate variability even in the absence of fetal distress. This drug-induced effect does not appear to be deleterious but may cause difficulty in the interpretation of fetal heart rate monitoring.

Early Decelerations

Early decelerations are characterized by slowing of the fetal heart rate that begins with the onset of the uterine contraction (Fig. 26-9).[14] This deceleration pattern is thought to be caused by vagal stimulation secondary to compression of the fetal head and is not indicative of fetal distress.

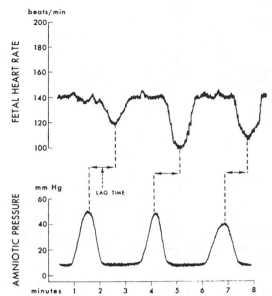

Figure 26-10. Late decelerations of the fetal heart rate are characterized by a delay between the onset of the uterine contraction and the beginning of fetal heart rate slowing. The fetal heart rate does not return to normal until after the contraction has ceased. Late decelerations indicate uteroplacental insufficiency. (Shnider SM. Diagnosis of fetal distress: fetal heart rate. In: Shnider SM, ed. Obstetrical anesthesia: current concepts and practice. © 1970 The Williams and Wilkins Co, Baltimore; 197–203.)

Late Decelerations

Late decelerations are characterized by slowing of the fetal heart rate that begins 10 to 30 seconds after the onset of the uterine contraction (Fig. 26-10).[14] This deceleration pattern is associated with fetal distress, most likely reflecting myocardial hypoxia secondary to uteroplacental insufficiency as produced by maternal hypotension. Determination of fetal scalp pH is indicated when this pattern persists.

Variable Decelerations

As the designation indicates, these deceleration patterns are variable in magnitude, duration, and time of onset (Fig. 26-11).[14] Variable decelerations are thought to

be caused by umbilical cord compression. Unless prolonged beyond 30 seconds or associated with bradycardia less than 70 beats/min, they are usually benign. Changing maternal position often lessens or abolishes this pattern.

EVALUATION OF THE NEONATE

The importance of assessment of the neonate immediately after birth is to promptly identify depressed infants who require active resuscitation (see Chapter 27). As a guide to identifying and treating the neonate, the Apgar score has not been surpassed.

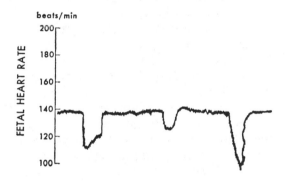
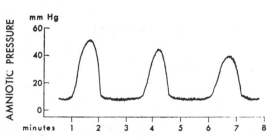

Figure 26-11. Variable decelerations of fetal heart rate are characterized by varying magnitudes and time of onset of heart rate slowing. This pattern is usually benign but if persistent may reflect compression of the umbilical cord. (Shnider SM. Diagnosis of fetal distress: fetal heart rate. In: Shnider SM, ed. Obstetrical anesthesia: current concepts and practice. © 1970 The Williams and Wilkins Co, Baltimore; 197–203.)

Table 26-7. Evaluation of the Neonate Using the Apgar Score

Variable	Score		
	Zero	One	Two
Heart rate (beats/min)	Absent	Below 100	Above 100
Respiratory effort	Absent	Slow	Irregular Crying
Reflex irritability	No response	Grimace	Cry
Muscle tone	Limp	Flexion of extremities	Active
Color	Cyanotic	Body pink and extremities cyanotic	Pink

Apgar Score

The Apgar score assigns a numerical value to five vital signs measured or observed in the neonate 1 and 5 minutes after delivery (Table 26-7). Of the five criteria, the heart rate and quality of the respiratory effort are the most important in identifying a depressed newborn. A heart rate less than 100 beats/min usually signifies arterial hypoxemia. When Apgar scores are above 7, neonates are either normal or have a mild respiratory acidosis. Mild to moderately depressed infants (scores 3 to 7) frequently improve in response to oxygen administered via mask, with or without positive pressure ventilation of the lungs. Intubation of the trachea and perhaps external cardiac massage are indicated when the score is less than 3.

Neurobehavioral Testing

Neurobehavioral testing is able to detect subtle or delayed effects of drugs administered during labor and delivery that are not appreciated by the Apgar score. This testing evaluates the neonate's state of wakefulness, reflex responses, muscle tone, and responses to sound. Neurobehavioral scores are depressed in infants born in the presence of a continuous lumbar epidural block with lidocaine but not bupivacaine.[1] There is concern that drugs administered during pregnancy can produce enduring behavioral deficits characterized by depressed development of cognitive, motor, and language skills. In man, the most vulnerable period may be from the seventh month of gestation to the second postnatal month corresponding to myelination in the central nervous system. Nevertheless, there is no evidence of significant or lasting adverse effects in infants manifesting a transient decrease in neurobehavioral performance attributed to drugs administered during labor and delivery. The neurologic and adaptive capacity score is an alternative to neurobehavioral testing for determining the impact on the neonate of drugs administered to the parturient.[15]

REFERENCES

1. Campbell C, Ravindran RS. The pregnant patient. In: Stoelting RK, Dierdorf SF, eds. Anesthesia and co-existing disease. New York, Churchill Livingstone 1983;683–739.
2. Morgan DJ, Blackman GL, Paull JD, Wolf LJ. Pharmacokinetics and plasma binding of thiopental. II: Studies at cesarean section. Anesthesiology 1981;54:474–80.
3. Palahniuk RJ, Shnider SM, Eger II EI. Pregnancy decreases the requirement of inhaled anesthetic agents. Anesthesiology 1974; 41:82–3.
4. Grundy EM, Zamora AM, Winnie AP. Comparison of spread of epidural anesthesia in pregnancy and nonpregnant women. Anesth Analg 1979;57:544–6.
5. Hodgkinson R, Glassenberg R, Joyce TH, Coombs DW, Ostheimer GW, Gibbs CP. Comparison of cimetidine (Tagamet) with antacid for safety and effectiveness in reducing gastric acidity before elective cesarean section. Anesthesiology 1983;59:86–90.

6. Ralston DH, Shnider SM, deLorimier AA. Effects of equipotent ephedrine, metaraminol, mephentermine, and methoxamine on uterine blood flow on the pregnant ewe. Anesthesiology 1974;40:354–70.

7. Shnider SM, Wright RG, Levinson G, Roizen MF, Wallis KL, Rolbin SH, Craft JB. Uterine blood flow and plasma norepinephrine changes during maternal stress in the pregnant ewe. Anesthesiology 1979;50:524–7.

8. Biehl D, Shnider SM, Levinson G, Callender K. Placental transfer of lidocaine. Effects of fetal acidosis. Anesthesiology 1978;48:409–12.

9. Friedman EA. Primigravid labor. A graphicostatistical analysis. Obstet Gynecol 1955;6:567–89.

10. Abboud TK, Shnider SM, Wright RG, Rolbin SH, Craft JB, Henriksen EH, Johnson J, Jones MJ, Hughes SC, Levinson G. Enflurane analgesia in obstetrics. Anesth Analg 1981;60:177–7.

11. Morishima HO, Pedersen H, Finster M, Tsuji A, Hiroka H, Feldman HS, Arthur GR, Covino BG. Is bupivacaine more cardiotoxic than lidocaine? Anesthesiology 1983;59:A409.

12. Ravindran RS, Bond VK, Tasch MD, Gupta CD, Luerssen TG. Prolonged neural blockade following regional analgesia with 2-chloroprocaine. Anesth Analg 1980;59:447–51.

13. Committee on Drugs of the American Academy of Pediatrics and the Committee on Obstetrics (Maternal and Fetal Medicine) of the American College of Obstetricians and Gynecologists: Effect of medication during labor and delivery on infant outcome. Pediatrics 1978;62:402–3.

14. Shnider SM. Diagnosis of fetal distress: fetal heart rate. In: Shnider SM, ed. Obstetrical anesthesia: current concepts and practice. Baltimore, The Williams and Wilkins Co 1979;197–203.

15. Amiel-Tison C, Barrier G, Shnider SM, Levinson G. Hughes SC, Stefani SJ. A new neurologic and adaptive capacity scoring system for evaluating obstetric medications in full term newborns. Anesthesiology 1982;56:340–50.

27

Pediatrics

Understanding the physiologic, anatomic, and pharmacologic differences between the neonate, infant, child, and adult permits principles utilized in adult anesthesia to be adapted to pediatric anesthesia. A neonate is defined as being 1 to 30 days in age, an infant is 1 to 12 months, and a child is 1 year to puberty.

PHYSIOLOGIC AND ANATOMIC DIFFERENCES

Cardiovascular

To compensate for an increased oxygen requirement (6 ml/kg/min vs. 3 ml/kg/min in an adult) and fetal hemoglobin which releases oxygen to the tissues less readily, the cardiac output of neonates and infants is 30 to 60 percent greater than that of adults. The fetal oxyhemoglobin dissociation curve is shifted to the left with the P_{50} (partial pressure at which hemoglobin is 50 percent saturated with oxygen) being 18 mmHg as compared to the adult P_{50} of 26 mmHg. Hemoglobin concentration is approximately 17 g/dl in the neonate, most of which consists of fetal hemoglobin. As fetal hemoglobin is replaced by adult hemoglobin, the hemoglobin concentration decreases to about 11 g/dl by 6 months of age. Thus, from ages 3 to 6 months, oxygen carrying capacity is significantly reduced.

Arterial blood pressure also increases with increasing age (Table 27-1). The cli-

nician must measure arterial blood pressure with the correct cuff size. The width of the blood pressure cuff should be greater than one-third of the circumference of the limb. If the cuff bladder is too large, a false low blood pressure will be recorded. Conversely, if the cuff bladder is too small, a false high blood pressure will be recorded.

Respiratory

Some common respiratory variables are compared in the neonate, infant, child, and adult in Table 27-2. When utilizing these data, it should be emphasized that there is considerable variability in each age group. In general, atelectasis may be more likely to occur in the infant as compared to the adult. The infant alveolus is smaller, intrapleural pressure is zero at end-expiration, and the chest wall is very compliant. For example, in the adult approximately one-half of the respiratory pressure required to provide adequate ventilation is utilized to expand the chest wall. In contrast, the more compliant chest wall of infants requires little pressure to expand it. Once the lungs are in a state of atelectasis, however, they may be difficult to reexpand because of increased chest wall compliance. Every time the infant tries to overcome atelectasis by deep breathing, the chest wall retracts inward, preventing an increase in airway pressure or tidal volume.

Table 27-1. Comparison of Circulatory Variables in Neonates, Infants, Children, and Adults

Age	Systolic Arterial Blood Pressure (mmHg)	Heart Rate (beats/min)	Hemoglobin (g/dl)	Oxygen Consumption (ml/kg/min)	Blood Volume (ml/kg)
Newborn	65	130	17	6	85
6 months	90	120	11	5	80
12 months	95	120	12	5	80
5 years	95	90	12.5	6	75
23 years	122	77	14	3	65

Temperature Regulation

To maintain normal body temperature, infants and children create heat by metabolizing brown fat, crying, and moving more vigorously but, unlike adults, rarely by shivering. Maintaining normal body temperature is more difficult in neonates and infants than adults because of a larger surface-to-volume ratio, increased metabolic rate (Table 27-1), and lack of sufficient body fat for insulation. Therefore, the neonate or infant is more likely than the adult to experience adverse reductions in body temperature when anesthetized in cold operating rooms.

Renal

The transition from fetal renal function to active neonatal function results in a kidney which has compromised abilities. The neonate kidney is characterized by decreased glomerular filtration rate, decreased sodium excretion, and decreased concentrating ability. Over the first 3 months of life, glomerular filtration rate increases two to three-fold. Thereafter, the rate of rise is slower until the adult values are reached by 12 to 24 months of age. Following fluid restriction, mean urine osmolarity for term neonates is 528 mOsm/kg. By 15 to 30 days of age, maximum urine osmolarity may be as high as 950 mOsm/kg. Still, it takes 6 to 12 months before infants are able to concentrate their urine as well as adults. Certainly, the therapeutic index for intravenous fluid and electrolyte therapy is rather narrow during the first 24 hours of life (Brett CM, San Francisco, CA, personal communication).

PHARMACOLOGIC DIFFERENCES

Because of differences in extracellular fluid volumes (40 percent of body weight in neonates vs. 20 percent in adults) and rates of metabolism and glomerular filtration, the pharmacokinetics of drugs should be different in neonates and infants as compared to adults. From a pharmacodynamic point of view, receptor maturation frequently has not been completed in the neonate or the infant, which may alter their sensitivity to various drugs as compared to adults.[1]

Table 27-2. Comparison of Respiratory Variables in Newborns, Infants, Children and Adults

Age	Weight (kg)	Respiratory Rate (breaths/min)	Tidal Volume (ml)	Minute Ventilation (ml/min)	FRC (ml)	VC (ml)	V_D (ml)
Newborn	3	35	15	525	70	90	7
6 months	6	30	30	900	150	200	14
12 months	10	24	70	1,680	260	470	21
5 years	18	20	135	2,700	660	1,100	49
23 years	70	12	500	6,000	3,000	4,600	150

Abbreviations: FRC, functional residual capacity, VC, vital capacity; V_D, respiratory dead space.

Inhaled Anesthetics

Both the uptake and distribution and potency of inhaled anesthetics differ in the neonate and infant as compared to the adult.[3] In general, the rate at which general anesthesia is induced is shortened in the neonate as compared to the adult. This is probably because of a smaller functional residual capacity per unit of body weight and a greater tissue blood flow, especially to vessel rich groups. For example, the vessel rich group (blood flow of the brain, heart, liver, and kidney) comprises approximately 10 percent of total body volume in the adult, whereas it comprises 22 percent of total body volume in the neonate.[2]

The minimum alveolar anesthetic concentration (MAC) is increased in the infant. For example, infants require approximately 40 percent more halothane than do adults to produce the same level of anesthesia (Fig. 27-1).[4] Conversely, anesthetic requirements for halothane in neonates are about 25 percent less than infants.[4] At comparable MAC values, the incidence of halothane-induced hypotension (greater than 30 percent decrease in systolic blood pressure from awake) was similar in neonates and infants.

Muscle Relaxants and Their Antagonists

The general conclusion with nondepolarizing muscle relaxants (e.g., d-tubocurarine, pancuronium, metocurine, vecuronium, and atracurium) is that the size of the dose should not differ from that of an adult on a body weight basis. Because of an increase in extracellular fluid volume, the volume of distribution of d-tubocurarine is larger in younger patients as compared to adults (Fig. 27-2).[5] Because infants have an increased sensitivity to d-tubocurarine (the blood concentration of d-tubocurarine required to produce a given neuromuscular blockade is lower in younger patients as compared to adults), the actual intravenous dose of d-tubocurarine required for a given

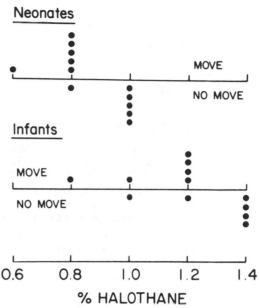

Figure 27-1. Data for an individual patient are given as a solid circle. The position of the circle along the horizontal line indicates the end-tidal halothane concentration immediately before skin incision. The position of the circle above or below the line indicates whether the patient moved or failed to move respectively. The greater sensitivity of neonates to halothane is apparent. (Lerman J, Robinson S, Willis MM, Gregory GA. Anesthetic requirement for halothane in young children 0–1 month and 1–6 months of age. Anesthesiology 1983;59:421–4.)

neuromuscular blockade is not altered. The increased volume of distribution means the blood concentration of d-tubocurarine that reaches the neuromuscular junction is less in the neonate as compared to the adult. This lower blood concentration produces the same effect that a higher blood concentration would in an adult, reflecting the increased sensitivity of the neonate to muscle relaxants. Because of a decreased glomerular filtration rate, the elimination half-time and, therefore, duration of action of a given dose of d-tubocurarine is longer in a neonate as compared to an adult (Fig. 27-3).[5] Likewise, decreased hepatic clearance results in prolongation of the duration of action of vecuronium in neonates.[6]

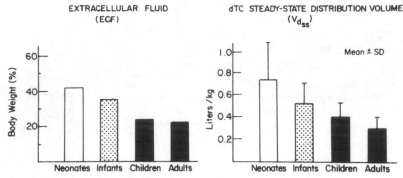

Figure 27-2. Comparison of known extracellular fluid values to the volume of distribution for d-tubocurarine. Note that the changes in extracellular fluid volume are mirrored by the differences in distribution volume. (Fisher DM, O'Keefe C, Stanski DR, Cronnelly R, Miller RD, Gregory GA. Pharmacokinetics and pharmacodynamics of d-tubocurarine in infants, children and adults. Anesthesiology 1982;57:203–7.)

From a clinical point of view, the pharmacology of neostigmine is not greatly different in infants and children as compared to adults. The time of onset and duration of antagonism are similar for infants, children, and adults. The dose of neostigmine required to antagonize a d-tubocurarine neuromuscular blockade is lower in infants and children. The ED_{50} (that dose of neostigmine which produces 50 percent antagonism of a d-tubocurarine induced neuromuscular blockade) is 13.1 µg/kg in infants, 15.5 µg/kg in children, and 22.9 µg/kg in adults.[7] Even though these are significant differences, it is not necessary to alter the dose of neostigmine administered to infants and children as compared to adults.

THE IMMEDIATE PREOPERATIVE PERIOD

Preoperative Evaluation

The purpose of the preoperative evaluation is to obtain a history, physical examination, and laboratory data, and to establish rapport with the child and his or her parents. Pediatric anesthesia differs from adult anesthesia in that the history frequently must be obtained from the parent rather than the patient. This requires coordination between the anesthesia team and the hospital ward to ensure that the parents are available during the preanesthetic evaluation. The history should elicit whether congenital anomalies, allergies, bleeding tendencies, or a recent exposure to a communicable disease exist. Also, the medications the child is taking should be determined. Lastly, experiences with previous anesthetics should be sought.

Physical examination includes evaluation of the heart, lungs, and evidence of upper respiratory infection (fever, coryza). A recent upper respiratory infection can be a reason for delaying elective surgery because of the secretions and increased airway reactivity. Also, the presence of loose teeth should be sought and dangerously loose teeth removed if necessary. The skin should be examined for evidence of dehydration or cyanosis (Table 27-3).

Laboratory data should seek evidence as to whether the infant is hypoglycemic, hypocalcemic, or has clotting disorders, which frequently occur in preterm infants or infants who have undergone asphyxia during birth. Also, if a history of vomiting or excessive fluid losses from diarrhea is

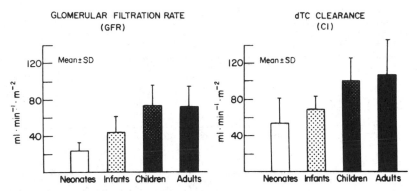

Figure 27-3. Known values of glomerular filtration are compared to values of clearance of d-tubocurarine. (Fisher DM, O'Keefe C, Stanski DR, Cronnelly R, Miller RD, Gregory GA. Pharmacokinetics and pharmacodynamics of d-tubocurarine in infants, children, and adults. Anesthesiology 1982;57:203–7.)

evident, serum electrolytes, pH and an assessment of extracellular fluid volume should be sought. If the hemoglobin is less than 10 g/dl, the reason for this should be determined. Although a hemoglobin below 10 g/dl per se is not a reason for delaying an elective operation, often a previously unknown abnormality will be detected.

Preoperative Medication

Obviously, the best preoperative medication scheme is a friendly, reassuring visit from the anesthesiologist. By answering questions and describing the operative pro-

Table 27-3. Changes Associated with Dehydration

Variable	Degree of Hydration (percent decrease in body weight)		
	5%	10%	15%
Skin turgor	↓	↓ ↓	↓ ↓ ↓
Sunken fontanelle	↓	↓ ↓	↓ ↓ ↓
Skin color	Pale	Gray	Mottled
Mucus membranes	Dry	Very dry	Parched
Urine	↓	↓ ↓	Anuria
Heart rate	No change	↑	↑ ↑

Symbols: ↓ = slight decrease; ↓ ↓ = moderate decrease; ↓ ↓ ↓ = severe decrease; ↑ = slight increase; ↑ ↑ = moderate increase.

cedure (sometimes with animated illustrations), the need for preoperative medication is markedly decreased. Still, barbiturates, narcotics, and sedative-hypnotics are frequently administered for preoperative medication. Intramuscular injections can be avoided by administering drugs orally with 30 ml of water, or rectally 1 to 2 hours prior to surgery. Oral administration of 0.25 ml/kg of a solution containing diazepam 0.2 mg/kg, meperidine 1.5 mg/kg, and atropine 0.02 mg/kg decreases the incidence of children crying on arriving in the operating room and does not delay recovery from anesthesia.[8] Rectally administered methohexital 10 to 25 mg/kg can be given in a 10 percent solution. An 8 French 15 cm long catheter can be inserted approximately 3 cm into the rectum. The parents can hold the child while the drug is being administered and until the child falls asleep, which is usually in 5 to 7 minutes. Once asleep, the patient can be transferred to the operating room.

Table 27-4 summarizes some commonly used drugs and their doses for preoperative medication of the pediatric patient. An anticholinergic is often recommended to attenuate the cardiac vagal reflex and to reduce secretions. It is our view, however,

Table 27-4. Some Drugs Used for Premedication and Suggested Doses

Age	Weight (kg)	Pentobarbital (mg)	Morphine (mg)	Meperidine (mg)	Diazepam[a] (mg)	Atropine (mg)
Newborn	3.2	—	—	—	—	0.1
6 months	7.0	15	0.7	7.0	1.5	0.2
1 year	9.5	20	1.0	10.0	2.0	0.2
6 years	21.0	40	2.0	20.0	4.5	0.4
12 years	39.0	90	6.0	60.0	9.0	0.6

[a] All drugs are usually administered intramuscularly, except diazepam, which is best given orally.

that these drugs frequently are unnecessary.

Pediatric Anesthetic Breathing Systems

The three most commonly utilized anesthetic breathing systems for pediatric anesthesia are the circle breathing system, the Ayre's T-piece, and the Bain system (see Chapter 11). Heated and humidified anesthetic gases can reduce operative heat loss and possibly postoperative respiratory complications in neonates undergoing major abdominal or thoracic surgery. Therefore, whatever anesthetic breathing system is chosen, heated, humidified gases probably should also be utilized.

INDUCTION AND MAINTENANCE OF ANESTHESIA

Although safety is of paramount importance, induction of anesthesia should be as rapid as possible. Having good rapport and resultant conversation with the patient often will facilitate induction of anesthesia. A constant monotone conversation is often conducive to a rapid induction of anesthesia. If an intravenous catheter is in place, anesthesia can be induced with thiopental 3 to 5 mg/kg, methohexital 1 to 2 mg/kg, or ketamine 1 to 2 mg/kg. If an intravenous catheter is not in place, ketamine can be given in doses of 4 to 6 mg/kg intramuscularly. Also, succinylcholine 1 to 2 mg/kg can be given in the same syringe with ketamine.

An inhalation induction of anesthesia is very common for elective procedures in children and is especially easy to perform with halothane as compared to enflurane or isoflurane because the former has a less pungent smell. Sometimes, the induction of anesthesia can be facilitated by initially breathing 70 percent nitrous oxide with the gradual introduction of the volatile anesthetic. Rapid increases in the anesthetic concentration should be avoided because it can be irritating to the respiratory tract, resulting in coughing and even laryngospasm.

Children are probably at a slightly greater risk for the development of aspiration of acidic gastric fluid than adults because of a greater gastric residual volume and lower pH. Cote et al.[9] found that the mean gastric residual volume in children ranging from 3 to 17 years was 0.78 ml/kg with a pH of 1.45. If cimetidine was given more than 1 hour and less than 4 hours before surgery, the amount of gastric fluid was significantly reduced. For example, in one group given 7.5 mg/kg of cimetidine orally in a cherry-flavored sorbitol solution 1.5 hours before the scheduled time of surgery, the volume of gastric fluid aspirate was only 0.15 ml/kg with a mean pH of 6.16[10]

Anesthesia should be maintained at a concentration which causes the fewest physiologic changes and still offers adequate surgical conditions, which is usually in the range of 1.1 to 1.4 MAC. The signs of anesthesia required for adequate surgical conditions for neonates, infants, and children are similar to those for adults, such as movement and an increase in heart rate and arterial pressure. Gregory[11] feels that a reasonable indication of anesthetic depth is loss of sucking reflex. This can be tested by placing a finger in the infant's mouth, which would normally elicit sucking. When the infant stops sucking, then the anesthetic concentration is usually sufficient for surgery.

When and How Should an Intravenous Infusion be Started?

Other than for very short surgical procedures, an intravenous infusion should be initiated in all children who are to be anesthetized. In many instances, it is difficult to start an intravenous infusion preoperatively. After induction of anesthesia, however, especially with an inhaled anesthetic, such as halothane, the peripheral veins dilate and movement of the child ceases, making placement of an intravenous catheter much easier. Fluids are ideally delivered from a calculated drip chamber in order to assure that an accidental overload of fluid given intravenously does not occur.

Monitoring

Monitoring of pediatric patients should be the same as for adult patients undergoing comparable types of surgery (see Chapter 16). Arterial blood pressure, electrocardiogram, heart and breath sounds with an esophageal or precordial stethoscope, and body temperature should be monitored routinely in all infants and children undergoing surgery. In seriously ill children who may be undergoing more extensive surgery, especially when hemorrhage or large shifts in extracellular fluid are expected, arterial blood pressure probably should be monitored continuously via a catheter inserted into a peripheral artery. Monitoring of central venous pressure may aid in determining the adequacy of intravascular fluid volume. Central venous pressure can be measured via an umbilical vein catheter in neonates and either the internal, external jugular or subclavian vein in infants or children. Catheterization of the bladder and monitoring of urinary output also are helpful when blood loss or shifts in extracellular fluid volume are expected. Urinary output should probably exceed 0.50 ml/kg/hr, and should have a specific gravity below 1.010.

Analysis of arterial blood gases is often helpful during extensive surgery. Acidosis is not uncommon during pediatric anesthesia. Also, the PaO_2 should be determined in premature infants since the risk of developing retrolental fibroplasia is increased until about 44 weeks postconception (see Chapter 31). Therefore, the preterm neonate born at 36 weeks gestation remains at risk until about 8 weeks of age. The PaO_2 should be maintained between 50 and 80 mmHg to minimize the possibility of retrolental fibroplasia developing. The inspired oxygen concentration can be reduced by adding either nitrous oxide or air to the inhaled gases. Arterial oxygen partial pressure can be measured transcutaneously. Technical difficulties with this technique include inaccuracies when arterial blood pressure falls and/or body temperature decreases below 35 Celsius. With improved technology, however, transcutaneous oxygen measurement will become a valuable adjunct in monitoring seriously ill neonates, infants, and children.

Hypoglycemia and hypocalcemia frequently occur in seriously ill infants. In these infants, blood glucose should be determined during surgery. If hypoglycemia occurs, 1 to 3 ml/kg of a 20 percent glucose solution should be infused intravenously over a 5 minute period. Blood glucose concentration then should be again determined 15 minutes later to ensure that adequate glucose has been given. Conversely, excessive glucose levels should be avoided because glucosuria and dehydration may result. Hypocalcemia can result in hypotension, poor peripheral perfusion, and cardiac failure, especially if the serum calcium level is below 4.5 mEq/L. If so, calcium gluconate,

Table 27-5. Basic Guidelines for Calculating Maintenance Fluid Requirements (5% Dextrose and 0.9% Saline)

Day	Neonate (ml/kg/hr)
1	0–2
2–3	2
4–6	3
7	4

Body Weight (kg)	Infants Greater than 10 Days (Amount and Rate)
0–10	4 ml/kg/hr
10–20	40 ml plus 2 ml/kg/hr
20	60 ml plus 1 ml/kg/hr

100 mg/kg, should be infused into a central vein while the electrocardiogram is being continuously monitored. Hopefully, measurement of ionized calcium levels will be more routine in the future.

Intubation of the Trachea (See Chapter 12)

Blood Loss and Fluid Maintenance and Replacement

Three questions should be asked in calculating any infant or child's intravenous fluid requirements intraoperatively (Brett CM, San Francisco CA, personal communication):

1. Does dehydration already exist?
2. Has the patient been without fluids for an unacceptable period of time?
3. Are the electrolytes, glucose, hematocrit, and acid-base status normal?

Intravenous fluid infusion rate should be calculated based on age, size, and body temperature (Table 27-5) (see Chapter 18). Ongoing intraoperative losses should be replaced, which includes urine, blood, nasogastric drainage, third-space losses, and respiratory tract losses. Estimation of ongoing losses intraoperatively is difficult because of losses into surgical drapes and concealed losses in sponges and into the surgical wound. Operative losses from exposed viscera and third-space extravasation can be estimated depending on the severity of surgery. In general, these losses are greater than 10 ml/kg/hr with extensive surgery, such as in infants with necrotizing entercolitis or during a gastroschisis repair. Guidelines for maintenance fluid infusion rates for mild surgery are 1 to 2 ml/kg/hr; moderate surgery 2 to 4 ml/kg/hr; and severe surgery 6 to 8 ml/kg/hr. Lactated Ringer's solution or 0.9 per cent saline is most often selected. An example of mild surgery is an inguinal hernia repair. Moderate surgery might include intestinal atresia or treatment of Hirschsprung's disease. Severe surgery might be exemplified by a gastroschisis repair.

Blood loss should be estimated based on weight of sponges, calibrated suction traps, and visual estimation of blood loss onto the operative field and on the drapes. The manner in which the patient is tolerating blood loss should be estimated by the vital signs and urinary output. In general, blood replacement should be considered when the hematocrit decreases to below 30 percent or when estimated blood loss has reached 10 percent of the calculated blood volume of 80 ml/kg. The following formula can be utilized to estimate the acceptable blood loss before hematocrit reaches 30 percent and replacement is necessary.[12]

$$\text{acceptable blood loss (ml)} = 3 \left(\begin{array}{c} \text{estimated erythrocyte mass} \\ - \text{estimated erythrocyte mass when hematocrit } 30 \text{ percent} \end{array} \right)$$

where erythrocyte mass

$$= \text{blood volume (80 ml/kg)} \times \text{hematocrit}$$

For example, if a 4 kg infant comes to the operating room with a hematocrit of 35 percent, approximately 50 ml of blood could be lost before the hematocrit would decrease to 30 percent. This formula, however, does not consider the dilutional aspect of crystalloid solution administration. Therefore, blood probably should be replaced when 30 to 35 ml of blood has been lost. If blood loss is to be replaced by crystalloid solution, then a volume of three times the estimated blood loss needs to be given, usually in the form of 0.9 percent saline or lactated Ringer's solution.

REGIONAL ANESTHESIA

Regional anesthesia is not popular in pediatric anesthesia. Nevertheless, caudal anesthesia has been given for lower abdominal and rectal procedures and for repair of myelomeningoceles. Also, intravenous and axillary blocks have been utilized for repair of tendon lacerations or fractures of one of the extremities. The administration of ketamine intramuscularly or intravenously may be utilized to facilitate the child's cooperation during regional anesthesia.

NEWBORN RESUSCITATION

In a severely depressed newborn immediate resuscitative efforts should take place. Although they are similar to adult resuscitative efforts, differences do exist which need to be emphasized (see Chapter 34).[13] In the immediate period of initial evaluation, the mouth and nose should be suctioned. Once breathing is established and the umbilical cord has stopped pulsating, the cord can be cut and the newborn taken to the resuscitative area. Stripping blood from the umbilical cord to the newborn increases blood volume, respiratory rate, and pulmonary artery pressure. Indeed, early clamping of the cord may deprive the newborn of up to 30 ml/kg of blood. The newborn should be placed in a radiantly heated resuscitation bed and the airway cleared by gentle suctioning of the mouth and nose.

Apgar Scores

The Apgar score (0 to 10) determined 1 minute following birth can be utilized to guide the extent to which resuscitation is necessary (see Chapter 26).

8 to 10. Most newborns fall into this category, which requires little treatment other than suctioning of the pharynx and wrapping in a warm blanket.

5 to 7. Usually, these newborns have suffered mild asphyxia prior to birth. They usually respond to vigorous stimulation and blowing of oxygen over the face. If they do not respond in 1 to 2 minutes, ventilation of the lungs should be instituted via a bag and mask.

3 to 6. These newborns are moderately depressed, cyanotic, and have poor respiratory efforts. Ventilation of the lungs should be controlled via a bag and mask. Ventilation of the lungs may be difficult because airway resistance is increased, which may cause gas to enter the esophagus, stomach, and gastrointestinal tract, leading to gastric distension and vomiting. If breathing has not started spontaneously the trachea should be intubated and blood obtained from a doubly clamped segment of the umbilical cord for analysis of arterial blood gases and pH. If the pH is below 7.2, blood gas analysis and pH should be obtained from a warmed heel (arterialized blood) or from a radial or temporal artery. If the pH in the sample is unchanged or lower in the second sample, sodium bicarbonate, 2 mEq/kg, should be given intravenously.

0 to 2. These newborns are severely asphyxiated and require immediate resuscitative efforts. The trachea should be immediately intubated and ventilation of the lungs controlled at a rate of 30 to 60 breaths per minute. An occasional breath should be held for 2 to 3 seconds to expand atelectatic areas. Also, positive end-expiratory pressure of 1 to 3 mmHg is often useful. The adequacy of ventilation of the lungs is best determined by physical examination and analysis of arterial blood gases. Both sides of the chest should rise equally and simultaneously. If one side rises before the other, the tip of the tracheal tube may have entered the bronchus, or pneumothorax or (rarely) a diaphragmatic hernia may be present. An airway pressure greater than 25 cm of water should not be utilized.

The trachea should be suctioned prior to ventilation of the lungs, especially in infants born with meconium staining of the amniotic fluid.[13] If meconium is distributed into the periphery of the lung, 16 percent of these infants will develop respiratory difficulties in the first few days of life.

Vascular Resuscitation

If the response to ventilation of the lungs and stimulation is not immediate, an umbilical artery catheter should be inserted to permit analysis of arterial blood gases, pH, and blood pressure, and to expand blood volume and administer drugs. The umbilical cord stump should be held straight up with a clamp and the abdomen and cord sterilized with an iodine-containing solution. The stump can then be tied near the base and the cord cleanly cut with a scalpel, leaving 1 to 2 cm of stump. The umbilical artery can then be dilated with a curved iris forcep. A 3.5 to 5.0 gauge French umbilical artery catheter is advanced into the dilated vessel and connected to a three-way stopcock. Before injecting anything from the catheter, blood must be withdrawn to clear air from the catheter.

Hypovolemic newborns are usually hypotensive (mean arterial pressure below 50 mmHg), pale, and have poor capillary filling and perfusion. Their extremities are cold and their pulses weak or absent. Hypovolemia is treated with blood, plasma, or crystalloid solutions. If hypovolemia is suspected at birth (any preterm and/or asphyxiated fetus), maternal blood can be crossmatched against O-negative, O-titer blood. One unit of packed erythrocytes and one unit of whole blood can be brought to the delivery room in a "cold pack." If no source of blood is available, 1.0 to 2.0 g of albumin, 10 ml/kg of plasma and/or lactated Ringer's solution can be given. At times, the volume of fluid required to raise blood pressure may be enormous and occasionally may exceed 50 percent of the blood volume, On the other hand, care must be taken not to over-expand the intravascular fluid volume and cause hypertension.

UNUSUAL DISEASES THAT AFFECT PEDIATRIC PATIENTS

Diaphragmatic Hernia

Diaphragmatic hernia results from incomplete embryologic closure of the diaphragm such that intestinal contents occupy the chest (most often the left thorax) with associated hypoplasia of the lung on that side. The incidence of this defect is about 1 in every 5000 live births. Manifestations at birth include a scaphoid abdomen and profound arterial hypoxemia. Pulmonary hypertension and congenital heart disease are common.

Immediate treatment of the neonate is decompression of the stomach via a gastric tube and administration of oxygen, most often via a tracheal tube. Pneumothroax on the side opposite the hernia is a hazard if airway pressures exceed 25 cm H_2O during controlled ventilation of the lungs. Nitrous oxide should be avoided during anesthesia for surgical correction, as this gas could diffuse into the loops of intestine in the chest (see Chapter 2). Arterial oxygenation should be monitored, as these neonates may be at risk for developing retrolental fibroplasia. After reduction of the hernia, attempts to expand the hypoplastic lung are not recommended, as damage to the normal lung can occur from excessive positive airway pressure.

Omphalocele

Omphalocele is characterized by external herniation of abdominal viscera covered by a hernia sac through the base of the umbilical cord. Associated congenital anomalies (heart defects, trisomy-21) are frequent. The incidence of this defect is about 1 in every 5000 to 10,000 live births.

Management of anesthesia for surgical correction emphasizes aggressive fluid administration and maintenance of body temperature. The use of nitrous oxide is questionable, as diffusion of this gas into the intestine may make primary abdominal closure more difficult. Arterial oxygenation should be monitored, as these often premature infants may be vulnerable for developing retrolental fibroplasia. Muscle relaxants must be used judiciously, as excessive skeletal muscle relaxation could make it difficult to determine if primary surgical closure of an already underdeveloped abdominal cavity is feasible. An excessively tight abdominal closure may interfere with adequate spontaneous ventilation postoperatively.

Gastroschisis

Gastroschisis is characterized by external herniation of abdominal viscera through a 2 to 5 cm defect in the anterior abdominal wall lateral to the umbilical cord. Unlike omphalocele, a hernia sac does not cover the exposed abdominal viscera and gastroschisis is rarely associated with other congenital anomalies. Management of anesthesia for surgical correction is as described for omphalocele.

Pyloric Stenosis

Pyloric stenosis occurs in about 1 of every 500 live births, and usually manifests at 2 to 5 weeks of age. Persistent vomiting results in loss of hydrogen ions with compensatory attempts by the kidney to maintain a normal pH by exchanging potassium for hydrogen. The result is a dehydrated infant with hypokalemic, hypochloremic metabolic alkalosis. Surgery is performed electively (not as an emergency) after 24 to 48

hours of intravenous fluid therapy including sodium and potassium chloride.

The likelihood of aspiration of gastric fluid is increased in these patients during induction of anesthesia. Therefore, the stomach should be emptied as completely as possible with a large-bore catheter before induction of anesthesia. Postoperative depression of ventilation (possibly due to cerebrospinal fluid alkalosis) is often seen in these patients, emphasizing the need for close monitoring in the early hours after surgery.

Trisomy-21 (Down's Syndrome)

Trisomy-21 occurs in about 0.15 percent of all live births. Correction of associated congenital anomalies (atrial or ventricular septal defects, duodenal atresia) or the need to provide dental care may be the reasons these patients undergo surgery. In this regard, the need to reduce excessive upper airway secretions with an anticholinergic and provide sedation for an often uncooperative patient must be considered in the preoperative medication. Patency of the upper airway may be difficult to maintain following the onset of unconsciousness, reflecting the short neck, small mouth, and large tongue characteristic of these patients. Intubation of the trachea, however, is usually not difficult.

Epiglottitis

Epiglottitis typically manifests as an acute onset of difficulty in swallowing, high fever, and inspiratory stridor in children 2 to 6 years old. Differentiation of epiglottitis from laryngotracheobronchitis (croup) may be difficult, but characteristically the latter occurs in younger patients, the onset is slower, the fever is lower, and airway obstruction less severe. It is mandatory that the child with suspected epiglottitis be admitted to the hospital, as sudden total upper airway obstruction can occur at any time. Treatment of epiglottitis is with antibiotics, such as ampicillin (causative bacteria is *Hemophilus influenzae*), and intubation of the trachea. An attempt to visualize the epiglottis should not be undertaken until the child is in the operating room and preparations are completed for intubation of the trachea and possible emergency tracheostomy. Induction and maintenance of anesthesia for intubation of the treachea is with a volatile anesthetic, most often halothane, in oxygen. Resolution of epiglottitis usually requires 48 to 96 hours. Extubation of the trachea is performed in the operating room only after direct laryngoscopy has confirmed the resolution of the swelling of the epiglottis.

Reye's Syndrome

Reye's syndrome is an acute encephalopathy and hepatic failure that typically develops in children under 10 years of age following a viral illness involving the respiratory or gastrointestinal tract. Treatment of severe Reye's syndrome (blood ammonia concentration greater than 100 $\mu M/L$) includes intubation of the trachea, mechanical ventilation of the lungs, and placement of an intracranial pressure monitor (see Chapter 32) during general anesthesia. Aggressive therapy to prevent damage from increased intracranial pressure, including barbiturate coma, and occasionally bifrontal craniectomy appears to have substantially reduced the mortality associated with this disease.

Bronchopulmonary Dysplasia

Bronchopulmonary dysplasia is a chronic pulmonary disorder characterized by recurrent pulmonary infections which typically afflicts infants and children who required increased concentrations of oxygen and mechanical ventilation of the lungs at birth to treat respiratory distress syndrome (see Chapter 31).

Malignant Hyperthermia

Malignant hyperthermia is an inherited disease that manifests most often, but not exclusively, in children. The incidence of this syndrome is approximately 1 in 15,000 pediatric anesthetics and 1 in 50,000 adult anesthetics. The pathophysiologic defect appears to be in the excitation-contraction coupling of skeletal muscle, and the concentration of calcium in the myoplasm. Exposure to a triggering agent, such as the volatile anesthetics, succinylcholine, or amide local anesthetics, results in sustained high levels of calcium in the myoplasm and persistent skeletal muscle contraction. This sustained skeletal muscle contraction results in signs of hypermetabolism including tachycardia, arterial hypoxemia, metabolic and respiratory acidosis, and profound elevations in body temperature. Intravenous dantrolene (up to 10 mg/kg) is the drug of choice for the treatment of malignant hyperthermia. Patients known to be susceptible to malignant hyperthermia should be pretreated with oral dantrolene (5 mg/kg/day in four divided doses for 1 to 3 days) and drugs known to trigger the syndrome avoided in the management of anesthesia. Although no anesthetic regimen is completely safe, drugs considered to be acceptable for use during anesthesia include narcotics, barbiturates, nitrous oxide, and ester local anesthetics. Pancuronium is an acceptable choice if a muscle relaxant is needed.

REFERENCES

1. Gregory GA. Pharmacology. In: Gregory GA, ed Pediatric anesthesia. New York, Churchill Livingstone 1983;315–39.
2. Eger EI II, Bahlman SH, Munson ES. The effect of age on the rate of increase of alveolar anesthesia concentration. Anesthesiology 1971;35:365–72.
3. Gregory GA, Eger EI II, Munson ES. The relationship between age and halothane re-

quirement in man. Anesthesiology 1969;30:488–91.

4. Lerman J, Robinson S, Willis MM, Gregory GA. Anesthetic requirements for halothane in young children 0–1 month and 1–6 months of age. Anesthesiology 1983;59:421–4.

5. Fisher DM, O'Keefe C, Stanski DR, Cronnelly, R, Miller RD, Gregory GA. Pharmacokinetics of d-tubocurarine in infants, children and adults. Anesthesiology 1982;57:203–7.

6. Fisher DM, Miller RD. Neuromuscular effects of vecuronium (ORG NC45) in infants and children during N_2O, halothane anesthesia. Anesthesiology 1983;58:519–23.

7. Fisher DM, Cronnelly R, Miller RD, Sharma M. The neuromuscular pharmacology of neostigmine in infants and children. Anesthesiology 1983;59:220–5.

8. Brzustowicz RM, Nelson DA, Betts EK, Rosenberry KR, Swedlow DB. Efficacy of oral premedication for pediatric outpatient surgery. Anesthesiology 1984;60:475–7.

9. Cote CJ, Goudsouzian NG, Liu LMP, Dedrick DF, Szyfelbein SK. Assessment of risk factors related to acid aspiration syndrome in pediatric patients: Gastric pH and residual volume. Anesthesiology 1982;56:70-2.

10. Cote CJ, Liu LMP, Dedrick DF. Dose-response effects of oral cimetidine on gastric pH and volume in children. Anesthesiology 1981;55:533–6.

11. Gregory GA. Pediatric anesthesia. In: Miller RD, ed. Anesthesia. New York, Churchill Livingstone 1981;1197–1230.

12. Furman EB, Roman DG, Lemmer LAS, Hairabet J, Jasinski M, Laver MB. Specific therapy in water, electrolyte and blood-volume replacement during pediatric surgery. Anesthesiology 1975;42:187–93.

13. Gregory GA. Resuscitation of the newborn. In: Miller RD, ed. Anesthesia. New York, Churchill Livingstone 1981;1175–96.

28

Elderly Patients

Elderly patients, who are arbitrarily defined as over 65 years of age, are becoming an increasingly important group, accounting for more than 10 percent of the population in the United States. These patients are particularly vulnerable to the adverse effects of anesthesia because of their reduced margin of safety. An important concept, which is often not appreciated, is to distinguish between the normal attrition of organ function that occurs in all patients with increasing age and the loss of function that marks the onset of pathologic changes from one or more of the diseases frequently encountered in elderly patients. Thus, the physiologic and pharmacologic changes that must be taken into account when anesthetizing elderly patients must be added to the concomitant disease processes that may also exist. Although the mortality and morbidity of surgery in elderly patients is higher than that for their younger counterparts, these problems are usually due to concomitant disease processes, such as infection or renal failure, rather than aging per se.[1]

PHYSIOLOGY

There is a progressive and irreversible deterioration in physiologic function with increasing age,[2] as summarized in Figure 28-1.

Cardiovascular

Cardiovascular reserve diminishes with increasing age. For example, after the third decade of life, cardiac output decreases at a rate of about 1 percent per year. As a result, cardiac output is decreased by about 50 percent in a 80-year-old individual as compared to a 30-year-old person. This decrease in cardiac output is probably secondary to several factors, including a decreased response to catecholamines, increased myocardial stiffness (due to increased interstitial fibrosis in the myocardium), progressive atheroscleroisis of the peripheral arteries leading to increased afterload of the heart, and increased amyloid deposits in the myocardium which predispose to cardiac failure often with conduction defects. Heart rate decreases with advancing age, suggesting an increase in the activity of the parasympathetic nervous system. Degenerative changes secondary to aging can involve the cardiac conduction system, contributing to bradycardia with or without significant degrees of atrioventricular heart block. Systolic blood pressure increases with aging, reflecting degenerative changes leading to poorly compliant arteries. The autonomic nervous system response to stress is attenuated, as reflected by diminished baroreceptor (carotid sinus) reflex activity. For example,

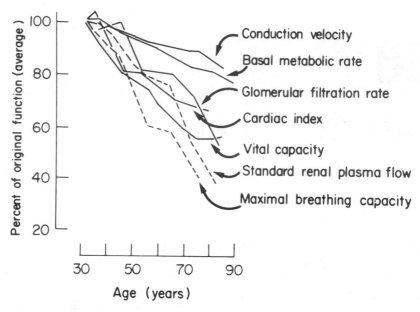

Figure 28-1. Changes in physiologic function with age in humans expressed as percentage of mean value at age 30 years. (Miller RD. Anesthesia for the elderly. In: Miller RD, ed. Anesthesia. New York, Churchill Livingstone 1981;1231–46.)

changes in heart rate elicited by arterial hypoxemia, hypercarbia, or alterations in blood pressure are reduced in elderly patients.

Ventilation

Pulmonary reserve decreases with increasing age. Despite a constant total lung capacity, vital capacity decreases about 25 ml/year starting at the age of 20 years. The functional residual capacity and residual volume increase. Although PAO_2 remains constant with increasing age, the PaO_2 progressively decreases. A rule of thumb is that the PaO_2 after the age of 20 years will decrease at a rate of 0.4 mmHg/year. The $PaCO_2$ is not influenced by aging per se. Also, there is a greater tendency for airways to collapse, as indicated by a progressive increase in the closing volume. This may contribute to a higher incidence of atelectasis postoperatively in such patients.

Although static lung compliance increases with age, dynamic lung compliance decreases and becomes more frequency-dependent in elderly patients. There is a 20 to 30 percent decrease in flow rates, including the forced expiratory volume in 1 second. This results in a decreased ability to generate normal expiratory pressures, as well as an increased resistance to exhalation due to early airway collapse. Maximum breathing capacity is reduced at least 50 percent at 70 years of age.

Elderly patients have an increased incidence of pneumonia compared with their younger counterparts. This probably relates to some general depression of the immune system, an increased incidence of aspiration of oral pharyngeal secretions, a decreased mechanical ability to clear the tracheobronchial tree by the mucociliary apparatus, and increased colonization in the oral pharynx because of poor oral hygiene.

Renal

Renal mass and function progressively decrease with increasing age. Reductions in blood flow parallel reductions in cardiac output. Because of a reduction in the number of glomeruli, there is an age-related decrease in glomerular filtration rate and creatinine clearance as depicted by the following equation:

creatinine clearance (ml/min)
$$= 135 - 0.84 \times age \text{ (years)}$$

A decrease in renal function has several implications for management of anesthesia. First, the ability of the kidney to regulate salt balance, especially under stress, is decreased with increasing age, making fluid and electrolyte balance more labile. Elderly patients are less able to concentrate urine after water deprivation, so the ability to excrete an acid load is reduced. Secondly, those drugs (especially muscle relaxants) which are dependent on renal excretion for their elimination will obviously be affected by the decreased renal function that occurs with aging. Thirdly, renal tubular function declines with increasing age, so that the maximum reabsorption of glucose follows a linear decrease with increasing age. Therefore, glucosuria may be misleading in the diagnosis and management of diabetes mellitus in elderly patients.

Despite the reduction in renal function, the serum creatinine concentration does not predictably increase in elderly patients. This unchanged concentration reflects the decreased production of creatinine which results from the decreased skeletal muscle mass that accompanies aging. Therefore, an increased serum concentration of creatinine in an elderly patient emphasizes the presence of severe renal dysfunction.

Hepatic

Hepatic blood flow decreases with aging in proportion to reductions in the cardiac output. Decreased activity of hepatic microsomal enzymes is predictable, but it is likely that reduced hepatic blood flow is more important in delayed drug clearance observed in elderly patients. Finally, the production of albumin by the liver decreases with aging, resulting in decreased plasma protein binding of drugs.

Gastrointestinal

There is a general decrease in esophageal and intestinal motility, which results in delayed gastric emptying. Also, gastroesophageal sphincter tone is frequently decreased. As a result of the delayed gastric emptying time and decreased gastroesophageal sphincter tone, the chances of vomiting and aspiration of gastric contents presumably are increased.

Musculoskeletal

Nerves, muscle, and neuromuscular junctions deteriorate with age. There is a reduction in the efficiency of coupling nerves to muscle and a reduction in the number of muscle cells innervated by an axon, which leads to denervation and atrophy of muscle with increasing age. Although the clinical importance has not been ascertained, conduction velocity also decreases in peripheral nerves.

Osteoporosis, which is characterized by a decrease in bone mass, is increased with aging. This, combined with an increased incidence of degenerative joint disease, makes positioning of the elderly patient during surgery crucial because fractures and dislocated joints are easier to induce.

Skin

Atrophy of the epidermis occurs with increasing age, especially in the exposed areas, such as the face, neck, and extensor surface of the hands and forearms. Furthermore, the turnover rate of cells in the stratum corneum decreases with aging. For example, in persons older than 65 years, it takes 50 percent longer to reepithelialize blistered skin than in young adults. The decrease in epidermal cell growth and division contributes to the increased incidence of decubitus ulcers in elderly patients. Obviously, elderly patients are more prone to damage from tape that the anesthesiologist might use during surgery, and undue pressure from incorrect positioning intraoperatively.

PHARMACOLOGY

Pharmacokinetics (distribution and elmination of drugs) and pharmacodynamic (sensitivity of the receptor) changes to drugs occur with increasing age.

Pharmacokinetics

There are at least four reasons why elderly patients may have different pharmacokinetic responses to drugs than their younger counterparts. First, renal function is decreased, which leads to increased blood levels and prolonged elimination half-times. Secondly, drug metabolism may be decreased in elderly patients because of decreased hepatic enzyme activity or reduced hepatic blood flow. Thirdly, protein binding of drugs is often decreased, resulting in higher blood levels of free drug. Lastly, there is a reduction in overall body weight reflecting decreased skeletal muscle mass and total body water content plus an increase in adipose tissue, all of which can alter the volume of distribution and elimination half-times of drugs in elderly patients.

Pharmacodynamics

Aging is associated with a decline in the number of receptors present in a given tissue. Yet, those receptors generally bind and respond to drugs in a normal fashion. Because of a reduced number of receptors, however, the blood level of drug required

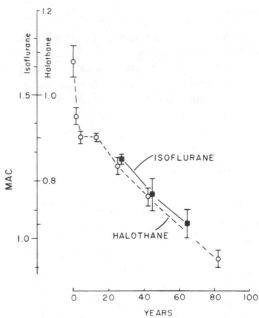

Figure 28-2. MAC for halothane and isoflurane decreases with increasing age. (Stevens WC, Dolan WM, Giffons RT, et al. Minimum alveolar concentrations (MAC) of isoflurane with and without nitrous oxide in patients of various ages. Anesthesiology 1975;42:197, as modified in Quasha AL, Eger EI. MAC. In: Miller RD, ed. Anesthesia. New York, Churchill Livingstone 1981;257–81.)

to achieve a given response may be reduced in elderly patients.

Specific Drugs

Inhaled Anesthetics. The minimum alveolar anesthetic concentration (MAC) has been shown with several inhaled anesthetics to decrease with increasing age (Fig. 28-2).[3] Nevertheless, because of decreased alveolar ventilation, the rate of induction of anesthesia may be slowed. In an attempt to hasten induction of anesthesia, the anesthesiologist must be careful to avoid doses of anesthetics which may be excessive and cause severe cardiovascular depression.

Sedative-Hypnotics. The doses of barbiturates and benzodiazepines should generally be reduced in elderly patients for both pharmacokinetic and pharmacodynamic reasons. For example, the dose of thiopental required to produce a state in which the patient is unable to be aroused is less in elderly patients as compared to their younger counterparts.[4] Diazepam has been studied extensively in elderly patients. The blood concentration required to achieve a state in which the patient will not respond verbally decreases with increasing age. Furthermore, the elimination half-time of diazepam is increased with increasing age. Thus, the increased effect of diazepam in elderly patients may be attributed to a change in distribution of the drug and/or receptor site sensitivity. The message is clear that the dose of these and presumably other similar drugs should be reduced and that their effect may be prolonged in elderly patients.[5,6]

Narcotics. The onset of analgesia from morphine and possibly other narcotics is often delayed in elderly patients. Furthermore, a smaller dose of narcotic is required to achieve a given level of analgesia, which may be based largely on pharmacokinetic changes. The volume of distribution of narcotics is smaller in elderly patients which results in initially higher plasma morphine concentrations in these patients as compared to their younger counterparts. Furthermore, the delayed onset of analgesia after an intravenous dose of morphine suggests that the narcotic receptors are in tissues which are not rapidly equilibrating with the drug in the blood.[7] Also, decreased plasma protein binding of narcotics may increase the free fraction of drug available to interact with the receptor. Finally, there is an increased incidence of nausea, depression of ventilation, and hypotension following administration of narcotics to elderly patients.[8,9]

Muscle Relaxants. Aging decreases the plasma clearance of pancuronium and vecuronium but not atracurium.[10] This most likely reflects Hofmann elimination and/or

plasma hydrolysis of atracurium which are independent of aging. Conversely, decreases in hepatic (pancuronium and vecuronium) and renal (pancuronium) function characteristic of aging interfere with elimination of pancuronium and vecuronium. Consequently the dose required for neuromuscular blockade and the speed of recovery will be decreased for pancuronium and vecuronium but not atracurium in elderly patients. In addition to pancuronium, other muscle relaxants known to be dependent on renal clearance (d-tubocurarine and metocurine) have a longer elimination half-time and therefore longer duration of action in elderly patients.[11,12]

ANESTHETIC MANAGEMENT

Preoperative

In addition to the normal process of aging which decreases the margin of safety, elderly patients are more likely to have hypertension, congestive heart failure, cardiac dysrhythmias, chronic obstructive airway disease, and diabetes mellitus.[13] Also, a drug history is particularly important because of the numerous abnormalities and drug interactions that may occur in elderly patients. Unfortunately, elderly patients can become confused and forget not only what drugs they are taking, but how much and when the last dose was taken. Close consultation with the family and physician is essential in these cases. Often, merely asking the patient to show you what drugs they are taking and how frequently they take them can alleviate some of the problems in taking an accurate history.

Although there are several drugs that elderly patients may be taking, diuretics, tricyclic antidepressants, and antihypertensives seem to present the more common problems (see Chapter 3). If diuretics are being taken, a careful evaluation of the intravascular fluid volume status and serum potassium concentration must be made. Tricyclic antidepressants may result in various degrees of heart block and the occurrence of adverse ineractions with drugs used in the perioperative period. Antihypertensives can interfere with the normal autonomic nervous system response to anesthetics. Generally, an attempt should be made to determine whether orthostatic hypotension is present as part of the routine preoperative evaluation of elderly patients. Although there may be many causes of orthostatic hypotension, autonomic nervous system dysfunction, usually from drugs or increasing age, and/or hypovolemia are the most common explanations. If orthostatic hypotension is not associated with an increase in heart rate, then the autonomic nervous system is probably not functioning properly.[14] If the hypotension is associated with tachycardia, then hypovolemia may be present.

Simplified bedside pulmonary function testing is often helpful in the preoperative evaluation of elderly patients. These values can determine whether chest physiotherapy might be beneficial preoperatively or can be used for comparison when assessing pulmonary function postoperatively. Because of the high incidence of pulmonary complications postoperatively, preoperative teaching of incentive spirometry and chest physiotherapy along with the use of bronchodilators may reduce the incidence of postoperative respiratory complications.

Preoperative medication in elderly patients should be used sparingly (see Chapter 10). Often, administration of diazepam, 2.5 to 10.0 mg orally, is the only preoperative medication necessary. Should the elderly patient request to be asleep on leaving the hospital room for the operating room, it should be explained that excessive preoperative medication can be dangerous.

Intraoperative

Several changes associated with aging cause mechanical problems during anesthesia (Table 28-1). In the edentulous pa-

Table 28-1. Mechanical Changes Associated with Aging which Can Cause Problems during Anesthesia

Edentulous or poor dental hygiene
Arthritis
Weak posterior membranous portion of trachea
Senile atrophy of skin
Less reactivity of airways
Decreased gastroesophageal sphincter tone

tient or the patient with poor dental hygiene, it is difficult to obtain a proper mask fit, and the chance of dislodging a loose tooth is enhanced. The presence of arthritis, especially in the cervical area, may make intubation of the trachea difficult. Furthermore, the weak posterior membranous portion of the trachea increases the possibility of tracheal trauma. The anesthesiologist should be especially careful in utilizing a stylet in performing an endotracheal intubation when the trachea is not easily visualized. Probing with the stylet in place can cause trauma and, in rare cases, create a false passage which will result in inadequate ventilation of the lungs and production of mediastinal emphysema. Senile atrophy makes the skin more sensitive to injury from adhesive tape and monitoring pads as used for the electrocardiogram. The combination of arthritis and sensitive skin makes the problems associated with poor positioning of the elderly patient particularly important so as to avoid pressure necrosis and neuropathies (see Chapter 15).

The reduced reactivity of the glottic opening and airways plus decreased tone of the gastroesophageal sphincter probably make regurgitation and aspiration of gastric contents more likely in the elderly patient. This possibility, however, does not routinely justify the rapid intravenous induction technique of anesthesia with drugs such as thiopental and succinylcholine. This approach may be particularly dangerous in elderly patients because of a decreased margin of safety, especially with respect to the circulatory system. On occasion an awake intubation of the trachea preceded by topical anesthesia and light sedation may be

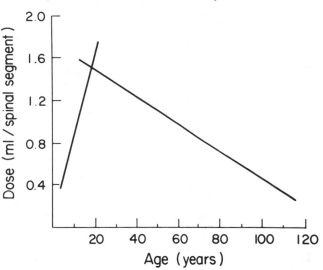

Figure 28-3. Segmental dose requirements related to age between 4 and 102 years. TBW = total body water; ICW = intracellular water. (Bromage PR: Aging and epidural dose requirements. Br J Anaesth 1969; 41:1016 as modified in Miller RD. Anesthesia for the elderly. In: Miller RD, ed. Anesthesia. New York, Churchill Livingstone 1981;1231–46.)

indicated (see Chapter 12). Regardless of the anesthetic technique chosen, it is especially important to titrate the dose of anesthetic so as to avoid adverse effects in vulnerable elderly patients.

Regional anesthesia is frequently useful in elderly patients. Although not precisely defined, the total dose of local anesthetic probably needs to be reduced to avoid toxic reactions. An advantage of regional anesthesia is that of maintaining consciousness, which allows the prompt recognition of angina pectoris, acute cerebral changes, and a body position which may be undesirable or even harmful. When using spinal anesthesia, elderly patients are probably more sensitive (e.g., higher sensory levels with a given dose) than their younger counterparts. Decreased blood flow to the vessels surrounding the subarachnoid space may explain the apparent longer duration of anesthesia in elderly arteriosclerotic patients. Elderly patients probably exhibit more hypotension than do their younger counterparts when equal levels of spinal anesthesia are induced. The incidence and severity of hypotension can be minimized by administering ephedrine, 50 mg intramuscularly, 5 to 10 minutes before institution of spinal anesthesia. Epidural anes-

thesia has the advantage that, although hypotensive effects are just as great as with spinal anesthesia, they appear more gradually. Also, the dose of local anesthetic required to achieve a given level of epidural anesthesia decreases with increasing age (Fig. 28-3).[2]

Because of the reduced margin of safety, adequate monitoring of elderly patients is essential. The well-known complications from monitoring, however, should be considered. For example, complications from insertion of a catheter into the radial artery may be more intense in elderly patients who have compromised circulation to the hand. Also, complications associated with a pulmonary artery catheter may induce cardiac dysrhythmias which may be more severe in elderly patients. The anesthesiologist must use his or her judgment in performing a risk/benefit analysis of each monitor selected.

REFERENCES

1. Harbrecht TJ, Garrison RN, Fry DE. Role of infection in increased mortality associated with age in laparotomy. Am Surg 1983;49:173–8.
2. Miller RD Anesthesia for the elderly. In: Miller RD, ed. Anesthesia. New York, Churchill Livingstone 1981;1231–46.

3. Quasha AL, Eger EI. MAC. In: Miller RD, ed. Anesthesia. New York, Churchill Livingstone 1981;257–81.

4. Muravchick S, Mandel J. Thiopental sleep dosages in geriatric patients. Anesthesiology 1982;57:A327.

5. Klotz U, Avant GR, Hoyumpa A. The effects of age and liver disease on the disposition and elimination of diazepam in adult man. J Clin Invest 1975;55:347–59.

6. Reidenberg MM, Levy M, Warner H, Coutinho CB, Schwartz MA, Yu G, Cheripko J. Relationship between diazepam dose, plasma level, age and central nervous system depression. Clin Pharmacol Ther 1978;23:371–4.

7. Owen JA, Sitar DS, Berger L, Brownell L, Duke PC, Metenko PA. Age-related morphine kinetics. Clin Pharmacol Ther 1983;34:364–8.

8. Chan K, Kendall MJ, Mitchard M. Wells WDE. The effect of ageing on plasma pethidine concentration. Br J Clin Pharmacol 1975;2:297–302.

9. Mather LE, Tucker GT, Pflug AE, Lindop MJ, Wilkerson C. Meperidine kinetics in man: Intravenous injection in surgical patients and volunteers. Clin Pharmacol Ther 1975;17:21–30.

10. D'Hollander AA, Luyckx C, Barvais L, DeVille A. Clinical evaluation of atracurium besylate requirement for a stable muscle relaxation during surgery: Lack of age-related effects. Anesthesiology 1983;59:237–40.

11. Matteo RS, Backus W, Abraham R, Diaz J. Pharmacodynamics of d-tubocurarine and metocurine in the elderly. Anesthesiology 1983;59:1268.

12. Duvaldestin P, Saada J, Berger JL, d'Hollander A, Desmonts JM. Pharmacokinetics, pharmacodynamics, and dose-response relationship of pancuronium in control and elderly subjects. Anesthesiology 1982;56:36–40.

13. Roizen MF. Preoperative evaluation of patients with disease that require special preoperative evaluation and intraoperative management. In: Miller RD, ed. Anesthesia. New York, Churchill Livingstone 1981;21–70.

14. Thompson PD, Melmon AL. Clinical assessment of autonomic function. Anesthesiology 1968;29:724–31.

29

Outpatient Surgery

Outpatient (ambulatory) surgery offers an alternative to the traditional sequence of hospitalization prior to elective operations requiring anesthesia. Approximately 20 to 40 percent of hospital inpatient surgery can be performed in an outpatient setting.[1] Compared with inpatient surgery, advantages of performing the same operation as an outpatient include a decrease in medical costs, increased availability of beds for patients who require hospitalization, protection from hospital-acquired infections, and avoidance of disruption of the family unit attendant upon hospitalization. Cost savings extend beyond the actual medical expenses as patients can return to daily activity sooner, reducing financial loss due to absence from work or need to provide for outside child care. Another cost saving results from the decreased need to build expensive hospital facilities, as existing beds become available for inpatients. The short separation time from family provided by outpatient surgery is especially important for children, as this reduces the number of postoperative psychological problems caused by separation-induced anxiety which may persist long after completion of surgery.

An alternative to the same-day admission and discharge outpatient surgery concept is a prospectively planned overnight admission to the hospital following surgery. This approach, which has been designated "come and stay surgery," preserves the advantages of the same-day admission but eliminates any physician concerns regarding the ability to optimally manage potential anesthetic or operative complications in the early postoperative period.

FACILITIES

Outpatient surgical facilities are either in a hospital or a free-standing clinic (Surgicenter). The free-standing clinic must have a transfer and admission agreement with a nearby hospital should unexpected hospitalization be required after surgery. Less than 2 percent of patients, however, will require hospitalization following outpatient surgery. Furthermore, the incidence of hospitalization because of life-threatening complications following outpatient surgery is very low, being estimated as 0.007 percent.[1]

The operating rooms, monitors, anesthetic equipment, and postoperative recovery room facilities used for outpatient surgery should not be different from those used for inpatients. The recovery room must be large enough to permit patients to remain for several hours following surgery without overtaxing the facilities. Outpatient surgical facilities should have a physician director, usually an anesthesiologist, who is responsible for the daily administrative decisions, including the final judgments regarding whether a given procedure should be done on an outpatient basis.

SELECTION OF PATIENTS

Selection of individuals for outpatient surgery is determined by the characteristics of the patient and the type of operation.

Characteristics of the Patient

The patient must desire to have surgery performed as an outpatient and be in otherwise good general health or have a systemic disease (diabetes mellitus, essential hypertension, congenital heart disease) that is medically controlled. The patient or a responsible adult must be reasonably intelligent and reliable to assure compliance with preoperative and postoperative instructions. Patients with a previous history of prolonged postoperative nausea and vomiting or in whom it is unlikely that pain will be relieved by oral analgesics are not likely candidates for outpatient surgery. Ideally, the driving distance to the outpatient facility should not exceed 1 hour to assure rapid return to the hospital should serious postoperative complications develop.

Patients prone to hospital-acquired infections (infants, immunosuppressed patients) may benefit from having their surgery performed as outpatients. For example, about 1 in 5 infants admitted as inpatients for elective inguinal hernia repair develop an upper respiratory tract or enteric infection.[1] The incidence of these types of infections is 50 to 70 percent less when the surgery is performed as an outpatient.

Age is usually not a factor in the selection of patients for outpatient surgery. Nevertheless, the pediatric patient probably benefits most from outpatient surgery. The prematurely born infant, however, is probably unsuitable for outpatient surgery because of the frequent presence of anemia in these patients plus the potential for immaturity of the respiratory center. Indeed, these infants are prone to become apneic in the perioperative period. For these reasons, it is often recommended that any prematurely born infant up to 6 months of age be admitted to the hospital for all types of surgery. These patients should be monitored on an apnea monitor for at least 18 hours postoperatively.[2] Other infants who may be at increased risk for outpatient surgery are those who required treatment of respiratory distress syndrome following birth. These infants often develop bronchopulmonary dysplasia associated with abnormal blood gases and an increased incidence of pulmonary infection in the first 6 to 12 months following termination of ventilator therapy (see Chapter 27). Despite these qualifications, performance of infant inguinal hernia repair is a well-accepted outpatient surgical procedure. In elderly patients, acceptability for outpatient surgery is influenced by physical status and the ability to be cared for by a competent adult at home.

Type of Operation

Operations that are best suited for outpatient procedures are those of short duration (ideally less than 2 hours) which are associated with minimal postoperative bleeding or physiologic derangements (Table 29-1). Nevertheless, there is no evidence that recovery time parallels anesthesia time. This suggests that arbitrary limits placed on the type of outpatient surgery permitted based on the anticipated duration of the procedure are unwarranted.[3] Finally,

Table 29-1. Examples of Operations that Can Be Performed as Outpatient Procedures

Extraocular muscle resection
Dental and oral surgical procedures
Bronchoscopy and esophagoscopy
Tonsillectomy and adenoidectomy
Nasal polypectomy
Rhinoplasty
Myringotomy
Breast biopsy
Augmentation mammoplasty
Laparoscopy with or without tubal ligation
Inguinal hernia repair
Dilation and curettage
Circumcision
Cystoscopy
Vasectomy
Superficial procedures on extremities

the surgery should not be associated with the risk of airway obstruction or interfere with early postoperative ambulation. These recommendations, however, are only guidelines as emphasized by the frequent performance, as outpatient procedures, of (1) tonsillectomy and adenoidectomy which may be accompanied by postoperative hemorrhage; and (2) laparoscopy which invades the peritoneal cavity. In one report, the incidence of bleeding following performance of tonsillectomy and adenoidectomy as an outpatient procedure was lower (1.73 percent) than the incidence of this complication when surgery was performed on inpatients (4.35 percent).[1]

Infected cases are rarely considered for outpatient surgery because of the need for separate operative and recovery facilities. Likewise, emergency surgery is not likely to be done as an outpatient procedure, as this would disrupt the elective schedule. Furthermore, it is difficult to adequately evaluate patients requiring emergency surgery as outpatients.

PREOPERATIVE PREPARATION AND INSTRUCTIONS TO THE PATIENT

The surgeon is responsible for scheduling outpatient surgery, obtaining a medical history, performing a physical examination, initiating the necessary preoperative laboratory studies, and providing instructions to the patient or responsible parent. It is not possible or convenient for the anesthesiologist to see every patient at the time of scheduling for outpatient surgery. Therefore, the surgeon must describe and explain the preoperative anesthetic requirements to the patient. If questions related to anesthesia arise that cannot be adequately answered by the surgeon, it is reasonable to ask the anesthesiologist for a consultation at this time. Otherwise, it is satisfactory for the patient to be seen by the anesthesiologist on the day of surgery.

Laboratory Data Required Preoperatively

The laboratory data required preoperatively will depend on the patient's age, history, physical examination, and current drug therapy (see Chapter 9). Most guidelines for outpatient surgery require a recent (within 30 days of surgery) hemoglobin determination. The hemoglobin concentration should exceed 10 g/dl. This minimum hemoglobin requirement is based on the concept that anemia is associated with medical diseases that could influence postoperative outcome. For patients over 40 years of age, it may be appropriate to determine the blood glucose concentration and blood urea nitrogen concentration preoperatively. Determination of the serum glutamic oxalacetic transaminase concentration as a routine screening test for the detection of unsuspected hepatocellular disease can be considered for adult patients. Serum potassium concentration should be measured routinely if the patient is being treated with potassium-losing diuretics. Routine urinalysis offers little or no new information and in many respects only duplicates the blood chemistry measurements. In the absence of positive findings on the history or physical examination, it is not necessary to obtain a routine preoperative electrocardiogram or radiograph of the chest in patients less than 40 years of age.

Written Instructions

Written instructions describing outpatient surgery requirements should be given to the patient or parent by the surgeon at the time of scheduling of the surgical procedure (Table 29-2). The reasons for these requirements should be explained verbally to the patient by the surgeon and the written instructions signed by the patient or parent. Explanation of the reasons for not eating or drinking prior to surgery is particularly important.

Table 29-2. Information Provided on Written Instruction Sheet Given to Patient when Outpatient Surgery Is Scheduled

1. Make sure requested laboratory tests are completed

2. Nothing to eat or drink up to 8 hours before surgery (traditionally NPO after midnight)

3. A child less than 1 year of age may receive clear liquids up to 4 hours before surgery

4. Wear minimal to no cosmetics or jewelry

5. Where and when to report for surgery and estimate of discharge time

6. Must be accompanied by an adult to provide transportation home

7. Notify surgeon if there is a change in the patient's medical condition before surgery

8. Following surgery resume eating when hungry, starting with clear liquids and progressing to soups and then regular diet

9. Do not drive an automobile or make important decisions for at least 24 to 48 hours following anesthesia

10. Telephone number to contact physician regarding significant postoperative complications

ARRIVAL ON THE DAY OF SURGERY

On arrival for outpatient surgery, the patient's compliance with the written instructions are verified particularly as they relate to fasting. It is especially important that clandestine liquid or food intake by pediatric patients be considered and confirmed not to have occurred. The anesthesiologist should review the patient's medical record and laboratory data at this time. In addition, the pertinent areas to be pursued by the anesthesiologist include questions regarding previous anesthetics, current drug therapy, allergies, and previous adverse responses such as postoperative vomiting. An examination of the upper airway including teeth and evaluation of the peripheral nervous system if regional anesthesia is anticipated are performed. Finally, the anesthesiologist should elicit any change in the medical condition (fever, cough, sputum, diarrhea) that may have developed since the outpatient surgery was scheduled. Pediatric patients must be thoroughly evaluated for any evidence of an upper respiratory tract infection that has manifested since scheduling. Indeed, rhinorrhea poses an enigma in the pediatric patient scheduled for outpatient surgery. Benign rhinorrhea is usually an allergic rhinitis that does not contraindicate elective surgery, assuming there is no associated history of asthma. If there is any doubt, the rhinorrhea should be assumed to be an upper respiratory tract infection and elective surgery cancelled. In this regard, the temperature pattern can be useful in differentiating between an infectious and noninfectious process. For example, a temperature above 38 Celsius in children is highly suggestive of an upper respiratory tract infection.

PREOPERATIVE MEDICATION

Preoperative medication with drugs to reduce anxiety or produce sedation prior to outpatient surgery is often avoided for fear of delaying the return to wakefulness following anesthesia and surgery. Indeed, recovery time is prolonged by narcotic premedication with morphine or meperidine but not by diazepam.[3] Reassurance by the anesthesiologist and surgeon is a potent antidote to preoperative anxiety in most patients (see Chapter 10). Nevertheless, pharmacologic premedication may be desirable in the mentally retarded or hyperactive patient. An oral barbiturate or benzodiazepine can be administered to these patients before they leave home. If this is not possible, the patient should arrive at the outpatient facility at least 2 hours before scheduled surgery to allow administration (ideally orally) of the preoperative medication and production of a desirable effect prior to induction of anesthesia.

Compared with adult inpatients, those scheduled for outpatient surgery have been

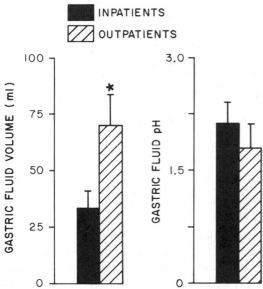

Figure 29-1. Gastric fluid volume and pH (mean ± SD) was determined for inpatients (N-21) and outpatients (N-21) undergoing minor surgery. Gastric fluid volume was significantly greater for outpatients (P<0.05) than inpatients despite similar periods (12 and 15 hours respectively) of fasting. Gastric fluid pH did not differ significantly between groups. (Based on data in Ong BY, Palahnuik J, Cumming M. Gastric volume and pH in out-patients. Can Anaesth Soc J 1978;25:36–9.)

shown to have increased volumes of acidic gastric fluid (Fig. 29-1).[4] Since inhalation of acidic gastric fluid is a major hazard associated with drug-induced depression or unconsciousness, it may be reasonable to administer drugs orally in the preoperative period in order to reduce gastric fluid volume (metoclopramide) and increase gastric fluid pH (antacids, H_2-antagonists). Nevertheless, the value or need for these drugs as a routine in the management of patients scheduled for inpatient or outpatient surgery has not been documented. More important than pharmacologic attempts to alter gastric fluid volume and pH is rapid and skillful protection of the airway by placement of a cuffed tube in the trachea of appropriate patients.

Routine intramuscular administration of an anticholinergic as preoperative medication is not necessary, with the possible exception of patients scheduled for oral endoscopies. In these patients, excessive oral secretions may interfere with the production of topical anesthesia. Otherwise, the discomfort of a dry mouth and throat and the possibility of residual mydriasis and difficulty focusing are undesirable in adult outpatients. Furthermore, pediatric patients may be susceptible to increases in body temperature secondary to anticholinergic effects on sweating. If bradycardia develops intraoperatively, atropine can be administered intravenously.

TECHNIQUE OF ANESTHESIA

All techniques of anesthesia and drugs used to produce anesthesia for inpatients can be considered for use in outpatients. However, use of a technique and/or drug that permits a prompt and nearly complete recovery with minimal side effects (absence of sedation, nausea, vomiting, orthostatic hypotension) is mandatory for optimal safety of patients who will be discharged from the hospital within a few hours following surgery. Local infiltration anesthesia is preferable when the planned operative procedure permits. Alternatives to local anesthesia are a general anesthetic, regional anesthetic, or peripheral nerve block (see Chapter 9). Regardless of the technique of anesthesia selected, a catheter should probably be inserted into a peripheral vein prior to the institution of anesthesia. This catheter is necessary to allow administration of fluids (5 to 7 ml/kg/hr of lactated Ringer's solution with 5 percent dextrose) to offset dehydration associated with preoperative fasting. The other important reason for placing an intravenous catheter is administration of drugs to produce anesthesia or treat adverse intraoperative events such as bradycardia, cardiac dysrhythmias or hypotension. Nevertheless, placement of an intravenous catheter in every patient may be unnecessary when technical difficulties outweight the advantages of having an intravenous infusion site and/or the surgery will be very short (less than 15 minutes) and only superficial tissues are involved.

General Anesthesia

General anesthesia is most frequently selected for outpatient surgery. Induction of anesthesia is pleasantly achieved with the intravenous administration of an ultrashort-acting barbiturate. Methohexital is alleged to have a shorter duration of action than thiopental or thiamylal, and for this reason is a popular drug for induction of anesthesia for outpatients. Nevertheless, it must be appreciated that repeated injection of any barbiturate can lead to cumulative effects and delayed postoperative awakening. Diazepam has been used for induction of anesthesia but is not popular for outpatient surgery because of its prolonged duration of action. Midazolam is a short-acting water soluble benzodiazepine but has not been documented to be superior to thiopental for induction of anesthesia.[5] Etomidate, like methohexital, is associated with rapid awakening but the increased incidence of myoclonic movements, nausea, and vomiting detracts from the use of this drug. Pediatric patients may prefer an inhalation induction to the needle stick required for an intravenous induction of anesthesia, but even this alternative should be discouraged as a small gauge catheter can be placed with minimal discomfort. Furthermore, the discomfort associated with local infiltration can be obviated by using a 30 gauge needle and wiping the alcohol prep solution from the site with a dry gauze before puncturing the skin. When an inhalation induction of anesthesia is planned, however, the most frequently selected drug is halothane. Compared with halothane, induction of anesthesia with enflurane or isoflurane is associated with more patient excitement, breath-holding, coughing, and laryngospasm. In uncontrollable patients, induction

Table 29-3. Myalgia 24 Hours Following Elective Dilation and Curettage

	Incidence
No succinylcholine (N-20)	Zero
Succinylcholine 1 mg/kg (N-20)	40 percent
d-Tubocurarine 0.04 mg/kg Succinylcholine 1 mg/kg (N-20)	Zero

(Data from Stoelting RK, Petersen C. Adverse effects of increased succinylcholine dose following d-tubocurarine pretreatment. Anesth Analg 1975;54:282–8.)

of anesthesia can be achieved with rectal methohexital (10 to 25 mg/kg) which produces unconsciousness in 7 to 10 minutes. The disadvantage of rectal methohexital is delayed awakening following surgery.

Intubation of the trachea should not be avoided because the surgery is being performed as an outpatient procedure. Use of a small diameter tube and care to avoid trauma, however, during direct laryngoscopy are particularly important for outpatients. Pediatric patients are probably the most vulnerable to airway edema following intubation of the trachea because of the small diameter of their glottic opening. Nevertheless, the incidence of laryngotracheal edema (croup) following 1 to 4 hours of tracheal intubation was only 5 percent in children 1 to 7 years of age.[7] Furthermore, symptoms of laryngotracheal edema are most likely to occur in the first hour following extubation of the trachea when the patient is still in the recovery room.

Placement of a tube in the trachea is facilitated by skeletal muscle relaxation produced by the intravenous administration of succinylcholine 1 mg/kg. Administration of intravenous gallamine 0.3 mg/kg or d-tubocurarine 0.04 mg/kg 3 minutes before succinylcholine prevents excessive heart rate slowing and greatly reduces the incidence of postoperative myalgia associated with this depolarizing muscle relaxant (Table 29-3).[8]

Maintenance of anesthesia is with nitrous oxide and a volatile anesthetic or a short-acting narcotic (fentanyl, sufentanil, alfentanil). There is no important difference between halothane, enflurane, and isoflurane with respect to awakening times, which are rapid following discontinuance of all three drugs. The dose of narcotic must be minimized to avoid prolonged postoperative effects. Ketamine is seldom used to anesthetize adults for outpatient surgery because of prolonged recovery and the occasional occurrence of unpleasant postoperative dreams. In contrast, ketamine has been extensively used for outpatient pediatric procedures without overt behavioral problems or hallucinations. Atropine should be administered as preoperative medication to avoid excessive salivation associated with ketamine anesthesia.

When nondepolarizing muscle relaxants are required, the dose administered is similar to that administered to inpatients. Likewise, residual neuromuscular block is appropriately antagonized by an anticholinesterase. At the conclusion of surgery, infiltration of the incision with a long-acting local anesthetic such as bupivacaine may decrease the need for postoperative analgesics.

Regional Anesthetic

A disadvantage of regional anesthesia (lumbar epidural or spinal block) for outpatient surgery is residual sympathetic nervous system blockade that produces orthostatic hypotension and prevents early postoperative ambulation. The possibility of headache following a spinal block further detracts from the use of this technique of anesthesia for outpatient surgery. Despite these disadvantages, regional anesthesia can be successfully utilized for outpatient surgery in selected patients. In younger patients or those in whom the potential for headache is unacceptably high, epidural block is a suitable alternative to spinal block.

Peripheral Nerve Block

Peripheral nerve blocks are ideal for operations on the extremities. An intravenous block is appropriate for superficial surgery on the extremities. When an intravenous block is selected, the duration of surgery must be considered, as adverse systemic reactions from entrance of the local anesthetic into the circulation are likely if the tourniquet is released before 45 minutes. Brachial plexus block is necessary when other than superficial surgery is performed on the arm. In the leg, any combination of sciatic, femoral, lateral femoral cutaneous, and obturator nerve blocks are appropriate for prolonged and involved surgery. Block of the brachial plexus by the supraclavicular approach or intercostal nerve block must be used cautiously, as an iatrogenic pneumothorax regardless of its size would be undesirable in an outpatient. Fentanyl, administered intravenously in 5 to 10 µg doses, attenuates patient discomfort associated with performance of the nerve block without interfering with patient cooperation or the elicitation of paresthesias.

DISCHARGE FROM RECOVERY ROOM

Discharge from the recovery room is based on documentation that residual effects of the anesthesia are dissipated. Recovery from anesthesia is evidenced by the presence of stable and normal vital signs, a level of consciousness similar to the preoperative status and the ability to ambulate without assistance. If regional anesthesia was employed, it is important to document complete return of both sensory and motor function. Nausea, vomiting, and vertigo should be absent and the patient should not be in excessive pain. The ability to tolerate fluids (water, carbonated drinks, popsicles) should be determined. Hoarseness or stridor in a patient in whom a tracheal tube was used must be watched carefully. Significant laryngeal edema typically manifests within the first hour following extubation of the trachea. Most of these patients respond to conservative measures and can be discharged without the need for overnight hospitalization. As a precaution, however, these patients should be observed for 3 to 4 hours following extubation of the trachea to assure that symptoms are not progressing. Otherwise, most patients are ready for discharge from the recovery room to an adult escort within 1.5 hours following surgery. The decision to discharge the patient is most often the responsibility of the anesthesiologist in consultation, when appropriate, with the surgeon.

The patient should be reminded that mental clarity and dexterity may remain impaired for as long as 24 to 48 hours despite an overall feeling of well-being. Therefore, important decisions, driving an automobile, or operation of complex equipment should not be attempted during this period (Table 29-2). Ingestion of alcohol or depressant drugs should be cautioned against, as additive responses with residual anesthetic effects are possible. Diet should initially consist of clear liquids progressing to soup, cereal, crackers, and ice cream as tolerated. An oral analgesic such as acetaminophen (Tylenol) should be provided for those likely to require such medication. Finally, patients should be provided with a telephone number of a physician familiar with their case as well as instructions for symptoms (bleeding, difficulty breathing, fever) that should be reported to the doctor as well as possible complications (sore throat, myalgia, incisional pain, headache) that do not require physician consultation. A telephone call the next day from a nurse or physician at the outpatient facility to the patient is important to assure that recovery is proceding without complications.

REFERENCES

1. Natof HE. Complications associated with ambulatory surgery. JAMA 1980;244:1116–8.
2. Liu LMP, Coté CJ, Goudsouzian NG, Ryan JF, Firestone S, Dedrick DF, Liu PL, Todres ID. Life-threatening apnea in infants recovering from anesthesia. Anesthesiology 1983; 59:506–10.
3. Meridy HW. Criteria for selection of ambulatory surgical patients and guidelines for anesthetic management: a retrospective study of 1553 cases. Anesth Analg 1982;61:921–6.
4. Ong BY, Palahniuk RJ, Cumming M. Gastric volume and pH in outpatients. Can Anaesth Soc J 1978;25:36–9.
5. Lebowitz PW, Cote ME, Daniels AL, Ramsey FM, Martyn JAJ, Teplick RS, Davison JK. Comparative cardiovascular effects of midazolam and thiopental in healthy patients. Anesth Analg 1982;61:771–5.
6. Steward DJ. A trial of enflurane for pediatric outpatient anesthesia. Can Anaesth Soc J 1977;24:603–8.
7. Smith FK, Deputy BS, Berry FA. Outpatient anesthesia for children undergoing extensive dental treatment. J Dis Child 1978;45:142–5.
8. Stoelting RK, Peterson C. Adverse effects of increased succinylcholine dose following d-tubocurarine pretreatment. Anesth Analg 1975;54:282–8.

Section V
Recovery Period

30

Recovery Room

The recovery room is that area designated for the monitoring and care of patients who are recovering from the immediate physiologic derangements produced by anesthesia and surgery. This room should be staffed with specially trained nurses skilled in the prompt recognition of postoperative complications. Location of the recovery room in close proximity to the operating rooms assures rapid access to physician consultation and assistance. Specifically, an anesthesiologist should be readily available and responsible for ensuring safe recovery from anesthesia. Equipment and drugs must be available to provide routine care (supplemental oxygen, suction, monitoring of vital signs, electrocardiogram) and advanced organ support (ventilators, transducers to monitor intravascular pressures, devices for continuous infusion of drugs). An electrical defibrillator and appropriate drugs to assist in the optimal provision of cardiopulmonary resuscitation must be available. The recovery room should have good access to radiographic and arterial blood gas services. The size of the recovery room is determined by the number and type of operative procedures, with approximately 1.5 recovery room beds being necessary for every operating room. Discharge of the patient from the recovery room is the responsibility of a physician, most often an anesthesiologist.

Administratively, an anesthesiologist usually serves as the medical director of the recovery room.

RECOVERY FROM ANESTHESIA

Recovery from anesthesia is usually uneventful and routine, beginning with discontinuation of the administration of anesthetic drugs and extubation of the trachea while the patient is still in the operating room. The rate of reduction in the alveolar concentration (partial pressure) of an inhaled anesthetic as a reflection of recovery is dependent on the patient's alveolar ventilation, the lipid solubility of the anesthetic drug, and the duration of anesthesia (Fig. 30-1).[1] Patients are likely to begin responding to verbal stimuli when the alveolar anesthetic concentration is reduced to about one-half the MAC value for the volatile drug.[2] This value is designated MAC awake. Recovery from the anesthetic effects of injected drugs depends on the dose administered, the time since the last injection, lipid solubility, hepatic inactivation, and/or renal excretion. If muscle relaxants have been administered, it is important to assess the residual activity of these drugs using a peripheral nerve stimulator. This assessment should be made in the operating room prior to allowing the return of spontaneous ventilation or considering extubation of the trachea.

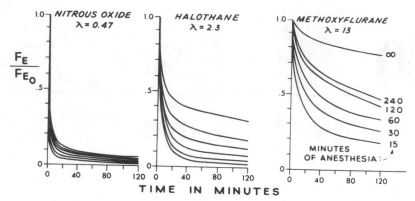

Figure 30-1. Recovery from anesthesia after varying lengths of drug administration is depicted by computer-derived curves plotting the rate of decrease in the alveolar concentration with time in minutes at a constant alveolar ventilation (4 L/min). The importance of duration of anesthesia decreases as the solubility (lambda) of the anesthetic in blood decreases. For example, the decline in the alveolar concentration (F_E/F_{Eo}) of poorly soluble nitrous oxide is rapid regardless of the duration of its administration. F_E/F_{Eo} is the ratio of alveolar gas concentration at each time in recovery divided by the alveolar gas concentration at the start of recovery. (Stoelting RK, Eger EI II. The effects of ventilation and anesthetic solubility on recovery from anesthesia: an in vivo and analog analysis before and after equilibrium Anesthesiology 1969;30:290-6.)

ADMISSION TO THE RECOVERY ROOM

Upon arrival in the recovery room the anesthesiologist provides the nurse with pertinent details of the patient's history, medical condition, anesthetic, and surgery (Table 30-1). Supplemental inspired oxygen is routinely provided in many instances regardless of the duration or type of surgery. Ideally, a nurse is responsible for the care of only one patient in the recovery room. Vital signs should be recorded at least every 15 minutes while the patient is in the recovery room. The vital signs and other pertinent information are recorded on a separate sheet that becomes part of the patient's medical record (Fig. 30-2). During the time in the recovery room, the patient is encouraged by the nurse to cough, breathe deeply, and change position. Prior to discharge from the recovery room, the patient is evaluated by a physician (usually an anesthesiologist), and a note describing perti-

nent aspects of the anesthetic and recovery room period is written in the patient's medical record by the physician. This note serves as a source of information to the anesthesiologist who may be responsible for administration of anesthesia to this patient in the future. Although criteria for discharge from the recovery room are not

Table 30-1. Information Given to Nurse at the Time of Admission to the Recovery Room

---

1. Patient's name and age
2. Surgical procedure
3. Preoperative medicatioans and anesthetic drugs used
4. Other intraoperative drugs—anticholinesterases, narcotic antagonists, diuretics, antidysrhythmics
5. Preoperative vital signs
6. Coexisting medical diseases and associated defects
7. Preoperative drug therapy
8. Allergies
9. Intraoperative estimated blood loss and measured urine output
10. Intraoperative fluid and blood replacement
11. Anesthetic and surgical complications
12. Special medications or procedures that will be necessary in the recovery room

---

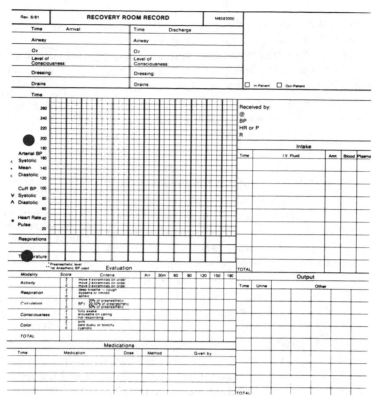

Figure 30-2. An example of a postanesthesia recovery room record.

standardized, they typically include (1) absence of adverse events associated with surgery, such as continued bleeding; (2) a level of consciousness consistent with the return of protective upper airway reflexes; (3) the ability to maintain a patent upper airway; (4) the presence of stable vital signs; and (5) acceptable cardiac, pulmonary, and renal function. A full description of the patient's intraoperative and immediate postoperative course should be given by the recovery room nurse to the ward nurse at the time the patient is returned to the ward.

PHYSIOLOGIC DISORDERS IN THE RECOVERY ROOM

Physiologic disorders that must be diagnosed and treated in the recovery room during emergence from the immediate effects of anesthesia and surgery include pulmonary complications, circulatory complications, agitation, pain, renal dysfunction,

bleeding abnormalities, and decreased body temperature.

Pulmonary Complications

Pulmonary complications associated with the early postoperative period include upper airway obstruction, arterial hypoxemia, alveolar hypoventilation, and inhalation (aspiration) of gastric contents.

Upper airway obstruction in the recovery room is most often due to occlusion of the pharynx by the tongue. Laryngeal obstruction is less common but can occur secondary to laryngospasm or due to direct airway injury. Obstruction of the pharynx or larynx can occur following head and neck surgery when the head cannot be positioned optimally to maintain a patent upper airway.

Physical examination of a patient with upper airway obstruction reveals flaring of the nares, retraction at the suprasternal notch (tracheal tug) and intercostal spaces and vigorous diaphragmatic and abdominal contractions. The most effective method of eliminating airway obstruction due to occlusion of the pharynx by the tongue is extension of the head with or without anterior displacement of the mandible (head tilt-jaw thrust method) (see Chapter 34). This maneuver stretches muscles attached to the tongue serving to pull the tongue away from the posterior pharyngeal wall. If upper airway obstruction is not immediately reversible by this maneuver, a nasopharyngeal or oropharyngeal airway can be inserted. A nasopharyngeal airway is better tolerated by patients awakening from general anesthesia and thus the preferred initial selection. An oropharyngeal airway placed in a semiconscious patient may stimulate gagging and vomiting as well as laryngospasm. Direct laryngoscopy and intubation of the trachea with a cuffed tube is indicated when upper airway obstruction persists despite proper head positioning and use of an artificial airway. Should intubation of the trachea be technically impossible, the placement of a 12 to 14 gauge extracath needle (catheter over-needle) through the cricothyroid membrane (cricothyroidotomy) will provide temporary oxygenation until a more definitive procedure such as tracheostomy can be performed. Laryngospasm during emergence from general anesthesia is usually caused by secretions or upper airway manipulation, as during placement of an oropharyngeal airway. Treatment is initially extension of the head and anterior displacement of the mandible plus application of positive airway pressure with a bag and mask delivering pure oxygen. If laryngospasm is incomplete, this treatment is satisfactory until the spasm spontaneously dissipates. Complete laryngospasm that persists despite the above maneuvers should be rapidly treated with intravenous administration of succinylcholine (0.15 to 0.3 mg/kg).

Table 30-2. Factors Leading to Postoperative Arterial Hypoxemia

Mismatching of ventilation to perfusion
Inhibition of reflex hypoxic pulmonary vasoconstriction
Decreased functional residual capacity
Perfusion of unventilated alveoli (atelectasis)
Decreased cardiac output
Alveolar hypoventilation due to residual effects of anesthetic and/or muscle relaxants
Inhalation of gastric contents (aspiration)
Pulmonary embolus
Pulmonary edema
Pneumothorax
Posthyperventilation hypoxia
Diffusion hypoxia
Increased oxygen consumption (shivering)
Elderly
Obese

Upper airway obstruction due to laryngeal edema may be treated by humidifying the inhaled gases and administering nebulized racemic epinephrine. Intravenous dexamethasone (0.15 mg/kg) has been utilized for treatment of laryngeal edema but the efficacy of this therapy has not been confirmed. In children, laryngeal edema can rapidly progress to complete upper airway obstruction, emphasing the importance of close surveillance in the recovery room.

Arterial hypoxemia in the immediate postoperative period most likely reflects the impact of anesthetic drugs and/or events occurring intraoperatively. Decreases in the PaO_2 are common, particularly following upper abdominal or thoracic surgery.[3] For example, the PaO_2 decreases about 20 mmHg following upper abdominal or thoracic surgery. The decrease in PaO_2 is much less after lower abdominal (10 mmHg) or peripheral surgery (6 mmHg).

Etiology. Factors leading to postoperative arterial hypoxemia are multiple (Table 30-2). Probably the most common cause of postoperative arterial hypoxemia is mismatching of ventilation to perfusion. An immediate postoperative cause of mismatching of ventilation to perfusion could be residual effects of anesthetic drugs that impair reflex hypoxic pulmonary vasoconstriction. Absence of this reflex vasoconstriction will exaggerate the impact of poorly ventilated areas of the lung on arterial oxygenation by preventing compensatory reductions in pulmonary blood flow to these regions. Reductions in the PaO_2 that persist beyond the early postoperative period most likely reflect mismatching of ventilation to perfusion due to mechanical abnormalities of the lung such as decreases in the functional residual capacity (FRC). Arterial hypoxemia postoperatively may also reflect perfusion of unventilated alveoli (right-to-left intrapulmonary shunt) due to atelectasis. Atelectasis may be segmental, due to bronchial obstruction with secretions, or diffuse, reflecting decreased lung volumes. Reductions in cardiac output can contribute to decreases in the PaO_2 in patients with mismatching of ventilation to perfusion or intrapulmonary shunts. In the absence of supplemental inspired oxygen, the accumulation of carbon dioxide in the alveoli due to drug-induced hypoventilation may lead to arterial hypoxemia. Inhalation of acidic gastric fluid results in rapid onset of profound arterial hypoxemia due to (1) reflex airway closure; (2) loss of surfactant activity, leading to atelectasis; and (3) loss of capillary integrity, manifesting as noncardiogenic pulmonary edema. A pulmonary embolus occurring in the immediate postoperative period can cause profound arterial hypoxemia, although the exact physiological explanation for the hypoxemia is unclear. This diagnosis should be suspected in any patient who develops acute dyspnea and tachypnea in the recovery room. Pulmonary edema due to left ventricular failure is usually preceded by systemic hypertension and typically occurs in the first hour following surgery.[4] Arterial hypoxemia due to a pneumothorax reflects compression of alveoli, producing a right-to-left intrapulmonary shunt. Patients undergoing radical neck dissection, mastec-

tomy, or nephrectomy are particularly vulnerable to the development of a pneumothorax. A pneumothorax of over 20 percent in a spontaneously breathing patient or any pneumothorax in the presence of mechanical ventilation of the lungs should be treated by insertion of a chest tube. If circulatory depression accompanies a tension pneumothorax, emergency treatment is placement of a 12 to 14 gauge extracath needle (catheter over-needle) into the second anterior intercostal space. Posthyperventilation hypoxia reflects compensatory hypoventilation in an attempt to replenish body stores of carbon dioxide that have been depleted by intraoperative hyperventilation.[3] Arterial hypoxemia due to this compensatory hypoventilation is prevented by increasing the inhaled concentration of oxygen. Diffusion hypoxia as a cause of arterial hypoxemia in the recovery room is unlikely, however, since the early dilutional effect of nitrous oxide on the alveolar partial pressure of oxygen is prevented by only a few breaths of oxygen at the conclusion of the anesthetic (see Chapter 2). Postoperative shivering can result in substantial increases in oxygen consumption but only rarely contributes to arterial hypoxemia.[5] Finally, advanced age and obesity are likely to be associated with an exaggerated reduction in arterial oxygenation in the postoperative period.

Diagnosis of arterial hypoxemia in the recovery room requires measurement of the PaO_2. Arterial hypoxemia is considered to be present when the PaO_2 is less than 60 mmHg. Clinical signs of arterial hypoxemia (hypertension, hypotension, tachycardia, bradycardia, cardiac dysrhythmias, agitation) are nonspecific. A lowered hemoglobin concentration may impair detection of cyanosis. Furthermore, circulatory and ventilatory responses to arterial hypoxemia are attenuated by the effects of residual anesthetics. For example, sedative concentrations of volatile anesthetics (0.1 MAC) nearly abolish the usual increase in ventilation produced by arterial hypoxemia (Fig. 30-3).[6] Thus, arterial hypoxemia is unlikely to stimulate ventilation in postoperative patients who have received a volatile anesthetic.

Treatment of arterial hypoxemia in the recovery room is with supplemental oxygen. Supplemental oxygen does not eliminate the cause of arterial hypoxemia but may symptomatically alleviate it while concomitant corrective measures are employed. For example, if arterial hypoxemia is due to hypoventilation from excessive residual effects of narcotics, specific pharmacologic antagonism with naloxone is indicated. Mismatching of ventilation to perfusion decreases with coughing, deep breathing, and eventually ambulation.

Indications for supplemental oxygen in the recovery room are not specific. Indeed, almost every patient demonstrates a reduction in PaO_2 following anesthesia and surgery and will therefore benefit from supplemental oxygen. Supplemental oxygen should never be withheld in the postoperative period for fear of abolishing the hypoxic drive to ventilation that may be present in patients with chronic obstructive airway disease. In the presence of chronic obstructive airway disease associated with carbon dioxide retention, graded doses of supplemental oxygen can be administered via an air-entrainment (Venturi) mask while following the patient's oxygenation with measurement of the PaO_2. Indeed, inhaled concentrations of oxygen of 24 to 28 percent are often sufficient to raise the patient's PaO_2 to an acceptable level. If arterial hypoxemia persists despite administration of pure oxygen or hypercapnia accompanies supplemental oxygen therapy, the trachea should be intubated and the patient's lungs mechanically ventilated. In such patients, ventilation of the lungs using positive end-expiratory pressure (PEEP) will increase the FRC and result in an increased PaO_2. Furthermore, ventilation of the lungs utilizing PEEP often allows a reduction in the inspired concentration of oxygen without a decrease in the PaO_2.

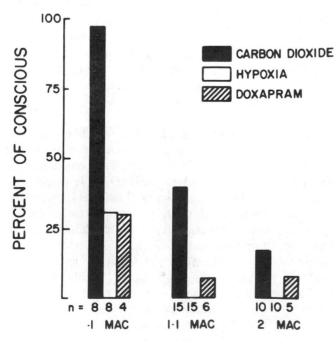

Figure 30-3. The ventilatory response (percent of conscious) to carbon dioxide, hypoxia, and doxapram was depressed in a dose-related manner by halothane administered to subjects without pulmonary disease. For example, 0.1 MAC halothane reduced the ventilatory response to hypoxia by about 75 percent as compared with the conscious response. The ventilatory response to hypoxia was absent at 1.1 MAC halothane. (Knill RL, Gelb AW. Ventilatory responses to hypoxia and hypercapnia during halothane sedation and anesthesia in man. Anesthesiology 1978;49:244–51.)

Table 30-3. Factors Leading to Postoperative Alveolar Hypoventilation

Drug-induced central nervous system depression
   Volatile anesthetics
   Injected anesthetics (narcotics)
Residual neuromuscular blockade
Suboptimal ventilatory muscle mechanics
Increased production of carbon dioxide
Coexisting chronic obstructive airway disease

Alveolar hypoventilation leading to hypercarbia is a frequent occurrence in the early postoperative period.

Etiology. Factors leading to postoperative alveolar hypoventilation are multiple (Table 30-3). A frequent cause, however, is inadequate central stimulation to ventilation due to residual effects of inhaled and/or injected anesthetic drugs. Anesthetic-induced depression of ventilation is evidenced by a shift of the carbon dioxide response curve to the right with or without a concomitant increase in the $PaCO_2$. Ventilatory depression produced by inhaled anesthetics decreases with time. In contrast, narcotics such as fentanyl can produce biphasic ventilatory depression. For example, drug-induced depression may dissipate with the increased external stimulation provided by the transport and admission to the recovery room, only to be followed by a second period of respiratory depression as external stimulation wanes (see Chapter 6).[7] Residual neuromuscular blockade may interfere with optimal activity of respiratory muscles, leading to accumulation of carbon dioxide. Persistent neuromuscular blockade may reflect (1) prior inadequate pharmacologic antagonism; (2) delayed excretion of the muscle relaxant due to renal disease; or (3) the potentiation of these drugs by other mechanisms (aminoglycoside antibiotics, hypermagnesemia, hypothermia). It should be appreciated that respiratory acidosis inhibits reversal of neuromuscular blockade with anticholinesterases as does hypokalemia. Conceivably,

alveolar hypoventilation in the recovery room could lead to respiratory acidosis and an unmasking of residual neuromuscular blockade, leading to further carbon dioxide retention. Evidence of residual neuromuscular blockade is best detected with a peripheral nerve stimulator. In addition, the ability to sustain head lift for at least 5 seconds, vigorous hand grasp, tongue protrusion for several seconds, vital capacity above 15 ml/kg, and maximal inspiratory force of at least minus 20 cm H_2O can be used as evidence of adequate recovery from the effects of the muscle relaxant. Suboptimal ventilatory mechanics may be related to the patient's position, obesity, gastric dilitation, and the site of the surgical incision. For example, the site of surgical incision affects the ability to take a deep breath as measured by vital capacity. Patients undergoing upper abdominal surgery have the greatest reduction in vital capacity, showing as much as a 60 percent reduction on the day of surgery. Postoperative pain can limit tidal volume. Increased production of carbon dioxide is rare but may be a consideration when hyperalimentation solutions are being administered or body temperature is elevated. Finally, chronic obstructive airway disease associated with preoperative hypercarbia is predictably accompanied by a similar finding postoperatively.

Diagnosis of alveolar hypoventilation in the recovery room requires measurement of the $PaCO_2$. Alveolar hypoventilation is considered to be present when the $PaCO_2$ exceeds 44 mmHg. Signs of carbon dioxide retention such as tachycardia and hypertension are not reliably present in the postoperative patient.

Measurement of the vital capacity and maximal inspiratory force are good guides to the ability of the postoperative patient to breathe spontaneously and maintain adequate alveolar ventilation. The vital capac-

Table 30-4. Factors Leading to Postoperative Hypotension

Hypovolemia
Decreased myocardial contractility
Sepsis
Pulmonary embolus
Pneumothorax
Cardiac tamponade

ity should be at least 15 ml/kg (about double the predicted tidal volume) and the inspiratory force greater than minus 20 cm H_2O. Inspiratory force can be tested in the absence of consciousness, while measurement of vital capacity requires patient cooperation. If these minimum values cannot be generated, ventilation of the lungs should be mechanically provided.

Treatment. If alveolar hypoventilation is due to residual effects of an inhaled anesthetic but the patient remains capable of generating an inspiratory force greater than minus 20 cm H_2O, it is permissible to allow spontaneous emergence from anesthesia combined with a regimen to keep the patient alert. If not, controlled ventilation of the lungs via a cuffed tube in the trachea will be necessary to maintain normocarbia and accelerate elimination of the inhaled drug. If alveolar hypoventilation is due to residual effects of a narcotic, the intravenous administration of naloxone (1 to 4 μg/kg) is an appropriate consideration. It must be appreciated, however, that the duration of naloxone is brief such that alveolar hypoventilation may recur. For this reason, intramuscular naloxone following an initial intravenous dose has been recommended.[8] Disadvantages of naloxone include sudden reversal of analgesia and associated activation of the sympathetic nervous system which has been associated with hypertension and cardiac dysrhythmias, particularly when a tracheal tube is in place. Irreversible ventricular fibrillation has also been reported following the administration of naloxone in the early postoperative period.[9] When residual neuromuscular blockade is responsible for alveolar hypoventilation, treatment is either mechanical ventilation of the lungs until the effect of the muscle relaxant spontaneously wanes or administration of an anticholinesterase.

Circulatory Complications

Circulatory complications associated with the early postoperative period include hypotension, hypertension, and cardiac dysrhythmias.

Hypotension

Etiology. Multiple causes must be considered in the differential diagnosis of hypotension in the recovery room (Table 30-4). The most likely cause of hypotension, however, is decreased venous return and reduced cardiac output due to hypovolemia. Indeed, residual effects of anesthetic drugs are likely to attenuate peripheral vasoconstrictor responses, leading to hypotension as an early manifestation of hypovolemia. Hypovolemia is usually a reflection of inadequately replaced blood loss or third space loss during surgery. Unrecognized continuing hemorrhage as a cause of hypovolemia and hypotension must also be considered. Reductions in myocardial contractility as a cause of hypotension in the recovery room may be due to residual effects of anesthetics, pre-existing ventricular dysfunction, or an acute myocardial infarction. Indeed, most patients with a confirmed postoperative myocardial infarction are found to have experienced a period of unexplained hypotension in the recovery room. Angina pectoris occurs in only about one-fourth of these patients, possibly reflecting masking of pain by residual analgesic effects of anesthetics. Sepsis leading to vasodilation and capillary fluid leakage may be responsible for hypotension, particularly following surgery on the genitourinary tract. Other causes of hypotension in the recovery room include pulmonary embolus, pneumothorax, and cardiac tamponade.

Diagnosis and Treatment. Before any therapy of hypotension is instituted, it is important to confirm the accuracy of the blood pressure measurement. Artifactual blood pressure readings can be due to an improperly placed or sized blood pressure cuff, an inaccurately calibrated transducer, or positioning of the transducer above the level of the right atrium (midaxillary line). For example, the transduced pressure is falsely reduced 0.7 mmHg for every cm the transducer is elevated above heart level in a supine patient.

Oliguria (less than 0.5 ml/kg/hr) is a useful guide to the presence of hypovolemia or decreased myocardial contractility. Increased urine output following a fluid challenge with 3 to 6 ml/kg of lactated Ringer's solution suggests the presence of hypovolemia rather than decreased myocardial contractility. A low hematocrit plus evidence of bleeding at the operative site should suggest inadequate surgical hemostasis. Elevation of the legs and administration of a sympathomimetic to maintain perfusion pressure until hypovolemia can be corrected is a prudent treatment.

If hypotension persists despite fluid replacement, an estimate of right atrial pressure is indicated. In the presence of normal left ventricular function, central venous pressure will be a reasonable reflection of intravascular fluid volume. In the presence of selective left ventricular dysfunction or co-existing chronic obstructive airway disease, the central venous pressure may not be an accurate guide and pressures measured via a pulmonary artery catheter are necessary for an accurate diagnosis. Hypovolemia as a cause of hypotension is suggested by a low pulmonary artery occlusion pressure (less than 10 mmHg), a normal to low cardiac index (normal 2.5 to 4 L/min/m^2), and a normal to elevated calculated systemic vascular resistance (normal 900 to 1400 dynes/sec/cm^{-5}). Decreased myocardial contractility as the etiology of hypotension is characterized by a high pulmonary artery occlusion pressure (above 15 mmHg) and a low cardiac output. After optimizing intravascular fluid volume, the treatment of hypotension due to decreased myocardial contractility is with an inotrope such as dopamine or dobutamine (see Chapter 3). Sepsis as a cause of hypotension is characterized by a low pulmonary artery occlusion pressure, elevated cardiac output, and decreased systemic vascular resistance. Replacement of fluid loss with crystalloid solutions (colloid can leak into tissues, drawing fluid with it) and maintenance of coronary perfusion pressure with an alpha agonist such as phenylephrine is indicated in the immediate treatment of hypotension due to sepsis.

Hypertension

Etiology. Hypertension that develops in the immediate postoperative period is most often due to the stimulation provided by sensation of pain as emergence from anesthesia occurs. When hypertension does develop during recovery from anesthesia, it usually manifests in the first 30 minutes following surgery.[10] Preoperative hypertension is present in over one-half of patients who develop hypertension in the recovery room. Postoperative hypertension can be exaggerated if antihypertensives are withdrawn preoperatively. Other causes to consider when hypertension occurs in the recovery room include fluid overload, arterial hypoxemia, and hypercarbia. Excessive and sustained elevations in blood pressure can lead to left ventricular failure with pulmonary edema, myocardial ischemia due to increased myocardial oxygen requirements, cardiac dysrhythmias, and cerebral hemorrhage.

Diagnosis and Treatment. Management of acute hypertension begins with identification and correction of the initiating cause.

When pain is the etiology of acute hypertension, the immediate treatment is the intravenous administration of a narcotic until adequate pain relief is achieved (see the section *Pain*). Hypertension that persists in the absence of a known etiology is best managed by the continuous intravenous infusion of a vasodilator such as nitroprusside. The blood pressure is titrated to a desired level by adjusting the infusion rate of nitroprusside. The infusion rate should not exceed 8 to 10 μg/kg/min or a total dose of 1.5 mg/kg for a 1 to 3 hour administration. Even when these dose recommendations are followed, it is important to measure the arterial pH hourly to detect the appearance of metabolic acidosis due to the metabolism of nitroprusside to cyanide. Should metabolic acidosis appear, nitroprusside must be discontinued immediately and an alternative vasodilator such as trimethaphan administered. Hydralazine in 2.5 to 5 mg increments administered intravenously is also an effective treatment for postoperative hypertension. Disadvantages of hydralazine include a delayed onset (5 to 15 minutes) and baroreceptor-mediated tachycardia when the blood pressure decreases. Regardless of the drug selected to produce normotension, it is important to reliably monitor blood pressure with a Doppler ultrasound transducer or via a catheter in a peripheral artery.

Cardiac Dysrhythmias

Etiology. Cardiac dysrhythmias in the immediate postoperative period have multiple causes (Table 30-5). Arterial hypoxemia should be the first cause considered when a cardiac dysrhythmia manifests for the first time in the recovery room. Sinus tachycardia is a common occurrence in the early postoperative period. This rhythm should suggest the possible presence of arterial hypoxemia, hypovolemia, or pain. Sinus bradycardia accompanies arterial hypoxemia,

Table 30-5. Factors Leading to Postoperative Cardiac Dysrhythmias

Arterial hypoxemia
Hypovolemia
Pain
Hypothermia
Anticholinesterase drugs
Myocardial ischemia
Electrolyte abnormalities
    Hypokalemia
    Hypocalcemia
Respiratory acidosis
Hypertension
Digitalis intoxication
Preoperative cardiac dysrhythmias

decreases in body temperature, and may reflect effects of an anticholinesterase administered earlier to reverse nondepolarizing neuromuscular blockade. The appearance of premature ventricular contractions should suggest the presence of arterial hypoxemia, myocardial ischemia, electrolyte abnormalities, or respiratory acidosis. Hypertension may increase myocardial irritability, leading to premature ventricular contractions. The appearance of cardiac dysrhythmias in patients receiving digitalis preparations should arouse suspicion of digitalis toxicity.

Treatment. Most cardiac dysrhythmias occurring in the recovery room do not require treatment other than correcting the underlying cause. Regardless of the type of cardiac dysrhythmia, the first priority is to assure the patency of the upper airway and the adequacy of arterial oxygenation. Specific drug therapies to treat hemodynamically significant cardiac dysrhythmias include intravenous administration of atropine (3 to 6 μg/kg) to increase heart rate, verapamil (75 to 150 μg/kg infused over 1 to 3 minutes) to slow heart rate, and lidocaine (1 to 1.5 mg/kg) to suppress premature ventricular contractions. Electrical cardioversion is necessary to treat atrial or ventricular tachydysrhythmias that are unresponsive to drug therapy.

Agitation (Emergence Delerium)

A small number of patients awaken from anesthesia in an agitated state which may require physical restraint. The incidence of this behavior seems to be increased in young patients who are apprehensive about the findings at operation as well as in individuals who fear pain. Arterial hypoxemia as a cause of agitation must be initially considered. The perception of pain in a patient who has not regained full consciousness and self-control may manifest as agitation. Other causes of agitation include unrecognized gastric dilitation, urinary retention, and pneumothorax. The incidence of postoperative agitation is increased in patients who have received scopolamine as preoperative medication, particularly when this drug is administered in the absence of a narcotic (see Chapter 10). Agitation can also follow the administration of atropine but the incidence is less than that associated with scopolamine. Intravenous physostigmine 15 to 45 μg/kg (often combined with glycopyrrolate to prevent peripheral cholinergic effects) will reverse agitation associated with an anticholinergic. Presumably, physostigmine (a tertiary amine anticholinesterase) crosses the blood brain barrier and acts to increase levels of acetylcholine which then displaces the anticholinergic from central receptor sites. Physostigmine has also been reported to reverse prolonged postoperative somnolence associated with diazepam and droperidol, but the mechanism for this effect is not know.[11]

Pain

Pain is a predictable response as the effects of anesthetic drugs wane in the early postoperative period.

Etiology. Many factors influence the incidence and severity of postoperative pain. The infant and elderly patient seem to experience less pain than middle-aged pa-

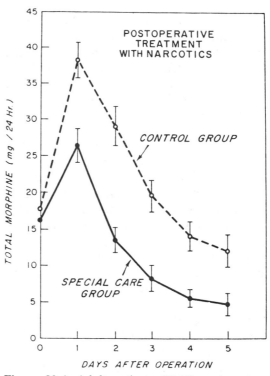

Figure 30-4. Adult patients (N-97) undergoing abdominal surgery were divided into two groups. Both groups were visited preoperatively by the anesthesiologist but only the special care group received a detailed explanation regarding the character, intensity, and management of pain in the postoperative period. The normal occurrence of postoperative pain was stressed to these patients. The value of this explanation was evidenced by the decreased total dose of morphine administered to the special care patients compared with the control group. (Egbert LD, Battit GE, Welch CE, Bartlett MK. Reduction of postoperative pain by encouragement and instruction of patients. A study of doctor-patient rapport. N Engl J Med 1964;270:825–7.)

tients. The need for postoperative pain medication is reduced when the anesthesiologist visits the patient preoperatively and provides a detailed explanation of postoperative events including the occurrence of pain (Fig. 30-4).[12] The inclusion of a narcotic in the preoperative medication or use of a narcotic during maintenance of anesthesia usually delays the first postoperative request for pain medication. Preoperative traits such as a neurotic personality or fear of pain tend to increase postoperative pain. The site of operation influences the severity of postoperative pain, with thoracotomy and upper abdominal and orthopedic surgery being the most painful.

Treatment of postoperative pain is usually with incremental doses of intravenous morphine (15 to 30 μg/kg) administered until adequate pain relief is achieved. Indeed, intravenous titration of narcotics often results in analgesia sooner than do larger doses administered intramuscularly. In the future, continuous intravenous infusion of a low dose of narcotic may be used to provide more consistent and optimal analgesia with minimal cardiorespiratory depression. Continuous thoracic or lumbar block with a long-acting local anesthetic such as bupivacaine is an effective method for providing postoperative analgesia, especially in patients with chronic pulmonary disease who may be vulnerable to narcotic-induced ventilatory depression. Disadvantages of the epidural block include skeletal muscle weakness and orthostatic hypotension due to peripheral sympathetic nervous system blockade. Both of these adverse effects interfere with early postoperative ambulation. Intercostal nerve blocks are particularly useful for management of postcholecystectomy pain. Pneumothorax is a rare but possible side effect of these blocks. In the future, placement of narcotics into the epidural space may find a useful role in providing prolonged postoperative analgesia. Most importantly, adequate analgesia regardless of how it is provided allows the patient to take deep breaths and cough, thus reducing the likelihood of postoperative atelectasis and pneumonia.

Renal Dysfunction

Oliguria (less than 0.5 ml/kg/hr) that manifests in the recovery room most likely reflects reduced renal blood flow due to hy-

Table 30-6. Patients at High Risk for Postoperative Renal Dysfunction

Coexisting renal disease
Major trauma
Sepsis
Advanced age
Multiple intraoperative blood transfusions
Prolonged intraoperative hypotension
Cardiac or vascular operations
Biliary tract surgery in presence of obstructive jaundice

povolemia or decreased cardiac output (see Chapter 22). An indwelling urinary catheter is important for the early recognition of oliguria in postoperative patients at high risk for renal failure (Table 30-6).

Bleeding Abnormalities

Bleeding abnormalities in the postoperative period most often reflect hemorrhage secondary to inadequate surgical hemostasis. Alternatively, postoperative bleeding may be due to a coagulopathy, which can be diagnosed utilizing specific laboratory tests (Table 30-7) (see Chapter 18). While awaiting the results of laboratory tests, the whole blood clotting test can be performed

Table 30-7. Laboratory Tests for Evaluation of Postoperative Bleeding Abnormalities

Test	Abnormal in Presence of
Platelet count	Dilutional thrombocytopenia Disseminated intravascular coagulation
Bleeding time	Platelet-inhibiting drugs (acetylsalicyclic acid-containing drugs)
Prothrombin time	Disseminated intravascular coagulation Vitamin K deficiency Hepatic disease Warfarin
Partial thromboplastin time	Deficiencies of factors V and/or VIII Heparin Hemophilia
Fibrinogen	Disseminated intravascular coagulation
Fibrin split products	Disseminated intravascular coagulation

at the bedside to evaluate both clot formation (forms in less than 12 minutes), retraction (platelet function), and lysis.

A platelet count is useful in evaluation of bleeding following massive transfusion of blood (see Chapter 18). A qualitative platelet defect may be due to drugs ingested preoperatively such as aspirin. This problem is recognized by demonstration of a prolonged bleeding time despite a normal platelet count. In these situations, the administration of platelets will reverse thrombocytopenia and also return the bleeding time to normal. Disseminated intravascular coagulation is suggested by thrombocytopenia, prolonged prothrombin time, reduced serum concentration of fibriongen, and increased circulating levels of fibrin split products. Decreased levels of factors V and VIII associated with massive transfusions of blood or inadequate reversal of heparin will manifest as a prolonged partial thromboplastin time.

Decreased Body Temperature

Decreased body temperature is a complication of operations performed in cold operating rooms. Compensatory mechanisms to offset heat loss (peripheral vasoconstriction, shivering) are prevented by anesthetics and muscle relaxants. Loss of body heat intraoperatively is minimized by maintaining the operating room temperature near 21 Celsius and warming of the inhaled gases. The reduced basal metabolic rate associated with decreased body temperature can manifest in the recovery room as slow awakening from anesthesia. When shivering develops in the postoperative patient, it is important to provide supplemental inspired oxygen to offset the marked increase (300 to 400 percent) in oxygen consumption that accompanies increased skeletal muscle activity.

PROPHYLACTIC VENTILATION

Following surgery, spontaneous ventilation is often rapid and shallow. Lung volumes are likely to be decreased, resulting in reduced pulmonary compliance, increased airway resistance, and an increased work of breathing. This restrictive pattern of breathing is accentuated by pain and the surgical incision which may interfere with normal chest and abdominal wall function. All these changes lead to the accumulation of secretions in the alveoli and often the development of atelectasis and pneumonia. For these reasons, postoperative mechanical ventilation of the lungs via a tracheal tube in selected patients at risk (especially those with co-existing chronic obstructive airway disease undergoing upper abdominal or thoracic operations) will serve to reduce the likelihood of significant pulmonary complications.

Criteria for extubation of the trachea following surgery must be individualized. Useful criteria include (1) state of consciousness; (2) vital capacity greater than 15 ml/kg; (3) inspiratory force greater than minus 20 cm H_2O; and (4) acceptable arterial blood gases and pH (see Chapter 32). The directional change of these measurements is more important than a single value. Extubation of the trachea is performed after suctioning the pharynx and trachea. The patient then inhales deeply or the lungs are passively expanded with oxygen, the cuff on the tracheal tube is deflated, and the tube removed from the trachea at maximum lung inflation. This sequence assures that the initial gas flow is outward and permits secretions to be forcefully exhaled rather than inhaled as the tracheal tube is removed.

REFERENCES

1. Stoelting RK, Eger EI II. The effects of ventilation and anesthetic solubility on recovery from anesthesia. An in vivo and analog analysis before and after equilibrium. Anesthesiology 1969;30:290–6.
2. Stoelting RK, Longnecker DE, Eger EI II. Minimum alveolar concentrations in man on awakening from methoxyflurane, halothane, ether and fluroxene anesthesia: MAC awake. Anesthesiology 1970;33:5–9.

3. Marshall BE, Wyche MQ. Hypoxemia during and after anesthesia. Anesthesiology 1972;37:178–209.
4. Cooperman LH, Price HR. Pulmonary edema in the operative and postoperative period: Review of 40 cases. Ann Surg 1970;172:883–91.
5. Bay J, Nunn JF, Prys-Roberts C. Factors influencing arterial PO_2 during recovery from anesthesia. Br J Anaesth 1968;40:398–407.
6. Knill RL, Gelb AW. Ventilatory responses to hypoxia and hypercapnia during halothane sedation and anesthesia in man. Anesthesiology 1978;49:244–51.
7. Becker LD, Paulson BA, Miller RD, Severinghaus JW, Eger EI II. Biphasic respiratory depression after fentanyl-droperidol or fentanyl alone used to supplement nitrous oxide anesthesia. Anesthesiology 1976; 44:291–6.
8. Longnecker DE, Grazis PA, Eggers GWN, Jr. Naloxone for antagonism of morphine-induced respiratory depression. Anesth Analg 1973;52:447–53.
9. Andree RA. Sudden death following naloxone administration. Anesth Analg 1980; 59:782–4.
10. Gal TJ, Cooperman LH. Hypertension in the immediate postoperative period. Br J Anaesth 1975;47:70–4.
11. Bidwai AV, Cornelius LR, Stanley TH. Reversal of Innovar-induced postanesthetic somnolence and disorientation with physostigmine. Anesthesiology 1976;44:249–52.
12. Egbert LD, Battit GE, Welch CE, Bartlett MK. Reduction of postoperative pain by encouragement and instruction of patients. N Engl J Med 1964;270:825–7.

Section VI
Consultant Anesthetic Practice

31

Respiratory Therapy

Respiratory therapy includes oxygen therapy, humidification and aerosol therapy, bronchial hygiene, and prophylaxis against the development of postoperative pulmonary complications. The anesthesiologist must possess a thorough knowledge of these various modalities of respiratory therapy, their efficacy, limitations, and potential complications. The value of respiratory therapy has been increased by an improved understanding of the pathophysiology of pulmonary disease and the predictable impact of anesthesia and operation on pulmonary function. In addition, the measurement of arterial blood gases and pH has provided a reliable means to both determine the need and assess the value of respiratory therapy.

OXYGEN THERAPY

Oxygen therapy administered as an increased inhaled concentration of oxygen (supplemental oxygen) is indicated when the PaO_2 decreases below 60 mmHg. The shape of the oxyhemoglobin dissociation curve is such that marked reductions in saturation of hemoglobin with oxygen occur with even small decreases in the PaO_2 below 60 mmHg (90 percent saturation). This marked reduction in saturation of hemoglobin with oxygen decreases the arterial content of oxygen and jeopardizes tissue oxygen availability.

The routine administration of supplemental oxygen to postoperative patients is often beneficial and seldom hazardous. Oxygen therapy is usually delivered by nasal cannula or face mask.

Nasal Cannula

Supplemental oxygen can be administered via a nasal cannula with minimal patient discomfort. A nasal cannula incorporates two prongs that extend about 1 cm into the nares and is held in place by an adjustable elastic head strap. The inhaled oxygen concentration achieved with a nasal cannula depends on the flow-rate of oxygen (L/min) as well as the patient's tidal volume, respiratory rate, inspiratory flow rate, and volume of the nasopharynx.[1] As a guideline, the inhaled oxygen concentration is increased about 4 percent for each L/min of oxygen delivered. Oxygen flow rates above 6 L/min (inhaled oxygen concentrations about 40 percent) do not predictably further increase the inhaled concentration of oxygen, since the volume of the nasopharynx is already filled. Excessive flow rates of oxygen may result in air swallowing and gastric distension. Mouth breathing does not ablate the effectiveness of oxygen therapy delivered by nasal cannula since inspiratory airflow through the posterior pharynx entrains (Bernoulli effect) oxygen from the nose.

Face Mask

Face masks used for oxygen therapy are categorized as simple, partial rebreathing, nonrebreathing, and air-entrainment (Fig. 31-1).[2]

Simple. A simple face mask contains no valve or oxygen reservoir bag. This mask can provide an inhaled concentration of oxygen between 35 and 60 percent with oxygen flow rates of 5 to 8 L/min (Fig. 31-1A).[2] Variations in the patient's ventilatory parameters alter the inhaled concentration of oxygen. In adults, the oxygen flow rate should always be at least 5 L/min to assure the absence of rebreathing of carbon dioxide. A simple face mask affords little, if any, advantage over a nasal cannula in terms of delivering a constant inhaled concentration of oxygen.

Partial Rebreathing. A partial rebreathing face mask is a valveless system that includes an oxygen reservoir bag (Fig. 31-1B).[2] With oxygen flows greater than 10 L/min, the inhaled concentration of oxygen is between 50 and 65 percent.

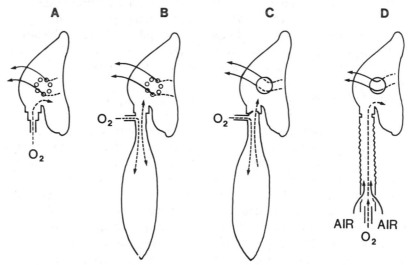

Figure 31-1. Examples of face masks used to provide supplemental oxygen. (A) Simple face mask. Oxygen flows directly into the mask and exhaled gases leave through holes at the side of the mask. (B) Partial rebreathing face mask. Since there are no valves, the initial portion of the exhaled gas which contains little or no carbon dioxide (dead space gas) is free to mix with the oxygen in the reservoir bag. As the reservoir bag fills and the pressure in the bag increases, the gas exhaled during the last part of exhalation which contains carbon dioxide (alveolar gas) is forced out through the holes at the side of the mask. This preferential loss of alveolar gas means that carbon dioxide rebreathing is unlikely. (C) Nonrebreathing face mask. A unidirectional valve prevents dilution of inhaled gases containing oxygen with room air or rebreathing of exhaled gases containing carbon dioxide. (D) Air-entrainment face mask. Oxygen flow through an air injector entrains varying volumes of room air producing predictable (24 to 40 percent) and unchanging inhaled concentrations of oxygen. (Inhalation therapy and pulmonary physiotherapy. In: Dripps RD, Eckenhoff JE, Vandam LD, eds., Introduction to anesthesia: The principles of safe practice. Philadelphia, WB Saunders, 1982;450–7.)

Table 31-1. Air Entrainment (Venturi) Face Masks

Inhaled Concentration of Oxygen (percent)	Oxygen Flows (L/min)	Air Entrainment (L/min)
24	2–4	50–100
28	4–6	40–60
31	6–8	56
35	8	40
40	8–12	24–36

Nonrebreathing. A nonrebreathing face mask includes a unidirectional valve plus an oxygen reservoir bag (Fig. 31-1C).[2] The inhaled concentration of oxygen can be increased to near 100 percent using this face mask. It is difficult, however, to provide a sufficiently tight mask fit to completely eliminate entrainment of room air. The flow rate of oxygen into this system should be sufficient to maintain an inflated reservoir bag.

Air-Entrainment. An air-entrainment (Venturi) face mask utilizes the Bernoulli principle to entrain large volumes of room air (up to 100 L/min) to mix with oxygen flowing through an injector (2 to 12 L/min) (Fig. 31-1D).[2] The resultant mixture of gases produces stable inhaled concentrations of oxygen between 24 and 40 percent, depending on the bore of the oxygen injector (Table 31-1).[3] Furthermore, the high flow of gas into the face mask results in a constant inhaled concentration of oxygen despite changes in the characteristics of the patient's ventilation.

Hazards of Oxygen Therapy

Hazards of oxygen therapy include retrolental fibroplasia, carbon dioxide retention, adsorption atelectasis, and pulmonary oxygen toxicity.

Retrolental fibroplasia is a hazard of oxygen therapy administered to neonates especially those of low birth weight (below 1500 g) and gestational age less than 44 weeks. Arterial hyperoxia causes vasoconstriction of immature retinal vessels leading to neovascularization, scarring, and in 10 to 20 percent of infants a permanent visual impairment. For this reason, it is recommended that inhaled concentrations of oxygen administered to neonates at risk for developing retrolental fibroplasia be titrated to maintain the PaO_2 between 50 and 80 mmHg.

Carbon dioxide retention may be exacerbated when patients with chronic obstructive airway disease dependent on hypoxic stimulation to maintain ventilation receive supplemental oxygen. In these patients, chronic elevation of the $PaCO_2$ has resulted in normalization of arterial and cerebrospinal fluid pH due to the active transport of bicarbonate ions. Such individuals may thus be insensitive to carbon dioxide as a respiratory stimulant. As a result, removal of the hypoxic stimulus to maintain ventilation by increasing the PaO_2 above 60 mmHg with supplemental inhaled oxygen can result in profound alveolar hypoventilation and hypercarbia. Nevertheless, supplemental oxygen should never be withheld when the PaO_2 is less than 50 mmHg remembering, however, there is little to gain by increasing the PaO_2 above 60 mmHg.

Adsorption atelectasis reflects oxygen uptake from the alveolus that exceeds delivery of oxygen by ventilation. Normally, the nitrogen in the alveolus is in equilibrium with that in the pulmonary capillary blood such that loss of nitrogen from the alveolus is unlikely. As a result, nitrogen maintains alveolar volume acting as an internal splint (Fig. 31-2A).[1] When high concentrations of oxygen (greater than 60 percent) are substituted for room air, the nitrogen is diluted or washed out of the alveoli and adsorption atelectasis occurs if oxygen uptake exceeds delivery (Fig. 31-2B).[1] Oxygen uptake in excess of delivery is likely to occur in selected alveoli that are poorly ventilated due to the

A

AIR

B

O_2

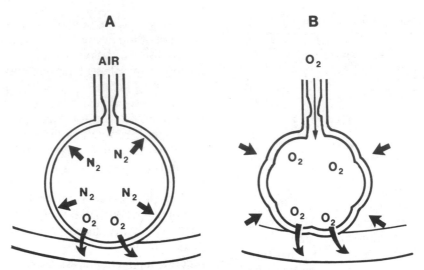

Figure 31-2. (A) Nitrogen remaining in a poorly ventilated alveolus after uptake of oxygen acts as a "splint" to prevent alveolar collapse. (B) When nitrogen is eliminated from the alveolus during inhalation of high concentrations of oxygen those alveoli with low ventilation due to peribronchiolar edema and/or secretions shrink in size as oxygen uptake exceeds delivery. The net effect of this discrepancy between oxygen uptake and delivery is adsorption atelectasis. (Adapted from Smith RA. Respiratory care. In: Miller RD, ed. Anesthesia. New York, Churchill Livingstone 1981;1379–1433.)

presence of peribronchiolar edema and/or secretions in the bronchioles supplying these alveoli.

Adsorption atelectasis is most common in the dependent regions of the lung because edema fluid and secretions tend to accumulate in these areas and the alveoli are relatively small. The impact on arterial oxygenation of low ventilation to these alveoli is exaggerated since gravity favors the distribution of pulmonary blood flow to dependent regions.

Pulmonary Oxygen Toxicity. It is well established that prolonged exposure of alveoli to high inhaled partial pressures of oxygen results in pulmonary damage. This damage is characterized by the formation of fibrin (hyaline) membranes, alveolar and septal thickening, endothelial destruction, and necrosis of membranous pneumocytes.

Other pulmonary effects of pure oxygen include depression of the ability of alveolar macrophages to kill phagocytosed bacteria, depression of mucociliary clearance, tracheitis after only 6 hours of exposure, decreased pulmonary compliance, increased airway resistance, and decreased diffusion capacity.

It is unlikely that pulmonary oxygen toxicity develops in man breathing less than 50 percent oxygen at 1 atmosphere even for prolonged periods.[4] Certainly, sufficient inspired oxygen should always be delivered to prevent the persistence of arterial hypoxemia. When greater than 50 percent inspired oxygen is needed, however, to maintain a satisfactory PaO_2, it is important to consider the use of positive end-expiratory pressure (PEEP) in an attempt to reduce the inhaled concentration of oxygen below 50 percent without adversely affecting PaO_2.

Bronchopulmonary dysplasia is characterized by acute and chronic changes involving alveoli, mucous membranes, and pulmonary vasculature in infants with previous respiratory distress syndrome whose lungs were mechanically ventilated after birth with high concentrations of oxygen. Speculated causes of bronchopulmonary dysplasia include pulmonary oxygen toxicity and damage due to high airway pressures (greater than 35 cm H_2O) during mechanical ventilation of the lungs. Infants receiving therapy for over 150 hours are likely to develop the chronic form of this syndrome, characterized by frequent pulmonary infections and abnormal arterial blood gases. With time, however, pulmonary function improves.

HUMIDIFICATION AND AEROSOL THERAPY

Absolute humidity is the mass of water vapor contained in a volume of gas at a given temperature. Relative humidity is the ratio of absolute humidity to the maximum mass of water vapor that a gas could contain at a given temperature expressed as a percent. At 37 Celsius and 100 percent relative humidity a liter of gas contains 43.8 mg of water which exerts a vapor pressure of 47 mmHg. Alveolar gases have a relative humidity of 100 percent at 37 Celsius. When the inhaled gases contain less than 43.8 mg of water per liter, the vapor pressure exerted by water is less than 47 mmHg and there is a vapor pressure gradient between the inhaled gases and respiratory mucosa. The amount of moisture given up by the mucosa is directly proportional to this gradient. For example, at 20 Celsius and 50 percent relative humidity, inhaled gases contain 9.3 mg of water per liter. For each liter of these gases inhaled, 34.5 mg of water (43.8 mg − 9.3 mg) must be vaporized from the airway mucosa to achieve 100 percent relative humidity in the alveoli at a body temperature of 37 Clesius. The resulting dehydration of the mucosa increases the viscosity of the mucous secretions and reduces the effectiveness of the mucociliary system in removing these secretions. Retained secretions produce an inflammatory response of the mucosa, while narrowing of small airways by partial obstruction with mucus results in increased airway resistance and maldistribution of ventilation to perfusion. Arterial hypoxemia may reflect maldistribution of ventilation to perfusion, while atelectasis is predictable with total occlusion of the bronchioles by mucus.

Warming, filtration, and humidification of inhaled gases normally occurs in the upper respiratory tract. When dry gases are inhaled or the natural conditioning system (nose) is bypassed by a tracheal tube or a tracheostomy tube, the lower airways must provide the additional moisture. In these situations, artificial humidifying devices such as humidifiers or nebulizers should be considered. Humidifiers are often used when dry gases are inhaled via a natural airway in an attempt to provide a water content similar to that normally present in room air. When the upper airway is bypassed, a humidifier is often inadequate and the water deficit must be made up by use of the more efficient nebulizer.

Humidifiers

Humidifiers are categorized as pass-over and bubble-through (cascade).

Pass-over humidifiers depend upon evaporation to add water vapor to gases that pass-over the water surface. Relative humidity of the effluent gases is dependent upon gas flow and the temperature of both the water and gases. Inability to predictably deliver 90 to 100 percent relative humidity at 37 Celsius limits the usefulness of these types of humidifiers.

Bubble-through humidifers that break up the delivered gases into small bubbles as they pass through a heated water reservoir are frequently used to humidify inhaled gases delivered by a mechanical ventilator. Heating the water is important, as the capacity of a gas to hold moisture is greatly increased when temperature is increased. The water in the humidifier can be heated to body temperature, but as gases travel through the delivery tubing, they cool and water collects ("rains out") in the tubing. Elevation of the water temperature above body temperature to assure delivery of gases at body temperature is acceptable. Temperature of the inhaled gases, however, should be monitored at the proximal airway in order to provide an early warning should these gases reach a temperature capable of producing a mucosal burn. Ideally, inhaled gases should be 36 to 37 Celsius so as to insure a relative humidity near 100 percent.

Nebulizers

An aerosol is a suspension of particles in a carrier gas. Devices used to generate aerosols are nebulizers. Nebulizers are categorized as jet (pneumatic) and ultrasonic.

Jet nebulizers are the most frequently used type of aerosol generators. High pressure gas enters the nebulizer chamber through a restricted orifice that produces a jet stream of high velocity. This jet stream is directed across one end of a small diameter tube that is immersed in the liquid to be nebulized and a subambient pressure (Bernoulli effect) immediately adjacent to the tube is produced, resulting in pulling of surface liquid into the tube. When the liquid reaches the top of the tube, it is aerosolized by the jet stream to particles usually less than 30 μm in diameter.

Jet nebulizers are used in respiratory therapy to humidify inhaled gases, decrease the viscosity of airway secretions, and deliver bronchodilator drugs directly to the airways.

Humidify Inhaled Gases. The particulate water produced by jet nebulizers evaporates as the inhaled gases are warmed in the respiratory tract. This evaporation reduces or eliminates the vapor pressure gradient for water between the inhaled gases and respiratory mucosa. In contrast to humidifers, jet nebulizers are more likely to provide sufficient relative humidity at 37 Celsius.

Decrease Viscosity of Airway Secretions. Aerosol administration of water is an efficient method used to decrease the viscosity of airway secretions and thus facilitate mucus clearance by normal mucociliary activity. In addition to aerosolized water, N-acetyl-L-cysteine (Mucomyst) and hypertonic saline have been utilized to enhance mucous clearance. Mucomyst is a mucolytic agent that disrupts the disulfide bonds in mucoproteins and reduces mucus viscosity. Mucomyst is extremely irritating to the airways and should always be administered with a bronchodilator to prevent or minimize bronchospasm. Hypertonic saline results in an osmotic flux that dilutes and increases the mucus volume and promotes expectoration. Like Mucomyst, saline aerosols increase airway resistance and are thus undesiarable in patients with chronic obstructive airway disease.

Deliver Bronchodilator Drugs. Bronchodilator drugs (racemic epinephrine, isoproterenol, isoetharine, salbutamol) are most often administered as aerosols to reduce airway resistance due to bronchoconstriction. Bronchodilation reflects beta-2 agonist effects of these drugs. Systemic absorption of racemic epinephrine and isoproterenol produces adverse beta-1 agonist effects (tachycardia, hypertension, cardiac dysrhythmias). Isoetharine and salbutamol have minimal beta-1 agonist effects and are thus attractive drug selections for patients with bronchoconstriction and underlying heart disease. Likewise, these drugs would be ideal for administration to the patient anesthetized with drugs such as halothane which can sensitize the heart to the arrhythmogenic effects of beta-adrenergic stimulation.

Racemic epinephrine is a mixture of the d and l-isomers of epinephrine. In theory, inhalation of the racemic mixture compared to the l-isomer (50 times more active than the d-isomer) is less likely to produce systemic effects. Therapeutic aerosols are most efficacious when particles of 0.5 to 3 μm in diameter are administered. Particles with a diameter less than 0.5 μm are so stable that they are exhaled, while those greater than 3 μm in diameter are likely to be deposited ("rain out") in the upper airways.

Aerosolized racemic epinephrine is used more for its alpha agonist (vasoconstrictive) than its beta agonist (bronchodilator) effect. For example, racemic epinephrine is effective in reducing laryngeal edema as follows intubation of the trachea, particularly in pediatric patients. The recommended dose is 0.25 to 0.5 ml of 2.25 percent racemic epinephrine in 5 ml of water or normal saline administered as an aerosol every 1 to 4 hours until stridor wanes.

Salbutamol is administered via a device placed in the inspiratory limb of the anesthesia delivery circuit. Each puff of salbutamol delivered into the breathing circuit provides about 100 μg of the drug, with 400 μg being the maximum dose usually necessary to produce a desirable effect on the airways.

Ultrasonic nebulizers convert alternating current into ultra-high frequency oscillations which are transmitted to the fluid container of the nebulizer, fragmenting the liquid into small particles. The mean particle diameter produced by an ultrasonic nebulizer is 2.8 μm (1 to 10 μm). Fluid overload is a potential problem, as the ultrasonic nebulizer can nebulize up to 6 ml of water per minute. Inhaled ultrasonic aerosols are also irritating to the airways, causing bronchoconstriction and increased airway resistance.

Nosocomial Pulmonary Infections

Sterile, pyrogen-free water should be used for all humidifiers and nebulizers so as to avoid the possibility of the water reservoir becoming a source of hospital acquired (nosocomial) infection. All aerosol and mechanical ventilator circuits should be changed every 24 hours. Most oxygen therapy humidifiers are now provided as sterile and disposable single patient units.

BRONCHIAL HYGIENE

Bronchial hygiene depends on optimal removal of secretions from the lungs by mucociliary clearance, coughing, tracheal suctioning, and chest physiotherapy.

Mucociliary Clearance

Cilia located on epithelial cells lining the respiratory mucosa are responsible for moving respiratory tract secretions (mucus) (10 to 100 ml daily) toward the glottic opening. Cilia beat in a whip-like manner at rates up to 20 times/sec and are able to move mucus cephalad at a rate of 2 cm/min. Depression of ciliary activity and an associated retention of secretions is produced by inhaled anesthetics, tracheal tubes, inhalation of cold and dry gases, high inhaled concentrations of oxygen, and pulmonary infections. Ciliary activity may be depressed up to 6 days postoperatively, depending upon the duration of the anesthetic.[6]

Coughing

Coughing is a major mechanism for removal of secretions from large airways. An effective cough requires a maximal inhalation followed by closure of the glottis and contraction of the muscles of the chest and abdomen to create subglottic pressures of up to 200 cm H_2O. As the glottis opens, the flow of exhaled air may exceed 600 L/min. High air-flow velocities necessary to propel secretions from the upper airways are generated most effectively at large lung volumes. Rapid shallow breathing patterns and decreased lung volumes characteristic of the postoperative patient with pain limit the effectiveness of coughing.

Tracheal Suctioning

Orotracheal or nasotracheal suctioning should be performed only when there is evidence during auscultation of the chest of retained secretions that do not clear with coughing. Tracheal suctioning should not be prophylactic or routine. For example, mechanical irritation by the catheter during tracheal suctioning may cause trauma to the respiratory mucosa and predispose to bacterial colonization. Mechanical stimulation of the trachea or carina by the catheter may evoke a vasovagal response with resultant bradycardia and hypotension.[7] Tracheal suctioning also predisposes to significant arterial hypoxemia because of aspiration of pulmonary gases with associated small airway closure and alveolar collapse. Arterial hypoxemia during tracheal suctioning is minimized by (1) administration of pure oxygen before suctioning, (2) selection of a suction catheter that is no greater than one-half the internal diameter of the trachea, (3) limitation of the duration of suctioning to less than 15 seconds, and (4) manual inflation of the lungs with oxygen after suctioning.

Chest Physiotherapy

Chest physiotherapy consists of postural drainage, percussion, vibration, deep breathing, and assisted coughing. These maneuvers aid in the removal of airway secretions and improve inflation of poorly ventilated alveoli. Indeed, improved ciliary clearance of airway secretions and a decreased incidence of postoperative atelectasis have been attributed to properly performed chest physiotherapy.

POSTOPERATIVE RESPIRATORY THERAPY

Postoperative respiratory therapy is designed to prevent events that lead to pneumonia and arterial hypoxemia that

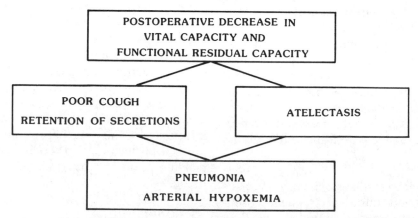

Figure 31-3. Pathogenesis of postoperative pulmonary complications. (LoSasso AM, Gibbs PS, Moorthy SS. Obstructive pulmonary disease. In: Stoelting RK, Dierdorf SF, eds. Anesthesia and co-existing disease. New York, Churchill Livingstone 1983;171–200.)

characterize postoperative pulmonary complications (Fig. 31-3).[8] The severity of postoperative pulmonary complications parallels the magnitude of reduction in lung volumes. Presumably, decreases in vital capacity (VC) and functional residual capacity (FRC) interfere with the generation of an effective cough as well as contributing to the collapse of alveoli. The net effect of these changes is a decreased clearance of secretions from the airways and atelectasis, leading to pneumonia and arterial hypoxemia. Atelectasis is likely to accompany shallow breathing ("splinting") that is a result of postoperative incisional pain. Likewise, a cough may be excruciatingly painful. Failure to prevent the postoperative reduction in FRC by totally relieving incisional pain with epidural analgesia suggests that trauma from the surgical procedure also interefers with the optimal function of the chest wall by changing the normal relation of the diaphragm, intercostal muscles, and abdominal muscles.[9]

The frequency of postoperative pulmonary complications is greatest after thoracic and upper abdominal surgery.[9] For example, significant postoperative atelectasis occurs in 20 to 40 percent of patients undergoing these types of surgery. This incidence parallels the 60 percent reduction of VC on the day after upper abdominal surgery. Lower abdominal surgery is associated with a lesser incidence of postoperative pulmonary complications and a smaller reduction in VC as compared with the observed decrease after upper abdominal surgery. In addition to the site of surgery, other factors that influence the incidence of postoperative pulmonary complications include coexisting pulmonary disease, a history of cigarette smoking, obesity, and increasing age. The choice of drugs or techniques used to produce anesthesia does not seem to alter predictably the incidence of postoperative pulmonary infections. A subcostal vs. transverse upper abdominal incision, as for a cholecystectomy, probably does not alter

the incidence of postoperative pulmonary complications.[10]

The identification of FRC as the most important lung volume in the postoperative period provides a specific goal for respiratory therapy following surgery. Specific therapies designed to increase FRC include voluntary deep breathing and ambulation, intermittent positive pressure breathing, incentive spirometry, and exhalation maneuvers.

Voluntary Deep Breathing and Ambulation

Voluntary deep breathing with maintenance of inspiration at peak inflation for 3 to 5 seconds creates a large transpulmonary presure gradient and facilitates re-expansion of collapsed alveoli and restoration of lung volumes. A motivated patient and adequate postoperative analgesia are necessary to assure optimal deep breathing.

Ambulation and the associated changes in position have great therapeutic benefit in the prevention of postoperative pulmonary complications. Presumably, this therapeutic benefit reflects increased lung volumes, particularly FRC.

Intermittent Positive Pressure Breathing

Intermittent positive pressure breathing (IPPB) as a method to reduce the incidence of postoperative pulmonary complications is controversial.[11] Certainly, postoperative IPPB therapy does not need to be routine. When IPPB is prescribed, the emphasis should be an achievement of an optimal tidal volume rather than creation of a peak airway pressure.

Patients scheduled for surgical procedures associated with a high incidence of postoperative pulmonary complications, such as upper abdominal or thoracic surgery, should have a preoperative measurement of inspiratory capacity (IC). Postoperatively, the IC should again be measured and if less than 80 percent of the preoperative value, IPPB therapy instituted. Ideally, the patient should inhale three to six times the predicted tidal volume for IPPB treatment to be effective. This inhaled tidal volume should be monitored with a spirometer placed at the exhalation valve of the IPPB delivery circuit. Nevertheless, there is no evidence that IPPB treatment is better than voluntary deep breathing and ambulation in altering the incidence or severity of postoperative pulmonary complications.

Incentive Spirometry

Incentive spirometry is a form of voluntary deep breathing in which the patient is given an inhaled volume as a goal to achieve. When the use of incentive spirometry is anticipated, a preoperative baseline IC should be obtained and the patient instructed in the use of the device. The preoperative IC should be the postoperative goal. Incentive spirometry therapy also emphasizes holding the inhaled volume to provide a sustained inflation important for expanding collapsed alveoli. The major disadvantage of this therapy is the need for patient cooperation which may be limited in the presence of postoperative pain.

Exhalation Maneuvers

Exhalation maneuvers such as inflating balloons, using blow-bottles, or performing a forced VC are not recommended, since their performance causes the patient to exhale below the FRC, leading to atelectasis and increased airway resistance. Indeed, the only therapeutic benefit elicited by exhalation maneuvers is the deep breath which must be taken initially.

REFERENCES

1. Smith RA. Respiratory care. In Miller RD, ed. Anesthesia. New York, Churchill Livingstone 1981;1379–1433.
2. Inhalation therapy and pulmonary physiotherapy. In: Dripps RD, Eckenhoff JE, Vandam LD, eds. Introduction to Anesthesia. The principles of safe practice. Philadelphia, WB Saunders 1982;450–7.
3. Cohen JL, Demers RR, Saklad M. Air-entrainment masks: A performance evaluation. Resp Care 1977;22:277–82.
4. Cheney FW Jr, Huang TW, Gronka R. The effects of 50% oxygen on resolution of experimental lung injury. Am Rev Resp Dis 1980;122:373–9.
5. Klein EF, Shah DA, Shah NJ, Modell JH, Desaultes D. Performance characteristics of conventional and prototype humidifiers and nebulizers. Chest 1973;64:690–6.
6. Gamsu G, Singer MM, Vincent HH. Postoperative impairment of mucus transport in the lung. Am Rev Resp Dis 1976;114:673–9.
7. Harken AH. A routine for safe, effective endotracheal suctioning. Am Surg 1975; 41:398–404.
8. LoSasso AM, Gibbs PS, Moorthy SS. Obstructive pulmonary disease. In: Stoelting RK, Dierdorf SF, eds. Anesthesia and coexisting disease. New York, Churchill Livingstone 1983;171–200.
9. Craig DB. Postoperative recovery of pulmonary function. Anesth Analg 1981;60:46–52.
10. Williams CD, Brenowitz JB. Ventilatory patterns after vertical and transverse upper abdominal incisions. Am J Surg 1975; 130:725–8.
11. Inverson LIG, Ecker RR, Fox HE, May IA. A comparative study of IPPB, the incentive spirometer, and blow bottles: The prevention of atelectasis following cardiac surgery. Ann Thoracic Surg 1978;25:197–200.

32

Critical Care Medicine

Evolution of critical care medicine as a legitimate and important area of specialization reflects the contributions of many clinicians, particularly anesthesiologists. Indeed, 10 of the 28 founding members of the Society of Critical Care Medicine (SCCM) were anesthesiologists.

The training of anesthesiologists in the management of anesthesia is an ideal beginning for subsequent development of additional skills required for the management of critically ill patients with multiple organ system dysfunction. For example, no other specialty provides day to day experience in airway management, ventilation of the lungs, intravenous administration of potent and rapidly acting drugs, blood and fluid administration, and both noninvasive and invasive monitoring of vital organ function.

Examples of organ system failure occurring alone or in combination in an intensive care unit and requiring treatment by specialists in critical care medicine (intensivists) include acute respiratory failure, congestive heart failure, septic shock, brain injury, acute renal failure, and acute liver failure.

ACUTE RESPIRATORY FAILURE

The treatment of acute respiratory failure is a major contribution of the intensivist. Acute respiratory failure is not a single disease entity but instead is a combination of pathophysiologic derangements that can arise from a variety of etiologic insults (Table 32-1).[1] Nevertheless, the manifestations of acute respiratory failure are sufficiently similar to be considered as a single entity designated the adult respiratory distress syndrome (ARDS).

Diagnosis

Arterial hypoxemia (PaO_2 below 60 mmHg) despite supplemental inhaled oxygen is an invariable accompaniment of ARDS. Mismatching of ventilation to perfusion is the most likely cause for arterial hypoxemia. In its most extreme form, this mismatching may be right-to-left intrapulmonary shunting in which unventilated alveoli continue to be perfused. Also contributing to this mismatching is a reduction in functional residual capacity (FRC) and decreased pulmonary compliance. Loss of pulmonary capillary integrity is reflected by pulmonary edema despite a pulmonary artery occlusion pressure less than 15 mmHg. Increased pulmonary vascular resistance and pulmonary hypertension are likely to develop when ARDs persists.

Acute respiratory failure is often distinguished from chronic respiratory failure on the basis of the relationship of the $PaCO_2$ to the arterial pH (pHa). For example, acute respiratory failure is associated with an abrupt increase in the $PaCO_2$ and a corre-

Table 32-1. Etiology of Acute Respiratory Failure

Primary pulmonary dysfunction
    Obstructive airway disease
    Restrictive pulmonary disease
    Pneumonia
    Inhaled toxins—gastric fluid, meconium, smoke
    Oxygen toxicity
    Embolization—blood, fat, amniotic fluid
    Pulmonary contusion
    Near-drowning
    Hyaline membrane disease

Cardiovascular dysfunction
    Hemorrhagic shock
    Sepsis
    Congestive heart failure
    Massive blood transfusion
    Disseminated intravascular coagulation
    Postcardiopulmonary bypass

Central nervous system dysfunction
    Hypothalamic injury
    Depressant drug overdose

Neuromuscular dysfunction
    Myasthenia gravis
    Spinal cord transection
    Guillain-Barré
    Tetanus
    Drug-induced—muscle relaxants, antibiotics

Miscellaneous
    Acute pancreatitis
    Uremia
    Morbid obesity

(Modified from LoSasso AM, Gibbs PS, Moorthy SS. Recognition and management of respiratory failure. In: Stoelting RK, Dierdorf SF, eds. Anesthesia and co-existing disease. New York, Churchill Livingstone 1983:209–25.)

sponding decrease in pHa. Conversely, in the presence of chronic respiratory failure, the pHa reflects compensation by virtue of renal tubular reabsorption of bicarbonate ions.

Serial measurement of arterial blood gases and pH is necessary to establish the diagnosis of ARDS, determine the need for mechanical support of ventilation, assess the effects of therapy, and confirm when the patient no longer needs mechanical support of ventilation.

Treatment

Treatment of ARDS is directed at supporting pulmonary function until the lungs can recover from the insult that initiated pulmonary dysfunction. In addition to administration of supplemental oxygen and maintenance of intravascular fluid volume, it is usually necessary to intubate the trachea and provide mechanical ventilation of the lungs, including the use of positive end-expiratory pressure (PEEP) or an end-inspiratory plateau.

Mechanical ventilation of the lungs is provided by machines known as ventilators. Ventilators may be classified as pressure-cycled, volume-cycled, or time-cycled, depending on the mechanism responsible for terminating the inspiratory phase of the mechanical breath. Mechanical ventilators may change from the expiratory to inspiratory phase by being set to deliver assisted ventilation, controlled ventilation, high frequency positive pressure ventilation (HFPPV), assisted-controlled ventilation, or intermittent mandatory ventilation (IMV).

Pressure-cycled ventilators such as the Bennett PR-1 terminate the inspiratory phase of the mechanical breath when a preselected pressure is achieved in the ventilator circuit. Therefore, tidal volume and inspiratory time are directly related to pulmonary compliance and inversely related to airway resistance. Significant leaks in the delivery circuit may prevent development of sufficient airway pressure to cycle the ventilator to exhalation. Conversely, decreased pulmonary compliance or increased airway resistance may result in attainment of the predetermined airway pressure before a sufficient tidal volume has been delivered to the patient. Most pressure-cycled ventilators are incapable of providing the constant tidal volume and unchanging inhaled concentration of oxygen necessary for the management of critically ill patients. Therefore, these types of ventilators are most often used for intermittent positive pressure breathing (IPPB) therapy and short term ventilatory support in the recovery room.

Volume-cycled ventilators such as the Bennett MA-1 terminate the inspiratory phase of the mechanical breath following delivery of preselected volume of gas to the delivery circuit. Flow generators maintain a uniform gas flow rate throughout the inspiratory phase that is independent of the airway pressure. Changes in the patient's pulmonary compliance or airway resistance are unlikely to alter the flow characteristics of the ventilator, insuring a more constant tidal volume with changing clinical conditions. For this reason, most ventilators used for critical care are volume-cycled.

It is a common misconception that the tidal volume delivered by a volume-cycled ventilator is constant regardless of changes in the patient's pulmonary compliance and airway resistance. In fact, a portion of the tidal volume generated by the ventilator is compressed within the ventilator breathing circuit and does not reach the patient. This lost compression volume is dependent upon the compliance of the entire ventilator-patient circuit and the peak inspiratory pressure. For most ventilators, the compression volume of the delivery circuit is 3 to 5 ml/cm H_2O. For example, a volume-cycled ventilator (equally true for all other types of ventilators) with a preset tidal volume of 700 ml, a peak inspiratory pressure of 20 cm H_2O, and a compression factor of 4 ml/cm H_2O will deliver 620 ml (700 ml minus compression volume) to the patient. If the patient's pulmonary compliance further decreases, the peak inflation pressure will increase and the delivered tidal volume will be further reduced. Compression volume is particularly important to consider in setting the tidal volume delivered to children. For example, a ventilator set to deliver a tidal volume of 10 ml/kg to a 10 kg child would deliver only 20 ml, assuming a peak inspiratory pressure of 20 cm H_2O and a compression factor of 4 ml/cm H_2O. Con-

sideration of compression volume loss may indicate the need to measure exhaled tidal volume with a spirometer in selected patients.

Time-cycled ventilators such as the Emerson IMV terminate the inspiratory phase of the mechanical breath after a preselected time interval has elapsed. The tidal volume delivered by time-cycled ventilators is determined by the inspiratory time and inspiratory flow rate.

Assisted Ventilation. Ventilators capable of assisted (patient-triggered) mechanical ventilation of the lungs respond to a decrease in airway pressure caused by the patient's spontaneous breathing effort which causes the ventilator to switch to the inspiratory mode. The magnitude of the decreased airway pressure necessary to trigger mechanical augmentation of a spontaneously initiated tidal volume is adjustable by means of a sensitivity control on the ventilator.

Controlled Ventilation. Controlled mechanical ventilation of the lungs provides automatic cycling of the ventilator at a preselected rate independent of the patient's effort to breathe. This mode of ventilation is used primarily to assure delivery of a predictable minute ventilation to patients being treated for ARDS. Initiation and/or maintenance of controlled ventilation of the lungs may require depression of the patient's own spontaneous ventilatory effort by the administration of sedatives or narcotics, muscle relaxants, or deliberate hyperventilation to lower the $PaCO_2$ below the apneic threshold. Deliberate hyperventilation produces respiratory alkalosis that may be physiologically deleterious (see Chapter 17).

The initial ventilator settings typically include a respiratory rate of 6 to 12 breaths/min, tidal volume 10 to 15 ml/kg, and an inhaled concentration of oxygen near 50 percent. A slow ventilator rate combined with a large tidal volume optimizes the distribution of ventilation relative to perfusion, particularly in the presence of regional differences in airway resistance. Subsequent adjustments of the ventilator settings and the inhaled concentration of oxygen are based on the measurement of arterial blood gases and pH. The goal is to achieve a PaO_2 between 60 and 100 mmHg, $PaCO_2$ between 36 and 44 mmHg and pHa between 7.36 and 7.44.

High frequency positive pressure ventilation (HFPPV) is an alternative mode of controlled ventilation that has been used to treat ARDS and manage patients with bronchopleural fistulas.[2] Characteristics of HFPPV include (1) ventilatory frequency 50 to 150 breaths/min, (2) small tidal volumes that result in a low mean positive airway pressure during inspiration, and (3) provision of continuous positive intratracheal pressure throughout the ventilator cycle. An important advantage ascribed to this form of ventilation is the failure of airway resistance and pulmonary compliance to influence the efficacy of ventilation. In addition, the maintenance of a low mean airway pressure results in minimal effects on cardiac output, and the likelihood of pulmonary barotrauma is reduced. Furthermore, it has been observed that HFPPV produces reflex suppression of spontaneous ventilation, allowing mechanical support without the use of drugs or deliberate hyperventilation. The mechanism by which HFPPV produces acceptable alveolar ventilation and arterial oxygenation delivering tidal volumes less than the patient's calculated anatomic dead space is unknown.

High frequency jet ventilation is similar to HFPPV, using ventilatory frequencies of 60 to 600 breaths/min. The distinguishing feature of this form of ventilation is gas entrainment such that the tidal volume and inhaled concentration of oxygen are difficult to quantitate. Also closely related to HFPPV is high frequency oscillation which uses ventilatory frequencies as high as 60 Hz or 3600 cycles/min.

Assisted-Controlled Ventilation. A ventilator used to provide assisted-controlled ventilation is set such that the cycling rate is slightly less than the patient's respiratory rate. If the patient stops breathing, the ventilator will convert to the controlled ventilation mode at the preset respiratory frequency.

Intermittent mandatory ventilation (IMV) is a ventilation mode that has been incorporated into many recently introduced ventilators. This mode of ventilation finds its greatest use during weaning (see the section *Cessation of Mechanical Inflation of the Lungs*).

Positive end-expiratory pressure (PEEP) is produced by applying positive pressure to the exhalation valve at the conclusion of the mechanical exhalation phase (Fig. 32-1). Alternatively, the exhalation valve can be depressurized gradually to provide resistance (retard) to exhalation (Fig. 32-2). Retardation of expiratory gas flow rate serves to maintain patency of peripheral airways.

Mechanism of Beneficial Effect. It is presumed that PEEP increases arterial oxygenation, pulmonary compliance, and the FRC by expanding previously collapsed but perfused alveoli. As a result, the matching of ventilation to perfusion is improved and the magnitude of right-to-left intrapulmonary shunting of blood is reduced. It should be recognized that PEEP is unlikely to improve the PaO_2 when arterial hypoxemia is due to hypoventilation or is associated with a normal or even increased FRC.

Institution of Positive End-Expiratory Pressure. Institution of PEEP is often recommended when the PaO_2 cannot be main-

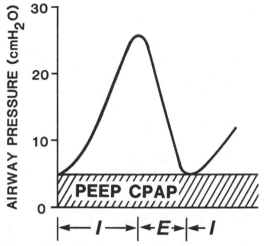

Figure 32-1. Schematic diagram of airway pressures during the inspiratory phase (I) and expiratory phase (E) of a mechanical breath. Airway pressure does not decrease below 5 cm H_2O during I and E reflecting positive end-expiratory pressure (PEEP). Spontaneous breathing in which airway pressure does not decrease to zero during I and E is commonly referred to as continuous positive airway pressure (CPAP).

tained above 60 mmHg despite inhaled concentrations of oxygen that exceed 50 percent. Short-term administration of greater than 50 percent oxygen to maintain adequate arterial oxygenation is acceptable, but it must be recognized that pulmonary oxygen toxicity is a hazard when in-

haled concentrations of oxygen exceed 50 percent for more than 24 hours.

Initially, PEEP is added in 2.5 to 5 cm H_2O increments until the PaO_2 is greater than 60 mmHg while the patient is breathing less than 50 percent oxygen. The goal is to deliver the amount of PEEP that maximally improves the PaO_2 without substantially reducing cardiac output or increasing the risk of pulmonary barotrauma. Typically, maximum improvement of PaO_2 is achieved with less than 15 cm H_2O of PEEP. Refractory arterial hypoxemia, however, may require PEEP up to 30 cm H_2O before improvement in arterial oxygenation is produced. Optimal levels of PEEP as reflected by maximal oxygen transport (arterial oxygen content times cardiac output) are also often associated with the best improvement in static lung compliance (Fig. 32-3).[3] The level of PEEP that produces maximal oxygen transport without overdistension of alveoli as reflected by the static lung compliance has been characterized as "best PEEP."[3]

Hazards of Positive End-Expiratory Pressure. Hazards of PEEP include (1) decreased cardiac output, (2) pulmonary barotrauma, (3) increased extravascular lung

Figure 32-2. Schematic diagram of airway pressures during the inspiratory phase (I) and expiratory phase (E) of a mechanical breath. The exhalation valve is depressurized slowly so as to "retard" or slow the rate at which airway pressure decreases towards zero during E.

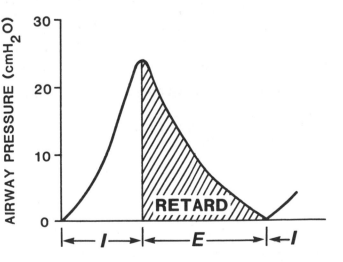

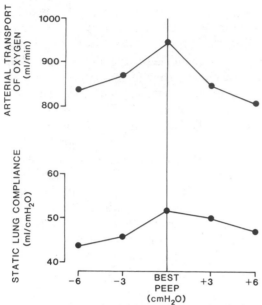

Figure 32-3. The arterial transport of oxygen (cardiac output times arterial content of oxygen) and static lung compliance were measured in patients with acute respiratory failure being treated with mechanical ventilation of the lungs and varying amounts of positive end-expiratory pressure (PEEP). "Best PEEP" was that amount of PEEP that resulted in the greatest arterial transport of oxygen and static lung compliance. PEEP that was 3 or 6 cmH$_2$O above or below "best PEEP" resulted in lower values for arterial transport of oxygen and static lung compliance. (LoSasso AM, Gibbs PS, Moorthy SS. Recognition and management of respiratory failure. In Stoelting RK, Dierdorf SF, eds, Anesthesia and co-existing disease. New York, Churchill Livingstone 1983; 209-25, with data from reference 3.)

water, and (4) redistribution of pulmonary blood flow.

The reduction in cardiac output produced by PEEP is due to interference with venous return and a leftward displacement of the ventricular septum which restricts filling of the left ventricle. It is conceivable that improvements in PaO$_2$ produced by PEEP could be offset by reductions in cardiac output. The potential for PEEP to reduce cardiac output is exaggerated in the presence of decreased intravascular fluid volume and/or normal lungs which permit maximal transmission of the increased airway pressure.[4] A pulmonary artery catheter is helpful in guiding fluid replacement and for monitoring the impact of PEEP on cardiac output. It must be recognized that levels of PEEP which exceed about 10 cm H$_2$O can interfere with the interpretation of the pulmonary artery occlusion pressure as a monitor of left atrial pressure. This reflects transmission of intraalveolar pressure to the pulmonary capillaries which is then measured as the pulmonary artery occlusion pressure.

Pneumothorax, pneumomediastinum, and subcutaneous emphysema are examples of barotrauma due to overdistension of alveoli by PEEP. An abrupt deterioration of PaO$_2$ and cardiovascular function during PEEP should arouse suspicion of pulmonary barotrauma, especially pneumothorax.

Increased intravascular lung water associated with PEEP may reflect obstruction to pulmonary lymph flow as well as alterations in permeability characteristics of the pulmonary capillaries.

The adverse effects of PEEP on distribution of pulmonary blood flow are complex but presumably reflect, in part, overdistension of alveoli. When overdistension of alveoli occurs, pulmonary blood flow is likely to be shunted to areas with less resistance to flow such as less distended or even collapsed alveoli. The net effect of this alveolar overdistension is increased mismatching of ventilation to perfusion, manifesting as a reduction of PaO$_2$.

End-inspiratory plateau (EIP) is characterized by sustained positive pressure for about 1.5 seconds at no flow (Fig. 32-4).[5] The rationale for EIP is to offset the impact of variations in pulmonary time constants (airway resistance times pulmonary compliance) between lung compartments that prevent homogeneity of gas distribution.

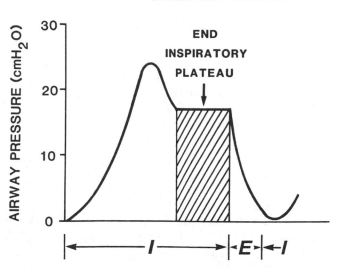

Figure 32-4. Schematic diagram of airway pressures during the inspiratory phase (I) and expiratory phase (E) of a mechanical breath. A sustained level of positive airway pressure for about 1.5 seconds at end-inspiration is designated on end-inspiratory plateau. (Adapted from Smith RA. Respiratory care. In: Miller RD, ed. Anesthesia. New York, Churchill Livingstone 1981;1379–1433.)

Presumably, EIP promotes distribution of gas to lung units with high resistance to flow. The net effect is an improved matching of ventilation to perfusion and inflation of collapsed alveoli in patients with ARDS. This inspiratory pattern may also be of benefit in the ventilator management of neonatal respiratory distress syndrome.

Monitoring of Treatment

Monitoring of treatment of ARDS depends on evaluation of pulmonary gas exchange and cardiac function. Measurements of arterial and venous blood gases, pHa, cardiac output, cardiac filling pressure and intrapulmonary shunt, and calculation of systemic and pulmonary vascular resistance are used to monitor the adequacy of treatment of ARDS. A pulmonary artery catheter is useful for making many of the measurements and calculations.

Arterial Oxygenation. The adequacy of treatment of ARDS that is directed toward relieving arterial hypoxemia is reflected by the PaO_2 (normal 60 to 100 mmHg). The efficiency of the exchange of oxygen across the capillary membrane is reflected by the difference between the calculated alveolar partial pressure of oxygen (PAO_2) and the measured PaO_2. Calculation of the alveolar-to-arterial difference for oxygen ($AaDO_2$) when the patient is breathing pure oxygen provides an estimate of the magnitude of right-to-left intrapulmonary shunting of blood (see Chapter 17). One of the difficulties with the use of the $AaDO_2$ is that the normal range changes with variations in the inhaled concentration of oxygen. With this in mind, a more useful calculation may be the ratio of the PaO_2 to PAO_2 which is not influenced by the inhaled concentration of oxygen (see Chapter 17).

Ventilation. The adequacy of alveolar ventilation during treatment of ARDS is monitored by measurement of the $PaCO_2$ (normal 36 to 44 mmHg). The efficiency of the transfer of carbon dioxide across the alveolar capillary membrane is reflected by the ratio of dead space ventilation to tidal volume (V_D/V_T) (see Chapter 17). Normally, the V_D/V_T is less than 0.3 but may increase to greater than 0.6 in the patient with ARDS.

Tissue Oxygenation. The mixed venous partial pressure of oxygen (PvO_2) as measured in blood obtained from the pulmonary artery reflects tissue extraction of oxygen (see Chapter 17). A PvO_2 below 30 mmHg indicates the need to increase cardiac output so as to assure adequate tissue oxygenation.

Acidemia. Measurement of pHa is necessary to detect metabolic and/or respiratory acidosis that commonly accompanies ARDS. For example, metabolic acidosis predictably accompanies arterial hypoxemia and inadequate delivery of oxygen to the tissues. Respiratory acidosis reflects alveolar hypoventilation and the resulting acute increase of the $PaCO_2$. Cardiac dysrhythmias, increased pulmonary vascular resistance, and decreased responsiveness to catecholamines are adverse effects of acidosis.

Cardiac Output and Filling Pressures. Measurement and maintenance of a normal cardiac output (above 4 L/min/m²) is essential for assuring adequate delivery of oxygen to tissues during treatment of ARDS. Cardiac output is most frequently measured by the thermodilution technique using a pulmonary artery catheter. Measurement of left and right atrial filling pressures combined with the value for cardiac output permits construction of ventricular function curves for use in guiding fluid administration and drug therapy. Likewise, systemic and pulmonary vascular resistance can be calculated utilizing appropriate pressure measurements and the cardiac output.

Cessation of Mechanical Support of Ventilation

Cessation of mechanical support of ventilation of the lungs in the patient being treated for ARDS can be considered in the presence of (1) measurements that are compatible with spontaneous ventilation, (2) cardiovascular stability, and (3) a favorable clinical impression of the patient's condition. Weaning can be considered to occur in three stages. The first step is cessation of mechanical inflation of the lungs (weaning) followed by removal of the tracheal

Table 32-2. Guidelines that Suggest the Likelihood of Successful Cessation of Mechanical Inflation of the Lungs

Vital capacity above 15 ml/kg
Alveolar-to-arterial difference for oxygen less than 350 mmHg ($F_1O_2 = 1.0$)
Arterial/alveolar partial pressure of oxygen above 0.75
Arterial partial pressure of oxygen above 60 mmHg (F_1O_2 below 0.5)
Arterial pH above 7.3
Arterial partial pressure of carbon dioxide below 50 mmHg
Maximal inspiratory pressure above -20 cmH$_2$O
Dead space/tidal volume less than 0.6
Conscious and oriented
Stable cardiac function
Optimal intravascular fluid volume and electrolyte status
Absence of infection
Good nutritional status

tube (extubation) and finally elimination of the need for supplemental oxygen.

Cessation of Mechanical Inflation of the Lungs. Guidelines that suggest the likely success of weaning include serial measurements and calculations of several parameters (Table 32-2). Ultimately, the decision to attempt weaning must be individualized considering not only the status of pulmonary function but also the co-existence of other organ system abnormalities (Table 32-2).

T-tube and intermittent mandatory ventilation (IMV) are the two methods employed in weaning the patient from mechanical support of ventilation of the lungs.

T-tube weaning is initiated by connecting the tube in the trachea of the patient to a device (T-tube) through which humidified and oxygen-enriched gases are delivered. In addition, 2.5 to 5 cm H$_2$O of continuous positive airway pressure (CPAP) is often delivered via the T-tube to the airway. The use of CPAP prevents the decrease in FRC associated with cessation of positive pressure ventilation of the lungs.[6] Indeed, incompetence of the glottic opening produced by the presence of a tracheal tube seems to interfere with the maintenance of a normal FRC. Initially, the patient is allowed to breathe spontaneously for 5 to 10 minutes each hour. Tachycardia, tachypnea (greater than 35 breaths/min), or alterations in the level of consciousness during the brief period of spontaneous ventilation confirm that weaning has been premature and mechanical support of ventilation is immediately reinstituted. When pulmonary function has recovered to the extent that weaning is appropriate, it will be possible to lengthen gradually the periods of spontaneous ventilation to 2 hours or longer.

Intermittent Mandatory Ventilation. Periodic mechanical inflation of the lungs during periods of spontaneous ventilation is described as IMV. The intermittent mechanical breath can be provided as a mandatory breath at a preset interval (nonsynchronous) or as a synchronized breath (SIMV) initiated by the spontaneous ventilatory effort of the patient. There is no evidence to substantiate an advantage of SIMV over IMV.

Weaning utilizing IMV is initiated by gradually decreasing the number of mechanical breaths delivered each minute. Ideally, the IMV rate is sequentially decreased as long as the $PaCO_2$ remains near the patient's normal level, the pHa is 7.36 to 7.44, and tachypnea is absent.

Removal of the Tracheal Tube. Extubation of the trachea should be considered when the patient tolerates 2 hours of spontaneous ventilation during T-tube weaning or an IMV rate of 1 to 2 breaths/min without deterioration of (1) arterial blood gases, (2) pHa, (3) consciousness, or (4) cardiac status. In addition, the patient should have active laryngeal reflexes and the ability to generate an effective cough so as to clear secretions from the airway.

Elimination of the Need for Supplemental Oxygen. Supplemental inhaled oxygen is often needed for a period of time despite recovery from ARDS sufficient to permit spontaneous ventilation. This need for supplemental oxygen most likely reflects persistence of mismatching of ventilation to perfusion. Weaning from supplemental oxygen is accomplished by the gradual reduction in the inhaled concentration of oxygen, as guided by monitoring the PaO_2. It is probably not necessary to increase the PaO_2 above 60 mmHg utilizing supplemental inhaled oxygen. Furthermore, a PaO_2 above 60 mmHg can eliminate the hypoxic stimulus to ventilation in patients with chronic obstructive airway disease associated with chronic carbon dioxide retention. This loss of hypoxic stimulation of ventilation in these patients could result in unacceptable hypercarbia despite an acceptable level of oxygenation.

CONGESTIVE HEART FAILURE

Congestive heart failure characterized by decreased cardiac output requires pharmacologic treatment with inotropes and/or vasodilators guided by information obtained from a pulmonary artery catheter. Drug-induced increases in cardiac output are reflected as reductions in atrial filling pressures, improved arterial oxygenation, and increased PvO_2. Dopamine and dobutamine are examples of inotropes that are used to increase myocardial contractility and cardiac output (see Chapter 3).

In certain patients, reduction in systemic vascular resistance produced by a vasodilator drug such as nitroprusside is used to improve forward left ventricular stroke volume. Reductions in systemic blood pressure with associated decreases in coronary perfusion pressure, however, limit the usefulness of vasodilator therapy of congestive heart failure. Maintenance of an optimal intravascular fluid volume as guided by cardiac filling pressures will minimize reductions in blood pressure produced by nitroprusside. Nitroglycerin is an alternative to nitroprusside and is particularly useful in patients with coronary artery disease, as it selectively redistributes coronary blood flow to subendocardial areas. Reductions in systemic vascular resistance are less predictable with nitroglycerin since this drug, in contrast to nitroprusside, acts predominately on venules.

Intra-aortic balloon counterpulsation may be helpful in some patients who develop cardiogenic shock following a myocardial infarction. The intra-aortic balloon is programmed to the electrocardiogram so as to deflate just prior to systole and to inflate during diastole. The presystolic deflation of the balloon diminishes systemic blood pressure and afterload which reduces cardiac work and myocardial oxygen requirements. Inflation of the balloon during diastole increases diastolic blood pressure and thus improves coronary blood flow and myocardial oxygen delivery.

SEPTIC SHOCK

Septic shock occurs most frequently after trauma or operative procedures on the genitourinary tract. About 70 percent of cases are due to gram-negative bacteremia. Septic shock can be divided into an early (hyperdynamic) and late phase.

Early Phase

The early phase (first 24 hours) of septic shock is characterized by vasodilation and hypotension associated with reductions in systemic vascular resistance and increased cardiac output. Fever and hyperventilation are frequently present.

Late Phase

After about 24 hours, vasoconstriction replaces vasodilation and lactic acidosis now accompanies a decreased cardiac output. Oliguria is characteristically present. Hematologic abnormalities suggestive of disseminated intravascular coagulation (decreased platelets, prolonged prothrombin and partial thromboplastin time, increased concentrations of fibrin split products) typically accompany the late phase of septic shock.

Treatment

Treatment of septic shock is with intravenous antibiotics, repletion of intravascular fluid volume, and administration of pharmacologic doses of corticosteroids. Antibiotics should be started immediately following the drawing of blood for culture and sensitivity. Most often two antibiotics are selected, with one (clindamycin) effective against gram-positive and another (aminoglycoside derivative) against gram-negative bacteria. Antibiotics can be changed if necessary following the results of the blood culture. Fluid replacement must be aggressive and guided by measurement of right or left atrial filling pressures and urine output. Pharmacologic doses of methylprednisolone (30 mg/kg) or dexamethasone (3 mg/kg) administered intravenously have also been recommended.[7] Nevertheless, firm evidence as to the efficacy of corticosteroids in the treatment of shock does not exist.[8] Dopamine is an effective inotrope when pharmacologic support of both cardiac output and renal function is necessary.

A role for endorphins in the manifestations of septic shock is suggested by reversal of endotoxin-induced hypotension and decreased mortality in animals treated with naloxone.[9] Likewise, naloxone (0.4 to 1.2 mg) administered intravenously to patients with sepsis often resulted in elevations of blood pressure which were accompanied by improved mentation and increased cardiac output.[10]

BRAIN INJURY

Critical care of the brain-injured patient is based on the recognition and treatment of hazardous elevations of the intracranial pressure (ICP). Cerebral protection and resuscitation have been most successful in pa-

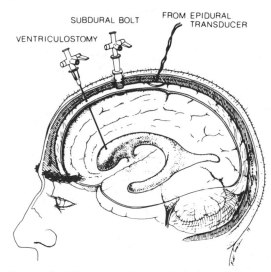

SUBDURAL BOLT

VENTRICULOSTOMY

FROM EPIDURAL
TRANSDUCER

Figure 32-5. Commonly employed techniques and sites for measurement of intracranial pressure. (Shapiro HM. Neurosurgical anesthesia and intracranial hypertension. In: Miller RD, ed. Anesthesia. New York, Churchill Livingstone 1981;1079–1132.)

tients who experience head injury. Institution of deliberate hyperventilation plus administration of diuretics and corticosteroids are the recommended initial interventions to reduce ICP. Administration of barbiturates is recommended when the ICP remains elevated despite traditional therapy.

Intracranial Pressure

A catheter placed through a burr hole into a cerebral ventricle or a transducer placed on the surface of the brain is used to monitor ICP (Fig. 32-5).[11] High risk patients including those with head injury, large brain tumors, cerebral aneurysms, and hydrocephalus should probably have their ICP monitored. A normal ICP pressure wave is pulsatile and varies with the cardiac impulse and respiration. The mean ICP should remain below 15 mmHg. An abrupt increase in the ICP observed during continuous monitoring is known as a plateau wave (Fig. 32-6).[12] Painful stimulation in an otherwise unresponsive patient can initiate a plateau

wave. Hence, the liberal use of analgesics to avoid pain is indicated even in the unresponsive patient.

Treatment

Methods to decrease ICP include posture, deliberate hyperventilation, and administration of osmotic and/or tubular diuretics, corticosteroids, barbiturates, and institution of cerebrospinal fluid drainage. A frequent recommendation is to treat sustained increases of ICP above 20 mmHg. Treatment may be indicated when ICP is less than 20 mmHg if the appearance of an occasional plateau wave suggests a low intracranial compliance.

Posture. Elevation of the head to about 30 degrees is essential in the care of the brain-injured patient so as to encourage venous outflow from the brain and thus lower ICP. It should also be appreciated that extreme flexion or rotation of the head can obstruct the jugular veins and restrict venous outflow from the brain. The head down position as utilized to place central catheters via the external or internal jugular vein must be avoided, as this position can markedly increase ICP.

Hyperventilation. Deliberate hyperventilation of adults to a $PaCO_2$ between 25 and 30 mmHg is an effective and rapid method to lower ICP. Further reductions in the $PaCO_2$ in a previously normocapnic patient do not provide additional benefit and excessive alkalosis might result in cerebral ischemia. Presumably, the beneficial effects of hyperventilation on ICP reflect decreased cerebral blood flow and resulting reductions in intracranial blood volume. Children with higher cerebral blood flows than adults are treated with more aggressive hyperventilation to lower the $PaCO_2$ to between 20 and 25 mmHg. The duration of the efficacy of hyperventilation for reducing ICP is unknown. In volunteers, however,

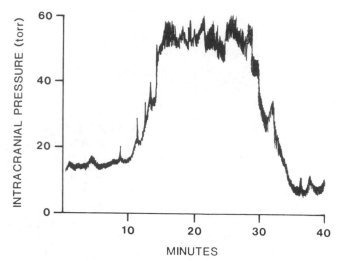

Figure 32-6. Schematic diagram of a plateau wave characterized by an abrupt and sustained (10 to 20 minutes) increase in intracranial pressure followed by a rapid reduction in pressure, often to levels below those present before the onset of the wave. (Defalque RJ, Musunuru VS. Diseases of the nervous system. In: Stoelting RK, Dierdorf SF, eds. Anesthesia and co-existing disease. New York, Churchill Livingstone 1983;239–325.

the effect of hyperventilation wanes with time as evidenced by a return of cerebral blood flow to normal after about 6 hours. Furthermore, if the cerebral vessels are damaged (e.g., trauma) or diseased (e.g., tumor), their reactivity may be diminished.

Osmotic Diuretics. Intravenous administration of a hyperosmotic drug such as mannitol (0.25 to 1 g/kg over 15 to 30 minutes) or urea (1 to 1.5 g/kg over 15 to 30 minutes) reduces ICP by producing a transient increase in the osmolarity of plasma which acts to draw water from tissues, including the brain. However, if the blood brain barrier is disrupted, these drugs may pass into the brain and cause cerebral edema by drawing water into the brain. The duration of the hyperosmotic effect of mannitol is about 6 hours. Importantly, mannitol is not associated with a high incidence of rebound increase in ICP after this time. In contrast, a rebound increase in ICP typically occurs 3 to 7 hours following the administration of urea. The brain eventually adapts to sustained elevations in plasma osmolarity, such that chronic use of hyperosmotic drugs is likely to become less effective.

Diuresis induced by mannitol or urea may result in acute hypovolemia and adverse electrolyte changes (hypokalemia, hyponatremia), emphasizing the need to replace intravascular fluid volume with infusion of crystalloid and colloid solutions. A rule of thumb is to replace urine output with an equivalent volume of crystalloid, most often lactated Ringer's solution. Glucose and water solutions are not recommended, since they are rapidly distributed in total body water including the brain. If the blood glucose concentration decreases more rapidly than brain glucose, the brain water becomes relatively hyperosmolar and water enters the central nervous system and exaggerates existing cerebral edema.

Tubular Diuretics. Intravenous administration of furosemide (0.5 to 1 mg/kg) is particularly useful in lowering an excessively elevated ICP that is associated with increased intravascular fluid volume. Advantages of furosemide compared with mannitol include the failure of furosemide to significantly increase serum osmolarity or decrease the plasma concentrations of potassium and sodium.

Corticosteroids such as dexamethasone or methylprednisolone are effective in lowering ICP and reducing mortality associated with acute head injury and intracranial tumors. The mechanism for the beneficial effect of corticosteroids is not known but may involve stabilization of capillary membranes and/or reductions in the production of cerebrospinal fluid.

Barbiturates. Administration of barbiturates may be recommended when the ICP remains elevated despite deliberate hyperventilation, drug-induced diuresis, and administration of corticosteroids. This recommendation is based on the predictable ability of these drugs to reduce ICP, presumably by decreasing cerebral blood volume secondary to cerebral vascular vasoconstriction and decreased cerebral blood flow. The goal of barbiturate therapy is to maintain the ICP below 20 mmHg without the occurrence of plateau waves. An effective regimen is the intravenous administration of an initial dose of pentobarbital (3 to 5 mg/kg) followed by a continuous rate of infusion to maintain the blood concentration of barbiturate between 3 to 6 mg/dl.[13] An alternative to measuring the blood concentration of pentobarbital every 12 to 24 hours is to adjust the infusion rate to maintain an isoelectric electroencephalogram, which confirms the presence of maximum drug-induced depression of cerebral metabolic requirements for oxygen. Discontinuation of barbiturate infusion can be considered when the ICP has remained in a normal range for 48 hours. Failure of barbiturates to lower the ICP is a grave prognostic sign. Even when barbiturates are effective, the overall morbidity and mortality in head trauma patients has not been shown to be improved by the use of these drugs as compared with patients treated aggressively with deliberate hyperventilation, drug-induced diuresis, and administration of corticosteroids.

A hazard of barbiturate therapy as used to lower the ICP is hypotension, which can jeopardize the maintenance of an adequate cerebral perfusion pressure. Such hypotension is particularly likely in the presence of decreased intravascular fluid volume. Dopamine or dobutamine may be necessary if barbiturate-induced hypotension due to myocardial depression occurs.

Cerebrospinal fluid drainage, either from the lateral cerebral ventricles or lumbar subarachnoid space, effectively reduces ICP and intracranial volume. Lumbar cerebrospinal fluid drainage, however, is not often recommended, since herniation of the cerebellum through the foramen magnum might occur.

ACUTE RENAL FAILURE

The best treatment of acute renal failure is prevention by maintenance of an optimal intravascular fluid volume and cardiac output (see Chapter 22). A pulmonary artery catheter is helpful in achieving these goals. A relative fluid overload resulting in pulmonary edema may be necessary to prevent oliguria and the risks of acute renal failure. Iatrogenic pulmonary edema which is treatable is an acceptable complication if the fluids responsible for this adverse response help prevent oliguric renal failure. When acute tubular necrosis develops, however, the only treatment is hemodialysis.

ACUTE HEPATIC FAILURE

Acute hepatic failure regardless of the etiology is associated with a poor prognosis. Hyperventilation is a constant feature of early hepatic failure and most likely reflects stimulation of ventilation by ammonia. Hypoglycemia is frequent. Cardiac output tends to be elevated, reflecting decreased systemic vascular resistance and increased arteriovenous shunting. Most patients with acute hepatic failure develop a bleeding diathesis resembling disseminated intravascular coagulation. Renal failure, arterial hypoxemia, hypotension, and hepatic encephalopathy accompanied by increased ICP are frequent terminal events. Treatment of acute hepatic failure is symptomatic and supportive including the use of neomycin and/or lactulose to decrease the production of ammonia.

REFERENCES

1. LoSasso AM, Gibbs PS, Moorthy SS. Recognition and management of respiratory failure. In: Stoelting RK, Dierdorf SF, eds. Anesthesia and co-existing disease. New York, Churchill Livingstone 1983;209–215.

2. O'Rourke PP, Crone RK. High frequency ventilation. JAMA 1983;250:2845–7.

3. Suter PM, Fairley HB, Isenberg MD. Optimum end-expiratory airway pressure in patients with acute pulmonary failure. N Engl J Med 1975;292:284–9.

4. Trichet B, Falke K, Togut A, Laver MB. The effect of preexisting pulmonary vascular disease on the response to mechanical ventilation with PEEP following open-heart surgery. Anesthesiology 1975;42:56–67.

5. Smith RA. Respiratory care. In: Miller RD, ed. Anesthesia. New York, Churchill Livingstone 1981;1379–1433.

6. Annest SJ, Gottlieb M, Paloski WH, Stratton H, Newell JC, Dutton R, Powers SR. Detrimental effects of removing end-expiratory pressure prior to endotracheal extubation. Ann Surg 1980;191:539–45.

7. Schumer W. Steroids in the treatment of clinical septic shock. Ann Surg 1976;184:333–9.

8. Sheagren JN. Septic shock and corticosteroids. N Engl J Med 1981;305:456–8.

9. Raymond RM, Harkema JM, Stoffs WV, Emerson TE. Effects of naloxone therapy on hemodynamics and metabolism following a sublethal dosage of Escherichia coli endotoxin in dogs. Surg Gynecol Obstet 1981;52:159–62.

10. Peters WP, Johnson MW, Friedman PA, Mitch WE. Pressor effects of naloxone in septic shock. Lancet 1981;1:529–32.

11. Shapiro HM. Neurosurgical anesthesia and intracranial hypertension. In: Miller RD, ed. Anesthesia. New York, Churchill Livingstone 1981;1079–1132.

12. Defalque RJ, Musunuru VS. Diseases of the nervous system. In: Stoelting RK, Dierdorf SF, eds. Anesthesia and co-existing disease. New York, Churchill Livingstone 1983;239–325.

13. Rockoff MA, Marshall LF, Shapiro HM. High dose barbiturate therapy in humans: a clinical review of 60 patients. Ann Neurol 1979;6:194–9.

14. Miller JD. Barbiturates and raised intracranial pressure. Ann Neurol 1979;6:189–93.

33

Management of Chronic Pain

Ironically, pain which is probably the most common symptom in medicine remains difficult to treat and poorly understood. Although cardiovascular disease and cancer are dramatic and life-threatening diseases, chronic pain can be the cause of months or years of discomfort with a resultant poor quality of life. Furthermore, chronic pain has the potential of interferring with an individual's livelihood and interaction with key people in his or her life, such as family members. Furthermore, although accurate statistics have not been accumulated, chronic pain probably costs society millions of dollars in medical services and loss of work productivity. Often patients are exposed to a high risk of iatrogenic complications from improper therapy, including narcotic addiction or multiple and often unsuccessful surgical procedures. Not surprising, a systematic, organized approach to the proper management of chronic pain rarely exists in the teaching of medical students or clinical practice of physicians.

ROLE OF THE ANESTHESIOLOGIST IN THE DIAGNOSIS AND TREATMENT OF CHRONIC PAIN

Depending on the level of commitment, at one extreme, an anesthesiologist may be a full time member of a pain clinic, or, at the other extreme, he or she may provide occasional diagnostic and therapeutic nerve blocks in the role of a consultant.

Pain Clinic

A pain clinic consists of a group of physicians from different specialties, including anesthesiology, who interact to solve the problem of chronic pain by evaluating the nociceptive and psychological aspects of chronic pain. Anesthesiologists are frequently directors of pain clinics. In such a pain clinic, patients are usually referred from their primary physician. Comprehensive records should be collected which document the activities and pain levels of the patient. When arriving at the pain clinic, patients will be given a conventional medical examination, followed by a psychological examination, in addition to a social worker evaluating and documenting significant social problems. When this information has been collected, the multidisciplinary pain clinic physicians will discuss the case and arrive at an appropriate diagnosis as to the most likely origin of the pain. A decision will then be reached as to what further evaluation or treatment is necessary, such as drug detoxification if drug dependency exists, referral to an orthopedic or neurosurgical physician if neural deficits are present, or performance of a nerve block by an anes-thesiologist.[1,2]

Consultant

The anesthesiologist whose primary com-mitment is in areas other than the diagnosis and treatment of chronic pain may be asked to perform a diagnostic or therapeutic nerve block. Those types of disease processes and nerve blocks with which all anesthesiolo-gists should be familiar are described below. Of prime importance is that the anes-thesiologist recognize his or her limitations. Expertise in performing a diagnostic or therapeutic nerve block in no way means that an equivalent amount of expertise ex-ists in the overall evaluation of chronic pain. For example, has a complete evaluation of a patient who has chronic back pain been performed prior to the epidural injection of steroid? Has a spinal cord tumor been ruled out? Diagnostic and therapeutic nerve blocks should only be performed after a thorough medical evaluation has been per-formed to ensure that some important dis-ease process is not being overlooked.

APPROACH TO THE PATIENT WITH CHRONIC PAIN

The initial contact of the patient with the anesthesiologist is an interview to deter-mine whether a nerve block or other pain-removing procedure will be helpful in the diagnosis or treatment of chronic pain. The interview should be constructed to answer the following types of questions:[1]

1. What has been the duration and con-sistency of pain?
2. What precipitates or exacerbates the pain?
3. How has the patient's daily activity, including his or her work, been altered as a result of the pain?
4. What medication is the patient taking?
5. Is there litigation or some form of fi-nancial compensation that would be lost if the pain were to be removed?

There are guidelines as to how satisfied a patient may be if the pain were removed. Patients who are happily married with ad-equate family support may continue their occupation despite the pain. These same pa-tients who are unhappy taking analgesics and who have had pain for several months, rather than years, are more likely to be mo-tivated to want to remove their pain.

Psychological Tests

Many clinics perform psychological screening tests prior to administration of a diagnostic or therapeutic nerve block. The Minnesota Multiphasic Personality Inven-tory is commonly utilized.[3]

Independent of sophisticated psycholog-ical testing, the clinician must resist the temptation to label patients with chronic pain as "crocks." Patients with chronic pain often are despaired, demoralized, wor-ried, and sometimes hostile. Neurotic be-havior is a natural and normal response to chronic pain. In fact, one may become sus-picious of a patient who has chronic debi-litating pain, and yet appears to be a happy, well-adjusted individual. Patients should not be excluded from treatment because of their personality profiles. Neurotic patients are entitled to the same pain relief as "nor-mal" patients.

Measurement of Pain

Although several methods of measuring pain exist, the "pain estimate" is probably the most useful method for the clinician who occasionally performs diagnostic or thera-peutic nerve blocks. With the pain estimate, the patient assigns a number to the intensity of the pain. The patient is asked to rank the pain on a scale of zero to 100, where "zero" refers to no pain and "100" refers to pain so severe that suicide may be considered. Several numbers may be assigned each day; for example, one number might be the av-erage pain per day, and another number might be the worse pain. Patients can record these numbers before and after a nerve block to assess the magnitude and duration of pain relief.

Physical Examination

A routine physical examination should be performed with special emphasis on a thorough neurological examination. In addition, the following areas require special attention during the physical examination.

Map Out the Painful Area. If the area is not too tender, the painful area can be outlined with a felt-tipped pen. If possible, the painful area should be identified according to the peripheral nerve or dermatome areas.

Skin. The characteristics of the skin often provide a clue as to sympathetic nervous system function. A warm, dry, smooth skin with coarse hair is evidence of vasodilation. Vasoconstricted skin is blanched, clammy, cool, thin and glistening, with thin or sparse hair.

Muscle and Joint. Evidence of guarding, wasting, deformity, swelling, and temperature changes should be noted and will give a clue as to how active a painful area has been. For example, a muscular hand and arm with a preliminary diagnosis of causalgia should be highly suspect because the evidence is that the patient has been using that arm extensively.

Maneuvers which Alter Pain. An assessment of maneuvers which relieve and cause the pain may include locally applied pressure (especially on a trigger point), leg raising to elicit lumbar root irritation, and changes in temperature.

DIAGNOSTIC NERVE BLOCKS

Diagnostic nerve blocks can be utilized to (1) anatomically define the pain pathway, (2) differentiate pharmacologically the size of the fibers that mediate the pain, (3) differentiate central pain from peripheral pain, and (4) determine whether a neurolytic block or surgical resection of a nerve should be performed.

If the specific pathway of pain can be localized, a neurolytic nerve block might be considered. Furthermore, the diagnostic block allows the patient to undergo a "trial run" without permanent change. Sometimes, the numbness or lack of sensation is more unpleasant for the patient than is the pain itself. Also, by utilizing different concentrations of local anesthetics, the size of the nerve fiber mediating the pain can be better defined (e.g., small diameter sympathetic nerve fibers versus larger somatic nerve fibers).

Nerve blocks can sometimes be used to detect drug addiction. If a patient with chronic pain still requires a normal dose of narcotic during the effective period of a successful nerve block, then addiction should be suspected.

Placebo

Placebo injection is the administration of a solution without known analgesia action. For example, a small amount of saline may be injected rather than a local anesthetic for a diagnostic nerve block. A naive clinician might assume that a patient does not have an organic basis for pain if a placebo relieves the discomfort. A placebo, however, may relieve pain 30 to 40 percent of the time in any one patient.[4] Therefore, a patient may have an organic basis for his or her pain, and yet still have partial relief of pain from a placebo injection. Accordingly, interpretation of a placebo response may be difficult, which limits its value to the clinician who occasionally attempts to evaluate the results of a diagnostic nerve block when a placebo has been injected.

Differential Nerve Block

Because fiber size is the primary factor which governs susceptibility of a nerve to be blocked by a local anesthetic, differential nerve blocks can be used to distinguish placebo, sympathetic, and somatic sensory sources of pain. The most common differential nerve block utilized is a graduated spinal block technique.[5] After a lumbar subarachnoid puncture is performed, the following solutions are injected in a four step procedure:

1. Several ml of "artificial cerebrospinal fluid" with no preservatives (placebo).
2. Seven ml of 0.2 percent procaine (sympathetic nerve blockade).
3. Seven ml of 0.5 percent procaine (sensory blockade).
4. Seven ml of 1.0 percent procaine (motor blockade).

Pain is judged to be psychogenic if relief occurs with the placebo injection. If relief occurs with a 0.2 percent procaine injection, a sympathetic nervous system pathway of transmission is usually assigned as the cause. If pain persists after 1.0 percent procaine has been administered, a more central origin, or psychogenic pain, should be considered.

Unfortunately, the differential spinal approach has many drawbacks. A patient cannot move during a differential spinal anesthetic to perform the maneuvers that elicit the pain. Insertion of an epidural catheter may provide more flexibility in this regard. Also, the placebo may itself cause relief of pain of organic basis. Hypotonic solutions injected into the cerebrospinal fluid are known to be able to result in blockade of pain conduction. Thus, a slow withdrawal of cerebrospinal fluid and then reinjection 5 minutes later is a preferable technique. Also, it is assumed is that 0.2 percent procaine only blocks sympathetic nerves without sensory involvement. Although the dominant block probably is sympathetic, sensory fibers are undoubtedly blocked to a limited extent. Thus, if a sympathetic nervous system origin for the pain is suspected, a more specific stellate ganglion or lumbar

sympathetic block can be performed (see Chapter 14).

DIAGNOSTIC AND THERAPEUTIC NERVE BLOCKS

Diagnostic and therapeutic nerve blocks may be performed with local anesthetics, neurolytics, or intraspinal placement of narcotics.

Local Anesthetics

Although nerve blocks with local anesthetics can be very valuable in a diagnostic manner, they also can be used in a therapeutic manner in patients with chronic pain. For example, reflex sympathetic dystrophy can be interrupted with a local anesthetic. Secondly, a temporary local anesthetic-induced nerve block may allow physical therapy to be performed in areas that are normally painful. Thirdly, the inflammatory response can be reduced by a local anesthetic nerve block, usually in combination with a steroid injection. Fourthly, occasionally chronic pain can be relieved with one or more local anesthetic nerve blocks on a prolonged, or even a permanent basis; however, these situations are very rare. Lastly, by performing a sympathetic nerve block with a local anesthetic, vascular supply in an ischemic area in patients with vascular disease can be improved.

Neurolytic

In those patients with persistent chronic pain, nerve destruction with neurolytics such as alcohol, phenol, or ammonium sulfate can be considered. Except for the use of ammonium sulfate in the treatment of intercostal neuralgia, the use of alcohol or phenol probably should be restricted to clinicians with special expertise and experience in the injection of these drugs. Furthermore, the use of neurolytics probably is only indicated in those patients with short life expectancy, such as those individuals with pain from terminal cancer. The use of alcohol or phenol on peripheral nerves is frequently followed by the appearance of a denervation hypersensitivity type of pain, which may be worse than the original pain. For this reason, injection of alcohol and phenol probably should be restricted to the epidural or subarachnoid space. Generally, alcohol is very painful during injection, but within a few minutes, produces neurolysis. On the other hand, phenol, usually mixed in saline or glycerine, takes several hours for its anesthetic effect to manifest.

One problem with neurolytics is that alcohol or phenol rarely produce as intense an analgesic state as did the diagnostic local anesthetic block. Therefore, patients are frequently disappointed that the neurolytic block has not produced as much pain relief as did the diagnostic local anesthetic block. The patient should, therefore, be cautioned about the effectiveness of a neurolytic block. Furthermore, "permanent" neurolytic blocks are really not permanent, and recovery of sensation of pain occurs in a matter of weeks or months, emphasizing their usefulness in patients with a short life expectancy. Furthermore, because neurolytics destroy surrounding tissue as well as the nerve, they should be injected in a very discriminating and accurate manner to avoid excessive tissue damage.

For somatic nerve blocks, 100 percent alcohol is utilized. For blockade of sympathetic nerves (e.g., those with a smaller diameter), 50 percent alcohol in saline can be used. Phenol is used in concentrations ranging from 5 to 20 percent for peripheral nerves. Ammonium sulfate is not as powerful a neurolytic as are alcohol or phenol. Accordingly, the success of analgesia with this drug is less, but the incidence of complications is also less. Basically, ammonium sulfate dehydrates the smaller diameter C fibers, while leaving the larger A and B fibers untouched. Therefore, if the pain is from the smaller diameter C fibers, ammonium sulfate will be effective, whereas with the larger somatic fibers, it will be ineffective.

Intraspinal Narcotics

Because of opiate receptors in the substantia gelatinosa of the spinal cord, very small doses of intraspinal narcotics (morphine, meperidine, fentanyl) administered into the subarachnoid or epidural space provide effective analgesia of sustained duration.[6,7] For example, morphine can produce long-lasting analgesia (6 to 24 hours) when administered into the subarachnoid (0.5 to 2 mg) or epidural (2 to 5 mg) space of an adult patient. This approach has been utilized most often in patients with acute postoperative pain, including that following cardiothoracic surgery and cesarean delivery.

The primary complication of this approach when used to treat acute postoperative pain is delayed depression of ventilation. The onset of ventilatory depression is typically from 1 to 10 hours after intraspinal administration of even low doses of narcotics. Based on carbon dioxide response curves, Kafer et al.[8] believe morphine administered into the epidural space causes early depression of ventilation (e.g., 1 to 2 hours) by absorption into the epidural veins and redistribution to the brain. Later depression (e.g., 6 to 10 hours) is a result of a cephalad movement of morphine in the cerebrospinal fluid such that vital medullary centers are bathed with narcotic. Whatever the cause, any patient who receives an epidural or subarachnoid administration of narcotics should be observed for at least 24 hours for signs of depression of ventilation.[9] Also, a small dose of naloxone (0.1 mg/70 kg) can be given intravenously to attenuate depression of ventilation, often without interferring with analgesia. Other complications of intraspinal narcotics include sedation, nausea and vomiting, pruritus, and urinary retention.[9] Interestingly, the pruritus can be relieved by the administration of naloxone.

Chronic pain has also been treated by subarachnoid or epidural administration of narcotics. Because relief of pain is usually less than 2 days, it is cumbersome to repetitively have to perform a spinal or epidural injection. Coombs et al.[10] have described the use of an implanted infusion device, which consists of a percutaneously-refillable reservoir for a narcotic and a mechanism for pumping the narcotic from the reservoir through the catheter into the subarachnoid or epidural space. This is still in an experimental stage, but if successful, will allow the continuous administration of narcotic for an extended period of time. Unfortunately, progressive tolerance to morphine develops when subarachnoid morphine has been administered over a 5 to 9 day period. Still, if these and other problems can be solved, the subarachnoid or epidural administration of narcotics may be a useful tool in the treatment of chronic pain.

EVALUATION OF A NERVE BLOCK

Especially to the clinician who only infrequently interacts with a patient with chronic pain, caution should be applied to the evaluation of a diagnostic and/or therapeutic nerve block. In fact, evaluation of a patient's physiologic and psychologic responses to a nerve block is often more difficult than the technical procedure required to produce the block. For example, the use of a local anesthetic block to predict the success of a neurolytic block or surgical resection of a nerve is difficult. To assume that if the diagnostic block relieves the pain, then a neurolytic block or a surgical resection certainly will be successful is incorrect. As indicated previously, local anesthetic blocks frequently produce a more intense relief of pain than neurolytics. Furthermore, if a surgical procedure is performed, the pain may return, either due to regeneration of the nerve or a denervation hypersensitivity type of reaction. Also, even though diagnostic nerve blocks allow the

patient to experience the numbness and side effects that could be permanent from nerve abelation techniques, they are not always accurate predictors of long term pain relief. For example, diagnostic nerve blocks provide little help in evaluating the influence of pain relief on psychological factors, such as family interactions and financial gain (e.g., litigation).

Evaluation of results from a therapeutic nerve block requires more thorough questioning than "Is your pain gone?" The following questions and list should be provided for the patient. First, the frequency and intensity of the pain should be recorded, including the number of hours in bed and the number of hours spent standing and reclining daily. The patient should record his or her estimate as to the ability to walk, bend, and work. Perhaps 20 to 30 activities (e.g., making the bed, washing the car) can be performed before and after a nerve block. Furthermore, the influence on recreational and social activities should be documented. Lastly, and perhaps most importantly, an accurate list of medications taken daily should be made. It is only after evaluation of this kind of record that the true effectiveness of this kind of nerve block can be evaluated.

COMMON PAIN PROBLEMS ALL ANESTHESIOLOGISTS SHOULD BE ABLE TO MANAGE

Although the clinician should refer most chronic pain problems to physicians who are involved with pain clinics on a full time basis, there are few pain problems with which all anesthesiologists should be capable of managing, at least in the initial stages of diagnosis and/or treatment.

Causalgia and Reflex Sympathetic Dystrophy

Causalgia occurs after nerve injury while reflex sympathetic dystrophy typically follows a trivial injury without apparent neurologic damage. Often, however, these terms are used interchangeably. Both are accompanied by similar manifestations which include chronic, severe burning pain, localized autonomic nervous system dysfunction, and atrophic changes. In addition, the pain is characterized as aching, intense, and/or agonizing and is usually enhanced by mechanical stimulation, movement, and application of heat or cold. Initially, vascular changes, probably resulting from altered sympathetic nervous system activity, lead to a warm, red, dry, swollen extremity. Later, the extremity will be cool, pale and/or cyanotic, and there will be atrophy of the skin, muscle, and decreased density of bones.

The diagnosis can be established and treatment initiated by performing a stellate ganglion block for causalgia of the upper extremity, or a lumbar sympathetic block for causalgia of the lower extremity (see Chapter 14). If sympathetic nerve blockade clearly produces relief of pain, then the diagnosis of causalgia is established.

Hopefully, the duration of pain relief will exceed the expected duration of local anesthetic action when performing a sympathetic block. Furthermore, subsequent blocks may provide progressively longer pain-free intervals. Up to five to seven stellate ganglion or lumbar sympathetic nerve blocks can be performed on alternate days with the hope that ultimately a prolonged period of pain relief will result, lasting several weeks or months.

Hannington-Kiff[11] has reported dramatic relief of pain and increase in skin temperature in several patients in whom sympathetic nerve blockade was performed by infusing a sympatholytic drug intravenously into an extremity isolated from the general circulation by a tourniquet. Specifically, guanethidine, 10 to 20 mg, or reserpine, 1 to 2 mg in 20 to 25 ml of normal saline, is injected through an indwelling needle into the extremity. The extremity is isolated from the circulation for 10 minutes to allow the binding of guanethidine or reserpine to the tissues. Then the tourniquet is slowly released. This intravenous regional sympathetic nerve block technique is utilized most often when stellate ganglion or lumbar sympathetic blocks have been ineffective. Furthermore, this approach appears to be useful in a patient who shows signs of returning sympathetic nervous system tone, despite apparently adequate surgical excision of the sympathetic ganglia.

Less common forms of therapy include physiotherapy, periodic perineural infiltration, surgical sympathectomy, and the oral administration of sympatholytics, such as guanethidine or propranolol.

Chronic Back Pain

Chronic back pain represents a significant health problem, with various conservative and surgical treatments frequently being ineffective. The result is chronic pain, loss of productivity, and occasionally disability. Patients who have a lumbar radiculopathy usually have pain as a result of inflammation of the nerve root or through compression of the dorsal root ganglion. Pain arising from inflammation surrounding the nerve root is frequently responsive to the epidural administration of steroids such as methylprednisolone. Before proceeding with this treatment, it is mandatory to rule out the presence of infection or a space occupying lesion. Lastly, an epidural injection of steroids should not be performed until a careful diagnostic evaluation (including consultation with a neurosurgeon or an orthopedic surgeon) has been performed and the patient is advised of the possible benefits and complications of a steroid injection, including the distinct possibility that no relief from the injection may occur. All information given and received should be recorded in the patient's chart.

Our technique is to place the patient in the lateral position and then, after a test dose of local anesthetic, 8 to 12 ml of 1 percent lidocaine (other local anesthetics could be used) is injected. The local anesthetic is injected to provide temporary relief of pain and to confirm that the tip of the needle is in the epidural space. Then, methylprednisolone, 80 to 100 mg, is injected. The patient is asked to remain in the lateral position for 15 minutes. If the radicular pain has been present for more than 6 months, the success of epidural steroids is markedly decreased. This is probably due to proliferation of scar and fibrous tissue around the damaged tissue surrounding the nerve root. Although epidural injection, either through the lumbar or caudal approach is most common, subarachnoid administration of steroids may be indicated for pantopaque arachnoiditis. Steroids with little or no neurolytic preservations should be used for subarachnoid injection.

Chymopapain is used for chemonucleolysis of herniated lumbar discs. In those patients in whom bed rest, analgesics, and heat have been ineffective, injection of chymopapain into the core of a herniated disc has led to 60 to 80 percent relief of pain. The primary problem with this approach is life-threatening allergic reactions in 0.5 to 1 percent of treated patients (Moss J et al. Boston MA, personal communication). Severe hypotension is the most common manifestation of an allergic reaction. Whether chymopapain injection is performed under local or general anesthesia, it is recomended that patients should receive cimetidine and diphenhydramine preoperatively so as to reduce the cardiopulmonary effects of histamine should an allergic reaction occur. Furthermore, monitoring of cardiopulmonary function should be such that rapid detection of signs of an allergic reaction are possible. A life-threatening allergic reaction may require treatment with intravenous epinephrine (0.1 to 0.3 mg).[12]

Intercostal Neuralgia

Intercostal neuralgia, following thoracotomy or rib fracture, is characterized by paresthesias and pain in response to touch or movement of the thorax. Although the pain usually subsides within 2 weeks, it can persist for several months or years, requiring active treatment. In most cases, destructive nerve blocks with alcohol or phenol, or surgical removal of a neuroma or rhizotomy offer little help. Alcohol or phenol injections are usually followed by a 10 to 50 percent incidence of post-block neuritis, in which the pain is worse than before the block. One approach is to perform local anesthetic intercostal or paravertebral nerve blocks. During the pain-free time, physical therapy can be performed. Repeated efforts of this kind occasionally will result in prolonged relief of pain. In severe cases, 10 percent ammonium sulfate has been used. While this is not effective in all cases, ammonium sulfate is not associated with complications, such as post-block neuritis.[13]

Posthepetic Neuralgia

Following an acute infection of herpes zoster, a syndrome called "posthepatic neuralgia" can exist for an extended period of time especially in elderly patients. Following the acute infective period in which the cutaneous lesions gradually disappear in 2 to 4 weeks, the pain usually subsides. Pain and scarring, however, may persist. Local anesthetic, alcohol and phenol intercostal nerve blocks are not predictably effective in relieving the pain. Early cases (less than 3 months) sometimes can be effectively treated with sympathetic nerve blocks with local anesthetic. Oral administration of a phenothiazine (fluphenazine) and a tricyclic antidepressant (amitriptyline) can occasionally relieve the pain. In elderly patients, however, complications such as postural hypotension can occur following the use of these drugs. Also, patients may become sleepy and loose their appetite, leading to increasing debilitation. Another approach has been the subcutaneous intralesional injection of a local anesthetic and steroids. Specifically, 20 to 30 ml of a solution of triamcinolone (2 mg/ml) and bupivacaine (0.25 percent) is injected, under the painful skin area. Although several clinicians are enthusiastic about this approach, our experience is that this has produced limited success. Hopefully, through the intralesional administration of steroids and local anesthetics, the epidural administration of steroids, sympathetic nerve blocks, and oral administration of the drugs indicated above, relief can be obtained. The approach is one of trial and error, of which the anesthesiologist can be a vital participant.

Myofascial Pain Syndrome

Many chronic pain states of obscure origin depend on feedback cycles from myofascial trigger points. The trigger point concept has been difficult for many physicians to accept, because the precise neuroanatomic connections between the trigger point and the pain are not understood. The clinician should always examine a patient with chronic pain for the possibility of a "trigger point." There often are multiple painful areas with multiple trigger points in the same patient. On examination of such patients, the painful muscular areas have been described as feeling like a rope. A positive "jump sign" has been described, whereby the trigger area is palpated, and the patient "jumps away" from the pain. Detection of a trigger point to palpation makes it relatively easy for a successful treatment regime to be instituted. For example, topical application of a vapor coolant and a follow-up of the localized analgetic effect with active and passive physiotherapy can be useful. Also, weak local anesthetic concentrations, such as 0.5 percent lidocaine or 0.25 percent bupivacaine, can be injected into the trigger point. By including a small dose of steroid with the local anesthetic mixture, more extended relief of pain can sometimes result.

SUMMARY

The use of nerve blocks in the diagnosis and therapy of chronic pain is an area where the anesthesiologist may be particularly helpful in the overall treatment of a patient. Use of a nerve block, however, represents only one of several approaches in dealing with a patient with chronic pain. Other areas, such as behavioral analysis, operant conditioning, biofeedback, transcutaneous nerve stimulation, acupuncture, neurosurgical techniques, such as percutaneous cordotomy, thermocoagulation of neural elements and alcohol injection of the pituitary, are examples of the additional approaches that can also be used in the treatment of chronic pain.

REFERENCES

1. Murphy TM. Treatment of chronic pain. In: Miller RD, ed. Anesthesia, New York, Churchill Livingstone 1981;1459–91.
2. Bonica JJ. Organization and function of a pain clinic. Adv Neur 1974;4:433–43.
3. Sternbach RA, Wolf SR, Murphy RW, Akeson WH. Traits of pain in patients: The low back looser. Psychosomatics 1973;14:226–9.
4. Taub A. Factors in the diagnosis and treatment of chronic pain. J Autism Child Schizophr 1975;5:1–12.
5. Miller RD, Munger WL, Power PE. Chronic pain and local anesthetic neural blockade. In: Cousins MJ, Bridenbaugh PO, eds. Neural blockade. Philadelphia, JB Lippincott Co 1981;616–37.
6. Stoelting RK. Opiate receptors and endorphins: Their role in anesthesiology. Anesth Analg 1980;59:874–80.
7. Wang JK, Naus LA, Thomas JE. Pain relief by intrathecally applied morphine in man. Anesthesiology 1979;50:149–51.
9. Kafer ER, Brown JT, Scott D, Findley JWA, Butz RF, Teeple E, Ghia JN. Biphasic depression of ventilatory response to CO_2 following epidural morphine. Anesthesiology 1983;58:418–27.
10. Coombs DW, Saunders RL, Gaylor MS, Pageau MG. Epidural narcotic infusion reservoir: Implantation techniques and efficacy. Anesthesiology 1982;56:469–73.

11. Hannington-Kiff G. Intravenous regional sympathetic block with guanethidine. Lancet 1974;1:1019–20.

12. Stoelting RK. Allergic reactions during anesthesia. Anesth Analg 1983;62:341–56.

13. Miller RD, Johnston RR, Hosobuchi Y. Treatment of intercostal neuralgia with 10 percent ammonium sulfate. J Thorac Cardiovas Surg 1975;69:476–8.

34

Cardiopulmonary Resuscitation

Cardiopulmonary resuscitation (CPR) applies many of the skills unique to the practice of anesthesiology. As a result, anesthesiologists are involved in the provision and teaching of all aspects of CPR (Table 34-1). Furthermore, new advances and concepts in CPR often reflect basic research by anesthesiologists.

CPR is categorized as Basic Life Support (BLS) and Advanced Cardiac Life Support (ACLS). BLS consists of provision of a patent upper airway (A-airway), exhaled air ventilation (B-breathing) and circulation of blood by closed chest cardiac compression (C-circulation). The A,B,C's of BLS may be instituted by trained lay persons as well as physicians without the need for specialized equipment. ACLS includes use of specialized equipment to maintain the airway, external defibrillation, drug therapy, and postresuscitation management. The highest survival rates as well as quality of survival are attained when BLS is initiated within 4 minutes from the time of cardiac arrest and when ACLS is initiated within 8 minutes.[1]

PROVISION OF A PATENT UPPER AIRWAY

Methods to provide a patent upper airway following a cardiac arrest are designed to relieve obstruction due to the tongue falling against the posterior pharynx. Extension of the head and displacement of the mandible anteriorly serves to stretch the muscles attached to the tongue and thus pull the tongue off the posterior pharynx. This maneuver is known as the head tilt-jaw thrust method and is identical to the recommended procedure for securing a patent airway in the patient rendered unconscious by anesthetic drugs (Fig. 34-1).[2] The jaw-thrust maneuver without head tilt is the recommended method for opening the upper airway in a victim with a suspected neck injury.

EXHALED AIR VENTILATION

Exhaled air ventilation (mouth-to-mouth) when performed properly provides adequate alveolar ventilation. However, the delivered oxygen concentration using this technique is only 16 to 17 percent such that the maximum alveolar PO_2 obtainable is predictably less than 80 mmHg. The arterial PO_2 will be even lower (e.g., arterial hypoxemia is predictable), reflecting increased venous admixture and low cardiac output present during CPR. Gastric distension often accompanies exhaled air ventilation particularly if high airway pressures due to an incompletely patent upper airway are required. Even with a patent upper air-

Table 34-1. Comparative Resuscitation Techniques

	Infant	Child (1 to 8 years old)	Adult
Ventilation method	Mouth-to-mouth and nose	Mouth-to-mouth and nose Mouth-to-mouth	Mouth-to-mouth
Ventilation rate	20/min	15/min	12/min
Check for pulse	Brachial artery at mid-forearm	Carotid artery	Carotid artery
Sternal depression method	Encircle chest with both hands and depress midsternum with thumbs	Depress sternum with three fingers	Depress sternum with heel of hand on lower third of sternum
Sternal depression depth	1.25 to 2.5 cm	2.5 to 3.5 cm	3.5 to 5 cm
Sternal depression rate	100/min	80/min	60/min
Sternal depression to ventilation ratio	5:1	5:1	15:2 if one rescuer 5:1 if two rescuers
Management of an obstructed upper airway due to a foreign body	Back blows followed by chest (not abdominal) thrust Finger probe under vision if unconscious	Same as infant	Back blows followed by abdominal or chest thrust Blind finger probe if unconscious

way, some gas is likely to enter the stomach when inflation pressures exceed 15 cm H_2O. Manual pressure applied over the victim's epigastrium to relieve gastric distension is not recommended, as this maneuver is likely to produce regurgitation of gastric contents.[3] Nevertheless, gastric distension that impairs ventilation of the lungs must be relieved by any method available including manual pressure over the epigastrium.

CLOSED CHEST CARDIAC COMPRESSION

Optimal blood flow produced by closed chest cardiac compression depends on the proper placement of the rescuer's hands on the victim's sternum, the position of the rescuer's body in relation to the victim, and the depth and the rate of depression of the sternum.

The heel of the rescuer's hand is placed over and parallel to the lower third of the adult victim's sternum so as to provide maximum compression of the underlying car-

diac ventricles (Fig. 34-2).[2] Pressure over the xyphoid process or rib cage must be avoided so as to minimize the likelihood of damage to abdominal organs, particularly the liver, or the production of rib fractures with damage to the heart and lungs. The rescuer should kneel next to the victim so that the upper body is over the victim's chest. The rescuer's elbows are kept straight and the shoulders positioned directly over the hands. This position enables the rescuer to use the weight of the upper body for compression which must depress the sternum of an adult victim 3.5 to 5 cm. Relaxation on the sternum must be complete at the end of each compression to permit the heart to fill. The rescuer's hands, however, must maintain contact with the victim's sternum or correct hand position may be lost. Optimum carotid blood flow occurs when the duration of sternal depression is 50 to 60 percent of the cycle length. When this ratio is maintained, systolic blood pressure and carotid blood flow produced by a sternal depression rate of 40/min

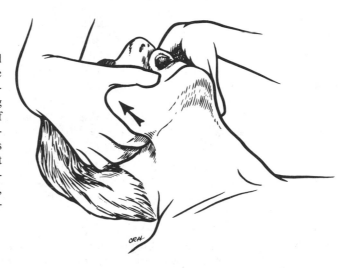

Figure 34-1. Extension of the head and displacement of the mandible anteriorly stretches the muscles attached to the tongue. Stretching these muscles pulls the tongue off the posterior pharynx creating a patent upper airway. This maneuver is known as the head tilt-jaw thrust method (Donegan JH. Cardiopulmonary resuscitation. In: Miller RD, ed. Anesthesia. New York, Churchill Livingstone 1981;1493–1529.

are not significantly different from those obtained at a depression rate of 60 to 80/min. Achievement of the proper ratio of compression time to relaxation time requires a pause at the point of maximal sternal depression. This is the reason for avoidance of quick, bouncing compressions. When a single rescuer is present, external cardiac compression and exhaled air ventilation are provided at a compression-to-breath ratio of 15:2 each minute. When two rescuers are available, the compression rate is 60/min and a breath is delivered during the upstroke of every fifth compression (a ratio of 5:1). The 15:2 or 5:1 ratio, depending on the number of rescuers, has become standard technique.[3]

Variations on the conventional techniques of CPR are being studied. For example, compared with the standard ratios, systolic blood pressure and carotid blood flow are increased when sternal depression is combined with simultaneous ventilation of the lungs using airway pressures of 60 to

Figure 34-2. Correct hand placement for external cardiac compression in an adult. The heel of one of the rescuer's hands is placed on and parallel to the lower third of the victim's sternum. The other hand of the rescuer is placed on top of the hand on the victim's sternum. The fingers of the hands are interlaced and held up off the chest (Donegan JH. Cardiopulmonary resuscitation. In: Miller RD, ed. Anesthesia. New York, Churchill Livingstone 1981; 1493–1529).

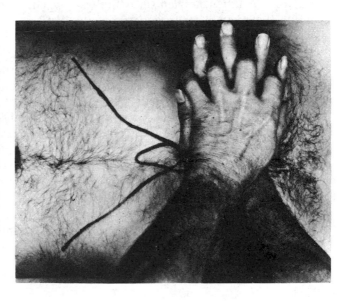

110 cm H_2O.[4] This technique has been termed "new CPR." In another report, the use of positive end-expiratory pressure (PEEP) improved oxygenation and ventilation but decreased systolic blood pressure and carotid blood flow.[5] Furthermore, even low levels of PEEP are hazardous in the presence of hypovolemia. The use of PEEP should not be confused with "new CPR" in which positive airway pressure is applied only during sternal depression and not during the relaxation phase. Finally, a technique which utilized the standard ratio but interposes abdominal compression between sternal depression has been shown to increase systolic blood pressure and cardiac output compared to techniques not utilizing alternating chest and abdominal compression.[6]

The mechanism responsible for blood flow during closed chest compression is traditionally attributed to compression of the cardiac ventricles between the sternum and the spine. In addition, the increase in intrathoracic pressure that results from depression of the sternum is important for producing antegrade flow. Conceptually, the heart is like a balloon in a closed box such that increases in intrathoracic pressure squeeze blood from the heart. Indirect evidence for this latter mechanism is the observation that patients who develop acute ventricular fibrillation remain conscious for a few seconds if they cough repeatedly.[7]

The potential exists for increases in intrathoracic pressure produced by CPR to elicit elevations in intracranial pressure (ICP), particularly in patients with co-existing decreases in intracranial compliance. If this is true, cerebral perfusion pressure (blood pressure minus ICP) may remain low despite apparently adequate CPR as reflected by systolic blood pressure. Indeed, data suggest that CPR is of limited effectiveness in providing cerebral blood flow.[8] Consistent with this observation is the extremely poor neurologic prognosis if adequate spontaneous cardiovascular function is not achieved within 15 minutes despite apparently adequate CPR.

SPECIALIZED EQUIPMENT TO MAINTAIN THE AIRWAY

Adjuncts for use in airway management are designed to assure control of the airway, improve ventilation and oxygenation, and isolate the trachea from the gastrointestinal tract. A pocket face mask is the simplest advancement beyond mouth-to-mouth ventilation. Exhaled air ventilation may be provided via this mask. Alternatively, a reservoir bag with a one-way valve may be attached to this mask to permit manual ventilation of the lungs. Another advantage of a reservoir bag is the ability to deliver oxygen for ventilation of the lungs. For example, a 10 L/min flow of oxygen will provide an inhaled oxygen concentration of about 50 percent. Finally, this mask should be transparent so that regurgitated gastric contents may be recognized promptly.

The best method for maintenance of a patent upper airway is placement of a cuffed tube in the trachea using direct laryngoscopy. This tracheal tube permits optimal adjustment of tidal volume and respiratory rate, reliable addition of supplemental oxygen to the inhaled gases, and, when the cuff is inflated with air, to provide a seal against the tracheal mucosa protection of the lungs from inhalation of gastric contents. An alternative to placement of a cuffed tube in the trachea is blind insertion of a solid cuffed tube known as an esophageal obturator airway (EOA) into the esophagus (Fig. 34-3A).[2] Inflation of the cuff on the EOA with 30 ml of air occludes the esophagus to reduce the likelihood of gastric regurgitation into the pharynx while openings in the proximal end of the tube, which remains in the pharynx, are a route for administration of oxygen and ventilation of the lungs. The length of the EOA has been standardized so insertion into the esophagus of an adult until the mask rests

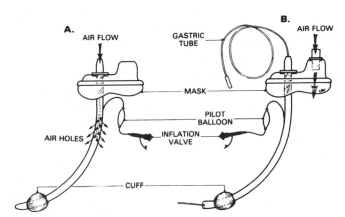

Figure 34-3. The esophageal obturator airway (EOA) (A) is an alternative to placement of a cuffed tube in the trachea. This airway is inserted blindly into the esophagus by lifting the tongue and mandible forward and inserting the obturator airway along the posterior wall of the pharynx. Inflation of the distal cuff with air occludes the esophagus while openings (air holes) in the proximal end of the tube which is in the pharynx are a route for administration of oxygen and ventilation of the lungs. The esophageal gastric tube airway (EGTA) (B) incorporates a lumen that allows passage of a gastric tube so as to permit the application of negative pressure to the stomach without interfering with ventilation of the lungs (Donegan JH. Cardiopulmonary resuscitation. In: Miller RD, ed. Anesthesia. New York, Churchill Livingstone 1981;1493–1529).

properly on the victim's face will result in positioning of the esophageal cuff below the carina. Thus, when the cuff is inflated with the proper amount of air, it will not compress the posterior membranous wall of the trachea. The major hazard of the EOA is esophageal perforation. In addition, regurgitation invariably follows removal of the EOA emphasizing the need to have a cuffed tube in the trachea prior to extubation of the esophagus. A modification of the EOA incorporates a lumen (esophageal gastric tube airway, EGTA) through which a gastric tube can be passed and the stomach suctioned without interfering with ventilation of the lungs (Fig. 34-3B).[2]

Mechanical ventilators are not reliably effective during CPR. For example, pressure-cycled ventilators will prematurely cease to deliver gas flow when the sternum is depressed while volume-cycled ventilators will not be able to deliver a reliable tidal volume during this time. Alternatively, manually triggered oxygen-powered breathing devices are available for ventilation of the lungs via a face mask, tracheal tube, or esophageal airways. Using these devices, the instantaneous development of a high flow rate of oxygen (100 L/min and maximum pressure of 50 cm H_2O) by manual depression of the control button allows the rescuer to interpose breaths at the desired time during external cardiac compression.

EXTERNAL DEFIBRILLATION

External defibrillation is the definitive treatment of ventricular fibrillation. The most important determinant of the success of external defibrillation is the length of the interval from cardiac arrest to application of countershock.[1] Current recommendations are to apply external defibrillation as soon as ventricular fibrillation is identified for the monitored patient or the victim who has been in cardiac arrest for less than 2 minutes.[3] When cardiac arrest has been present for an undetermined period, the recommendation is to apply BLS for 2 minutes followed by external defibrillation. The initial energy level setting on the external defibrillator for delivery to an adult regardless of body weight is 200 to 300 joules using paddles greater than 8 cm in diameter. If this initial attempt is unsuccessful, a second attempt should be made utilizing the same energy setting, remembering that thoracic impedance decreases after the first shock such that a second attempt at the same energy level will deliver the same or even more current to the heart than with the first attempt. It is important to minimize the current delivered to the heart to reduce the likelihood of damage to the myocardium. If more than two attempts at external defibrillation are required, it is important to continue BLS and precede the third attempt at external defibrillation with supplemental oxygen, intravenous epinephrine, and sodium bicarbonate. In addition, the energy setting for the third and subsequent attempts at external defibrillation should be increased to 360 joules.

DRUG THERAPY

Goals of drug therapy during CPR include (1) treatment of arterial hypoxemia with oxygen, (2) increase of perfusion pressure and myocardial contractility with epinephrine, and (3) reversal of metabolic acidosis with sodium bicarbonate (Table 34-2). Recurrent or persistent ventricular fibrillation despite external defibrillation may be treated with lidocaine, procainamide, or bretylium. A persistent slow heart rate following successful external defibrillation may require administration of atropine or isoproterenol.

The preferred route of administration of these drugs is intravenously. Drugs including epinephrine, lidocaine, atropine, and isoproterenol, however, are absorbed from the tracheobronchial tree after injection via a tracheal tube. The effectiveness of tracheal absorption emphasizes the importance of early intubation of the trachea, as this procedure can often be accomplished more rapidly than the placement of a catheter in a vein.

Epinephrine

Epinephrine is effective in the treatment of cardiac arrest because this drug produces peripheral vasoconstriction. As a result, external cardiac compression produces increased blood pressure. The increased perfusion pressure leads to improved

Table 34-2. Drug Therapy During CPR

Drug	Indications	Dose
Oxygen	Hypoxemia	100
Epinephrine	Ventricular fibrillation Cardiac asystole Electromechanical dissociation	5 µg/kg IV 1 mg in 10 ml trachael tube (TT)
Sodium bicarbonate	Metabolic acidosis	1 mEq/kg IV initially 0.5 mEq/kg IV every 15 minutes of continued cardiac arrest or as dictated by pHa
Lidocaine	Recurrent or refractory ventricular fibrillation Ventricular tachycardia	1 mg/kg IV or TT, then continuous IV infusion of 15 to 60 µg/kg/min (1 to 4 mg/min to a 70 kg adult)
Procainamide	When lidocaine not effective	1.5 mg/kg IV over 5 minutes not to exceed 1 g in an adult
Bretylium	When lidocaine and procainamide not effective	5 mg/kg IV every 5 minutes not to exceed 30 mg/kg in an adult
Atropine	Bradycardia Third degree atrioventricular heart block Cardiac asystole	70 µg/kg IV or TT not to exceed 3 mg in an adult
Isoproterenol	When atropine not effective	0.03 µg to 0.3 µg/kg/min (2 to 20 µg/min to a 70 kg adult)
Calcium chloride	Cardiac asystole Electromechanical dissociation	5 to 10 mg/kg IV

myocardial blood flow. Evidence of improved myocardial blood flow and myocardial oxygenation is conversion of fine ventricular fibrillation to coarse ventricular fibrillation as manifested on the electrocardiogram (ECG). Coarse ventricular fibrillation reflects a well-oxygenated myocardium which is more susceptible than fine ventricular fibrillation to termination with external defibrillation.

Ideally, epinephrine is administered intravenously in a dose of 5 µg/kg. Epinephrine may also be given via the tracheal tube but the systemic blood level achieved is only about one-tenth that achieved with intravenous injection.[2] Intracardiac injection of epinephrine is recommended only when the intravenous or tracheal route are not available. Hazards of intracardiac injection of epinephrine include pneumothorax, coronary artery laceration, cardiac tamponade, and interruption of external cardiac compression. Furthermore, inadvertent injection of the epinephrine into the cardiac muscle can produce intractable ventricular fibrillation.

Sodium Bicarbonate

Accumulation of lactic acid and the development of metabolic acidosis during cardiac arrest reflects anaerobic metabolism due to arterial hypoxemia. At the same time, respiratory acidosis may be superimposed on metabolic acidosis if elimination of carbon dioxide is impaired by inadequate alveolar ventilation. Adverse effects of acidosis include (1) depression of myocardial contractility, (2) suppression of spontaneous cardiac activity, (3) reduced threshold for ventricular fibrillation, and (4) impaired cardiac responsiveness to catecholamines.

Treatment of respiratory acidosis is increased alveolar ventilation, while metabolic acidosis is best treated by the intravenous administration of sodium bicarbonate. Sodium bicarbonate buffers the hydrogen ion of lactic acid, ultimately resulting in the formation of carbon dioxide and water. Alveolar ventilation must be adequate to remove the additional carbon dioxide formed by this reaction. Ideally, the administration of sodium bicarbonate is guided by measurement of arterial pH (pHa). Indeed, pHa can be kept within acceptable limits during CPR by providing adequate alveolar ventilation assuming metabolic acidosis did not exist prior to cardiac arrest. When pHa measurements are not available, sodium bicarbonate should be administered initially in a dose of 1 mEq/kg followed by 0.5 mEq/kg every 15 minutes if cardiac arrest persists. Adverse effects of excessive administration of sodium bicarbonate include (1) hypercarbia, (2) hypernatremia, (3) hyperosmolarity, and (4) metabolic alkalosis.

Lidocaine

The rapid onset and absence of adverse effects on myocardial contractility or conduction of the cardiac impulse make lidocaine the drug of choice for suppression of ventricular dysrhythmias in patients with refractory or recurrent ventricular tachycardia or fibrillation. Lidocaine may suppress ventricular dysrhythmias by (1) slowing the rate of spontaneous depolarization to decrease automaticity, (2) elevating the fibrillation threshold, (3) inhibition of reentry pathways. Prevention of re-entry is probably the most important mechanism by which lidocaine prevents ventricular dysrhythmias. It should be appreciated that administration of lidocaine to a patient with third degree atrioventricular heart block is hazardous, as drug-induced suppression of the ectopic ventricular pacemaker could cause ventricular arrest.

Therapeutic blood levels of lidocaine (1.5 to 6 µg/ml) are most predictably obtained with an initial rapid intravenous injection of 1 mg/kg followed by a continuous infusion of 15 to 60 µg/kg/min. Lidocaine is metabolized by the liver and its rate of metabolism is dependent on hepatic blood flow. When an intravenous route of administration is not immediately available, it should be remembered that lidocaine injected via a tracheal tube will undergo significant systemic absorption from the tracheobronchial mucosa.

Procainamide

Procainamide may be effective in suppressing ventricular ectopy when lidocaine is not effective. Phase 4 depolarization is slowed and re-entry pathways are blocked but, unlike lidocaine, this drug depresses interventricular conduction of the cardiac impulse. The dose of procainamide is 1.5 mg/kg intravenously over 5 minutes until the ventricular dysrhythmia is suppressed or signs of toxicity (hypotension, widening of the QRS on the ECG) occur. The maximum recommended dose of procainamide is 1 gram.

Bretylium

Bretylium is indicated for treatment of (1) refractory ventricular dysrhythmias unresponsive to lidocaine or procainamide and (2) persistent ventricular defibrillation despite multiple attempts at external defibrillation. This drug has effects on the autonomic nervous system (stimulation of norepinephrine release) and cell membranes (elevation of the ventricular fibrillation threshold, increased duration of the cardiac action potential, and prolonged effective refractory period). Prolongation of the cardiac action potential and effective refractory period of normal cardiac muscle makes it less likely that irritable foci in ischemic myocardium will initiate reentry circuits. Bretylium, in contrast to lidocaine or procainamide, does not slow phase 4 depolarization.

The initial intravenous dose of bretylium is 5 mg/kg infused over 5 minutes followed by attempted external defibrillation. If ventricular fibrillation persists, additional doses can be administered every 15 to 30 minutes to a total dose not to exceed 30 mg/kg to an adult. Bretylium can also be administered as a continuous intravenous infusion at a rate of 1 to 2 mg/min. An adverse effect of bretylium is hypotension, presumably due to block of the sympathetic nervous system. The dose of bretylium should be reduced in patients with severe renal disease, since most of this drug is excreted unchanged by the kidneys.

Atropine

Atropine is the initial drug for treatment of hemodynamically significant bradycardia or atrioventricular heart block. The parasympatholytic action of atropine is responsible for acceleration of conduction of the cardiac impulse through the atrioventricular node. Atropine 70 μg/kg should be given intravenously every 5 minutes until the desired heart rate is achieved or until a total dose of 3.0 mg has been administered. Single doses of less than 70 μg/kg may accentuate heart rate slowing as a result of atropine-induced peripheral and/or central vagal stimulation. Atropine is also absorbed into the systemic circulation when administered via the tracheal tube into the trachea.

Isoproterenol

Isoproterenol administered as a continuous intravenous infusion of 0.03 to 0.3 μg/kg/min is indicated for the treatment of atropine-refractory bradycardia or third degree atrioventricular heart block associated with hemodynamic depression. Beta agonist effects of isoproterenol are responsible for the desirable increases in systolic blood pressure, heart rate, and myocardial contractility produced by this drug. These advantages, however, may be offset by the associated increase in myocardial oxygen requirements. Furthermore, vasodilation due to beta stimulation of peripheral vascular receptors leads to decreased diastolic blood pressure which decreases coronary blood flow and myocardial oxygen delivery. For these reasons, isoproterenol should be administered only until a transvenous artificial cardiac pacemaker can be inserted.

CARDIAC ASYSTOLE

Cardiac asystole is less frequent than ventricular fibrillation as a cause of cardiac arrest, but the initial treatment is BLS. Specific drug therapy of cardiac asystole includes intravenous administration of epinephrine, atropine, and calcium. If epinephrine fails to restore cardiac activity, intravenous atropine (up to 3.0 mg) and/or calcium chloride (5 to 10 mg/kg) is administered. Calcium increases myocardial contractility and stimulates myocardial cells to fire spontaneously, making this a logical drug for the treatment of cardiac asystole. Calcium chloride provides a more rapid increase in the ionized calcium concentration than does the gluconate salt, making the chloride salt the recommended drug for use during CPR. Persistent cardiac asystole despite drug therapy may respond to the intracardiac injection of epinephrine or insertion of a transvenous artificial cardiac pacemaker. Despite aggressive and prompt treatment, the prognosis for successful resuscitation in patients who develop cardiac asystole is poor.

ELECTROMECHANICAL DISSOCIATION

Electromechanical dissociation is present when a normal ECG persists in the absence of an effective stroke volume, as evidenced by the disappearance of peripheral pulses and blood pressure. The cause of electromechanical dissociation is most likely an impairment of calcium transport. Treatment of electromechanical dissociation includes BLS and administration of epinephrine, sodium bicarbonate, isoproterenol, and calcium chloride.

Conditions which mimic electromechanical dissociation include (1) severe hypovolemia, (2) cardiac tamponade, (3) compression of the vena cava, (4) massive pulmonary embolus, and (5) dissecting aneurysm of the thoracic aorta. The appropriate and successful treatment of these disorders depends upon their prompt diagnosis facilitated by a high index of suspicion.

MANAGEMENT OF THE OBSTRUCTED AIRWAY

An airway that is obstructed due to the lodgement of a foreign body in the glottic opening will not be effectively managed by maneuvers such as the head-tilt jaw thrust method that is designed to pull the tongue away from the posterior pharynx (Fig. 34-1).[2] In this situation, the recommended treatment in both conscious and unconscious victims is delivery of back blows (Fig. 34-4).[3] If unsuccessful, back blows should be followed by manual maneuvers applied to the abdomen or chest to increase airway pressure. For example, manual inward and upward depression over the victim's epigastrium (abdominal thrust, external subdiaphragmatic compression, or Heimlich maneuver) forces the diaphragm cephalad, compressing the lungs and raising the airway pressure.[9] The increased airway pressure produced by the abdominal thrust forces ("pops") the obstructing particle out of the glottic opening into the pharynx. The abdominal thrust maneuver can be utilized in awake as well as unconscious victims and is equally effective in the supine or standing position. Complications of this maneuver include rib fractures and rupture of the stomach. An equally effective alternative to the abdominal thrust is manual compression over the mid or lower sternum (chest thrust) of the victim. In the unconscious victim, delivery of a precordial thump (see the section *Precordial Thump*) or external cardiac compression creates airway pressures similar to those produced by chest thrust. Fi-

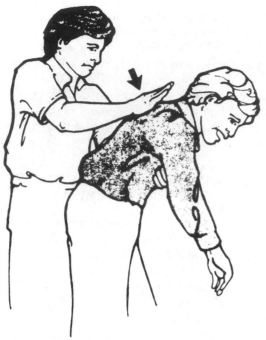

Figure 34-4. The delivery of a back blow is the recommended first step in the treatment of an obstructed airway due to lodgement of a foreign body in the glottic opening (Reprinted from the Supplement to Journal of the American Medical Association, August 1, 1980. Copyright 1980, the American Medical Association. Reprinted with permission from the American Heart Association.)

nally, in the unconscious victim, a blind finger examination of the pharynx is indicated if these previous maneuvers have not been successful.

Transtracheal catheter ventilation via percutaneous insertion of an extracath needle with its associated catheter through the cricothyroid membrane (cricothyrotomy) may be the only way to provide oxygen in a severely obstructed airway. This catheter can be connected to a high pressure oxygen source but it must be appreciated that excessive intrapulmonary pressure may develop if passive exhalation cannot occur through the glottis. In fact, the elevated airway pressure may cause a partially obstructing foreign body to be expelled from the glottic opening.

PRECORDIAL THUMP

A precordial thump is a forceful blow delivered with the fleshy part of the rescuer's fist to the midportion of the victim's sternum. This maneuver is recommended only for initial treatment of monitored (1) ventricular fibrillation or tachycardia and (2) cardiac asystole due to third degree atrioventricular heart block.[3] The precordial thump may serve as mechanical defibrillation or cardioversion or as a mechanism to produce cardiac contraction until a transvenous artificial cardiac pacemaker can be inserted. Precordial thump is not recommended for pediatric patients.

RESUSCITATION OF INFANTS AND CHILDREN

Techniques of CPR as applied to infants (less than 1 year old) differ in some instances from those of the child (1 year to puberty) or the adult (Table 34-1). These differences relate to airway management, ventilation of the lungs, closed chest cardiac compression, external debrillation, and drug therapy. Furthermore, the most readily palpable pulse in infants is the brachial artery at the mid-upper arm, in contrast to the carotid artery in children and adults.

Airway Management and Ventilation of the Lungs

Excessive extension of the infant's head may obstruct the upper airway. The infant's tongue is large, however, in relation to the mouth such that moderate extension of the head is useful for opening the upper airway. The rescuer seals his or her mouth over the mouth and nose of the infant to provide exhaled air ventilation. This approach is easier than mouth-to-mouth ventilation because of the disparate sizes of the structures involved. In addition, the infant under 9 months of age is more easily ventilated through the nose than through the mouth due to the cephalad position of the infant larynx (C1 to C3) and the proximity of the epiglottis to the palate. After 1 year of age, mouth-to-mouth ventilation is acceptable.

Airway obstruction due to lodgement of a foreign body in the glottic opening of the infant is initially treated by back blows followed by chest thrusts (Table 34-2). If obstruction persists and the patient is unconscious, the pharynx should be visually inspected for a foreign body. In contrast to adults, blind finger probes are not recommended as they may push the material further into the larynx. Likewise, abdominal thrusts should not be performed in infants and children because of the increased potential for traumatizing the liver in this age group.

Airway adjuncts for adults are available in smaller sizes for infants and children with the exception of the EOA and EGTA which are not recommended for victims less than 16 years old. Tracheal tubes without cuffs are used in children less than 5 years of age.

Closed Chest Cardiac Compression

Differences in size and anatomy of the infant, child, and adult dictate differences in the technique of external cardiac compression for these various age groups. In infants, the cardiac ventricles are positioned more cephalad in the chest such that external compression is performed on the midsternum rather than the lower sternum. The recommended rate of sternal depression is 100/min and the depth of sternal depression is 1.25 to 2.5 cm.[3] The rescuer's hands should encircle the infant's chest and the thumbs are used to depress the sternum against the heart. Depression of the sternum may be achieved with three fingers in the young child and the heel of one hand in the older child.

External Defibrillation and Drug Therapy

The energy setting for successful external defibrillation in children is directly related to body weight.[2] An initial energy setting of

Table 34-3. Postresuscitation Drug Therapy

Drug	Indications
Lidocaine	Cardiac ventricular irritability
Dopamine	Decreased myocardial contractility associated with oliguria
Dobutamine	Same as dopamine but not specific for increasing renal blood flow
Furosemide	Increased intracranial pressure
Barbiturates Diazepam Phenytoin	CNS seizure activity
Nitroprusside	Systemic hypertension

2 joules/kg should be selected and if this is unsuccessful a second attempt may be made using 4 joules/kg. If a second attempt is unsuccessful, the recommendation is to reevaluate the adequacy of BLS and the possible need for drug therapy rather than increasing the energy setting above 4 joules/kg. Paddles 4.5 cm in diameter are suitable for infants and those 8 cm in diameter are used for children.

POSTRESUSCITATION MANAGEMENT

Postresuscitation management begins following the establishment of a spontaneous cardiac output in the victim of a cardiac arrest. The patient who is awake and breathing spontaneously needs only to be monitored closely in an intensive care unit. Supplemental oxygen and a radiograph of the chest should be routine after CPR. Drug therapy may be necessary to optimize vital organ fuction and survival (Table 34-3). For example, a continuous intravenous infusion of lidocaine is often maintained for the first 24 hours. Optimal adjustment of the intravascular fluid volume and support of the circulation is facilitated by monitoring with a pulmonary artery catheter. Renal failure may necessitate hemodialysis.

Restoration of a spontaneous cardiac output after 12 or more minutes of cerebral ischemia is accompanied by an initial hyperperfusion of the brain followed within 15 to 90 minutes by profound reductions of cerebral blood flow to levels (5 to 40 percent of normal) incompatible with neuronal viability.[10] This "no reflow phenomenon" is not accompanied by intravascular clotting or changes in intracranial pressure. Presumably, a massive increase in cerebral small vessel resistance, possibly due to the accumulation of vasoconstrictor prostaglandins, is responsible for the decreased cerebral blood flow. Furthermore, ischemia is accompanied by decay of the normal calcium gradient across the cell membrane. Rapid shifts of calcium into arterial walls can also result in vascular spasm and possible neuronal damage. For this reason, there is interest in exploring the use of calcium blockers to ameliorate postischemic brain injury. Moreover, the routine administration of calcium during management of cardiac arrest may not be beneficial if neuronal calcium overloading is a result of cellular ischemia.

The ability of barbiturate therapy to reduce ICP is accepted (see Chapter 32). The efficacy of barbiturate therapy, however, for improving brain survival following cardiac arrest is unproven. A study performed in cats demonstrated that thiopental, 60 mg/kg given 5 minutes following successful CPR, reduced the incidence of neurologic deaths but failed to improve the neurologic function of survivors as compared with controls.[11] In another study, high dose thiopental following 16 minutes of complete global ischemia failed to produce any brain-damage ameliorating effect in monkeys.[12] Possibly, the most beneficial effect of barbiturates or other drugs such as diazepam or phenytoin is to suppress seizure activity and associated increases in the cerebral oxygen requirements in the postresuscitation period. Advantages of nonbarbiturate therapy (diazepam, phenytoin) would be less cardiovascular depression, which often limits the total dose of barbiturate that can be administered particularly if hypovolemia is present. Certainly, there is no evidence to support the routine administration of barbiturates to patients who have been resuscitated from a cardiac arrest. Furthermore, there is no evidence that hypothermia or corticosteroids instituted after cardiac arrest improve survival or neurologic outcome. Mild hypothermia present at the time of cardiac arrest, however, may offer some degree of cerebral protection.

Monitors specific for the central nervous system in the cardiac arrest victim with residual neurologic dysfunction include (1) ICP monitoring devices, (2) the electroencephalogram, (3) computed tomography of the cerebral ventricles, (4) cortical evoked potentials, (5) measurement of total and/or regional cerebral blood flow, and (6) frequent neurologic examination. Resuscitation and protection of the brain that has experienced potential ischemic damage includes (1) maintenance of systemic blood pressure at normal levels, (2) prevention of increased ICP by mild hyperventilation ($PaCO_2$ 25 to 30 mmHg), (3) drug-induced diuresis, (4) avoidance of hyperthermia, and (5) elevation of the head 30 degrees to increase cerebral venous drainage (see Chapter 32).

REFERENCES

1. Eisenberg MS, Bergner L, Hallstrom A. Cardiac resuscitation in the community: importance of rapid provision and implications for program planning. JAMA 1979; 241:1905–7.
2. Donegan JH. Cardiopulmonary resuscitation. In: Miller RD, ed. Anesthesia. New York, Churchill Livingstone 1981;1493–1529.
3. Standards and guidelines for cardiopulmonary resuscitation (CPR) and emergency cardiac care (ECC). JAMA 1980;244:453–78.
4. Chandra N, Rudikoff M, Weisfeldt ML. Simultaneous chest compression and ventilation at high airway pressure during cardi-

opulmonary resuscitation. Lancet 1980; 1:175–8.

5. Hodgkin BC, Lambrew CT, Larence FH, Angelakos ET. Effects of PEEP and of increased frequency of ventilation during CPR. Crit Care Med 1980;8:123–6.

6. Ralston RH, Babbs CF, Niebauer MJ. Cardiopulmonary resuscitation with interposed abdominal compression in dogs. Anesth Analg 1982;61:645–51.

7. Neimann JT, Rosborough J, Hausknecht M, Brown D, Criley JM. Cough-CPR. Documentation of systemic perfusion in man and in an experimental model: a "window" to the mechanism of blood flow in external CPR. Crit Care Med 1980;8:141–6.

8. Rogers MC, Weisfeldt ML, Traystan RJ. Cerebral blood flow during cardiopulmon-

ary resuscitation (Editorial). Anesth Analg 1981;60:73–5.

9. Heimlich HJ. A life-saving maneuver to prevent food-choking. JAMA 1975;234:398–401.

10. White BC, Wiegenstein JG, Winegar CD. Brain ischemic anoxia. Mechanisms of injury. JAMA 1984;251:1586–90.

11. Todd MM, Chadwick HS, Shapiro HM, Dunlop BJ, Marshall LF, Dueck R. The neurologic effects of thiopental therapy following experimental cardiac arrest in cats. Anesthesiology 1982;57:76–86.

12. Gisvold SE, Safar P, Hendrickx HHL, Rao G, Moossy J, Alexander H. Thiopental treatment after global brain ischemia in pigtailed monkeys. Anesthesiology 1984; 60:86–90.

Index

Page numbers followed by f represent figures; page numbers followed by t represent tables.